Minimally Invasive Cardiac Surgery

CONTEMPORARY CARDIOLOGY

CHRISTOPHER P. CANNON, MD
SERIES EDITOR

Coronary Disease in Women: *Evidence-Based Diagnosis and Treatment,* edited by *Leslee J. Shaw, PhD and Rita F. Redberg, MD, FACC, 2004*

Complementary and Alternative Medicine in Cardiovascular Disease, edited by *Richard A. Stein, MD and Mehmet C. Oz, MD, 2004*

Nuclear Cardiology, The Basics: *How to Set Up and Maintain a Laboratory,* by *Frans J. Th. Wackers, MD, PhD, Wendy Bruni, CNMT, and Barry L. Zaret, MD, PhD, 2004*

Minimally Invasive Cardiac Surgery, Second Edition, edited by *Daniel J. Goldstein, MD, and Mehmet C. Oz, MD, 2003*

Cardiovascular Health Care Economics, edited by *William S. Weintraub, MD, 2003*

Platelet Glycoprotein IIb/IIIa Inhibitors in Cardiovascular Disease, Second Edition, edited by *A. Michael Lincoff, MD, 2003*

Heart Failure: *A Clinician's Guide to Ambulatory Diagnosis and Treatment,* edited by *Mariell L. Jessup, MD, and Evan Loh, MD, 2003*

Management of Acute Coronary Syndromes, Second Edition, edited by *Christopher P. Cannon, MD, 2003*

Aging, Heart Disease, and Its Management: *Facts and Controversies,* edited by *Niloo M. Edwards, MD, Mathew S. Maurer, MD, and Rachel B. Wellner, MPH, 2003*

Peripheral Arterial Disease: *Diagnosis and Treatment,* edited by *Jay D. Coffman, MD, and Robert T. Eberhardt, MD, 2003*

Cardiac Repolarization: *Bridging Basic and Clinical Science,* edited by *Ihor Gussak, MD, PhD, Charles Antzelevitch, PhD, Stephen C. Hammill, MD, Win K. Shen, MD, and Preben Bjerregaard, MD, DMSc, 2003*

Essentials of Bedside Cardiology: *With a Complete Course in Heart Sounds and Murmurs on CD, Second Edition,* by *Jules Constant, MD, 2003*

Primary Angioplasty in Acute Myocardial Infarction, edited by *James E. Tcheng, MD, 2002*

Cardiogenic Shock: *Diagnosis and Treatment,* edited by *David Hasdai, MD, Peter B. Berger, MD, Alexander Battler, MD, and David R. Holmes, Jr., MD, 2002*

Management of Cardiac Arrhythmias, edited by *Leonard I. Ganz, MD, 2002*

Diabetes and Cardiovascular Disease, edited by *Michael T. Johnstone, MD and Aristidis Veves, MD, DSC, 2001*

Blood Pressure Monitoring in Cardiovascular Medicine and Therapeutics, edited by *William B. White, MD, 2001*

Vascular Disease and Injury: *Preclinical Research,* edited by *Daniel I. Simon, MD, and Campbell Rogers, MD, 2001*

Preventive Cardiology: *Strategies for the Prevention and Treatment of Coronary Artery Disease,* edited by *JoAnne Micale Foody, MD, 2001*

Nitric Oxide and the Cardiovascular System, edited by *Joseph Loscalzo, MD, PhD, and Joseph A. Vita, MD, 2000*

Annotated Atlas of Electrocardiography: *A Guide to Confident Interpretation,* by *Thomas M. Blake, MD, 1999*

Platelet Glycoprotein IIb/IIIa Inhibitors in Cardiovascular Disease, edited by *A. Michael Lincoff, MD, and Eric J. Topol, MD, 1999*

Minimally Invasive Cardiac Surgery, edited by *Mehmet C. Oz, MD, and Daniel J. Goldstein, MD, 1999*

Management of Acute Coronary Syndromes, edited by *Christopher P. Cannon, MD, 1999*

MINIMALLY INVASIVE CARDIAC SURGERY

Second Edition

Edited by

DANIEL J. GOLDSTEIN, MD

Newark Beth Israel Medical Center, Newark, NJ

and

MEHMET C. OZ, MD

New York Presbyterian Hospital, New York, NY

SPRINGER SCIENCE+BUSINESS MEDIA, LLC

Originally published by Humana Press Inc. in 2004
Softcover reprint of the hardcover 1st edition 2004

Due diligence has been taken by the publishers, editors, and authors of this book to assure the accuracy of the information published and to describe generally accepted practices. The contributors herein have carefully checked to ensure that the drug selections and dosages set forth in this text are accurate and in accord with the standards accepted at the time of publication. Notwithstanding, as new research, changes in government regulations, and knowledge from clinical experience relating to drug therapy and drug reactions constantly occurs, the reader is advised to check the product information provided by the manufacturer of each drug for any change in dosages or for additional warnings and contraindications. This is of utmost importance when the recommended drug herein is a new or infrequently used drug. It is the responsibility of the treating physician to determine dosages and treatment strategies for individual patients. Further it is the responsibility of the health care provider to ascertain the Food and Drug Administration status of each drug or device used in their clinical practice. The publisher, editors, and authors are not responsible for errors or omissions or for any consequences from the application of the information presented in this book and make no warranty, express or implied, with respect to the contents in this publication.

Cover illustrations: *EndoWrist*® Robotic Surgical Instruments © 2003 Intuitive Surgical, Inc. CORx System® ©2003 CardioVention, Inc. Figure 14 from "Minimally Invasive Conduit Harvesting" by K. D. Accola, et al. (Chapter 14). Figure 2 from "Thoracoscopic Pericardial Surgery" by P. M. McFadden (Chapter 23).

Cover design by Patricia F. Cleary.

This publication is printed on acid-free paper. ∞
ANSI Z39.48-1984 (American National Standards Institute) Permanence of Paper for Printed Library Materials.

10 9 8 7 6 5 4 3 2 1
ISBN 978-1-61737-400-5 ISBN 978-1-59259-416-0 (eBook)
DOI 10.1007/978-1-59259-416-0

Library of Congress Cataloging-in-Publication Data
Minimally invasive cardiac surgery / edited by David J. Goldstein and Mehmet C. Oz.--2nd ed.
p.;cm. -- (Contemporary cardiology)
Includes biblioographical references and index.

1. Heart–Surgery–Miscellanea. 2. Coronary artery bypass–Miscellanea. 3. Operations, Surgical–Miscellanea. I. Goldstein, David J., MD II. Oz, Mehmet, 1960- III. Contemporary cardiology (Totowa, N.J.: Unnumbered)
[DNLM: 1. Cardiac Surgical Procedures. 2. Surgical Procedures, Minimally Invasive. WG 169 M665 2003]
RD598.M525 2003
617.4'12–dc21 2003040673

Preface

In 1962, Thomas Kuhne coined the term "paradigm shift" while arguing that human knowledge advances by quantum leaps with interspersed smaller steps. Preparation for the major advance is generally not a concerted effort by thought leaders. Rather, a few (or one) visionaries gain insights into a process and are able to definitely demonstrate the accuracy of their worldview. Often, the epiphany does not occur during the intellectual lifetime of the discoverers. Medicine has had numerous such "paradigm shifts" including the compelling reworking of Galen's concepts of the body. Of note, the scientific world of the time explained the new views by arguing that the human body must have changed between the time of ancient Greece and modern Europe.

The inauguration of cardiac surgery itself required profound shifts in medicine's view of physiology. Yet, over the ensuing 40 years, the field was fine tuned so we could provide greater than 95% success rates in elective surgery with low cost and short hospital stays. In some parts of the world, the procedures were viewed as commodities and prices dropped as providers were unable to differentiate the quality of their work. As patients and their physicians became more demanding, the desire to make the procedures "minimally invasive" grew. In effect, what we were really searching for was a life saving procedure that also preserved quality of life. In short, "minimally invasive" has really been a code phrase for procedures that disrupt our quality of life the least. We will use this definition as we explain the constant trade-offs between incision size and location, cardiopulmonary bypass time, and expensive new technologies. The constant bottom line is our need to bring value to the health care system and our patients, recognizing that the early forays may not reflect longer term potential.

Our first edition argued that this evolution was really a revolution, as stunning reports from countries outside North America, the birthplace of cardiac surgery, revealed that heart surgery could be successfully performed without arresting the heart. In fact, these investigators were able to export these radical concepts more readily to heart surgeons around the globe because many in the field perceived the stagnation that arises when a field has been mastered. Heart surgeons, generally a restless breed, often choose our demanding field because they enjoy the challenge and the opportunity to engage these new procedures was alluring. Many took the bait, not realizing the costs incurred, and in some areas the pendulum of growth has swung back towards the status quo. If for no other reason than to provide medium term updates, a second edition was warranted.

In addition, the overall rapid growth in the range and volume of minimally invasive procedures since the first edition mandated an update. In this evolutionary cycle, some procedures have become extinct even as others have become mainstays. New approaches, unthinkable even three years ago, are being presented at our most prestigious national meetings. In particular, the invasion of robotic technologies into the traditionally conservative cardiac operating theatre paralleled the stunning growth of laparoscopic cholecystectomy once it was discovered in the rural southeastern United States. Once the possibility of this radically new approach was comprehended, new generations of procedures were inaugurated. Surgeons do not just perform the old operation with new tools. We should create new procedures that are adapted to the new tools.

Finally, the fictitious border between different specialties focusing on atherosclerosis, especially cardiac surgery, cardiology, and invasive radiology, has blurred. Our different lineages are less important than our current procedural needs and the evolution of minimally invasive heart surgery will demand a reworking of training programs and mindsets —a healthy process that will mature over the next decade.

Daniel Goldstein, MD
Mehmet Oz, MD

Contents

Preface v

Contributors xi

Part I Physiology of Coronary Bypass Grafting With and Without Cardiopulmonary Bypass

1 Pathophysiology of Cardiopulmonary Bypass 3
Ron G. H. Speekenbrink, Wim van Oeveren, Charles R. H. Wildevuur, and León Eijsman

2 Endothelial Injury During Minimally Invasive Bypass Grafting 27
Robert J. Dabal, Craig R. Hampton, and Edward D. Verrier

Part II Minimally Invasive Coronary Bypass Grafting

3 Minimally Invasive Bypass Grafting: *A Historical Perspective* 45
Enio Buffolo and Luís Roberto Gerola

4 Tailoring Minimal Invasive Coronary Bypass to the Patient 53
Michael A. Borger and M. Anno Diegeler

5 OPCAB: *A Primer on Technique* 67
John D. Puskas

6 Mechanical Stabilization: *The Medtronic Octopus System* 75
Michael Gibson, Robert B. Beauford, and Daniel J. Goldstein

7 Mechanical Stabilization Systems: *The Genzyme-OPCAB Elite System* 89
William E. Cohn and Marc Ruel

8 Mechanical Stabilization Systems: *The Guidant OPCAB System* 105
Marc W. Connolly and Valavanur A. Subramanian

9 The MIDCAB Operation 113
Mercedes K. C. Dullum and Albert J. Pfister

10 Minimally Invasive Coronary Artery Bypass Grafting on the Beating Heart: *The European Experience* 129
Antonio M. Calafiore, Michele Di Mauro, Alessandro Pardini, Antonio Bivona, and Stefano D'Alessandro

11 Minimally Invasive Coronary Artery Bypass Grafting: *The South American Experience* 147
Federico J. Benetti and Maximo Guida

12 Reoperative Off-Pump CABG 157
Valavanur A. Subramanian, James D. Fonger, and Nilesh U. Patel

13 Perioperative Evaluation of Graft Patency in OPCAB 179
Vinod H. Thourani and John D. Puskas

14 Minimally Invasive Conduit Harvesting 193
Kevin D. Accola, Mike Butkus, and Brenda Dickey

15 Hybrid Revascularization 207
Uwe Klima and Axel Haverich

16 Neurocognitive Issues in Off-Pump CABG 217
Ronald M. Lazar and Daniel F. Heitjan

17 Multivessel Off-Pump Revascularization in High-Risk Patients: *Severe Left Ventricular Dysfunction* 229
Daniel J. Goldstein, Robert B. Beauford, Patricia Garland, and Craig R. Saunders

18 Multivessel Off-Pump Revascularization in High-Risk Populations: *Octogenarians* 241
Frederic Sardari, Robert B. Beauford, and Daniel J. Goldstein

Part III Minimally Invasive Valvular Surgery

19 Minimally Invasive Mitral Valve Surgery 255
Victor F. Chu, L. Wiley Nifong, and W. Randolph Chitwood, Jr.

20 Port-Access Mitral Valve Surgery 273
Ashish S. Shah and Donald D. Glower

21 Minimally Invasive Aortic Valve Surgery 293
Jerome Sepic and Lawrence H. Cohn

Part IV Minimally Invasive Congenital, Pericardial, and Arrhythmia Surgery

22 Strategies for Reducing Trauma in Congenital Heart Surgery 311
Redmond P. Burke and Robert L. Hannan

23 Thoracoscopic Pericardial Surgery 327
P. Michael McFadden

24 Less Invasive Surgical Treatment of Atrial Fibrillation 343
Mathew R. Williams and Michael Argenziano

Part V Miscellaneous Aspects of Minimally Invasive Cardiac Surgery

25 The Economic Impact of Minimally Invasive Cardiac Surgery 361
Aftab R. Kherani, Elizabeth H. Burton, and Mehmet C. Oz

26 Minimally Invasive Cardiac Surgery: *Quality-of-Life Issues* 369
Giulio Pompilio, Francesco Alamanni, and Paolo Biglioli

27 Experimental Percutaneous Mitral Valve Repair 383
Juan P. Umaña and Peter Fitzgerald

28 Alternative Anastomotic Techniques 393
David A. D'Alessandro and Mehmet C. Oz

29 Making Cardiopulmonary Bypass Less Invasive 411
James R. Beck, Linda B. Mongero, and A. Kenneth Litzie

Part VI Robotic Surgery

30 Robotics and Telemanipulation: *The Zeus™ System* 429
Hersh S. Maniar, Sunil M. Prasad, and Ralph J. Damiano, Jr.

31 Robotics and Telemanipulation: *The da Vinci™ System* 445
Volkmar Falk, Thomas Walther, and Friedrich W. Mohr

32 Totally Endoscopic Atrial Septal Defect Repair with Robotic Assistance 461
Michael Argenziano, Mehmet C. Oz, and Craig R. Smith, Jr.

Index 471

Contributors

Kevin D. Accola, md, *Florida Heart Institute, Florida Hospital, Orlando, FL*

Francesco Alamanni, md, *Department of Cardiovascular Surgery, University of Milan, Centro Cardiologico Monzino IRCCS, Milan, Italy*

Michael Argenziano, md, *Assistant Professor of Surgery, Director, Cardiac Robotics and Arrhythmia Surgery, Division of Cardiothoracic Surgery, Columbia Presbyterian Medical Center, New York, NY*

Robert B. Beauford, md, *Surgical Resident, Department of General Surgery, Brookdale University Hospital Medical Center, Brooklyn, NY*

James R. Beck, bs, ccp, *Co-Director, Perfusion Services, Columbia Presbyterian Medical Center, New York, NY*

Federico J. Benetti, md, PhD, *Fundacion Benetti, Buenos Aires, Argentina*

Paolo Biglioli, md, *Department of Cardiovascular Surgery, University of Milan, Centro Cardiologico Monzino IRCCS, Milan, Italy*

Antonio Bivona, md, *Department of Cardiology and Cardiac Surgery, "G. D'Annunzio" University, S. Camillo de' Lellis Hospital, Chieti, Italy*

Michael A. Borger, md, PhD, *Division of Cardiovascular Surgery, Toronto General Hospital, Toronto, Ontario, Canada*

Enio Buffolo, md, PhD, *Escola Paulista Medicina, São Paulo, Brazil*

Redmond P. Burke, md, *Chief, Division of Cardiovascular Surgery, Miami Children's Hospital, Miami, FL*

Elizabeth H. Burton, ba, *Research Assistant, Division of Cardiothoracic Surgery, Columbia University, College of Physicians and Surgeons, New York, NY*

Mike Butkus, p.a.-c., *Florida Heart Institute, Florida Hospital, Orlando, FL*

Antonio M. Calafiore, md, *Professor and Chairman, Department of Cardiology and Cardiac Surgery, "G. D'Annunzio" University, S. Camillo de' Lellis Hospital, Chieti, Italy*

W. Randolph Chitwood, Jr., md, *Professor and Chairman, Department of Surgery, The Brody School of Medicine, East Carolina University, Greenville, NC*

Victor F. Chu, md, *Fellow in Minimally Invasive and Robotic Surgery, Department of Surgery, The Brody School of Medicine, East Carolina University, Greenville, NC*

Lawrence H. Cohn, md, *Virginia and James Hubbard Professor of Surgery, Harvard Medical School, and Chief, Division of Cardiac Surgery, Brigham and Women's Hospital, Boston, MA*

William E. Cohn, md, *Department of Cardiothoracic Surgery, Beth Israel Deaconess Medical Center, Boston, MA*

Marc W. Connolly, md, *Department of Cardiothoracic Surgery, St. Michael's Medical Center, Newark, NJ*

Robert J. Dabal, md, *Cardiothoracic Resident, Division of Cardiothoracic Surgery, University of Washington, Seattle, WA*

David A. D'Alessandro, md, *Division of Cardiothoracic Surgery, Columbia Presbyterian Medical Center, New York, NY*

Stefano D'Alessandro, md, *Department of Cardiology and Cardiac Surgery, "G. D'Annunzio" University, S. Camillo de' Lellis Hospital, Chieti, Italy*

Ralph J. Damiano, Jr., md, *Chief, Division of Cardiothoracic Surgery, Washington University School of Medicine, St. Louis, MO*

BRENDA DICKEY, RN, *Florida Heart Institute, Florida Hospital, Orlando, FL*
M. ANNO DIEGELER, MD, PhD, *Department of Cardiothoracic Surgery, University of Leipzig, Bad Neustadt, Germany*
MICHELE DI MAURO, MD, *Department of Cardiology and Cardiac Surgery, "G. D'Annunzio" University, S. Camillo de' Lellis Hospital, Chieti, Italy*
MERCEDES K. C. DULLUM, MD, *Washington Regional Cardiac Surgery P.C., Washington Hospital Center, Washington, DC*
LEÓN EIJSMAN, MD, PhD, *Department of Thoracic Surgery, Onze Lieve Vrouwe Gasthius, Amsterdam, The Netherlands*
VOLKMAR FALK, MD, PhD, *Department of Cardiac Surgery, Heartcenter, University of Leipzig, Leipzig, Germany*
PETER FITZGERALD, MD, *Associate Professor of Medicine, Department of Cardiothoracic Surgery, Stanford University School of Medicine, Palo Alto, CA*
JAMES D. FONGER, MD, *Division of Cardiovascular and Thoracic Surgery, Lenox Hill Hospital, New York, NY*
PATRICIA GARLAND, RN, *Heart Hospital of New Jersey, Newark Beth Israel Medical Center, Newark, NJ*
LUÍS ROBERTO GEROLA, MD, PhD, *Escola Paulista Medicina, São Paulo, Brazil*
MICHAEL GIBSON, MD, *Cardiothoracic Surgery Resident, Department of Cardiothoracic Surgery, Newark Beth Israel Medical Center, Newark, NJ*
DONALD D. GLOWER, MD, *Duke University Medical Center, Durham, NC*
DANIEL J. GOLDSTEIN, MD, *Surgical Director of Cardiac Transplantation and Mechanical Assistance, Department of Cardiothoracic Surgery, Heart Hospital of New Jersey, Newark Beth Israel Medical Center, Newark, NJ*
MAXIMO GUIDA, MD, *Department of Cardiovascular Surgery, Hospital Mendez de Valencia, Venezuela*
CRAIG R. HAMPTON, MD, *Cardiothoracic Research Fellow, Division of Cardiothoracic Surgery, University of Washington, Seattle, WA*
ROBERT L. HANNAN, MD, *Attending Physician, Division of Cardiovascular Surgery, Miami Children's Hospital, Miami, FL*
AXEL HAVERICH, MD, *Professor of Surgery, Division of Cardiothoracic and Vascular Surgery, Hannover Medical School, Hannover, Germany*
DANIEL F. HEITJAN, PhD, *Professor of Biostatistics, Joseph P. Mailman School of Public Health, Columbia University, New York, NY*
AFTAB R. KHERANI, MD, *Resident in General Surgery, Duke University Medical Center, Durham, NC*
UWE KLIMA, MD. *Associate Professor of Surgery, Division of Cardiothoracic and Vascular Surgery, Hannover Medical School, Hannover, Germany*
RONALD M. LAZAR, PhD, *Associate Professor of Clinical Neuropsychology, Columbia University College of Physicians & Surgeons, and Director, Cerebral Localization Laboratory, Neurovascular Service, Neurological Institute of New York, Columbia-Presbyterian Medical Center, New York, NY*
A. KENNETH LITZIE, *Director, Clinical Development, Cardiovention, Santa Clara, CA*
HERSH S. MANIAR, MD, *Division of Cardiothoracic Surgery, Washington University School of Medicne, St. Louis, MO*

P. Michael McFadden, md, *Surgical Director Lung Transplantation, Ochsner Clinic Foundation, Clinical Professor of Surgery, Tulane University School of Medicine, New Orleans, LA*

Friedrich W. Mohr, md, PhD, *Department of Cardiac Surgery, Heartcenter, University of Leipzig, Leipzig, Germany*

Linda B. Mongero, bs, ccp, *Co-Director, Perfusion Services, Columbia Presbyterian Medical Center, New York, NY*

L. Wiley Nifong, md, *Assistant Professor of Surgery, Department of Surgery, and Director, Minimally Invasive and Robotic Surgery, The Brody School of Medicine, East Carolina University, Greenville, NC*

Mehmet C. Oz, md, *Associate Professor of Surgery, Director of the Cardiovascular Institute, Columbia Presbyterian Medical Center, New York, NY*

Alessandro Pardini, md, *Department of Cardiology and Cardiac Surgery, "G. D'Annunzio" University, S. Camillo de' Lellis Hospital, Chieti, Italy*

Nilesh U. Patel, md, *Division of Cardiovascular and Thoracic Surgery, Lenox Hill Hospital, New York, NY*

Albert J. Pfister, md, *Washington Regional Cardiac Surgery P.C., Washington Hospital Center, Washington, DC*

Giulio Pompilio, md, PhD, *Department of Cardiovascular Surgery, University of Milan, Centro Cardiologico Monzino IRCCS, Milan, Italy*

Sunil M. Prasad, md, *Division of Cardiothoracic Surgery, Washington University School of Medicne, St. Louis, MO*

John D. Puskas, md, MSc, *Carlyle Fraser Heart Center, Division of Cardiothoracic Surgery, Department of Surgery, Emory University School of Medicine, Atlanta, GA*

Marc Ruel, md, mph, *Department of Cardiothoracic Surgery, Beth Israel Deaconess Medical Center, Boston, MA*

Frederic Sardari, md, *Department of Cardiothoracic Surgery, Saint Barnabas Hospital, Heart Hospital of New Jersey, Newark, NJ*

Craig R. Saunders, md, *Chairman, Department of Cardiothoracic Surgery, Heart Hospital of New Jersey, Newark, NJ*

Jerome Sepic, md, *Cardiac Surgery Research Fellow, Harvard Medical School, Brigham and Women's Hospital, Boston, MA*

Ashish S. Shah, md, *Duke University Medical Center, Durham, NC*

Craig R. Smith, Jr., md, *Calvin Barber Professor of Surgery, Chief, Division of Cardiothoracic Surgery, Columbia Presbyterian Medical Center, New York, NY*

Ron G. H. Speekenbrink, md, PhD, *Department of Thoracic Surgery, Onze Lieve Vrouwe Gasthius, Amsterdam, The Netherlands*

Valavanur A. Subramanian, md, *Chairman, Department of Surgery, Lenox Hill Hospital, New York, NY*

Vinod H. Thourani, md, *Carlyle Fraser Heart Center, Division of Cardiothoracic Surgery, Department of Surgery, Emory University School of Medicine, Atlanta, GA*

Juan P. Umaña, md, *Chairman, Division of Cardiovascular Surgery, Fundacion Cardioinfantil, Instituto de Cardiologia, Bogota, Columbia*

WIN VAN OEVEREN, PhD, *The Center for Blood Interaction Research, Department of Cardiothoracic Surgery, University Hospital Groningen, Groningen, The Netherlands*

EDWARD D. VERRIER, MD, *William K. Edmark Professor of Cardiovascular Surgery, Vice Chairman, Department of Surgery, Chief, Division of Cardiothoracic Surgery, University of Washington, Seattle, WA*

THOMAS WALTHER, MD, PhD, *Department of Cardiac Surgery, Heartcenter, University of Leipzig, Leipzig, Germany*

CHARLES R. H. WILDEVUUR, MD, *Department of Thoracic Surgery, Onze Lieve Vrouwe Gasthius, Amsterdam, The Netherlands*

MATHEW R. WILLIAMS, MD, *Surgical Arrhythmia Program, Division of Cardiothoracic Surgery, Columbia Presbyterian Medical Center, New York, NY*

I

Physiology of Coronary Bypass Grafting With and Without Cardiopulmonary Bypass

1 Pathophysiology of Cardiopulmonary Bypass

Ron G. H. Speekenbrink, MD, PHD,
Wim van Oeveren, PHD,
Charles R. H. Wildevuur, MD, PHD,
and León Eijsman, MD, PHD

CONTENTS

Introduction
Material-dependent Activation
Methods To Attenuate Material-dependent Activation
Material-independent Activation
Future Developments
References

INTRODUCTION

From the earliest clinical experiences with cardiopulmonary bypass (CPB) for cardiac operations, it was apparent that significant morbidity and even mortality were associated with the CPB procedure itself *(1)*. Often, only the contact of blood to the foreign material of the extracorporeal circuit was held responsible. However, cardiopulmonary bypass implies more than just connecting the circulation of the patient to an extracorporeal circuit, resulting in the material-dependent activation of blood. With cardiopulmonary bypass, a number of other nonphysiological events are introduced, including hemodilution, hypothermia, nonpulsatile blood flow, retransfusion of shed blood, and exclusion of the metabolic function of the lung resulting in material-independent activation. Together, these events cause the massive and systemic activation of the patient's defense mechanisms, with repercussions on nearly every end-organ system. Signs of this "whole-body inflammatory reaction" can be observed in every postoperative patient. In a number of patients, especially neonates, the elderly, and those undergoing large procedures or

From: *Contemporary Cardiology: Minimally Invasive Cardiac Surgery, Second Edition*
Edited by: D. J. Goldstein and M. C. Oz © Humana Press Inc., Totowa, NJ

those with severe comorbidities, this phenomenon can escalate into the so-called postperfusion syndrome, which is characterized by elevated cardiac output with decreased vascular resistance, capillary leak, and renal function impairment, a constellation of factors that is associated with increased mortality *(2)*.

In this chapter, we discuss the various biochemical mechanisms that underlie the deleterious effects of cardiopulmonary bypass, methods to mitigate these effects, and guidelines for future developments.

MATERIAL-DEPENDENT ACTIVATION

In the past, activation of the contact system by the nonbiocompatible surface of the extracorporeal circuit was considered to be the initiating factor in blood activation in CPB and to be responsible for most of the detrimental effects of CPB. Because the contact system is linked to the other humoral defense systems, its activation would result in subsequent activation of the kallikrein, fibrinolytic, and coagulation systems. The active products of these systems would cause, directly or indirectly via activation of leukocytes, platelets, and endothelium, a part of the detrimental effects of CPB *(3)*. This concept is supported by studies in simulated bypass models showing activation of the contact system by the extracorporeal circuit *(4)*. However, clinical observations of patients with a deficiency in contact system proteins have undermined this concept. Indeed, patients with a severe deficiency of the primary factor of contact activation, factor XII, were shown to have similar patterns of thrombin generation as healthy patients *(5,6)*. Moreover, data from recent clinical investigations have shown no change in the marker for contact-activation kallikrein–C1 esterase inhibitor complex between prebypass and bypass levels, and no increase of factor XIIa levels during cardiopulmonary bypass *(7,8)*. Furthermore, the levels of a second marker for contact activation factor XIIa–C1 esterase inhibitor complex during cardiopulmonary bypass remained below the detection limit in the majority of patients *(7)*. Coagulation studies have shown that factor X activation and thrombin generation precede factor IX activation during cardiopulmonary bypass (**Fig. 1**), which indicates activation through the extrinsic (tissue factor) pathway and not through the intrinsic (contact-phase) pathway *(8,9)*. From these data it appears justified to conclude that the role of the contact system in cardiopulmonary bypass needs to be redefined.

It is undisputed that the contact of blood with foreign materials results in the activation of the complement system. Complement is activated through one of two pathways, the "classical" or the "alternative" pathway (**Fig. 2**). The latter is predominantly involved in complement activation by biomaterials because it can be activated in the absence of specific antibodies *(10)*. Both pathways form complexes named "C3 convertases," which cleave the third component of complement, C3, generating the anaphylatoxin C3a and a major cleavage fragment C3b. Accumulation of C3b molecules onto the surface in the vicinity of C3 convertases changes the specificity of the C3-cleaving enzyme into a C5 convertase, resulting in the cleavage of C5, generation of the leukocyte-activating C5a, and recruitment of the terminal complement complex (TCC) C5–C9 *(11)*. During CPB, C3a appears in the circulation after 10–20 min, followed by C5a and TCC *(12)*.

Although the composition of the artificial surfaces plays a predominant role in complement activation during cardiopulmonary bypass, nonbiomaterial-dependent triggers can also activate complement. Contact of air with blood as it occurs in bubble oxygenators and in the cardiotomy suction line activates complement *(13)*. This advantage of the membrane oxygenator, having no direct blood–air contact, may be nullified by its larger

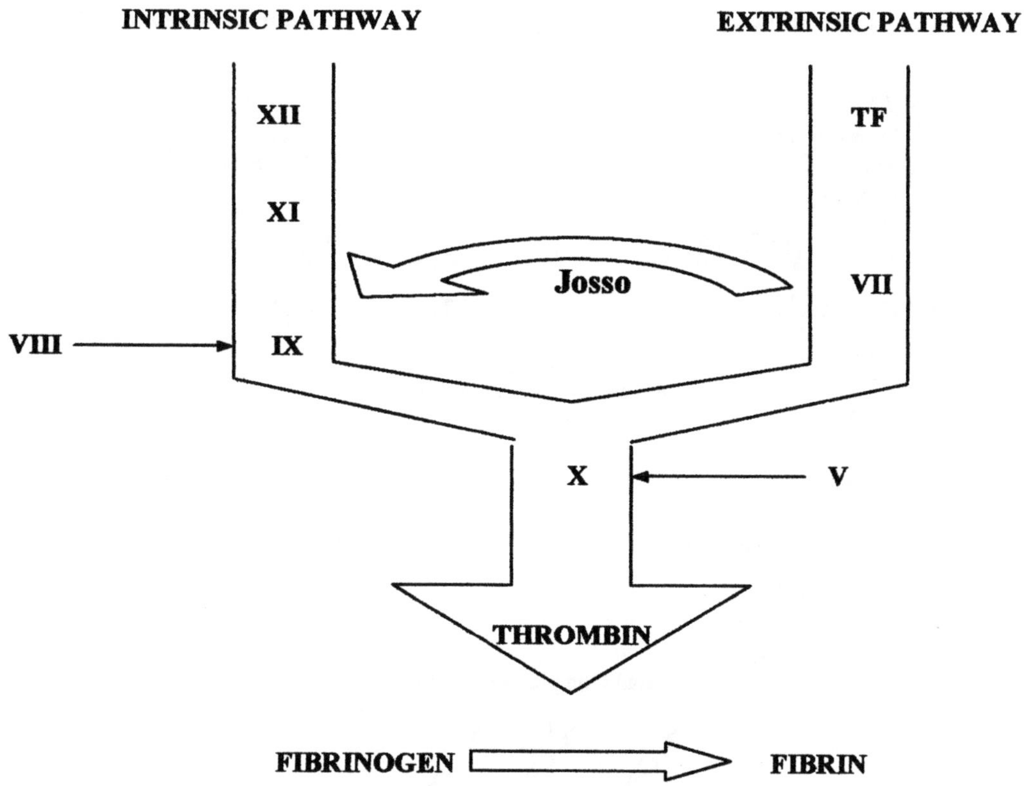

Fig. 1. Relation between the intrinsic (contact) pathway and the extrinsic pathway to the common pathway of coagulation. Josso indicates the Josso loop, which links the extrinsic to the intrinsic pathway. TF = tissue factor. Roman numerals represent coagulation factors.

surface *(14)*. Dextran 70 and, to lesser extent, polygeline induce complement activation *(15)*. Classical pathway activation is also initiated on interaction of C1 with antigen–antibody complexes and, in some instances, with other activators, including some bacterial and viral surfaces and bacterial endo- or exotoxins *(16,17)*. Furthermore, activation of the classical pathway occurs after administration of protamine through formation of heparin–protamine complexes *(18,19)*.

The effects of complement activation are mediated by the products C3a, C5a, and TCC. TCC, also called the membrane attack complex, deposits on erythrocytes and leukocytes to augment cell lysis and cell activation *(20)*. We recently found that TCC concentrations formed during pediatric CPB correlated with postoperative fever and gain in body weight *(21)*. C3a and C5a are also called the anaphylatoxins. The anaphylatoxins have chemotactic activity for neutrophils and monocytes *(22)* and induce cytokine release. Binding of C5a and C5a desArg to specific receptors on neutrophils induces:

1. Aggregation of the cells and their adherence to endothelial cells *(23,24)*
2. Release of reactive oxygen species, which may damage the endothelium to which activated neutrophils have bound *(25,26)*
3. Release of lysosomal enzymes *(27)*
4. Neosynthesis and release of leukotrienes *(28,29)*

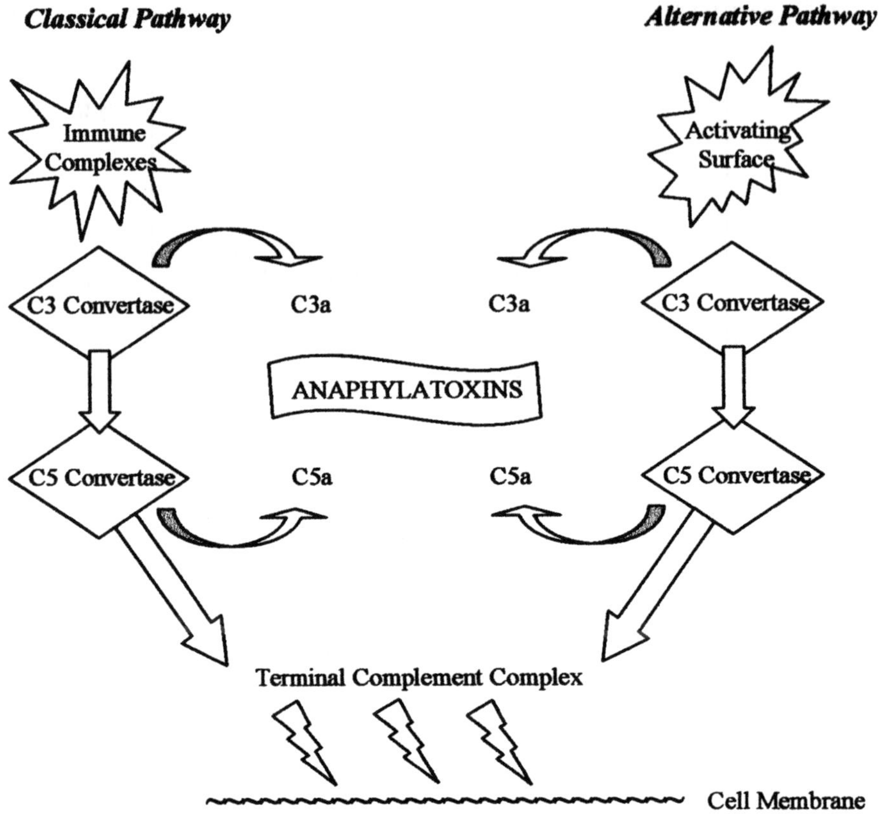

Fig. 2..Schematic of the complement system. Immune complexes or activating surfaces activate the first step of the classic and alternative pathway respectively. This results in the formation of pathway-specific C3 and C5 convertases and finally formation of the terminal complement complex, which damages the cell membranes.

Special attention has been paid to the lysosomal enzyme elastase, which affects the endothelial junctions *(30)* and enhances vascular permeability for blood proteins *(31)*. The appearance of proteins, including elastase, in the alveolar space may be an important cause for surfactant dysfunction and decreased lung compliance, resulting in pulmonary dysfunction and possibly in adult respiratory distress syndrome *(32)*.

Cytokines (Table 1) are released by monocytes, macrophages, endothelium, and other cells on stimulation with the anaphylatoxins or the lipopolysaccharide endotoxin, a constituent of the cell wall of Gram-negative bacteria. A number of acute and chronic adverse consequences, such as hypotension and an increased body temperature after extracorporeal circulation, may be attributed to the cytokine interleukin-1 (IL-1) *(33)*. IL-1 is an essential component of the inflammatory reaction and the immune response by its ability to stimulate neutrophil degranulation *(34)* and to activate T- and B-cells *(35,36)*. The cytokine tumor necrosis factor (TNF), a mediator of the host response in sepsis, is derived from monocytes and macrophages *(37)*. It has some common properties with IL-1, such as induction of fever *(38)*. TNF induces procoagulant activity *(39)* and IL-1 release *(38,40)* from endothelial cells by interaction with specific receptors. TNF generation has been measured in CPB patients and was assumed to be associated with endotoxin release

Table 1
Properties of the Most Well Known Cytokines Released During and After Cardiac Surgery

	Main Source	*Main Target*	*Main Effects*
TNF-α	Monocytes, macrophages	TNF receptors on neutrophils, monocytes, endothelial cells, hepatocytes, chondrocytes, astrocytes, fibroblasts, osteoclasts	Hypotension, fever, cytokine + APP synthesis/release ↑, plasma albumin ↓, neutrophil/endothelial interaction ↑
Il-1	Monocytes, macrophages	Il-1 receptors	Hypotension, fever
Il-6	Fibroblasts, monocytes,	Il-6 receptors on macrophages, T-lymphocytes	Hypotension, fever, hepatocytes APP synthesis/release ↑, tissue iNOS expression↑, Il-1-RA ↑,TNF-RA ↑
Il-8	Monocytes, macrophages	Chemokine receptors on T-cells, fibroblasts, monocytes, and neutrophils	Chemoattraction and activation of neutrophils
Il-10	Monocytes, macrophages, T- and B-lymphocytes	Il-10 receptor on macrophages and monocytes in the liver	Soluble TNF receptor ↑, TNF/Il-1/Il-6 ↓, Th1-lymphocyte response ↓

TNF-α = tumor necrosis factor α , Il = interleukin, APP = acute-phase response, iNOS = inducible nitric oxide synthase, RA = receptor antagonist, Th1 = T-helper type 1. (Adapted from P. Bruins. Changes in the inflammatory response during and after cardiac surgery. Thesis, University of Amsterdam, 2000.)

(41,42). Interleukin-6 (IL-6) is produced by activated monocytes, endothelial cells, fibroblasts, and T- and B-cells. It is therefore a general marker of blood and tissue damage, observed in a variety of surgical interventions and diseases. Il-6 levels after off-pump coronary bypass grafting (OPCAB) are similar to levels after conventional on-pump CABG *(43,44)*. In CPB, IL-6 is of interest by its correlation with the ischemic time during crossclamping *(45)*: 4 h after CPB, peak levels of IL-6 are observed *(46)*. Next to its function as a marker for inflammation, IL-6 generated in the ischemic myocardium appears to induce intercellular adhesion molecule-1 (ICAM-1) on the myocyte surface, which could be held responsible for granulocyte adhesion in the myocardial tissue after reperfusion of the ischemic heart *(47)*. IL-8, similar to IL-6, is produced in several cell types, including alveolar macrophages, fibroblasts, lymphocytes, and endothelial cells. IL-8 plays an important role in leukocyte activation and contributes to myocyte reperfusion injury. Its responses have been reported to be at maximum during or 2 h after CPB *(45,48)*, which is faster than other proinflammatory cytokines. IL-8 release is thought to be dependent on C5a generation *(49)*. IL-10 was recently reported as an anti-inflammatory cytokine that deactivates monocytes and macrophages and thus likely reduces release of IL-6, IL-8, and TNF. Its rapid release within 1 h after CPB might offer important negative feedback to further TNF production *(45)*.

Adhesion molecules (Table 2) play a major role in the recruitment of neutrophils to the site of inflammation. Multiple steps are involved in this process. Each step is characterized by the participation of a different family of adhesion molecules. The rolling phase of neutrophils over the endothelial layer is mediated by the selectin family, the E-, L-, and P- selectins and their ligands. The next step, the activation and adhesion of the neutrophils to the endothelium, is regulated by the integrin family and their ligands. The final step of transendothelial migration is mediated by these two families of adhesion molecules, the selectins and integrins. It has been demonstrated that soluble isoforms of these adhesion molecules can be found in circulation. In addition, these soluble isoforms appear to be useful markers of disease activity, and they have physiological effects *(50)*.

E-selectin is a specific marker for endothelial activation. The soluble form is biologically active in its capacity to bind to neutrophils. High concentrations of (recombinant) E-selectin can inhibit neutrophil adhesion. L-selectin is produced by leukocytes after stimulation with chemotactic peptides, IL-8, or endotoxin. It enhances the binding of leukocytes to (inflammed) endothelium. P-selectin is produced by platelets and endothelium and mediates the interaction with neutrophils and some lymphocyte subsets. It has been suggested that P-selectin has anti-inflammatory effects, shown by reduced oxygen radical production by neutrophils and inhibition of integrin-mediated adhesion of neutrophils *(50)*. However, blocking of P-selectin during experimental CPB with specific monoclonal antibodies resulted in reduced levels of IL-6, IL-8, and metabolites of nitric oxide. The most extensively studied integrin in the field of cardiopulmonary bypass surgery is CD11b/CD18, previously called Mac-1 or CR3 *(51,52)*. The increased adhesiveness of neutrophils following incubation with C5a and C5a desArg is dependent on the enhancement of membrane expression of the adhesion-promoting glycoprotein Mac1 on the cells *(53)*. The integrins bind to the ECAM-1, ICAM-1, and VCAM-1, which are constitutionally expressed ligands on endothelium *(54)*.

The expressions of CD11b/CD18 and L-selectin have been used as markers for neutrophil activation during cardiopulmonary bypass *(55)*. CD18 expression increased immediately at the start of CPB, while L-selectin was shed from the neutrophil surface,

Table 2
Specific Ligands and Cell Membrane Adhesion Molecules

Group/Type	*Expressed by*	*Ligand*
Ig-like		
ICAM-1	Endothelial cells, leukocytes	CD11a/CD18
CD11b/CD18		
ICAM-2	Endothelial cells, leukocytes	CD11a/CD18
ICAM-3	Endothelial cells, leukocytes	CD11a/CD18
VCAM	Endothelial cells	VLA-4
PECAM	Platelets	
Selectins		
E-selectin (ELAM-1)	Endothelial cells, leukocytes	L-selectin, ESL-1
L-selectin	Leukocytes	P-selectin
P-selectin (GMP-140)	Endothelial cells, platelets	L-selectin
β2-Integrins		
CD11a/CD18 (LFA-1)	Leukocytes	ICAM-1, -2, and -3
CD11b/CD18 (MAC-1)	Leukocytes	ICAM-1, ICAM-2
CD11c/CD18	Monocytes	
β1-Integrin		
CD49d/CD29 (VAL-4)	Endothelial cells	VCAM/fibronectin

Ig = immunoglobulin; ICAM = intercellular adhesion molecule; PECAM = platelet-endothelial cell adhesion molecule; VCAM = vascular cell adhesion molecule; VLA = very late antigen; LFA = leukocyte function associated antigen; ESL = endothelial sialyl Lewis antigen. (Reproduced with permission from P. Bruins. Changes in the inflammatory response during and after cardiac surgery. Thesis, University of Amsterdam, 2000.)

shown by a gradual loss during 60 min of CPB. Similarly, instant activation of platelets, reflected by a decreased expression of the adhesive receptor Gp1b after initiation of cardiopulmonary bypass has been reported *(56)*. Markers for activation of the complement, coagulation, or fibrinolytic systems do not show such rapid increases at the onset of cardiopulmonary bypass, but rather increase slowly during the procedure. Therefore, the stimulus for this rapid activation of platelets and neutrophils is unclear. It is possible that direct activation by the foreign surface is involved. Another explanation could be the production of trace amounts of activators, not distinguishable systemically, on the surface of the extracorporeal circuit *(57)*. Based on the observations of fast cellular responses to extracorporeal circulation the generally used activation scheme, contact activation → activation of humoral defense systems → activation of cells, probably needs to be revised. Most likely, the activated cell membranes and the cell constituents form major triggers for activation of the hemostatic and inflammatory reactions to CPB.

The endothelium plays an important role in the regulation of vascular tone. Two systems are involved in this regulation: the nitric oxide (NO)/endothelin and the prostacyclin/thromboxane system. Both systems are affected by the inflammatory response after CPB. NO was formerly known as endothelium-derived relaxing factor. It is formed by two synthases, a constitutive form, which produces NO in picomolar quantities, and an inducible form, which produces nanomolar amounts of NO *(58)*. The activity of the inducible form is increased by endotoxin, TNF, and IL-1. Increased NO concentrations are found during and after cardiopulmonary bypass, and might have a role in the vasoplegic syndrome affecting some patients after cardiac procedures *(58)*. The cardiodepressive effect of IL-6 and TNF was shown to result from increased NO production through inducible synthase activation *(59)*. Moreover, NO in high concentrations has been implicated in vascular, lung, and bowel injury *(60)*. The counterpart of NO is endothelin, a small peptide with potent vasoconstrictive capacities that is produced by endothelium, macrophages, and the hypothalamus *(61,62)*. Institution of CPB results in a rapid increase of endothelin, which is likely the result of a neurohumoral response to decreased blood pressure. During CPB, a slow increase of endothelin concentrations can be observed that correlates with endotoxin concentrations *(63)*. Inappropriate endothelin concentrations can cause pulmonary hypertension and myocardial ischemia, are associated with increased inotrope requirements and ICU stay, and might have a role in perioperative gut ischemia *(63–66)*.

Prostacyclin and thromboxane are byproducts of the cyclooxygenase pathway located in platelets and endothelium. Prostacyclin (PGI_2) is produced by endothelial cyclooxygenase. It is a potent vasodilator and inhibits platelet adhesion to endothelium in synergy with NO. Thromboxane B2 (TXB_2) is produced by activated platelets and results in irreversible platelet aggregation and vasoconstriction. The balance between prostacyclin and TXB_2 can be modified with acetylsalicylic acid, which irreversibly inhibits platelet cyclooxygenase. This is a common therapy in patients with coronary heart disease. During cardiopulmonary bypass prostacyclin levels are increased due to the presence of heparin. Following platelet activation, TXB_2 levels are increased during and after cardiopulmonary bypass *(67)*. This results in a disturbed balance between prostacyclin and TXB_2 in the immediate postoperative period, which might have an influence on graft patency. It has been advocated to continue acetylsalicylic acid therapy in the perioperative period, but fear for increased postoperative bleeding discouraged many centers to adopt this policy. Because treatment with aprotinin effectively inhibits the increased bleeding in acetylsalicylic acid-treated patients, but maintains the effect of acetylsalicylic acid on platelets, this policy is no longer warranted *(68)*.

METHODS TO ATTENUATE MATERIAL-DEPENDENT ACTIVATION

Surface Coating of Extracorporeal Circuits

A large improvement in the biocompatibility of the extracorporeal circuit was expected with the development of extracorporeal circuits that were lined with a more biocompatible coating. The first and most extensively studied coating is heparin coating. Promising recent developments include coatings of poly-2-methoxyethyl acrylate *(69)* synthetic protein *(70)* and phosphorylcholine *(71)*. The concept behind heparin coating is to mimic the endothelial surface that contains heparan sulfate. Currently two types of heparin coating are commercially available for extracorporeal circuits. In the first coating heparin is ionically bound to the polymeric surface of the extracorporeal circuit (Duraflo II, Baxter, Muskegon, MI). The second type of coating uses covalently bound heparin (Carmeda, Medtronic, Minneapolis, MN; Bioline, Jostra, Hirrlingen, Germany). Both coatings have been studied extensively during the past decade. The most striking effect of heparin-coated circuits is the reduction of complement activation, which has been estimated at 45% *(72)*. Another study comparing Duraflo II with Carmeda coatings demonstrated a 25% reduction with both coatings *(73)*. The reductions are most prominent in C5a and TCC levels, probably owing to their slower clearance. Secondary to the reduced complement activation, the inflammatory responses of leukocytes, platelets, and endothelium are attenuated, resulting in reduced lactoferin and myeloperoxidase levels *(74,75)*, IL-6, IL-8, and E-selectin *(76,77)*, oxygen free-radical production *(78)*, integrin and selectin response of platelets *(79)*, and platelet β-thromboglobulin release *(80)*. Although heparin coating is effective in reducing complement activation through the alternative pathway, classical pathway activation after protamine infusion was also shown to be reduced *(81)*. This might indicate that a key component of the complement system is inactivated or bound by the coating *(82)*.

The levels of kallikrein–C1 esterase inhibitor complex, a marker for contact activation, were shown to be reduced during cardiopulmonary bypass with heparin-coated circuits, but remained unchanged when uncoated circuits were used *(7)*. Binding of FXII to the coating could be responsible for this observation *(83)*.

Contrary to initial expectations, thrombin generation and the activity of the fibrinolytic system are not reduced with heparin coating *(84,85)*. Improved hemostasis, reflected by a decrease in perioperative blood loss and transfusions with the use of coated circuits has only been reported anecdotally. These results were obtained when heparin coating was combined with a lower dose of systemic heparin *(86,87)*. However, the use of a decreased dose of heparin in conjunction with heparin-coated circuits is not considered to be safe and is indicated only in special circumstances *(88)*.

Although substantial reductions in blood activation can be obtained with heparin-coated circuits, it has proven difficult to translate these into improved clinical outcomes. In one study, a decreased intrapulmonary shunt with improved respiratory index was found after cardiopulmonary bypass with heparin-coated circuits. However, intubation time and ICU stay were not affected *(89)*. A composite score, consisting of intubation time, the central–peripheral temperature difference, and postoperative fluid balance, was significantly reduced with heparin-coated circuits *(90)*. Similarly, a composite score of adverse events after coronary surgery was improved by using heparin-coated circuits *(91,92)*. In a multicenter European trial, a significantly better postoperative recovery was found in females and in patients with crossclamp times exceeding 60 min when heparin-coated circuits were used *(93)*.

Aprotinin

Aprotinin is a polypeptide processed from bovine lung that acts as an inhibitor of serine proteases such as plasmin, trypsin, and kallikrein *(94)*. It was first introduced into cardiac surgery in an attempt to reduce complement activation during cardiopulmonary bypass. Although this attempt failed, "bone-dry" operative fields with significantly reduced postoperative blood loss and perioperative homologous blood product use were noted *(95)*. Since these initial reports, use of aprotinin has become widespread as an adjunct in blood-saving programs in cardiac surgery. Two dosage regimens with aprotinin have evolved, the low Groningen and the high Hammersmith dose, which have similar effectiveness in reducing blood loss and transfusion requirements *(96–98)*. More recently, encouraging results were obtained with aprotinin administered topically to the pericardial sac *(99)*.

Owing to its nonspecific mode of action, aprotinin has a number of effects. Most notably, aprotinin, in either dose, preserves platelet function by preventing the acute loss of the Gp1b adhesive receptor expression on platelets that occurs at the onset of cardiopulmonary bypass *(56)*. The mechanism underlying this protective effect has not been elucidated. Possibly, aprotinin inhibits the activity or production of trace amounts of agonists on the surface of the extracorporeal circuit, or interferes with the interaction between the platelet and the foreign surface. Inhibition of hyperfibrinolysis is a second mechanism by which aprotinin reduces bleeding in cardiopulmonary bypass, and probably explains the efficacy of topically administered aprotinin and other antifibrinolytic agents *(100–102)*. Aprotinin has also been shown to protect platelets against the inhibitory effect of heparin, a phenomenon present in 30% of patients that is not clarified *(103)*.

A number of anti-inflammatory effects of aprotinin have been demonstrated. In simulated bypass, aprotinin inhibited contact, complement, and neutrophil activation *(104)*. In vitro aprotinin inhibits ICAM-1 and VCAM expression on endothelial cells *(105)* and inhibits shedding of L-selectin of leukocytes *(106)* and neutrophil transmigration *(107)*. In a murine bronchial epithelial cell line, aprotinin inhibited expression of the cytokine-inducible form of nitric oxide synthase *(108)*, which could account for the decreased airway NO levels found during CPB in aprotinin-treated patients *(109)*. During CPB, aprotinin inhibits CD11b expression *(110–112)*, and after CPB, reduced levels of TNF *(110)*, IL-8 *(113)*, and IL-6 and increased IL-1 receptor antagonist *(114)* were found. In a comparative study, the effects of aprotinin on CD11b expression and TNF levels were comparable to those of methylprednisolone *(110)*. Bronchoalveolar lavage fluid obtained after CPB contained less neutrophils and less IL-8 in aprotinin-treated patients *(115)*, and lung tissue contained reduced levels of malondialdehyde, a marker of oxygen free radical damage, higher glutathione peroxidase levels, and reduced leukocyte sequestration *(116)*.

Although use of aprotinin in cardiac surgery is considered efficacious and safe *(117)*, many clinicians caution against liberal use of aprotinin, arguing that the inhibition of fibrinolysis might increase thromboembolic complications, particularly the occlusion of thrombogenic de-endothelialized vein grafts *(118–120)*. Others have implicated inhibition of activated protein C, a pivotal factor in the regulation of coagulation, by aprotinin as a cause for thromboembolic complications *(121)*. Although thromboembolic complications after aprotinin treatment have been reported anecdotally, it appears to be safer to use the lowest effective dose of aprotinin during CPB. Currently, the low-dosage regimen and topical aprotinin meet this criterion. As for the inhibition of activated protein C, we demonstrated that aprotinin treatment, either low or high dose, does not change the pattern of activation of the protein C system *(122)*.

Corticosteroids

Administration of high-dose corticosteroids has been shown to attenuate the inflammatory response induced by cardiopulmonary bypass and to improve the postoperative course *(41)*. Although inhibition of the alternative pathway by methylprednisolone has been demonstrated *(123)*, C3a and elastase levels during cardiopulmonary bypass were not influenced by high-dose corticosteroids *(124,125)*. The cytokine response during cardiopulmonary bypass is markedly modulated by high-dose corticosteroids. Increase of the inflammatory cytokines Il-6, Il-8, and TNF is prevented, whereas concentrations of the anti-inflammatory Il-10 increase 10-fold *(126–130)*. Reduced cytokine-mediated activation of neutrophils results in reduced CD11b expression and leukotriene B4 release *(125,131)*. Moreover, leukocyte adhesion to endothelium is reduced because glucocorticoids inhibit the expression of ICAM-1 to which CD11b adheres *(132)*. The attenuated inflammatory response with high-dose corticosteroids has been associated with enhanced myocardial recovery, reduced pulmonary damage, and an overall better clinical recovery after cardiopulmonary bypass *(123,133,134)*.

MATERIAL-INDEPENDENT ACTIVATION

Cardiotomy Suction

Recently, it became clear that blood collected in the pericardium is highly activated by tissue factor and t-PA and is rich in the highly procoagulant microparticles derived from damaged platelets and erythrocytes *(135–137)*. Tissue factor is not expressed by pericardium, but enters the pericardium from the surgical wounds *(138)*. Being a mesothelial surface, pericardium is rich in t-PA *(139)*. In vitro experiments have indicated that the activation of pericardial blood is triggered by the extrinsic (tissue factor) coagulation system and that the activation of fibrinolysis is secondary *(135)*. Retransfusion of the activated blood introduces fibrin(ogen) degradation products into the circulation, which interfere with platelet receptors, fibrinogen binding to platelets, and clot formation *(140,141)*. Moreover, activators are retransfused, which can result in further systemic activation and impaired hemostasis *(142)*. Similarly, retransfusion of mediastinally shed blood after operation was shown to result in a dose-dependent inflammatory response, impaired hemostasis, and increased bleeding *(143)*. Nevertheless, with a limited amount of retransfusion, reductions in blood use could be achieved *(144)*.

There are several ways to reduce the activation of pericardial blood. Use of a controlled suction device, which incorporates a level sensor that is activated when blood accumulates in the pericardium, minimizes superfluous suctioning and air entering the suction line, and thus the formation of activating air–blood interfaces *(145)*. Reduction of the contact time between blood and pericardium might have additional effects.

Topical administration of aprotinin into the surgical wound and the pericardium can inhibit the hyperfibrinolysis that occurs in the pericardial blood and improve hemostasis *(99)*. Because heparin levels in pericardial blood were shown to be lower than systemic levels, topical administration of heparin might also reduce the activation of pericardial blood, by reducing thrombin activity *(135)*.

Ischemia and Reperfusion

Cooling and cardioplegia have been shown to attenuate the negative effects of ischemia on the heart after crossclamping of the aorta by reducing the metabolic demand of the myocardium. Nevertheless, ischemia will occur or is already present owing to the disease process that is being treated. This ischemia will reduce high-energy phosphate content of cells and may cause a degree of reversible and irreversible myocardial damage. Proposed mediators of reperfusion injury following ischemia involve the generation of oxygen free radicals, which are produced via the xanthine oxidase reaction *(146)* and by activated neutrophils *(147)*. Exposure of the ischemic endothelium to oxygen free radicals induces a rapid upregulation of P-selectin and integrin expression *(148)*. At reperfusion, this will result in the accumulation of more activated neutrophils, which shed their cytotoxic enzymes, cytokines, and oxygen free radicals on the endothelium, leading to tissue injury. Damage to receptors involved in the activation of constitutive NO synthase will reduce nitric oxide production and as a consequence coronary spasm and the no-reflow phenomenon can occur *(149)*. Possible ways to reduce reperfusion damage include oxygen-radical scavengers *(150)*, maintenance of physiological oxygen concentrations during CPB *(151)*, inhibition of xanthine oxidase by allopurinol *(152)*, or prevention of ischemia by using continuous blood cardioplegia techniques *(153)*.

Respiratory dysfunction is a well-recognized side effect of cardiac operations. One-quarter of uncomplicated CPB patients still have a significant respiratory impairment 1 wk after operation *(154)*. A proportion of these impairments can be attributed to deteriorated breathing mechanics as a result of surgical factors (e.g., wound pain, drains, effusions). The effects of cardiopulmonary bypass primarily involve the gas flow and gas exchange owing to parenchymal damage *(155)*.

The bronchial circulation might be expected to prevent ischemia of the lungs during CPB and crossclamping. However, in a piglet study a 10-fold decrease in bronchial artery blood flow during CPB was demonstrated *(156)*. Thus, low or absent flow in the pulmonary circulation during aortic crossclamping is likely to occur and will result in similar reperfusion phenomena as in the myocardium. This is supported by the salutary role of inhaled NO, intravenous NO donors, and endothelin-1 antagonists in the treatment of postperfusion pulmonary dysfunction *(157–159)*. Apart from reperfusion injury, other factors unique to the lung render it more susceptible to damage by cardiopulmonary bypass. First, the lung is the filter of the venous circulation, meaning that all active or activating substances and cells generated during CPB transit the pulmonary circulation. Second, the lung capillaries are smaller in diameter than the average systemic capillaries, resulting in preferential trapping of aggregates in the lung. Third, a considerable pool of neutrophils is present in the lungs *(160)*. The importance of neutrophils in inducing lung damage is illustrated by the correlation of postoperative shunt fraction and respiratory index with elastase levels *(161)*. Animal experiments demonstrated that leukocyte depletion by filtration reduced heart and lung reperfusion injury *(162)*. Clinically, the use of leukocyte filters transiently improved the pulmonary shunt fraction and the mean arterial pressure *(163)*. In another study, post-bypass filtration of 2 L heart–lung machine blood significantly improved the postoperative lung function *(164)*. Maintenance of some pulmonary flow during aortic crossclamping, as is achieved with the use of two-stage venous canulas, was shown to prevent the increase in extravascular lung water content and preserve endothelin clearance *(165,166)*. This concept is expanded by using the Drew perfusion technique, in which no oxygenator is used but the patient's lungs provide oxygenation through separate perfusion of the systemic and pulmonary circulations *(167)*. Use of this technique resulted in reduced pulmonary leukocyte sequestration and complement activation *(168)*.

Hemodilution

At the initiation of CPB, mixing of the patient's blood with the relatively large asanguineous pump prime results in a sudden hemodilution. Although moderate hemodilution is considered beneficial in the setting of CPB, unwanted side effects do occur, and dilution to hematocrits below 0.23 during CPB are associated with increased mortality *(169)*. Next to the apparent effect on oxygen delivery, hemodilution can reduce the plasma colloid oncotic pressure to borderline values, resulting in a transcapillary oncotic imbalance. Consequently, important fluid shifts toward the interstitial tissue take place, contributing to edema formation, hypovolemia, and impaired oxygen delivery to vital organs such as the digestive tract *(170,171)*. Reduction of the priming volume of the extracorporeal circuit was demonstrated to attenuate the hyperdynamic response to CPB, as measured by fluid load, arterial pressure, cardiac index, vascular resistance, and oxygen delivery *(172)*. Furthermore, endotoxin levels, likely derived from ischemic intestines, were reduced in these patients. Increasing the colloid oncotic pressure of the priming solution by replacement of crystalloids with colloids similarly improved the postoperative course and resulted in reduced hospital stay *(173)*.

Reduction of priming volumes also results in important savings in the use of donor blood by two mechanisms *(172)*. First, the reduction of hemodilution will allow for predonation of relatively large volumes of blood in the majority of patients while maintaining a sufficiently high hematocrit during perfusion. Retransfusion of predonated blood after perfusion has been shown to improve hemostasis *(174)*. Second, the attenuated hyperdynamic response will reduce the need for fluid administration and thus further hemodilution during and after perfusion *(173)*. Other methods to prevent or treat excessive hemodilution during extracorporeal circulation, such as the use of blood cardioplegia or perioperative hemofiltration, were shown to further reduce the need for blood transfusions in coronary surgery *(175)*.

Hypothermia

Hypothermic perfusion has for a long time been a standard procedure during CPB. In addition to its effect on cell metabolism, a reduction of the inflammatory reaction can be anticipated. Indeed, IL-1, IL-6, and TNF production appeared higher at 37°C during in vitro experiments and in clinical CPB *(176)*. Similarly, elastase levels were higher after normothermic perfusion *(177)*. Also, the production of E-selectin was reduced, and CD11b upregulation was delayed at low temperature, which could account for reduced leukocyte adherence to the vasculature after reperfusion *(178,179)*. Other researchers have found a similar release of cytokines at normothermia (>36.5°C) compared to hypothermia *(180)*.

Although normothermic cardiopulmonary bypass appears to induce a more severe inflammatory reaction on a biochemical level, this is not reflected in clinical parameters. No difference in adverse events such as perioperative infarctions, use of an intra-aortic balloon pump, length of ICU stay, or mortality was observed *(181)*. However, vasopressors are used more frequently in normothermic perfusion, probably as a result of reduced endothelial endothelin-1 release, or an increased production of nitric oxide *(181–183)*. Other studies reported improved pulmonary function with shorter intubation times and a reduced incidence of postoperative atrial fibrillation after normothermic CPB *(184–186)*.

When considering normothermic CPB, neuroprotection is of special interest. Cognitive impairment can be identified in up to 45% patients who undergo CPB and focal deficits in 1–3% *(187,188)*. The cerebral damage is caused mainly by emboli. Focal defects are the result of large emboli that originate from surgical manipulation of the heart and aorta. Microemboli are thought to be responsible for the more subtle neurological defects detected in neuropsychological testing *(189)*. With the use of a particle counter, it was found that a bubble oxygenator produced more 15–80 μm microemboli than a membrane oxygenator, but that 80% of all particles were produced in the blood circulation owing to cardiotomy suction *(190)*. The small capillary and arteriolar dilatations (SCADs) that are caused by diffuse depositions of acellular fatty material found postmortem in the brains of patients who have recently undergone CPB might be the result of these microemboli *(191)*. In a dog study, use of a cell saver instead of cardiotomy suction reduced the number of SCADs by more than 50% *(192)*.

Several studies have addressed the issue of perfusion temperature and cerebral protection, often with the use of an impressive battery of neuropsychological tests *(193–200)*. The results of these studies vary greatly. Some found a protective effect of hypothermia, others of normothermia or of "tepid" perfusion. A meta-analysis by the Cochrane Collaboration could only demonstrate a trend toward fewer strokes with hypothermic perfusion, but this was offset by a trend toward increased incidence of non-stroke-related mortality and morbidity *(201)*. The current knowledge is far from conclusive and in many centers an intermediate course with temperatures between 32 and 35°C is followed. Recently, specific markers for cerebral damage such as the S-100 protein and neuron-specific enolase have become available *(202,203)*. A correlation of CPB time with levels of S-100 could be explained by intensified suction in these patients *(204)*. Similarly, intracardiac operations appeared to be associated with higher S-100 levels than CABG operations and the use of an arterial filter with reduced S-100 levels in CABG operations *(205,206)*. In OPCAB, 10-fold reductions in S-100 levels compared to on-pump CABG were observed *(207)*. These assays will be of aid in the development of improved neuroprotective strategies in cardiopulmonary bypass.

Heparin

Because blood will clot in an extracorporeal circuit, strict anticoagulation is mandatory. Traditionally, heparin is used for this purpose because of its easy dosage, control of effectivity and the availability of an antidote. However, heparin does have side effects. Despite adequate heparin levels, thrombin generation can be detected during cardiopulmonary bypass. Moreover, heparin administration results in a rapid release of t-PA from its body sources, which may induce fibrinolysis *(208,209)*. Recently, in vitro inhibition of platelet function by heparin was reported *(210)*. This inhibition, which was present in more than 30% of the study population, was associated with an increased postoperative blood loss. Heparin also has proactivating properties on granulocytes and platelets *(211,212)*. With the neutralization of heparin with protamine, complexes are formed that activate the complement system through the classical pathway. This classical pathway activation correlates with postoperative pulmonary shunt fraction *(213)*. The recombinant form of platelet factor 4, a polypeptide present in platelets that binds and inhibits heparin, could become an attractive alternative to protamine *(214,215)*.

The disadvantages related to heparin and protamine have prompted a search for better anticoagulants. Hirudin, a selective thrombin inhibitor derived from leeches, is frequently mentioned as an attractive alternative. Animal studies comparing recombinant hirudin with heparin demonstrated good clinical results without increased bleeding tendency *(216)*. Unlike heparin, however, hirudin only inhibits thrombin; it does not prevent its formation. This could result in the escape of small amounts of thrombin, as was demonstrated in vitro *(217)*. The absence of an inhibitory effect of hirudin on components higher in the coagulation cascade will not prevent an ongoing activation at this level and might result in depletion of these factors *(218)*. Finally, an antidote to hirudin is not available. Based on these considerations, replacement of heparin with hirudin is not advised. Perhaps there is a role for hirudin as an adjunct to heparin.

FUTURE DEVELOPMENTS

From the previous sections it is clear that many factors are involved in the detrimental effects of cardiopulmonary bypass. Therefore, substantial improvements in the procedure of cardiopulmonary bypass can only be obtained when a multifactorial approach is followed, directed at both material-dependent and -independent factors. Thus, biocompatibility of material surfaces has to be improved, and material-independent sources of blood activation should be controlled by adaptation of perfusion techniques and, when necessary, pharmacological intervention.

Based on current insights and available technologies, we propose a novel system for CPB aimed at minimal disturbance of the patient's homeostasis. Primary in this system is a newly designed low-prime, closed-volume, and hemocompatible extracorporeal circuit. The basic principle of this circuit is to abandon the use of gravity drainage and use a venoarterial blood pump instead *(219)*. An alternative is the use of vacuum-assisted drainage *(220)*. Both techniques allow for the use of smaller cannulae and tubings and placement of the extracorporeal circuit close to the patient. Together with a low-prime oxygenator with an integrated arterial filter, a drastic reduction of the prime volume will be achieved. Hemodilution can be further minimized by using the technique of retrograde autologous priming, in which a substantial portion of the priming volume can be extracted from the extracorporeal circuit by controlled exsanguination of the patient into the circuit while simultaneously draining priming solution *(221)*. Handling of air in such a system is more complicated and will require an advanced air-trapping mechanism. The cardiotomy reservoir will be connected to a controlled suction or a cell-saving device. All components of the circuit will be coated with heparin and primed with aprotinin.

The described system is expected to provide a more physiological perfusion. The reduced prime volumes will avoid hemodilution, hypooncotic pressures, and fluid shifts, ensuring improved preservation of the patient's autoregulatory mechanisms and better hemodynamic stability and organ perfusion. The use of controlled suction will minimize the contact time between blood and nonendothelialized tissues, thus avoiding activation of the coagulation and fibrinolytic systems. Addition of heparin, hirudin, or aprotinin to the pericardial sac can be of further aid to achieve this goal. An alternative to controlled suction might be the use of a cell-saving device, which separates red cells from the fluid in the pericardial sac. In the proposed system, heparin coating is used. However, it should be emphasized that this coating results in only a 25–45% reduction in complement activation and, to a lesser extent, inhibits contact activation. Although contact activation can be inhibited by the addition of aprotinin to the pump prime, the problem of complement activation will persist. Because the mechanism of heparin coating is probably the result of absorption of an essential factor of the complement system, it does not seem to be pragmatic to improve the efficacy of the heparin coating. Instead, research should be focused at the development of biologically active coatings that actually prevent the activation of the humoral and cellular components of blood.

The use of improved perfusion equipment and techniques should be accompanied by improved methods for monitoring the quality of the perfusion. Traditionally, perfusion is guided by the values of flow, pressures, diuresis, and a limited number of laboratory results. These do not adequately monitor the primary goal of perfusion, i.e., maintenance of adequate microcirculation, but mainly reflect the macrocirculation. Moreover, the target values for flow, perfusion pressure, and their interactions with temperature management and hematocrits resulted more from assumptions than from (patho)physiological studies.

Direct monitoring of the microcirculation is possible with the technique of orthogonal polarization spectral imaging *(222)*. With this technique the microcirculation on mucous membranes can be visualized up to the level of individual traveling erythrocytes. Currently this technique is in an experimental phase. Difficulties in the interpretation and processing of data preclude its routine use. Furthermore, probes for measurement of the microcirculation in the intestine, which is affected earliest during CPB, are not yet available. Alternatively, the adequacy of the microcirculation can be monitored by measurement of biochemical markers for ischemic organ damage. These markers should be sensitive and specific, be measurable by simple assays that can be performed on a routine basis with results available during or shortly after the perfusion. Obviously, if beating heart revascularization proves to be as safe and effective as conventional bypass grafting in the short and long term, off-pump approaches will circumvent many of the pathophysiological derangements associated with extracorporeal circulation.

REFERENCES

1. Kirklin JW. Open-heart surgery at the Mayo Clinic: the 25th anniversary. Mayo Clin Proc 1980;55:339–341.
2. Westaby S. Organ dysfunction after cardiopulmonary bypass. A systemic inflammatory reaction initiated by the extracorporeal circuit. Intensive Care Med 1987;13:89–95.
3. Edmunds LH Jr. Blood-surface interactions during cardiopulmonary bypass. J Card Surg 1993;8: 404–410.
4. Wachtfogel YT, Harpel PC, Edmunds LH Jr, Colman RW. Formation of C1s-C1-inhibitor, kallikrein-C1-inhibitor and plasmin-alpha 2-plasmin-inhibitor complexes during cardiopulmonary bypass. Blood 1989;73:468–471.
5. Burman JF, Chung HI, Lane DA, Philippou H, Adami A, Lincoln JC. Role of factor XII in thrombin generation and fibrinolysis during cardiopulmonary bypass. Lancet 1994;344:1192–1193.
6. Moorman RM, Reynolds DS, Communale ME. Management of cardiopulmonary bypass in a patient with congenital factor XII deficiency. J Cardiothorac Vasc Anesth 1993;7:452–454.
7. te Velthuis H, Baufreton C, Jansen PG, et al. Heparin coating of extracorporeal circuits inhibits contact activation during cardiac operations. J Thorac Cardiovasc Surg 1997;114:117–122.
8. Boisclair MD, Lane DA, Philippou H, et al. Mechanisms of thrombin generation during cardiopulmonary bypass. Blood 1993;82:3350–3357.
9. Philippou H, Adami A, Boisclair MD, Lane DA. An ELISA for factor X activation peptide: application to the investigation of thrombogenesis in cardiopulmonary bypass. Br J Haematol 1995;90:432–437.
10. Kazatchkine MD, Nydegger UE. The human alternative pathway. Biology and immunopathology of activation and regulation. Prog Allergy 1982;30:193–234.
11. Müller-Eberhard HJ. Complement: Chemistry and pathways. In Gallin JI, Goldstein IM, Snyderman R. Inflammation: Basic Principles and Clinical Correlates. New York: Raven Press, 1988:21–54.
12. Chenoweth DE, Cooper SW, Hugli TE, Stewart RW, Blackstone EH, Kirklin JW. Complement activation during cardiopulmonary bypass. N Engl J Med 1981;304:497–503.
13. Parker DJ, Cantrell JW, Karp RB, Stroud RM, Digerness SB. Changes in serum complement and immunoglobins following cardiopulmonary bypass. Surgery 1972;71:824–827.
14. Videm V, Fosse E, Mollnes TE, Garred P, Svennevig JL. Complement activation with bubble and membrane oxygenators in aortocoronary bypass grafting. Ann Thorac Surg 1990;50:387–391.
15. Videm V, Mollnes TE. Human complement activation by polygeline and dextran 70. Scand J Immunol 1994;39:314–320.
16. Cooper NR. The classical complement pathway: activation and regulation of the first complement component. Adv Immunol 1985;37:151–216.
17. Loos M, Wellek B, Thesen R, Opferkuch W. Antibody-independent interaction of the first component of complement with gram-negative bacteria. Infect Immun 1978;22:5–9.
18. Fehr J, Rohr H. In vivo complement activation by polyanion-polycation complexes: Evidence that C5a is generated intravascularly during heparin-protamine interaction. Clin Immunol 1983;29:7–14.
19. Kirklin JK, Chenoweth DE, Naftel DC, et al. Effects of protamine administration after cardiopulmonary bypass on complement, blood elements, and the hemodynamic state. Ann Thorac Surg 1986;41: 193–199.

20. Salama A, Hugo F, Heinrich D, et al. Deposition of terminal C5b-9 complement complexes on erythrocytes and leukocytes during cardiopulmonary bypass. N Engl J Med 1988;318:408–414.
21. Schreurs HH, Wijers MJ, Gu YJ, et al. Heparin coated bypass circuits: effects on inflammatory response in paediatric cardiac surgery. Ann Thorac Surg 1998;66:166–171.
22. Hugli TE, Müller-Eberhard HJ. Anaphylatoxins C3a and C5a: Adv Immunol 1978;26:1–53.
23. Charo IF, Yuen C, Perez HD, Goldstein IM. Chemotactic peptides modulate adherence of human polymorphonuclear leukocytes to monolayers to monolayers of cultured endothelial cells. J Immunol 1986;136:3412–3419.
24. Tonnesen MG, Smedly LA, Henson PM. Neutrophil-endothelial cell interactions. J Clin Invest 1984;74:1581–1592.
25. Bender JG, van Epps DE. Stimulus interactions in release of superoxide anion (O_2^-) from human neutrophils. Inflammation 1985;9:67–86.
26. Bender JG, Mc Phail LC, van Epps DE. Exposure of human neutrophils to chemotactic factors potentiates activation of the respiratory burst enzyme. J Immunol 1983;130:2316–2323.
27. Henson PM, Zanolari B, Schwartzman NA, Hong SR. Intracellular control of human neutrophil secretion. I. C5a-induced stimulus-specific desensitisation and the effects of cytochalasin B. J Immunol 1978;121:851–855.
28. Clancy RM, Dahinden CA, Hugli TE. Arachidonate metabolism by human polymorphonuclear leukocytes stimulated by N-formyl-Met-Leu-Phe or complement component C5a is independent of phospholipase activation. Proc Natl Acad Sci USA 1983;80:7200–7204.
29. Palmer RMJ, Salmon JA. Release of leukotriene B4 from human neutrophils and its relationship to degranulation induced by *n*-formyl-methionyl-leucyl-phenylalanine, serum-treated zymosan and the ionophore A23187. Immunology 1983;50:65–73.
30. Cochrane CG, Spragg RG, Revak SD. Studies on the pathogenesis of the adult respiratory distress syndrome: evidence of oxidants in the broncheoalveolar lavage fluid. J Clin Invest 1983;71:754–761.
31. Royston D, Minty BD, Higenbottam TW, Wallwork J, Jones GJ. The effect of surgery with cardiopulmonary bypass on alveolar-capillary barrier function in human beings. Ann Thorac Surg 1985;40:139–143.
32. Rinaldo JE, Rogers RM. Adult respiratory distress syndrome. Changing concepts of lung injury and repair. N Engl J Med 1982;306:900–909.
33. Dinarello CA. Interleukin-1. Rev Infect Dis 1984;6:51–95.
34. Smith RJ, Speziale SC, Bowman BJ. Properties of interleukin-1 as a complete secretagogue for human neutrophils. Biochem Biophys Res Commun 1982;130:1233–1240.
35. Mizel SB. Interleukin 1 and T cell activation. Immunol Rev 1982;63:51–72.
36. Falkoff RJM, Muraguchi A, Hong JX, Buttler JL, Dinarello CA, Fanci AS. The effects of interleukin 1 on human B cell activation and proliferation. J Immunol 1983;131:801–805.
37. Old LJ. Tumor necrosis factor (TNF). Science 1985;230:630–632.
38. Dinarello CA, Cannon JG, Wolff SM, et al. Tumor necrosis factor (cachectin) is an endogenous pyrogen and induces production of interleukin 1. J Exp Med 1986;163:1433–1450.
39. Nawroth PP, Stern D. Modulation of endothelial cell hemostatic properties by tumor necrosis factor. J Exp Med 1986;164:740–745.
40. Nawroth PP, Bank I, Handley D, Cassimeris J, Chess L, Stern D. Tumor necrosis factor/cachectin interacts with endothelial cell receptors to induce release of interleukin 1. J Exp Med 1986;163: 1363–1375.
41. Jansen NJ, van Oeveren W, van de Broek L, et al. Inhibition by dexamethasone of the reperfusion phenomena in cardiopulmonary bypass. J Thorac Cardiovasc Surg 1991;102:515–525.
42. Jansen NJ, van Oeveren W, Gu YJ, van Vliet MH, Eijsman L, Wildevuur CR. Endotoxin release and tumor necrosis factor formation during cardiopulmonary bypass. Ann Thorac Surg 1992;54:744–748.
43. Fransen E, Maessen J, Dentener M, Senden N, Geskes G, Buurman W. Systemic inflammation present in patients undergoing CABG without extracorporeal circulation. Chest 1998;113:1290–1295.
44. Schulze C, Conrad N, Schutz A, et al. Reduced expression of systemic proinflammatory cytokines after off-pump versus conventional coronary artery bypass grafting. Thorac Cardiovasc Surg 2000;48: 364–369.
45. Wan S, Marchant A, DeSmet JM, et al. Human cytokine responses to cardiac transplantation and coronary artery bypass grafting. J Thorac Cardiovasc Surg 1996;111:469–477.
46. Butler J, Chong GL, Baigrie RJ, Pillai R, Westaby S, Rocker GM. Cytokine responses to cardiopulmonary bypass with membrane and bubble oxygenation. Ann Thorac Surg 1992;53:833–838.

47. Kukielka GL, Smith CW, Manning AM, Youker KA, Michael LH, Entman ML. Induction of interleukin-6 synthesis in the myocardium. Potential role in postreperfusion inflammatory injury. Circulation 1995;92:1866–1875.
48. Jorens PG, de Jongh R, de Backer W, et al. Interleukin-8 production in patients undergoing cardiopulmonary bypass. The influence of pre-treatment with methylprednisolone. Am Rev Respir Dis 1993;148:890–895.
49. Ivey CL, Williams FW, Collins PD, Jose PJ, Williams TJ. Neutrophil chemoattractants generated in two phases during reperfusion of ischemic myocardium in the rabbit. Evidence for a role for C5a and interleukin-8. J Clin Invest 1995;95:2720–2728.
50. Gearing AJH, Newman W. Circulating adhesion molecules in disease. Immunol Today 1993;14: 506–512.
51. Gu YJ, van Oeveren W, Boonstra PW, de Haan J, Wildevuur CR. Leukocyte activation with increased membrane expression of CR3 receptors induced by cardiopulmonary bypass. Ann Thorac Surg 1992;53:839–844.
52. Gillinov AM, Bator JM, Zehr KJ, et al. Neutrophil adhesion molecule expression during cardiopulmonary bypass with bubble and membrane oxygenators. Ann Thorac Surg 1993;56:847–853.
53. Arnaout MA, Hakim RM, Todd RF III, Dana N, Colten HR. Increased expression of an adhesion-promoting surface glycoprotein in the granulocytopenia of hemodialysis. N Engl J Med 1985;312:457–462.
54. Etzioni A. Adhesion molecules—their role in health and disease. Pediatr Res 1996;39:191–198.
55. Dreyer WJ, Michael LH, Millman EE, Berens KL. Neutrophil activation and adhesion molecule expression in a canine model of open heart surgery with cardiopulmonary bypass. Cardiovasc Res 1995;29:775–781.
56. van Oeveren W, Eijsman L, Roozendaal KJ, Wildevuur CR. Platelet preservation by aprotinin during cardiopulmonary bypass. Lancet 1988;19:644.
57. Moncada S, Higgs A. The L-arginine-nitric oxide pathway. N Engl J Med 1993;329:2002–2012.
58. Speziale G, Ruvolo G, Marino B. A role for nitric oxide in the vasoplegic syndrome. J Card Surg (Torino) 1996;37:301–303.
59. Finkel MS, Oddis CV, Jacob TD, et al. Negative inotropic effects of cytokines on the heart mediated by nitric oxide. Science 1992;257:387–389.
60. Alican I, Kubes P. A critical role for nitric oxide in intestinal barrier function and dysfunction. Am J Physiol 1996;270:G225–G237.
61. Yanagisawa M, Kurihara H, Kimura S, et al. A novel potent vasoconstrictor peptide produced by vascular endothelial cells. Nature 1988;332:411–415.
62. Yoshizawa T, Osamu S, Giaid A, et al. Endothelin, a novel peptide in the posterior pituitary system. Science 1989;247:462–464.
63. te Velthuis H, Jansen PG, Oudemans-van Straaten HM, et al. Circulating endothelin in cardiac operations: influence of blood pressure and endotoxin. Ann Thorac Surg 1996;61:904–908.
64. Dorman BH, Bond BR, Clair MJ, et al. Temporal synthesis and release of endothelin within the systemic and myocardial circulation during and after cardiopulmonary bypass: relation to postoperative recovery. J Cardiothorac Vasc Anesth 2000;14:540–545.
65. Kirshbom PM, Tsui SS, Di Bernardo LR, et al. Blockade of endothelin-converting enzyme reduces pulmonary hypertension after cardiopulmonary bypass and circulatory arrest. Surgery 1995;118: 440–444.
66. Matheis G, Haak T, Beyersdorf F, Baretti R, Polywka C, Winkelmann BR. Circulating endothelin in patients undergoing coronary artery bypass grafting. Eur J Cardiothorac Surg 1995;9:269–274.
67. Nakamura H, Kim DK, Philbin DM, et al. Heparin-enhanced plasma phospholipase A2 activity and prostacyclin synthesis in patients undergoing cardiac surgery. J Clin Invest 1995;95:1062–1070.
68. Tabuchi N, Gallandat Huet RC, Sturk A, Eijsman L, Wildevuur CR. Aprotinin effects on aspirin treated platelets and hemostasis during cardiopulmonary bypass. Ann Thorac Surg 1994;58:1036–1039.
69. Suhara H, Sawa Y, Nishimura M, Oshiyama H, Yokoyama K, Saito N, Matsuda H. Efficacy of a new coating material, PMEA, for cardiopulmonary bypass circuits in a porcine model. Ann Thorac Surg 2001;71:1603–1608.
70. Wimmer-Greinecker G, Matheis G, Martens S, Oremek G, Abdel-Rahman U, Moritz A. Synthetic protein treated versus heparin coated cardiopulmonary bypass surfaces: similar clinical results and minor biochemical differences. Eur J Cardiothorac Surg 1999;16:211–217.
71. De Somer F, Francois K, van Oeveren W, et al. Phosphorylcholine coating of extracorporeal circuits provides natural protection against blood activation by the material surface. Eur J Cardiothorac Surg 200;18:602–606.

72. Videm V, Svennevig JL, Fosse E, Semb G, Osterud A, Mollnes TE. Reduced complement activation with heparin-coated oxygenator and tubings in coronary bypass operations. J Thorac Cardiovasc Surg 1992;103:806–813.
73. Ovrum E, Mollnes TE, Fosse E, et al. Complement and granulocyte activation in two different types of heparinized extracorporeal circuits. J Thorac Cardiovasc Surg 1995;110:1623–1632.
74. Lundblad R, Moen O, Fosse E. Endothelin-1 and neutrophil activation during heparin-coated cardiopulmonary bypass. Ann Thorac Surg 1997;63:1361–1367.
75. Moen O, Fosse E, Brockmeier V, et al. Disparity in blood activation by two different heparin-coated cardiopulmonary bypass systems. Ann Thorac Surg 1995;60:1317–1323.
76. Steinberg BM, Grossi EA, Schwartz DS, et al. Heparin bonding of bypass circuits reduces cytokine release during cardiopulmonary bypass. Ann Thorac Surg 1995;60:525–529.
77. Weerwind PW, Maessen JG, van Tits LJ, et al. Influence of Duraflo II heparin-treated extracorporeal circuits on the systemic inflammatory response in patients having coronary bypass. J Thorac Cardiovas Surg 1995;110:1633–1641.
78. Bozdayi M, Borowiec J, Nilsson L, Venge P, Thelin S, Hansson HE. Effects of heparin-coating of cardiopulmonary bypass circuits on in vitro oxygen free radical production during coronary bypass surgery. Artif Organs 1996;20:1008–1016.
79. Moen O, Hogasen K, Fosse E, et al. Attenuation of changes in leukocyte surface markers and complement activation with heparin-coated cardiopulmonary bypass. Ann Thorac Surg 1997;63:105–111.
80. Fukutomi M, Kobayashi S, Niwaya K, Hamada Y, Kitamura S. Changes in platelet, granulocyte and complement activation during cardiopulmonary bypass using heparin-coated equipment. Artif Organs 1996;20:767–776.
81. Gu YJ, van Oeveren W, Akkerman C, Boonstra PW, Huyzen RJ, Wildevuur CR. Heparin-coated circuits reduce the inflammatory response to cardiopulmonary bypass. Ann Thorac Surg 1993;55:917–922.
82. te Velthuis H, Jansen PGM, Hack CE, Eijsman L, Wildevuur CR. Specific complement inhibition by heparin-coated extracorporeal circuits. Ann Thorac Surg 1996;61:1153–1157.
83. van der Kamp KW, van Oeveren W. Contact, coagulation and platelet interaction with heparin treated equipment during heart surgery. Int J Artif Organs 1993;16:836–842.
84. Gorman RC, Ziats N, Rao AK, et al. Surface-bound heparin fails to reduce thrombin formation during clinical cardiopulmonary bypass. J Thorac Cardiovasc Surg 1996;111:1–12.
85. Ovrum E, Brosstad F, Am Holen E, Tangen G, Abdelnoor M. Effects on coagulation and fibrinolysis with reduced versus full heparinization and heparin coated cardiopulmonary bypass. Circulation 1995;92:2579–2584.
86. von Segesser LK, Weiss BM, Garcia E, von Felten A, Turina MI. Reduction and elimination of systemic heparinization during cardiopulmonary bypass. J Thorac Cardiovasc Surg 1992;103:790–799.
87. Ovrum E, Holen EA, Tangen G, et al. Completely heparinized cardiopulmonary bypass and reduced systemic heparin: clinical and hemostatic effects. Ann Thorac Surg 1995;60:365–371.
88. Edmunds LH Jr. Surface-bound heparin; panacea or peril? Ann Thorac Surg 1994;85:285–286.
89. Ranucci M, Cirri S, Conti D, et al. Beneficial effects of Duraflo II heparin-coated circuits on post-perfusion lung dysfunction. Ann Thorac Surg 1996 61:76–81.
90. Jansen PG, te Velthuis H, Huybrechts RA, et al. Reduced complement activation and improved post-operative performance after cardiopulmonary bypass with heparin-coated circuits. J Thorac Cardiovasc Surg 1995;110:829–834.
91. Jansen PG, Baufreton C, Le Besnerais P, Loisance DY, Wildevuur ChRH. Heparin-coated circuits and aprotinin prime for coronary artery bypass grafting. Ann Thorac Surg 1996;61:1363–1366.
92. Baufreton C, Le Besnerais P, Jansen P, et al. Clinical outcome after coronary surgery with heparin-coated extracorporeal circuits for cardiopulmonary bypass. Perfusion 1996;11:437–443.
93. Wildevuur CR, Jansen PG, Bezemer PD, et al. Clinical evaluation of Duraflo II treated extracorporeal circuits (2nd version). The European Working Group on heparin coated extracorporeal circulation circuits. Eur J Cardiothorac Surg 1997;11:616–623.
94. Verstraete M. Clinical application of inhibitors of fibrinolysis. Drugs 1985;29:236–261.
95. van Oeveren W, Jansen NJ, Bidstrup BP, et al. Effects of aprotinin on hemostatic mechanisms during cardiopulmonary bypass. Ann Thorac Surg 1987;44:640–645.
96. Wildevuur CR, Eijsman L, Roozendaal KJ, Harder MP, Chang MP, van Oeveren W. Platelet preservation during cardiopulmonary bypass with aprotinin. Eur J Cardiothor Surg 1989;3:533–538.
97. van Oeveren W, Harder MP, Roozendaal KJ, Eijsman L, Wildevuur CR. Aprotinin protects platelets against the initial effect of cardiopulmonary bypass. J Thorac Cardiovasc Surg 1990;99:788–797.

98. Speekenbrink RG, Wildevuur CR, Sturk A, Eijsman L. Low-dose and high-dose aprotinin improve hemostasis in coronary surgery. J Thorac Cardiovasc Surg 1996;112:523–530.
99. Tatar H, Cicek S, Demirkilic U, et al. Topical use of aprotinin in open heart operations. Ann Thorac Surg 1993;55:659–661.
100. Speekenbrink RG, Vonk AB, Wildevuur CR, Eijsman L. Hemostatic efficacy of dipyridamole, tranexamic acid and aprotinin in coronary bypass grafting. Ann Thorac Surg 1995;59:438–442.
101. Maquelin KN, Nieuwland R, Lentjes EG, et al. Aprotinin administration in the pericardial cavity does not prevent platelet activation. J Thorac Cardiovasc Surg 2000:120:552–557.
102. Horrow JC, Hlavacek J, Strong MD, et al. Prophylactic tranexamic acid decreases bleeding after cardiac operations. J Thorac Cardiovasc Surg 1990;99:70–74.
103. John LC, Rees GM, Kovacs IB. Reduction of heparin binding to and inhibition of platelets by aprotinin. Ann Thorac Surg 1993;55:1175–1179.
104. Wachtfogel YT, Kucich U, Hack CE, et al. Aprotinin inhibits the contact, neutrophil, and platelet activation systems during simulated extracorporeal perfusion. J Thorac Cardiovasc Surg 1993;106:1–10.
105. Asimakopoulos G, Lidington EA, Mason J, Haskard DO, Taylor KM, Landis RC. Effect of aprotinin on endothelial cell activation. J Thorac Cardiovasc Surg 2001;122:123–128.
106. Asimakopoulos G, Taylor KM, Haskard DO, Landis RC. Inhibition of neutrophil L-selectin shedding: a potential anti-inflammatory effect of aprotinin. Perfusion 2000;15:495–499.
107. Asimakopoulos G, Thompson R, Nourshargh S, et al. An anti-inflammatory property of aprotinin detected at the level of leukocyte extravasation. J Thorac Cardiovasc Surg 2000;120:361–369.
108. Hill GE, Taylor JA, Robbins RA. Differing effects of aprotinin and e-aminocaproic acid on cytokine-induced inducible nitric oxide synthase expression. Ann Thorac Surg 1997;63:74–77.
109. Hill GE, Springal DR, Robbins RA. Aprotinin is associated with a decrease in nitric oxide production during cardiopulmonary bypass. Surgery 1997;121:449–455.
110. Hill GE, Alonso A, Spurzem JR, Stammers AH, Robbins RA. Aprotinin and methylprednisolone equally blunt cardiopulmonary bypass-induced inflammation in humans. J Thorac Cardiovasc Surg 1995;110:1658–1662.
111. Asimakopoulos G, Kohn A, Stefanou DC, Haskard DO, Landis RC, Taylor KM. Leukocyte integrin expression in patients undergoing cardiopulmonary bypass. Ann Thorac Surg 2000;69:1192–1197.
112. Alonso A, Whitten CW, Hill GE. Pump prime only aprotinin inhibits cardiopulmonary bypass-induced neutrophil CD11b up-regulation. Ann Thorac Surg 1999;67:392–395.
113. Isbir CS, Dogan R, Demircin M, Yaylim I, Pasaoglu I. Aprotinin reduces the IL-8 after coronary artery bypass grafting. Cardiovasc Surg 2001;9:403–406.
114. Tassani P, Augustin N, Barankay A, Braun SL, Zaccaria F, Richter JA. High-dose aprotinin modulates the balance between proinflammatory and anti-inflammatory responses during coronary artery bypass graft surgery. J Cardiothorac Vasc Anesth 2000;14:682–686.
115. Hill GE, Pohorecki R, Alonso A, Rennard SI, Robbins RA. Aprotinin reduces interleukin-8 production and neutrophil accumulation after cardiopulmonary bypass. Anesth Analg 1996;83:696–700.
116. Rahman A, Ustunda B, Burma O, Ozercan IH, Cekirdekci A, Bayar MK. Does aprotinin reduce lung reperfusion damage after cardiopulmonary bypass? Eur J Cardiothorac Surg 2000;18:583–588.
117. Rich JB. The efficacy and safety of aprotinin use in cardiac surgery. Ann Thorac Surg 199;66:S6–S11.
118. van Oeveren W, van Oeveren B, Wildevuur CR. Anticoagulation policy during use of aprotinin in cardiopulmonary bypass. J Thorac Cardiovasc Surg 1992;104:210–211.
119. Feindt P, Seyfert U, Volkmar I, Huwer H, Kalweit G, Gams E. Is there a phase of hypercoagulability when aprotinin is used in cardiac surgery? Eur J Cardiothor Surg 1994;8:308–314.
120. Bidstrup BP, Underwood SR, Sapsford RN. Effect of aprotinin (Trasylol) on aorta-coronary bypass graft patency. J Thorac Cardiovasc Surg 1993;105:147–153.
121. Westaby S. Aprotinin in perspective. Ann Thorac Surg 1993;55:1033–1041.
122. Speekenbrink RG, Bertina RM, España F, Wildevuur CR, Eijsman L. Activation of the protein C anticoagulant system during cardiopulmonary bypass and the influence of aprotinin. Ann Thorac Surg 1998;66:1998–2002.
123. Weiler JM, Packard B. Methylprednisolone inhibits the alternative and amplification pathways of complement. Infect Immun 1982;38:122–126.
124. Boscoe MJ, Yewdall VM, Thompson MA, Cameron JS. Complement activation during cardiopulmonary bypass: quantitative study of effects of methylprednisolone and pulsatile flow. Br Med J (Clin Res Ed) 1983;287:1747–1750.

125. Jansen NJ, van Oeveren W, van Vliet M, Stoutenbeek CP, Eijsman L, Wildevuur CR. The role of different types of corticosteroids on the inflammatory mediators in cardiopulmonary bypass. Eur J Cardiothorac Surg 1991;5:211–217.
126. Hill GE, Snider S, Galbraith TA, Forst S, Robbins RA. Glucocorticoid reduction of bronchial epithelial inflammation during cardiopulmonary bypass. Am J Respir Crit Care Med 1995;152:1791–1795.
127. Kawamura T, Inada K, Okada H, Okada K, Wakusawa R. Methylprednisolone inhibits increase of interleukin 8 and 6 during open heart surgery. Can J Anaesth 1995;42:399–403.
128. Teoh KH, Bradley CA, Gauldie J, Burrows H. Steroid inhibition of cytokine-mediated vasodilation after warm heart surgery. Circulation 1995;92:347–353.
129. Tabardel Y, Duchateau J, Schmartz D, et al. Corticosteroids increase blood interleukin-10 levels during cardiopulmonary bypass in men. Surgery 1996;119:76–80.
130. Tassani P, Richter JA, Barankay A, et al. Does high-dose methylprednisolone in aprotinin-treated patients attenuate the systemic inflammatory response during coronary artery bypass grafting procedures? J Cardiothorac Vasc Anesth 1999;13:165–172.
131. Hill GE, Alonso A, Thiele GM, Robbins RA. Glucocorticoids blunt neutrophil CD11b surface glycoprotein upregulation during cardiopulmonary bypass in humans. Anesth Analg 1994;79:23–27.
132. Cronstein BN, Kimmel SC, Levin RI, Martiniuk F, Weissman G. A mechanism for the anti-inflammatory effects of corticosteroids: the glucocorticoid receptor regulates leukocyte adhesion to endothelial cells and expression of endothelial-leukocyte adhesion molecule 1 and intercellular adhesion molecule 1. Proc Natl Acad Sci USA 1992; 89:9991–9995.
133. Busuttil RW, George WJ, Hewitt RL. Protective effect of methylprednisolone on the heart during ischemic arrest. J Thorac Cardiovasc Surg 1975;70:955–965.
134. Hill DG, Aguilar MJ, Kosek JC, Hill JD. Corticosteroids and prevention of pulmonary damage following cardiopulmonary bypass in puppies. Ann Thorac Surg 1976;22:36–40.
135. Tabuchi N, de Haan J, Boonstra PW, van Oeveren W. Activation of fibrinolysis in the pericardial cavity during cardiopulmonary bypass. J Thorac Cardiovasc Surg 1993;106:828–833.
136. Nieuwland R, Berckmans RJ, Rotteveel-Eijkman RC, et al. Cell-derived microparticles generated in patients during cardiopulmonary bypass are highly procoagulant. Circulation 1997;96:3534–3541.
137. Philippou H, Adami A, Davidson SJ, Pepper JR, Burman JF, Lane DA. Tissue factor is rapidly elevated in plasma collected from the pericardial cavity during cardiopulmonary bypass. Thromb Haemost 2000;84:124–128.
138. Chung JH, Gikakis N, Rao AK, Drake TA, Colman RW, Edmunds LH Jr. Pericardial blood activates the extrinsic coagulation pathway during clinical cardiopulmonary bypass. Circulation 1996;93: 2014–2018.
139. van Hinsbergh VW, Kooistra T, Scheffer MA, van Bockel JH, van Muijen GN. Characterization and fibrinolytic properties of human omental tissue mesothelial cells. Comparison with endothelial cells. Blood 1990;75:1490–1497.
140. Adelman B, Michelson AD, Loscalzo J, Greenberg J, Handin RI. Plasmin effect on platelet glycoprotein Ib-von Willebrand's factor interaction. Blood 1985;65:32–40.
141. Coller BS. Platelet and thrombolytic therapy. N Engl J Med 1990;99:518–527.
142. de Haan J, Boonstra PW, Monnink SH, Ebels T, van Oeveren W. Retransfusion of suctioned blood during cardiopulmonary bypass impairs hemostasis. Ann Thorac Surg 1995;59:901–907.
143. Schönberger JP, van Oeveren W, Bredee JJ, Everts PA, de Haan J, Wildevuur CR. Systemic blood activation during and after autotransfusion Ann Thorac Surg 1994;57:1256–1262.
144. Schönberger JP, Bredee JJ, Speekenbrink RG, Everts PA, Wildevuur CR. Autotransfusion of shed blood contributes additionally to blood saving in patients receiving aprotinin (2 million KIU). Eur J Cardiothorac Surg 1993;7:474–477.
145. Boonstra PW, van Imhoff GW, Eijsman L, et al. Reduced platelet activation and improved hemostasis after controlled cardiotomy suction during clinical membrane oxygenator perfusions. J Thorac Cardiovasc Surg 1985;89:900–906.
146. Menasché P, Piwnica A. Free radicals and myocardial protection: a surgical viewpoint. Ann Thorac Surg 1989;47:939–945.
147. Royston D, Fleming JS, Desar JB, Westaby S, Taylor KM. Increased production of peroxidation products associated with cardiac operations. J Thorac Cardiovasc Surg 1986;91:759–766.
148. Lefer AM. Role of selectins in myocardial ischemia-reperfusion injury. Ann Thorac Surg 1995;60:773–777.
149. Seccombe JF, Schaff HV. Coronary artery endothelial function after myocardial ischemia and reperfusion. Ann Thorac Surg 1995;60:778–788.

150. Menasché P, Grousset C, Gauduel Y, Piwnica A. A comparative study of free radical scavengers in cardioplegic solutions. Improved protection with peroxidase. J Thorac Cardiovasc Surg 1986;92: 264–271.
151. Kaneda T, Ku K, Inoue T, Onoe M, Oku H. Postischemic reperfusion injury can be attenuated by oxygen tension control. Jpn Circ J 2001;65:213–218.
152. Bochenek A, Religa Z, Spyt TJ, Mistarz K, Bochenek Ad, Zembala M, Grzybek H. Protective influence of pretreatment with allopurinol on myocardial function in patients undergoing coronary artery surgery. Eur J Cardiothorac Surg 1990;4:538–542.
153. Lichtenstein SV, Kassam AA, El Dalati H, Cusimano RJ, Panos A, Slutsky AS. Warm heart surgery. J Thorac Cardiovasc Surg 1991;101:269–274.
154. Taggart DP, El-Fiky MM, Carter R, Bowman A, Wheatley DJ. Respiratory dysfunction after uncomplicated cardiopulmonary bypass. Ann Thorac Surg 1993;56:1123–1128.
155. Ratcliff NB, Young WG Jr, Hackel DB, et al. Pulmonary injury secondary to extracorporeal circulation: an ultrastructural study. J Thorac Cardiovasc Surg 1973;65:425–432.
156. Schlensak C, Doenst T, Preusser S, Wunderlich M, Kleinschmidt M, Beyersdorf F. Bronchial artery perfusion during cardiopulmonary bypass does not prevent ischemia of the lung in piglets: assessment of bronchial artery blood flow with fluorescent microspheres. Eur J Cardiothorac Surg 2001;19: 326–331.
157. Hillman ND, Cheifetz IM, Craig DM, Smith PK, Ungerleider RM, Meliones JN. Inhaled nitric oxide, right ventricular efficiency, and pulmonary vascular mechanics: selective vasodilation of small pulmonary vessels during hypoxic pulmonary vasoconstriction. J Thorac Cardiovasc Surg 1997;113: 1006–1013.
158. King RC, Binns OA, Kanithanon RC, et al. Low-dose sodium nitroprusside reduces pulmonary reperfusion injury. Ann Thorac Surg 1997;63:1398–1404.
159. Pearl JM, Wellmann SA, McNamara JL, et al. Bosentan prevents hypoxia-reoxygenation-induced pulmonary hypertension and improves pulmonary function. Ann Thorac Surg 1999;68:1714–1721.
160. MacNee W, Selby C. Neutrophil kinetics in the lungs. Clin Sci 1990;79:97–107.
161. Tönz M, Mihaljevic T, von Segesser LK, Fehr J, Schmid ER, Turina MI. Acute lung injury during cardiopulmonary bypass: are the neutrophils responsible? Chest 1995;108:1551–1556.
162. Bando K, Pillai R, Cameron DE, et al. Leukocyte depletion ameliorates free radical-mediated lung injury after cardiopulmonary bypass. J Thorac Cardiovasc Surg 1990;99:873–877.
163. Johnson D, Thomson D, Mycyk T, Burbridge B, Mayers I. Depletion of leucocytes transiently improves postoperative cardiorespiratory status. Chest 1995;107:1253–1259.
164. Gu YJ, Vries AJ de, Boonstra PW, van Oeveren W. Leukocyte depletion results in improved lung function and reduced inflammatory response after cardiac surgery. J Thorac Cardiovasc Surg 1996;112;494–500.
165. Boldt J, Zickmann B, Dapper F, Hempelmann G. Does the technique of cardiopulmonary bypass affect lung water content? Eur J Cardiothorac Surg 1991;5:22–26.
166. Matheis G, Haak T, Beyersdorf F, Baretti R, Polywka C, Winkelmann BR. Circulating endothelin in patients undergoing coronary artery bypass grafting. Eur J Cardiothorac Surg 1995;9:269–274.
167. Dobell AR, Bailey JS. Charles Drew and the origins of deep hypothermic circulatory arrest. Ann Thorac Surg 1997;63:1193–1199.
168. Bochenek A, Religa Z, Kokot F, et al. Biocompatibility of extracorporeal circulation with auto-oxygenation. Eur J Cardiothorac Surg 1992;6:397–402.
169. DeFoe GR, Ross CS, Olmstead EM, et al. Lowest hematocrit on bypass and adverse outcomes associated with coronary artery bypass grafting. Ann Thorac Surg 2001;71:769–776.
170. Beattie HW, Evans G, Garnett ES, Webber CE. Sustained hypovolemia and extracellular fluid volume expansion following cardiopulmonary bypass. Surgery 1972;71:891–897.
171. Utley JR, Wachtel C, Cain RB, Spaw AE, Collins JC, Stephens DB. Effects of hypothermia, hemodilution, and pump oxygenation on organ water content, blood flow, and oxygen delivery, and renal function. Ann Thorac Surg 1981;31:121–133.
172. Jansen PG, te Velthuis H, Bulder ER, et al. Reduction in prime volume attenuates the hyperdynamic response after cardiopulmonary bypass. Ann Thorac Surg 1995;60:544–550.
173. Jansen PG, te Velthuis H, Wildevuur WR, et al. Cardiopulmonary bypass with modified fluid gelatin and heparin-coated circuits. Br J Anaesth 1996;6:13–19.
174. Schönberger JP, Bredee JJ, Tjian D, Everts PA, Wildevuur CR. Intraoperative predonation contributes to blood saving. Ann Thorac Surg 1993;56:893–898.

175. Schönberger JP, Woolley S, Tavilla G, et al. Efficacy and safety of a blood conservation program including low-dose aprotinin in routine myocardial revascularization. J Cardiovasc Surg (Torino) 1996;37:35–44.
176. Menasché P, Haydar S, Peynet J, et al. A potential mechanism of vasodilation after warm heart surgery. J Thorac Cardiovasc Surg 1994;107:293–299.
177. Menasché P, Peynet J, Lariviere J, et al. Does normothermia during cardiopulmonary bypass increase neutrophil-endothelium interactions? Circulation 1994;90:II275–II279.
178. Haddix TL, Pohlman TH, Noel RF, Sato TT, Boyle EM Jr, Verrier ED. Hypothermia inhibits human E-selectin transcription. J Surg Res 1996;64:176–183.
179. Menasché P, Peynet J, Haeffner-Cavaillon N, et al. Influence of temperature on neutrophil trafficking during clinical cardiopulmonary bypass. Circulation 1995;92(suppl):II334–II340.
180. Frering B, Philip I, Dehoux M, Rolland C, Langlois JM, Desmonts JM. Circulating cytokines in patients undergoing normothermic cardiopulmonary bypass. J Thorac Cardiovasc Surg 1994;108:636–641.
181. Birdi I, Regragui I, Izzat MB, Bryan AJ, Angelini GD. Influence of normothermic systemic perfusion during coronary artery bypass operations: a randomized prospective study. J Thorac Cardiovasc Surg 1997;114:475–481.
182. Tonz M, Mihaljevic T, von Segesser LK, Shaw S, Luscher TF, Turina M. Postoperative hemodynamics depend on cardiopulmonary bypass temperature: the potential role of endothelin-1. Eur J Cardiothorac Surg 1997;11:157–161.
183. Ohata T, Sawa Y, Kadoba K, Kagisaki K, Suzuki K, Matsuda H. Role of nitric oxide in a temperature dependent regulation of systemic vascular resistance in cardiopulmonary bypass. Eur J Cardiothorac Surg 2000;18:342–347.
184. Ranucci M, Soro G, Frigiola A, et al. Normothermic perfusion and lung function after cardiopulmonary bypass: effects in pulmonary risk patients. Perfusion 1997;12:309–315.
185. Ohata T, Sawa Y, Kadoba K, Masai T, Ichikawa H, Matsuda H. Effect of cardiopulmonary bypass under tepid temperature on inflammatory reactions. Ann Thorac Surg 1997;64:124–128.
186. Adams DC, Heyer EJ, Simon AE, et al. Incidence of atrial fibrillation after mild or moderate hypothermic cardiopulmonary bypass. Crit Care Med 2000;28:574–545.
187. Vingerhoets G, Van Nooten G, Vermassen F, De Soete G, Jannes C. Short-term and long-term neuropsychological consequences of cardiac surgery with extracorporeal circulation. Eur J Cardiothorac Surg 1997;11:424–431.
188. Sotaniemi KA. Long-term neurologic outcome after cardiac operation. Ann Thorac Surg 1995;59:1336–1339.
189. Blauth CI. Macroemboli and microemboli during cardiopulmonary bypass. Ann Thorac Surg 1995;59:1300–1303.
190. Liu JF, Su ZK, Ding WX. Quantitation of particulate microemboli during cardiopulmonary bypass: experimental and clinical studies. Ann Thorac Surg 1992;54:1196–1202.
191. Moody DM, Brown WR, Challa VR, Stump DA, Reboussin DM, Legault C. Brain microemboli associated with cardiopulmonary bypass: a histologic and magnetic resonance imaging study. Ann Thorac Surg 1995;59:1304–1307.
192. Kincaid EH, Jones TJ, Stump DA, et al. Processing scavenged blood with a cell saver reduces cerebral lipid microembolization. Ann Thorac Surg 2000;70:1296–1300.
193. Plourde G, Leduc AS, Morin JE, et al. Temperature during cardiopulmonary bypass for coronary artery operations does not influence postoperative cognitive function: a prospective, randomized trial. J Thorac Cardiovasc Surg 1997;114:123–128.
194. Engelman RM, Pleet AB, Rousou JA, et al. What is the best perfusion temperature for coronary revascularization? J Thorac Cardiovasc Surg 1996;112:1622–1632.
195. Regragui I, Birdi I, Izzat MB, et al. The effects of cardiopulmonary bypass temperature on neuropsychologic outcome after coronary artery operations: a prospective randomized trial. J Thorac Cardiovasc Surg 1996;112:1036–1045.
196. Mora CT, Henson MB, Weintraub WS, et al. The effect of temperature management during cardiopulmonary bypass on neurologic and neuropsychologic outcomes in patients undergoing coronary revascularization. J Thorac Cardiovasc Surg 1996;112:514–522.
197. McLean RF, Wong BI, Naylor CD, et al. Cardiopulmonary bypass, temperature, and central nervous system dysfunction. Circulation 1994;90:II250–II255.
198. Martin TD, Craver JM, Gott JP, et al. Prospective, randomized trial of retrograde warm blood cardioplegia: myocardial benefit and neurological threat. Ann Thorac Surg 1994;57:298–304.

199. Engelman RM, Pleet AB, Rousou JA, et al. Influence of cardiopulmonary bypass perfusion temperature on neurologic and hematologic function after coronary artery bypass grafting. Ann Thorac Surg 1999;67:1547–1555.
200. Grimm M, Czerny M, Baumer H, et al. Normothermic cardiopulmonary bypass is beneficial for cognitive brain function after coronary artery bypass grafting—a prospective randomized trial. Eur J Cardiothorac Surg 2000;18:270–275.
201. Rees K, Beranek-Stanley M, Burke M, Ebrahim S. Hypothermia to reduce neurological damage following coronary artery bypass surgery (Cochrane Review). Cochrane Database Syst Rev 2001;1:CD002138.
202. Johnsson P, Lundqvist C, Lindgren A, Ferencz I, Alling C, Stahl E. Cerebral complications after cardiac surgery assessed by S-100 and NSE levels in blood. J Cardiothorac Vasc Anesth 1995;9:694–699.
203. Ali MS, Harmer M, Vaughan R. Serum S100 protein as a marker of cerebral damage during cardiac surgery. Br J Anaesth 2000;85:287–298.
204. Westaby S, Johnsson P, Parry A, et al. Serum S100 protein: a potential marker for cerebral events during cardiopulmonary bypass. Ann Thorac Surg 1996;61:88–92.
205. Taggart DP, Mazel JW, Bhattacharya K, et al. Comparison of serum S-100ß levels during CABG and intracardiac operations. Ann Thorac Surg 1997;63:492–496.
206. Taggart DP, Bhattacharya K, Meston N, et al. Serum S-100 protein concentration after cardiac surgery: a randomized trial of arterial line filtration. Eur J Cardiothorac Surg, 1997;11:645–649.
207. Anderson RE, Hansson LO, Vaage J. Release of S100B during coronary artery bypass grafting is reduced by off-pump surgery. Ann Thorac Surg 1999;67:1721–1725.
208. Khuri SF, Valeri CR, Loscalzo J. Heparin causes platelet dysfunction and induces fibrinolysis before cardiopulmonary bypass. Ann Thorac Surg 1995;60:1008–1014.
209. Upchurch GR, Valeri CR, Khuri SF, et al. Effect of heparin on fibrinolytic activity and platelet function in vivo. Am J Physiol 1996;271:528–534.
210. John LCH, Rees GM, Kovacs IB. Inhibition of platelet function by heparin. J Thorac Cardiovasc Surg 1993;105:816–822.
211. Wahba A, Black G, Koksch M, et al. Cardiopulmonary bypass leads to a preferential loss of activated platelets. A flow cytometric assay of platelet surface antigens. Eur J Cardiothorac Surg 1996;10:768–773.
212. Videm V. Heparin in clinical doses "primes" granulocytes to subsequent activation as measured by myeloperoxidase release. Scand J Immunol 1996;43:385–390.
213. Shastri KA, Logue GL, Stern MP, Rehman S, Raza S. Complement activation by heparin-protamine complexes during cardiopulmonary bypass: effect of C4a null allele. J Thorac Cardiovasc Surg 1997;114:482–488.
214. Levy JH, Cormack JG, Morales A. Heparin neutralization by recombinant platelet factor 4 and protamine. Anesth Analg 1995;81:35–37.
215. Dehmer GJ, Fisher M, Tate DA, Teo S, Bonnem EM. Reversal of heparin anticoagulation by recombinant platelet factor 4 in humans. Circulation 1995;91:2188–2194.
216. Riess FC, Potsch B, Behr I, et al. Recombinant hirudin as an anticoagulant during cardiac operations: experiments in a pig model. Eur J Cardiothorac Surg 1997;11:739–745.
217. Bernabei A, Rao AK, Niewiarowski S, Colman RW, Sun L, Edmunds LH Jr. Recombinant desulphatohirudin as a substitute for heparin during cardiopulmonary bypass. J Thorac Cardiovasc Surg 1994;108:381–382.
218. Edmunds LH Jr. HIT, HITT and desulphatohirudin: look before you leap. J Thorac Cardiovasc Surg 1995;110:1–3.
219. Jegger D, Tevaearai HT, Horisberger J, et al. Augmented venous return for minimally invasive open heart surgery with selective caval cannulation. Eur J Cardiothorac Surg 1999;16:312–316.
220. Nakanishi K, Shichijo T, Shinkawa Y, et al. Usefulness of vacuum-assisted cardiopulmonary bypass circuit for pediatric open-heart surgery in reducing homologous blood transfusion. Eur J Cardiothorac Surg 2001;20:233–238.
221. Rosengart TK, DeBois W, O'Hara M, et al.Retrograde autologous priming for cardiopulmonary bypass: a safe and effective means of decreasing hemodilution and transfusion requirements. J Thorac Cardiovasc Surg 1998;115:426–438.
222. Groner W, Winkelman JW, Harris AG, et al. Orthogonal polarization spectral imaging: a new method for study of the microcirculation. Nat Med 1999:10;1209–1213.

2 Endothelial Injury During Minimally Invasive Bypass Grafting

Robert J. Dabal, MD, *Craig R. Hampton,* MD, *and Edward D. Verrier,* MD

CONTENTS

INTRODUCTION
OVERVIEW OF ENDOTHELIAL FUNCTION
ACUTE ENDOTHELIAL INJURY
CHRONIC ENDOTHELIAL INJURY
CONCLUSION
REFERENCES

INTRODUCTION

Over the last few decades, the vascular endothelium has emerged as a central mediator of the biochemical events that underlie the preoperative, operative, and postoperative course of nearly all patients who undergo cardiovascular interventional procedures and cardiovascular surgery. While initially felt to be a passive bystander of the whole-body response to cardiac surgery, it is now clear that the endothelium is a dynamic organ which is a central regulator of vascular tone, vasomotor function, coagulation, and cellular interactions. Although in the physiologically unstressed state the role of the endothelium is to maintain intravascular homeostasis, it also serves a critical role in the response to injury. Specifically, in terms of cardiovascular surgery, the endothelium modulates the systemic inflammatory response, changing vasomotor tone, impacting coagulation responses, initiating the intimal hyperplastic response, and mediating the chronic changes leading to atherosclerosis.

Enhanced understanding of these complex biochemical cascades has suggested a causal role in the morbidity and mortality of cardiovascular operations with cardiopulmonary bypass (CPB). Accordingly, in order to blunt the systemic and myocardial consequences of these biochemical alterations and improve clinical outcome, surgical techniques and

From: *Contemporary Cardiology: Minimally Invasive Cardiac Surgery, Second Edition*
Edited by: D. J. Goldstein and M. C. Oz © Humana Press Inc., Totowa, NJ

management strategies have been altered. Recognizing that the utilization of CPB has been considered a primary stimulator of endothelial cell activation in the myocardial, pulmonary, and systemic vasculature, there has been a major shift toward the use of minimally invasive techniques and the elimination of CPB. However, off-pump minimally invasive surgery employs novel techniques, such as vessel snaring, intraluminal shunts, rotation of the heart, and high-frequency gas insufflation, which can disrupt the endothelium acutely and lead to short- and long-term consequences *(1,2)*. With the increasing use of off-pump techniques, recent investigations have attempted to characterize the cellular and biochemical consequences of eliminating CPB. More important, increased understanding of these cellular events, and their causal relationship to clinical outcomes, will allow a more precise characterization of the relative advantages and disadvantages of off-pump techniques in cardiovascular surgery. This chapter highlights the current understanding of the role of the vascular endothelium in cardiovascular surgery, with emphasis on the effects of eliminating CPB. Moreover, the endothelial effects of some unique aspects of off-pump surgical techniques (e.g., target vessel snaring) will be discussed.

OVERVIEW OF ENDOTHELIAL FUNCTION

While it was initially felt to be a passive barrier between the intravascular compartment and the body's tissues, it is now clear that the endothelium is a critical regulator of inflammation, hemostasis, thrombosis, and fibrinolysis. It is important to note that the endothelium regulates membrane permeability, lipid transport, vasomotor tone, coagulation, fibrinolysis, and inflammation, and maintains vascular wall structure (**Fig. 1**). The endothelium performs these functions by numerous mechanisms, including (1) the expression of biologically active agents such as surface proteins and soluble factors; (2) homeostatic regulation of the coagulation and fibrinolytic cascades with a dynamic phenotype that can be thromboresistant or prothrombotic; (3) the regulation of cellular trafficking at the blood–endothelium interface, including the recruitment of cellular elements to the interstitial space; and (4) the alteration of the arterial wall, including the intima and media, through the release of growth factors and extracellular matrix *(3)*.

In the inactivated state, the endothelium serves to promote blood flow. However, the quiescent endothelium may become activated upon exposure to myriad stimuli, including oxidative stress from ischemia, proinflammatory cytokines (interleukins, tumor necrosis factor [TNF]), infectious stimuli (lipopolysaccharide [LPS]), increased shear forces, and physical injury. This activation alters the endothelial cell phenotype. It disrupts the barrier function of the endothelium, causes enhanced vasoconstriction, alters coagulation, and stimulates leukocyte adhesion and smooth muscle cell proliferation. The net effect of this phenotypic shift, if excessive and unbalanced, includes severe tissue damage, impaired organ function, and an abnormal fibroproliferative response *(3)*. Moreover, in addition to the local consequences, endothelial activation may also affect distant tissue beds through activation of systemic cascades. Thus, the vascular endothelium is a central regulator of a wide variety of humoral and cellular processes, which are important in nonpathological and pathological states. Accordingly, the importance of understanding the molecular details and consequences of activated endothelium in minimally invasive off-pump cardiovascular surgery is clear.

Vasomotor Function

Vascular tone is controlled largely by the endothelium, which produces a variety of vasoactive substances that can cause both relaxation and contraction of the affected blood

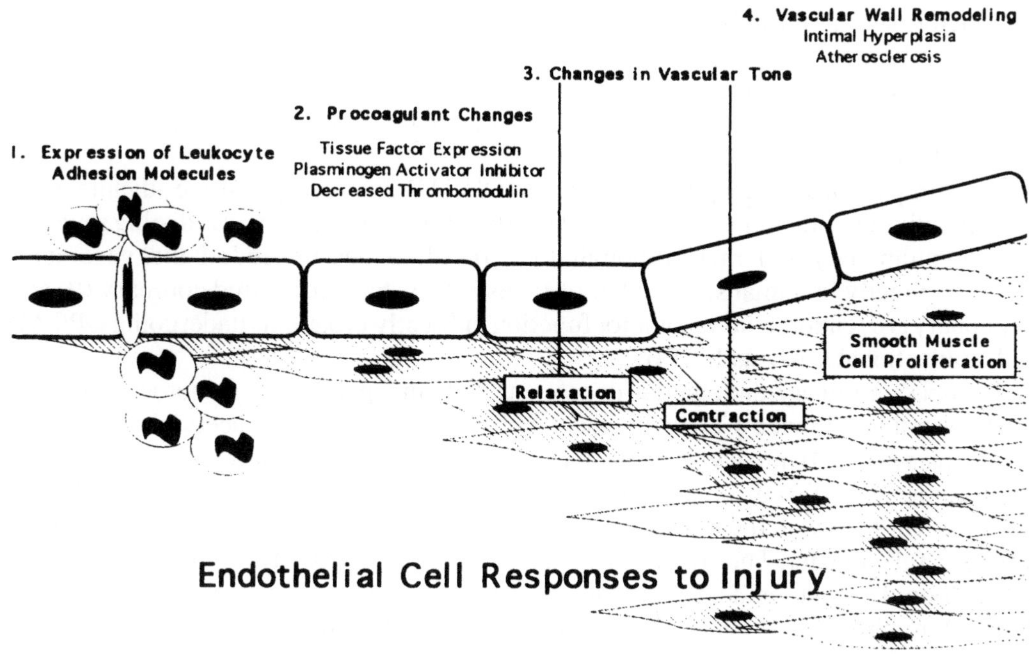

Fig. 1. Endothelial cell responses to injury.

vessels. While nitric oxide (NO) is perhaps the best-known relaxant factor produced by the endothelium, prostacyclin (PGI_2), bradykinin, endothelium-derived hyperpolarizing factor, and adenosine are also produced, resulting in vessel dilation and prevention of thrombosis.

Derived from L-arginine by a family of nitric oxide synthases, NO, formerly called endothelium-derived relaxing factor, is a vasodilator and potent inhibitor of platelet and monocyte activation. In the resting state, there is a continuous basal release of NO from the endothelium. Activation of the endothelium by either platelets or the coagulation cascade results, however, in increased NO production, which prevents vasoconstriction, platelet aggregation, and thrombus formation *(4)*.

These vasorelaxing factors are balanced by a group of vasconstrictive substances including arachidonic acid metabolites including prostanoids (e.g., thromboxane A_2, prostaglandin H_2) and the leukotrienes, oxygen free radicals, endothelin, angiotensin II, and cytokines, including tumor necrosis factor-alpha (TNF-α) and interleukin-1. In particular, endothelin (ET), working through membrane ET receptors and G-protein-linked cell-signaling pathways, causes vasoconstriction at both low and high doses. While intramyocardial vessels are particularly sensitive to endothelin, the epicardial coronary vessels also respond to endothelin by regulating blood flow.

In patients undergoing cardiovascular surgery with CPB, the finely controlled balance between vasoconstriction and vasorelaxation is frequently tipped toward a state of impaired vasomotor control. A variety of conditions commonly seen in the cardiac surgical patient population may contribute to altered endothelial vasomotor function, including advanced age, diabetes mellitus, hypertension, chronic nicotine use, hypercholesterolemia, and atherosclerosis *(5,6)*—all of which may predispose the patient to thrombosis, hypertension, and atherogenesis. This predisposition reflects both a lack of baseline vasorelaxation with decreases in NO production and an overproduction of potent vasoconstrictors such as thromboxane A_2, endothelin, and angiotensin II. These alterations in vasomotor function are particularly deleterious in the patient undergoing cardiovascular surgery because they can lead to coronary spasm, spasm of the internal mammary conduit, and microcirculatory no-reflow leading to acute myocardial ischemia, arrhythmias, and death *(4,7,8)*.

Off-pump coronary artery bypass grafting (OPCAB) may provide some advantages to postoperative endothelial vasomotor function by eliminating CPB and reducing myocardial and pulmonary ischemia. Although it is difficult to measure endothelial vasomotor function directly in humans, a number of investigators have measured coronary *(9)* and pulmonary *(10)* endothelial vasomotor function indirectly in patients undergoing OPCAB and conventional CAB with CPB.

To assess coronary endothelial-dependent and -independent vasomotor responses, Lockowandt and Franco-Cereceda gave a bolus injection of either acetylcholine (Ach) or adenosine (ADO) into a vein graft anastomosed to a coronary target vessel in patients undergoing OPCAB and compared them to a case-matched cohort undergoing CAB with CPB *(9)*. Then, flow in the vein graft was measured, as an indirect indicator of coronary target vessel diameter. They demonstrated that elimination of CPB significantly reduced dysfunction of coronary endothelium as measured by endothelium-dependent vasorelaxation. Since there was no true negative control group, the extent to which OPCAB, via brief periods of target vessel occlusion, impairs endothelium-dependent vasorelaxation was not determined. In a separate study, these same investigators assessed endothelium-dependent vasorelaxation in an animal model following 10 min of vessel occlusion, and demonstrated impairment of endothelium-dependent vasorelaxation after this brief period of ischemia *(11)*. Taken together, these results suggest that occlusion of the target vessel during OPCAB may result in some impairment of endothelium-dependent vasorelaxation, although it seems to be significantly reduced when CPB is eliminated.

Recognizing that CPB results in little or no flow in the pulmonary circulation with subsequent impaired endothelium-dependent vasorelaxation *(12)*, Angdin et al. assessed the effect of OPCAB on pulmonary endothelial vasomotor function following CAB. In a similar study design comparing OPCAB to a case-matched cohort undergoing CAB with CPB, they demonstrated significantly improved endothelial function when CPB was eliminated. Compared to preoperative response to Ach (control), there was attenuated endothelial-dependent vasorelaxation in both groups undergoing CAB. These data are consistent with the aforementioned coronary endothelium data—that OPCAB significantly attenuates, but does not eliminate, endothelial vasomotor dysfunction of the coronary and pulmonary vascular beds following CAB. More important, the long-term consequences of these observations are not known. It is tempting to postulate that a reduction in vasomotor dysfunction following CAB may reduce the risk of thrombosis and vasospasm following coronary revascularization, thus improving both short- and long-term patency, but this remains unproven.

Coagulation

The vascular endothelium is a master regulator of hemostasis and thrombosis. To this end, it is strategically positioned at the interface of the blood and the tissues and is the source, either directly or indirectly, of the majority of regulatory molecules of the hemostatic and thrombotic cascades. As a result, quiescent endothelium maintains the fluidity of blood and promotes flow, while activated endothelium potently causes coagulation, through activation of platelets and the coagulation cascades. In this regard, the endothelium finely orchestrates the pro- and anti-thrombotic effector molecules in the vascular space, which has been reviewed in detail elsewhere *(13,14)*.

Prostacyclin (PGI_2) and NO are two of the best-characterized endothelial-derived inhibitors of platelet aggregation and thrombosis *(13)*. Both potently inhibit platelet aggregation and simultaneously cause vasodilation, thus serving to limit the extent of intravascular thrombus formation at sites of endothelial injury or stress. Moreover, PGI_2 and NO may act synergistically to inhibit platelet aggregation *(15)*. Taken together, normal functioning of PGI_2 and NO are critical for normal hemostasis, and abnormal function of either may predispose to excessive platelet aggregation and thrombosis.

An additional endothelial-derived molecule important in suppressing platelet activation is ecto-adenosine diphosphatase (ADPase) *(13,14)*. In contrast to NO and PGI_2, which are secreted to act in a paracrine fashion, ADPase is expressed on the cell surface, where it enzymatically degrades ADP, a potent potentiator of platelet recruitment and activation, thereby limiting the extent of platelet activation *(16)*.

In addition to the endothelial-derived antiplatelet molecules listed above, the endothelium also antagonizes the coagulation cascade through synthesis of multiple molecules, including (1) surface-expressed thrombomodulin, (2) heparin-like molecules, (3) protein S, and (4) tissue-factor pathway inhibitor (TFPI) *(17)*.

Thrombomodulin is a cell surface protein that is present in all endothelial cells, and, by competing with catalytic activity of thrombin, inhibits the procoagulant effects of thrombin. Furthermore, thrombomodulin binds factor Xa and inhibits subsequent activation of prothrombin. Taken together, thrombomodulin inhibits coagulation at multiple regulatory steps in the coagulation cascade.

The expression of heparin-like proteoglycans on the surface of the endothelium provides another endothelial-generated anticoagulant mechanism. Heparin-like molecules on endothelium serves as a cofactor for the anticoagulant antithrombin III (ATIII), thereby increasing its activity and inhibition of the coagulation factors thrombin, factor Xa, IXa, and XIIa.

Protein S is a vitamin K-dependent glycoprotein that is a cofactor for activated protein C, thereby enhancing inactivation of factor Va and inhibiting coagulation. Protein S is synthesized by the vascular endothelium, in addition to the liver and megakaryocytes.

An additional mechanism whereby the endothelium inhibits coagulation is through tissue factor pathway inhibitor (TFPI), which antagonizes the factor VIIa/tissue factor complex, the main initiator of the extrinsic coagulation cascade. It is important to note that, unlike other extravascular cells (e.g., mononuclear phagocytes), endothelial cells do not normally express tissue factor, the primary trigger of the coagulation cascade. Upon exposure to various stresses, tissue factor is expressed on the surface of endothelial cells, thereby promoting coagulation *(18–22)*. TFPI is constitutively expressed by endothelial cells and is present in low concentrations in the circulation. As mentioned, TFPI inhibits factor VIIa/tissue factor, and does so much more efficiently when TFPI is complexed with factor Xa *(23)*.

Indeed, in addition to the regulation of platelet activity and the coagulation system, the vascular endothelium also modulates the fibrinolytic cascade. The vascular endothelium is the primary source of tissue-type plasminogen activator (tPA), required for initiation of fibrinolysis. When bound to fibrin, tPA efficiently generates plasmin from its precursor, plasminogen, effectively localizing plasmin formation to sites of clot. In addition to constitutive expression and release, tPA is synthesized and released in response to thrombin, shear stress, vasopressin, acidosis, and hypoxia *(13,14,24)*. The endothelium also synthesizes the major inhibitor of tPA, plasminogen activator inhibitor-1 (PAI-1), which is usually present in significant excess relative to tPA. Like other procoagulant molecules, PAI-1 synthesis is increased in response to inflammation, hormones, and cytokines, while tPA levels change very little. In clinical situations where cytokine release may be significant (e.g., sepsis, SIRS following coronary artery bypass [CAB + CPB]), it has been suggested that this disparate activation of PAI-1, compared to tPA, may provide a biochemical basis toward an early procoagulant state *(25,26)*.

In summary, the vascular endothelium plays an active role in resisting adherence and activation of platelets, and inhibiting activation of the coagulation cascade, resulting in a thromboresistant barrier between the blood and tissues. To these ends, there is a complex interplay between a variety of endothelial-derived antiplatelet factors, anticoagulant mediators, and modulators of fibrinolysis. However, the quiescent thromboresistant phenotype of the endothelium can rapidly change upon exposure to cellular stresses including hypoxia, mechanical trauma, and proinflammatory cytokines, among others. Many of these cellular stresses are integral to cardiac surgery with CPB, leading to profound endothelial cell activation.

There is a vast literature, including recent reviews, describing the effects of coronary revascularization with cardiopulmonary bypass (CPB) on the coagulation and fibrinolytic cascades, as well as on platelet function *(27–29)*. Abnormalities of these systems may contribute to significant morbidity and mortality following cardiovascular operations with CPB, including postoperative hemorrhage and tendency for thromboembolic complications. The biochemical alterations are complex and likely result from simultaneous activation of coagulation, fibrinolysis, and platelets. Following CPB, thrombin is generated in significant amounts, as measured by prothrombin fragments 1+2 (F1 + 2) and by thrombin–antithrombin complex (TAT) levels *(30)*. Although initially thought to be produced primarily by activation of the intrinsic coagulation cascade, when factor XII becomes activated after contacting the CPB circuit, recent evidence suggests that coagulation is initiated via the tissue factor pathway of the extrinsic coagulation cascade *(31,32)*. Activated vascular endothelium is likely a significant modulator of these alterations, given its upregulation of tissue factor and TFPI in response to proinflammatory mediators (e.g., C5a) known to be increased after CAB with CPB *(33)*. Platelet activation also contributes to the hemostatic disturbances following CAB with CPB, resulting, at least in part, from endothelial cell activation.

There are both qualitative and quantitative platelet defects following cardiac surgery with CPB, with various causes, including endothelial-derived substances *(27)*. The vascular endothelium responds to humoral mediators elaborated during CAB with CPB, such as thrombin, by releasing von Willebrand factor (vWF), P-selectin, and other proinflammatory mediators, such as IL-8 *(34)*. The net effect of these endothelial-derived mediators is to activate and aggregate platelets at sites of tissue injury. If this process is widespread in multiple vascular beds, such as following CAB with CPB, then thrombocytopenia may result and the remaining platelets are qualitatively abnormal, as demonstrated by prolonged bleeding time in patients after CPB *(35)*. The observation that von Willebrand factor, as a marker of endothelial cell activation, increases after cardiac surgery with CPB provides evidence of in vivo endothelial cell activation and injury *(36)*.

Finally, activation of the fibrinolytic cascade, further disturbing the coagulation abnormalitites, has been documented in numerous studies following CPB *(37,38)*. Moreover, it has been demonstrated that following cold cardioplegia administration for CPB, the coronary circulation releases tPA *(39)*, thus supporting the notion of endothelial cell activation and initiation of fibrinolysis.

Taken together, these data provide compelling evidence for a critical role of the vascular endothelium in modulating platelets, coagulation, and fibrinolysis in cardiovascular surgery. Although these abnormalities have been well documented with the use of CPB, much less is known about these systems when CPB is eliminated in OPCAB.

Casati and colleagues assessed changes in biochemical markers of coagulation, fibrinolysis, and platelets in patients undergoing OPCAB and compared them to a case-matched cohort undergoing CAB with CPB *(40)*. To account for the reduced hemodilution in OPCAB patients, they adjusted the biochemical results for hemodilution. In both groups, there was a comparable consumption of prothrombin and fibrinogen, consistent with activation of the coagulation cascade via the tissue factor/VII pathway, independent of the CPB circuit and contact activation of factor XII. When CPB was used, there was a transient reduction in platelet counts, with plasminogen activation, and increased D-dimer formation (reflecting fibrinolysis)—an effect that was not seen in the OPCAB group. By 24 h postoperatively, the hemostatic profiles were similar between groups.

Although there is a paucity of data examining the coagulation disturbances following OPCAB, multiple studies have demonstrated reduced bleeding and transfusion requirements when CPB is eliminated *(41,42)*. Additional studies are warranted to better characterize the benefits of OPCAB with respect to disturbances of coagulation.

Cell–Cell Interactions

Under normal physiological conditions, inflammatory cells in the bloodstream do not adhere to the endothelium. Endothelial cell activation, however, can result in the expression of a variety of inflammatory mediators and cell adhesion molecules. These adhesion molecules, including the selectins, the integrins, and the immunoglobulin supergene family (e.g., ICAM-1), lead to interactions of neutrophils, monocytes, platelets, and lymphocytes with the endothelium. Following adherence, these cells are able to invade the internal elastic lamina and release a variety of substances that act on the cellular milieu and promote chemotaxis, thereby defining the vessel's response to injury.

Monocytes and platelets have classically been the two cell types most intimately linked with the regulation of the inflammatory response. The monocyte is able to transmigrate across vessel walls and transform into tissue macrophages or foam cells. In addition to the elaboration of inflammatory mediators, these cells are able to ingest lipids and scavenge oxidized low-density lipoproteins, producing free radicals in the process. Platelets, via elaboration of platelet-derived growth factor, stimulate vascular smooth muscle cell proliferation after adhering to collagen in the basement membrane.

While the various cell types involved in inflammation are important, an understanding of the mediators produced by these cells is also critical. A complex network of cytokines and growth factors regulates the inflammatory state via autocrine and paracrine signaling. Classically, these mediators are divided into growth factors, chemokines, and pro- or anti-inflammatory factors. However, most factors have multiple roles that are influenced by the setting in which they are expressed. The redundancy and complexity of this system of inflammatory mediation makes it challenging to target any single component this system to improve clinical endpoints.

A final mediator of the inflammatory response that is critical in the setting of endothelial damage is nitric oxide (NO). With endothelial damage, there are decreases in NO, prostacyclin, and adenosine—all of which have been shown to be potent antiadhesive mediators. It has therefore been suggested that NO or NO-donor therapy may be beneficial in protecting the myocardium from endothelial injury by inhibiting neutrophil adherence and accumulation *(43)*.

ACUTE ENDOTHELIAL INJURY

While the whole-body inflammatory response to CPB is largely avoided with off-pump techniques *(44)*, several mechanisms by which endothelial cell damage can occur remain. Furthermore, despite the attenuation of systemic inflammation, OPCAB can lead to regional myocardial injury with localized effects, such as endothelial dysfunction or myocardial stunning *(9,45)*. The endothelial stress response during OPCAB is likely regional, rather than widespread as seen in after CAB with CPB *(29)*, and results from the novel techniques employed during OPCAB including target vessel snaring, intraluminal shunts, and high-frequency gas insufflation *(1,46,47)*. Loosely categorized, these etiologies may be divided into mechanical trauma of the vasculature and ischemia reperfusion injury.

Mechanical Trauma

The most obvious source of damage in minimally invasive cardiac surgery comes from the temporary disruption of coronary blood flow during completion of the distal anastomosis. A variety of clamps and stabilization devices have been employed with the end result of stabilization of the target coronary artery in a hemostatic field. The full effects of these types of occlusion have been shown both in animal models and, more recently, in human studies *(47–52)*. However, the evidence regarding the acute impact of operative control of the coronary arteries on endothelial function is somewhat conflicting, as other reports have shown no endothelial dysfunction with ischemic periods up to 1 h in a swine model *(51)*. Finally, it has been shown that the type of technique used (i.e., bulldog occluders, prolene sutures, vascular snares) has an impact on the degree of endothelial disruption present *(50,52)*. Local microthrombus *(50)* or acute vasospasm *(53)* may then result from this endothelial disruption.

High-flow gas insufflation is another technique used to maintain coronary arteriotomy visualization during minimally invasive techniques for coronary revascularization. The effects of this insufflation on the coronary vascular endothelium have not been fully elucidated. However, it has been suggested that gas insufflation results in almost complete denudation of the exposed endothelium *(46,54)*. Humidification of the insufflated gas may attenuate but not alleviate this type of endothelial injury *(46)*.

Ischemia/Reperfusion

Minimally invasive techniques, which avoid CPB and cardiac arrest, may not cause global myocardial ischemia, but local myocardial ischemia does still occur. Moreover, patients with coronary artery disease often suffer from myocardial ischemia at baseline, and the main goal in correction of this problem is the restoration of oxygenated blood to the ischemic myocardium. Interventional procedures in the cardiac catheterization lab as well as surgical procedures, by necessity, incur a period of superimposed complete ischemia on a background of chronic low-grade ischemia. Reperfusion of this ischemic myocardium results in further but necessary myocardial injury that can be either reversible or irreversible. The key determinant of irreversible damage is the length of the ischemic time, with 20 min accepted as the maximal length for reversible defects. Beyond

20 min, myocardial necrosis is inevitable, with concomitant endothelial cell damage. Elevation of lactate levels indicating anaerobic metabolism occur within 10 min of coronary occlusion in both animals and humans *(55)*. The role of apoptosis, or programmed cell death, in the setting of acute myocardial ischemia is less clear *(56)*.

Although the exact mechanism of ischemia/reperfusion injury is not known, a simplified paradigm suggests that oxidative stress initiates numerous cell-signaling cascades that result in transcriptional activation of multiple stress-responsive gene products, which, in total, result in tissue injury *(57,58)*. In addition, with a shift to anaerobic metabolism, endothelial hypoxic stress induces transcriptional activation of multiple stress-response gene products *(59)*. Although this stress response likely involves multiple transcriptional regulators, NF-κB has received the most attention and is the best characterized *(60,61)*.

NF-κB, a redox-sensitive transcription factor, exists in a latent form in the cytoplasm and upon activation translocates to the nucleus with binding of the protein to DNA in target genes, thus promoting transcription and translation *(62)*. This molecule has been shown—through deletional and mutational analyses—to be necessary for activation of many of the genes involved in ischemia/reperfusion injury including IL-1, IL-8, E-selectin, VCAM-1, ICAM-1, MCP-1, inducible nitric oxide synthase, and tissue factor *(61)*. This transcriptional activation in turn leads to activation of endothelial and other cells, including platelets and leukocytes. Taken together, injury is potentiated upon reperfusion with oxygenated blood at the completion of coronary revascularization *(63)*. In particular, the phenomenon of neutrophil adherence to the endothelium following ischemia/reperfusion is mediated via a variety of substances including the cytokine IL-1 *(64)* and the cell adhesion markers E-selectin and P-selectin *(65,66)*.

While localized ischemia would seem to be less deleterious than global ischemia from CPB, there are studies that show that the endothelial response is similar. Indeed, in patients undergoing OPCAB there is a comparable increase in serum vascular endothelial growth factor (VEGF) compared to those undergoing CAB with CPB *(67)*. Recognizing that vascular endothelium responds to hypoxic stress with transcriptional activation of myriad genes, including VEGF *(58)*, these data imply that OPCAB may cause a profound response of the vascular endothelium despite elimination of cardioplegia and CPB.

The increased use of minimally invasive techniques of cardiac surgery has led to interest in techniques to avoid or reduce the amount of ischemia/reperfusion injury. Emphasis has been placed on ischemic preconditioning (IP) of the myocardium as a mechanism of inducing cardioprotection against ischemia. Ischemic preconditioning of the myocardium is a phenomenon whereby brief periods of sublethal ischemia protect the heart against subsequent prolonged ischemia *(68)*. There are two phases, or windows, of protection against ischemia—a classic, or early, window of protection that begins within minutes of the preconditioning stimulus and lasts up to 4 h, which is followed by a late, or second, window of protection that ensues 24 h after preconditioning, and lasts up to 4 d *(69)*. In contrast to the early phase of protection, which is effective against both necrotic and apoptotic cell death, the second window of protection is also effective against myocardial stunning *(70)*. As a result of its longer duration of action and its efficacy against myocardial stunning, the second window of protection may ultimately have greater translational potential in cardiac surgery. While there is some evidence that IP may reduce postoperative myocardial dysfunction in patients undergoing OPCAB, the clinical utility of either phase of IP is not known at this time *(71)*. Other techniques that may be useful in protecting against myocardial ischemia/reperfusion injury include hypothermia *(72,73)* and the use of aprotinin *(74)*.

CHRONIC ENDOTHELIAL INJURY

While the acute damage to the endothelium is somewhat different with minimally invasive techniques, the chronic endothelial response to injury is quite similar and may limit the long-term patency of bypass grafts. Both the development of intimal hyperplasia at the sites of vessel injury and the progression of underlying atherosclerotic disease lead to reductions in coronary blood flow over time, which may lead to the need for further procedures *(47,75)*. In support, Hangler et al. examined CAB grafts in patients undergoing cardiac transplantation who had previously been revascularized with OPCAB *(50)*. Examination of coronary target vessels occluded with snares revealed focal endothelial denudation, local microthrombosis, atherosclerotic plaque rupture, and injury to target-vessel side branches. These data support a chronic endothelial response following OPCAB that may affect long-term graft patency and clinical course. To assess this postulate, Gundry et al. compared long-term (7-yr) intervention-free outcome in patients subjected to OPCAB vs a case-matched cohort subjected to CAB with CPB *(76)*. In this study, twice as many patients revascularized with OPCAB (30% vs 16%) required repeat catheterization during the observation period, and nearly three times as many patients in the OPCAB group required a second intervention (20% vs 7%). While it has been suggested that use of newer stabilizing devices and occlusion techniques may attenuate endothelial damage with improved long-term patency rates following OPCAB, there are limited data to make this determination *(47,77)*. Moreover, recognizing that OPCAB results in comparable levels of endothelial-derived vascular mitogens such as VEGF *(67)* that are thought to be important mediators in the vascular response to injury, additional investigation is warranted into the endothelial effects of OPCAB surgical techniques, with an emphasis on long-term graft patency and clinical outcome.

Intimal Hyperplasia

During the course of cardiovascular revascularization, there is damage to both the conduit being harvested and the native vessel, which results in fibroproliferation and the formation of a neointima *(78)*. The intimal response to arterial injury can be divided into three phases. Beginning within 24 h of injury, there is vascular smooth muscle proliferation. With denudation of the endothelium, platelets become adherent to the vessel wall and become activated. These activated platelets are responsible for the release of a variety of substances that stimulate smooth muscle division and migration into the intima. Smooth muscle proliferation is also stimulated in the media by substances such as fibroblast growth factor. Over the period from 1 to 2 wk after injury, there is a gradual relocation of smooth muscle cells from the media to the intima with formation of a neointima. This neointima then expands via further smooth muscle cell proliferation, which can eventually result in luminal obstruction.

Clearly, the vascular smooth muscle cell is the central cell type involved in neointimal hyperplasia. These cells are critical in modulating vascular tone with their contractile properties and are also the principal manufacturers of the extracellular matrix, including proteoglycans and collagen. Regulation of smooth muscle cell proliferation is quite variable, however, and is subject to fluctuations related to interactions with inflammatory mediators such as tumor necrosis factor and interferon *(78)*.

One interesting factor that influences the degree of neointimal hyperplasia is the choice of bypass conduit, which has important implications for postoperative vascular tone. The patency of mammary grafts is clearly superior to that of vein grafts. This difference is likely secondary to differences in endothelial function. Mammary grafts are sensitive to relaxation from acetylcholine, bradykinin, thrombin, and adenosine diphosphate. Vein grafts are not sensitive to thrombin or adenosine diphosphate and only weakly sensitive to acetylcholine. In fact, vein grafts exhibit a converse effect from thrombin or adenosine diphosphate from platelets, including contraction and release of growth factors, which stimulate smooth muscle cell proliferation. Also, mammary grafts produce more NO and prostacyclin than vein grafts *(4)*.

Atherosclerosis

Since the early 1970s it has been recognized that atherosclerosis results from an endothelial response to chronic injury characterized by neutrophil, lymphocyte, platelet, and macrophage adhesion and migration into the subendothelium *(79)*. Multiple risk factors exist in cardiac surgical patients that predispose them to this chronic type of endothelial injury, including nicotine abuse, hypertension, diabetes, and hypercholesterolemia.

The underlying pathophysiology of chronic endothelial injury and atherosclerosis is complex and not completely defined. Chronic injury leads to disruption of the normal endothelial monolayer via a loss of endothelial cell ability to replicate. This, in turn, exposes the subendothelium to a variety of activated inflammatory cells including activated monocytes, platelets, and T-lymphocytes, which stimulate smooth muscle cell proliferation and coverage of the denuded area *(80,81)* via the elaboration of multiple growth factors. These growth factors in combination with locally expressed cytokines stimulate the smooth muscle cells to allow for deposition of extracellular matrix with the establishment of a fibrous plaque.

One of the key substances implicated in the progression of atherosclerosis is NO. Dysregulation of NO has been shown to result in an impairment of endothelium-dependent relaxation that causes vascular spasm with increased shear stress, increased smooth muscle cell proliferation from the loss of NO antimitogenic effects, increased platelet adherence, and even thrombosis *(82)*.

Endothelin has also been demonstrated to play a key role in atherosclerotic vascular disease. Low-density lipoproteins stimulate increased endothelin production from the endothelium via increased gene transcription. Also, there is a down-regulation of endothelin receptor expression and increased production of endothelin from vascular smooth muscle cells. As a result, endothelin levels correlate with the extent of atherosclerosis present *(83)*.

While the underlying pathophysiology of atherosclerosis is less clearly defined, the natural history and progression of atherosclerosis are quite well established. Beginning as lipid deposits in the intima, there is further accumulation of intracellular lipids in foam cells. Following this, there is the gradual buildup of extracellular pools of lipid that eventually becomes clinically evident and leads to distortion of blood vessel architecture. Further smooth muscle cell proliferation and collagen deposition leads to greater surface defects from the fibroatheroma, which can result in vessel occlusion from either hemorrhage or thrombosis *(82)*. The end clinical result of this plaque rupture can be acute myocardial infarction and sudden death *(84)*.

CONCLUSION

The endothelium plays a central role in cardiovascular function. It helps to regulate vasomotor function, resists intravascular thrombosis by maintaining a state of anticoagulation, and works to prevent the activation of a variety of intravascular inflammatory cells. Cardiovascular surgery, however, results in damage of the endothelium that impairs normal function and alters homeostasis, with the balance tipped toward tissue injury. A recent trend toward minimally invasive techniques of cardiovascular revascularization has led to the avoidance of endothelial damage from extracorporeal circulation. However, elimination of CPB has not abrogated the problem of endothelial damage. Indeed, minimally invasive techniques cause acute endothelial injury by employing new techniques such as vessel snaring, intraluminal shunts, and trauma from high-flow gas insufflation. Certainly, these new techniques have not mitigated the chronic response to endothelial injury, intimal hyperplasia, or the progression of atherosclerosis.

As techniques of minimally invasive surgery for cardiac revascularization evolve, it will be increasingly important to further delineate the endothelial response to injury and to employ techniques that minimize this trauma and maximize endothelial preservation. A thorough understanding of endothelial biology will enable the cardiovascular surgeon to greatly improve the long-term success of cardiac revascularization.

REFERENCES

1. Perrault LP, Menasche P, Wassef M, et al. Endothelial effects of hemostatic devices for continuous cardioplegia or minimally invasive operations. Ann Thorac Surg 1996;62(4):1158–1163.
2. Chavanon O, Perrault LP, Menasche P, Carrier M, Vanhoutte PM. As originally published in 1996: Endothelial effects of hemostatic devices for continuous cardioplegia or minimally invasive operations. Updated in 1999. Ann Thorac Surg 1999;68(3):1118–1120.
3. Verrier ED, Boyle EMJ. Endothelial cell injury in cardiovascular surgery: an overview. Ann Thorac Surg 1997;64(4):S2–S8.
4. Ruschitzka FT, Noll G, Luscher TF. The endothelium in coronary artery disease. Cardiology 1997;88(suppl 3):3–19.
5. Vita JA, Treasure CB, Nabel EG, et al. Coronary vasomotor response to acetylcholine relates to risk factors for coronary artery disease. Circulation 1990;81(2):491–497.
6. Ludmer PL, Jelwyn AP, Shook TL, et al. Paradoxical vasoconstriction induced by acetylcholine in atherosclerotic coronary arteries. N Engl J Med 1986;315(17):1046–1051.
7. Pearson PJ, Evora PR, Schaff HV. Bioassay of EDRF from internal mammary arteries: implications for early and late bypass graft patency. Ann Thorac Surg 1992;54(6):1078–1084.
8. Nonami Y. The role of nitric oxide in cardiac surgery. Surg Today 1997;27(7):583–592.
9. Lockowandt U, Franco-Cereceda A. Off-pump coronary bypass surgery causes less immediate postoperative coronary endothelial dysfunction compared to on-pump coronary bypass surgery. Eur J Cardiothorac Surg 2001;20(6):1147–1151.
10. Angdin M, Settergren G, Vaage J. Better preserved pulmonary endothelium-dependent vasodilation with off- pump coronary surgery. Scand Cardiovasc J 2001;35(4):264–269.
11. Lockowandt U, Liska J, Franco-Cereceda A. Short ischemia causes endothelial dysfunction in porcine coronary vessels in an in vivo model. Ann Thorac Surg 2001;71(1):265–269.
12. Angdin M, Settergren G. Acetylcholine reactivity in the pulmonary artery during cardiac surgery in patients with ischemic or valvular heart disease. J Cardiothorac Vasc Anesth 1997;11(4):458–462.
13. Pearson JD. Endothelial cell function and thrombosis. Baillieres Best Pract Res Clin Haematol 1999;12(3):329–341.
14. Wu KK, Thiagarajan P. Role of endothelium in thrombosis and hemostasis. Annu Rev Med 1996;47:315–331.
15. Radomski MW, Palmer RM, Moncada S. Comparative pharmacology of endothelium-derived relaxing factor, nitric oxide and prostacyclin in platelets. Br J Pharmacol 1987;92(1):181–187.
16. Marcus AJ, Safier LB. Thromboregulation: multicellular modulation of platelet reactivity in hemostasis and thrombosis. FASEB J 1993;7(6):516–522.
17. Wu C. Heat shock transcription factors: structure and regulation. Annu Rev Cell Dev Biol 1995;11:441–469.
18. Ogawa S, Gerlach H, Esposito C, Pasagian-Macaulay A, Brett J, Stern D. Hypoxia modulates the barrier and coagulant function of cultured bovine endothelium. Increased monolayer permeability and induction of procoagulant properties. J Clin Invest 1990;85(4):1090–1098.

19. Camera M, Giesen PL, Fallon J, et al. Cooperation between VEGF and TNF-alpha is necessary for exposure of active tissue factor on the surface of human endothelial cells. Arterioscler Thromb Vasc Biol 1999;19(3):531–537.
20. Lyberg T, Galdal KS, Evensen SA, Prydz H, et al. Cellular cooperation in endothelial cell thromboplastin synthesis. Br J Haematol 1983;53(1):85–95.
21. Bevilacqua MP, Pober JS, Majeau GR, Cotran RS, Gimbrone MA. Interleukin 1 (IL-1) induces biosynthesis and cell surface expression of procoagulant activity in human vascular endothelial cells. J Exp Med 1984;160(2):618–623.
22. Brox JH, Osterud B, Bjorklid E, Fenton JW 2nd. Production and availability of thromboplastin in endothelial cells: the effects of thrombin, endotoxin and platelets. Br J Haematol 1984;57(2):239–246.
23. Bajaj MS, Birktoft JJ, Steer SA, Bajaj SP. Structure and biology of tissue factor pathway inhibitor. Thromb Haemost 2001;86(4):959–972.
24. Emeis JJ, vanden Eijnden-Schrauwen Y, vanden Hoogen CM, de Priester W, Westmuckett A, Lupu F. An endothelial storage granule for tissue-type plasminogen activator. J Cell Biol 1997;139(1):245–256.
25. Colucci M, Paramo JA, Collen D. Generation in plasma of a fast-acting inhibitor of plasminogen activator in response to endotoxin stimulation. J Clin Invest 1985;75(3):818–824.
26. van der Poll T, Levi M, Buller HR, et al. Fibrinolytic response to tumor necrosis factor in healthy subjects. J Exp Med 1991;174(3):729–732.
27. Weerasinghe A, Taylor KM. The platelet in cardiopulmonary bypass. Ann Thorac Surg 1998;66(6):2145–2152.
28. Raymond PD, Marsh NA. Alterations to haemostasis following cardiopulmonary bypass and the relationship of these changes to neurocognitive morbidity. Blood Coagul Fibrinolysis 2001;12(8):601–618.
29. Boyle EM Jr, Verrier ED, Spiess BD. Endothelial cell injury in cardiovascular surgery: the procoagulant response. Ann Thorac Surg 1996;62(5):1549–1557.
30. Boisclair MD, Lane DA, Philippou H, Sheikh S, Hunt B. Thrombin production, inactivation and expression during open heart surgery measured by assays for activation fragments including a new ELISA for prothrombin fragment F1 + 2. Thromb Haemost 1993;70(2):253–258.
31. Boisclair MD, Lane DA, Philippou H, et al. Mechanisms of thrombin generation during surgery and cardiopulmonary bypass. Blood 1993;82(11):3350–3357.
32. Philippou H, Adami A, Boiselair MD, Lane DA. An ELISA for factor X activation peptide: application to the investigation of thrombogenesis in cardiopulmonary bypass. Br J Haematol 1995;90(2):432–437.
33. Ikeda K, Nagasawa K, Horiuchi T, Tsuru T, Nishizaka H, Niho Y. C5a induces tissue factor activity on endothelial cells. Thromb Haemost 1997;77(2):394–398.
34. van Mourik JA, Romani De Wit T, Voorberg J. Biogenesis and exocytosis of Weibel-Palade bodies. Histochem Cell Biol 2002;117(2):113–122.
35. Harker LA, Malpass TW, Branson HE, Hessel EA 2nd, Slichter SJ. Mechanism of abnormal bleeding in patients undergoing cardiopulmonary bypass: acquired transient platelet dysfunction associated with selective alpha-granule release. Blood 1980;56(5):824–834.
36. Holdright DR, Hunt BJ, Parratt R, et al. The effects of cardiopulmonary bypass on systemic and coronary levels of von Willebrand factor. Eur J Cardiothorac Surg 1995;9(1):18–21.
37. Hunt BJ, Parratt RN, Segal HC, Sheikh S, Kallis P, Yacoub M. Activation of coagulation and fibrinolysis during cardiothoracic operations. Ann Thorac Surg 1998;65(3):712–718.
38. Tabuchi N, de Haan J, Boonstra PW, van Oeveren W. Activation of fibrinolysis in the pericardial cavity during cardiopulmonary bypass. J Thorac Cardiovasc Surg 1993;106(5):828–833.
39. Valen G, Eriksson E, Risberg B, Vaage J. Fibrinolysis during cardiac surgery. Release of tissue plasminogen activator in arterial and coronary sinus blood. Eur J Cardiothorac Surg 1994;8(6):324–330.
40. Casati V, Gerli C, Franco A, et al. Activation of coagulation and fibrinolysis during coronary surgery: on-pump versus off-pump techniques. Anesthesiology 2001;95(5):1103–1109.
41. Nader ND, Khadra WZ, Reich NJ, Bacon DR, Salerno TA, Panos AL. Blood product use in cardiac revascularization: comparison of on- and off-pump techniques. Ann Thorac Surg 1999;68(5):1640–1643.
42. Ascione R, Williams S, Lloyd CT, Sundaramoorthi T, Pitsis AA, Angelini GD. Reduced postoperative blood loss and transfusion requirement after beating-heart coronary operations: a prospective randomized study. J Thorac Cardiovasc Surg 2001;121(4):689–696.
43. Vinten-Johansen J, Sato H, Zhao ZQ. The role of nitric oxide and NO-donor agents in myocardial protection from surgical ischemic-reperfusion injury. Int J Cardiol 1995;50(3):273–281.
44. Ascione R, Lloyd CT, Underwood MJ, Lotto AA, Pitsis AA, Angelini GD. Inflammatory response after coronary revascularization with or without cardiopulmonary bypass. Ann Thorac Surg 2000;69(4):1198–1204.

45. Grubitzsch H, Ansorge K, Wollert GH, Eckel L. Stunned myocardium after off-pump coronary artery bypass grafting. Ann Thorac Surg 2001;71(1):352–355.
46. Okazaki Y, Takarabe K, Murayama J, et al. Coronary endothelial damage during off-pump CABG related to coronary-clamping and gas insufflation. Eur J Cardiothorac Surg 2001;19(6):834–839.
47. Perrault LP, Nickner C, Desjardins N, Carrier M. Effects on coronary endothelial function of the Cohn stabilizer for beating heart bypass operations. Ann Thorac Surg 2000;70(3):1111–1114.
48. Walia AS, Kole SD. Clamp for coronary artery operations. Ann Thorac Surg 1998;65(5):1475–1476.
49. Bandyopadhyay A, Kapoor L, Gan M. Bulldog with spikes: clamp for coronary artery operations. Ann Thorac Surg 1999;67(2):594–595.
50. Hangler HB, Pfaller K, Antretter H, Dapunt OE, Bonatti JO. Coronary endothelial injury after local occlusion on the human beating heart. Ann Thorac Surg 2001;71(1):122–127.
51. Perrault LP, Menasche P, Biolouard JP, et al. Snaring of the target vessel in less invasive bypass operations does not cause endothelial dysfunction. Ann Thorac Surg 1997;63(3):751–755.
52. Sokullu O, Karabulut H, Gercekoglu H, et al. Coronary artery stabilization causes endothelial damage: an electron microscopic study on dogs. Cardiovasc Surg 2001;9(4):407–410.
53. Fonger JD, Yang XM, Cohen RA, Haudenschild CC, Shemin RJ. Human mammary artery endothelial sparing with fibrous jaw clamping. Ann Thorac Surg 1995;60(3):551–555.
54. Burfeind WR Jr, Duhaylongsod FG, Annex BH, Samuelson D. High-flow gas insufflation to facilitate MIDCABG: effects on coronary endothelium. Ann Thorac Surg 1998;66(4):1246–1249.
55. Hall RI, O'Regan N, Gardner M. Detection of intraoperative myocardial ischaemia—a comparison among electrocardiographic, myocardial metabolic, and haemodynamic measurements in patients with reduced ventricular function. Can J Anaesth 1995;42(6):487–494.
56. Elsasser A, Suzuki K, Lorenz-Meyer S, Bode C, Schaper J. The role of apoptosis in myocardial ischemia: a critical appraisal. Basic Res Cardiol 2001;96(3):219–226.
57. Boyle EM Jr, Canty TG Jr, Morgan EN, Yun W, Pohlman TH, Varrier ED. Treating myocardial ischemia-reperfusion injury by targeting endothelial cell transcription. Ann Thorac Surg 1999;68(5):1949–1953.
58. Faller DV. Endothelial cell responses to hypoxic stress. Clin Exp Pharmacol Physiol 1999;26(1):74–84.
59. Pohlman TH, Harlan JM. Adaptive responses of the endothelium to stress. J Surg Res 2000;89(1):85–119.
60. Parry GCN, Mackman N. NF-kB mediated transcription in human monocytic cells and endothelial cells. Trends Cardiovasc Med 1998;8:138–142.
61. De Martin R, Hoeth M, Hofer-Warbinek R, Schmid JA. The transcription factor NF-kappa B and the regulation of vascular cell function. Arterioscler Thromb Vasc Biol 2000;20(11):E83–E88.
62. Collins T, Read MA, Neish AS, Whitley MZ, Thanos D, Maniatis T. Transcriptional regulation of endothelial cell adhesion molecules: NF-kappa B and cytokine-inducible enhancers. FASEB J 1995;9(10):899–909.
63. Johnson M, Pohlman TH, Verrier ED. Neutrophil antiadhesion therapy for myocardial ischemia: clinical potential. Clin Immunother 1995;3:8–14.
64. Shreeniwas R, Koga S, Karakurum M, et al. Hypoxia-mediated induction of endothelial cell interleukin-1 alpha. An autocrine mechanism promoting expression of leukocyte adhesion molecules on the vessel surface. J Clin Invest 1992;90(6):2333–2339.
65. Shen I, Verrier ED. Expression of E-selectin on coronary endothelium after myocardial ischemia and reperfusion. J Card Surg 1994;9(3 suppl):437–441.
66. Winn RK, Liggitt P, Vedder NB, Paulson JC, Harlan JM. Anti-P-selectin monoclonal antibody attenuates reperfusion injury to the rabbit ear. J Clin Invest 1993;92(4):2042–2047.
67. Burton PB, Owen VJ, Hafizi S, et al. Vascular endothelial growth factor release following coronary artery bypass surgery: extracorporeal circulation versus "beating heart" surgery. Eur Heart J 2000;21(20):1708–1713.
68. Murry CE, Jennings RB, Reimer KA. Preconditioning with ischemia: a delay of lethal cell injury in ischemic myocardium. Circulation 1986;74(5):1124–1136.
69. Baxter GF, Goma FM, Yellon DM. Characterisation of the infarct-limiting effect of delayed preconditioning: timecourse and dose-dependency studies in rabbit myocardium. Basic Res Cardiol 1997;92(3):159–167.
70. Sun JZ, Tang XL, Knowlton AA, Park SW, Qiu Y, Bolli R. Late preconditioning against myocardial stunning. An endogenous protective mechanism that confers resistance to postischemic dysfunction 24 h after brief ischemia in conscious pigs. J Clin Invest 1995;95(1):388–403.
71. Laurikka J, Wu ZK, Iusalo P, et al. Regional ischemic preconditioning enhances myocardial performance in off-pump coronary artery bypass grafting. Chest 2002;121(4):1183–1189.

72. Hale SL, Kloner RA. Myocardial hypothermia: a potential therapeutic technique for acute regional myocardial ischemia. J Cardiovasc Electrophysiol 1999;10(3):405–413.
73. Dave RH, Hale SL, Kloner RA. Hypothermic, closed circuit pericardioperfusion: a potential cardioprotective technique in acute regional ischemia. J Am Coll Cardiol 1998;31(7):1667–1671.
74. Hendrikx M, Rega F, Jamaer L, Valkenborgh T, Gutermann H, Mecs U. Na(+)/H(+)-exchange inhibition and aprotinin administration: promising tools for myocardial protection during minimally invasive CABG. Eur J Cardiothorac Surg 2001;19(5):633–639.
75. Allaire E, Clowes AW. Endothelial cell injury in cardiovascular surgery: the intimal hyperplastic response. Ann Thorac Surg 1997;63(2):582–591.
76. Gundry SR, Romano MA, Shattuck OH, Razzouk AJ, Bailey LL. Seven-year follow-up of coronary artery bypasses performed with and without cardiopulmonary bypass. J Thorac Cardiovasc Surg 1998;115(6):1273–1277; discussion 1277–1278.
77. Jansen EW, Borst C, Lahpor JR, et al. Coronary artery bypass grafting without cardiopulmonary bypass using the octopus method: results in the first one hundred patients. J Thorac Cardiovasc Surg 1998;116(1):60–67.
78. Schwartz SM, deBlois D, O'Brien ER. The intima. Soil for atherosclerosis and restenosis. Circ Res 1995;77(3):445–465.
79. Ross R, Glomset JA. Atherosclerosis and the arterial smooth muscle cell: proliferation of smooth muscle is a key event in the genesis of the lesions of atherosclerosis. Science 1973;180(93):1332–1339.
80. Ross R. The pathogenesis of atherosclerosis: a perspective for the 1990s. Nature 1993;362(6423):801–809.
81. Ross R. Cell biology of atherosclerosis. Annu Rev Physiol 1995;57:791–804.
82. Billiar TR. Nitric oxide. Novel biology with clinical relevance. Ann Surg 1995;221(4):339–349.
83. Lerman A, Edwards BS, Hallett JW, Heublein DM, Sandberg SM, Burnett JC Jr. Circulating and tissue endothelin immunoreactivity in advanced atherosclerosis. N Engl J Med 1991;325(14):997–1001.
84. Selzman CH, Miller SA, Harken AH. Therapeutic implications of inflammation in atherosclerotic cardiovascular disease. Ann Thorac Surg 2001;71(6):2066–2074.

II

Minimally Invasive Coronary Bypass Grafting

3 Minimally Invasive Bypass Grafting

A Historical Perspective

Enio Buffolo, MD, PHD
and Luís Roberto Gerola, MD, PHD

After some isolated cases of direct myocardial revascularization performed by Goetz *(1)* in 1961 and years later by Kolessov *(2)*, myocardial revascularization was standardized by Favaloro *(3)* and others using cardiopulmonary bypass and cardioplegic arrest.

In 1975, Trapp and Bisarya *(4)* published for the first time a consecutive series of 63 patients who were operated on without cardiopulmonary bypass. In this series, the right coronary artery and left anterior descending (LAD) artery were grafted with saphenous vein graft or internal mammary artery. The authors reported no deaths related to the cardiac operation and only one death due to stroke. In this landmark paper, the authors presented the bases of beating-heart revascularization technique including a system to maintain myocardial perfusion with a perfusion catheter and some maneuvers to stabilize the heart to perform the distal anastomosis (**Fig. 1**). At that time, it was considered dangerous and/or impossible to completely occlude the coronary artery without perioperative myocardial infarction.

A similar study was done by Ankeney *(5)* in the same year with satisfactory results, but these isolated studies were soon abandoned due to technical difficulties, the ease of performing a delicate anastomosis in a quiet arrested heart, and the belief that distal coronary perfusion was imperative to avoid myocardial infarction, even for short periods of coronary occlusion.

In 1981, our group *(6)* and Benetti *(7)* in Argentina, working independently, began the clinical application of beating-heart revascularization. These were the first reports describing coronary revascularization without cardiopulmonary bypass on consecutive

From: *Contemporary Cardiology: Minimally Invasive Cardiac Surgery, Second Edition*
Edited by: D. J. Goldstein and M. C. Oz © Humana Press Inc., Totowa, NJ

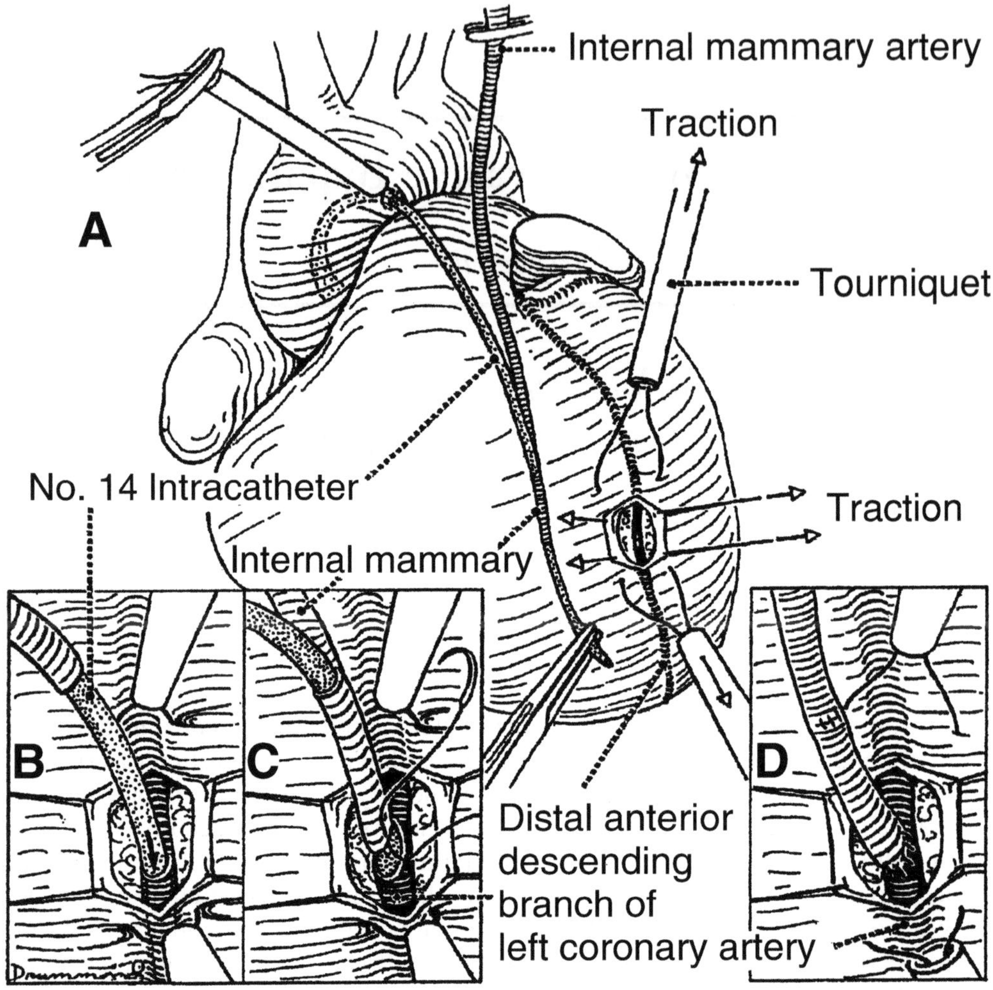

Fig. 1. Original method of distal coronary perfusion and maneuvers to stabilize the heart. The distal perfusing catheter is passed through the side of the internal mammary artery **(A)** prior to being led into the distal left anterior descending artery **(B)**. With this technique, perfusion of the distal coronary artery is carried out to support the heart up until the moment the three interrupted sutures are placed in the side of the internal mammary artery **(C,D)**.

patients after the techniques of myocardial revascularization with extracorporeal circulation and cardiac arrest had been established.

In our series of 80 patients operated on without cardiopulmonary bypass, and paralleling the experience of Trapp et al., only atherosclerotic disease of the right coronary artery and left anterior descending artery were treated. The technique was premised on the use of pharmacological manipulation with intravenous calcium-channel antagonist (verapamil) before coronary occlusion. This created a situation of controlled hypotension and reduction of myocardial metabolic need, permitting occlusion of the coronary arteries without myocardial injuries. To our knowledge, this represented the first stabilization maneuver used to facilitate coronary suturing.

Encouraged by this early experience, we initiated a program of myocardial revascularization without extracorporeal circulation with the goal of employing it in all applicable patients and, indeed, it became our routine procedure for patients with one- or two-vessel disease that did not include the circumflex artery circulation.

Naturally, many questions remained unanswered at that time. The first issue we addressed was whether the snaring of the coronary arteries caused damage to the coronary arterial wall. In an experimental study in human cadavers *(8)*, we evaluated the potential for local trauma to the native coronary artery caused by the snaring tourniquets. We applied both 5-0 polypropylene and 2-0 polyester snares to the proximal and distal right coronary and LAD arteries in 25 isolated fresh human cadaver hearts. A total of 100 points of snare application to the native coronary vessel were induced and then investigated histologically.

The results suggested a direct relationship between the severity of the arterial lesion, induced by the snares, and the degree of local atherosclerotic disease in the native coronary artery. Compression and bucking of elastic lamellae with medial fracture were seen when snares were applied to a region with marked atherosclerotic disease *(9)* (**Fig. 2**).

Based on these findings, we developed a surgical technique employing very soft snares to avoid damage in the coronary wall. Nowadays, we avoid the use of tourniquets altogether in the distal portion of the target coronary artery, as they are unnecessary in most instances.

It is important to note that issues surrounding the quality of the anastomosis, its short- and long-term patency, neurological effects, impact on blood use, and costs needed to be investigated before widespread use of beating-heart revascularization could be supported.

Patency of the coronary anastomosis was analyzed in an unpublished study from our group. Sixty patients with single-vessel disease (LAD lesion) were randomized to receive a left internal thoracic artery-to-LAD graft by conventional cardiopulmonary bypass and cardioplegic arrest or using our off-pump techniques. All patients were submitted to coronary arteriograms before hospital discharge. Early patency of left internal thoracic artery to LAD artery was 96% for each group without any statistical difference. This experience convinced us that two-vessel bypass grafting (LAD and right coronary arteries) could be performed effectively with low morbidity and mortality.

With this conviction, we began to study whether more difficult patients could safely undergo off-pump myocardial revascularization. Our first objective was to evaluate patients with acute myocardial infarction who successfully received intravenous streptokinase in the early era of thrombolytic therapy. Twenty-five such patients were submitted to off-pump myocardial revascularization. The time from acute myocardial infarction to operation ranged from 1 to 21 d (mean 8 d). There was no in-hospital mortality, and no patients had hemorraghic complications *(10)*. These results showed that in the burgeoning era of thrombolytic therapy, it was possible to operate in the subset of patients with evolving myocardial infarction after thrombolysis.

Another focus of interest was the application of off-pump revascularization to the elderly, a subject that is covered in more contemporary fashion in Chapter 18. In 1994, we presented our results in 265 patients older than 70 years of age who underwent coronary revascularization. Of these, 204 were operated on with conventional bypass grafting and 61 patients were operated on with beating-heart techniques. The hospital mortality was 7.8% in patients operated with cardiopulmonary bypass and 1.6% in patients operated off-pump. Moreover, length of stay and the need for blood transfusion were lower in patients operated without extracorporeal circulation *(11)*.

A particularly attractive concept of beating-heart techniques was the potential benefit to postoperative neurological function. To this effect, we undertook a study in which

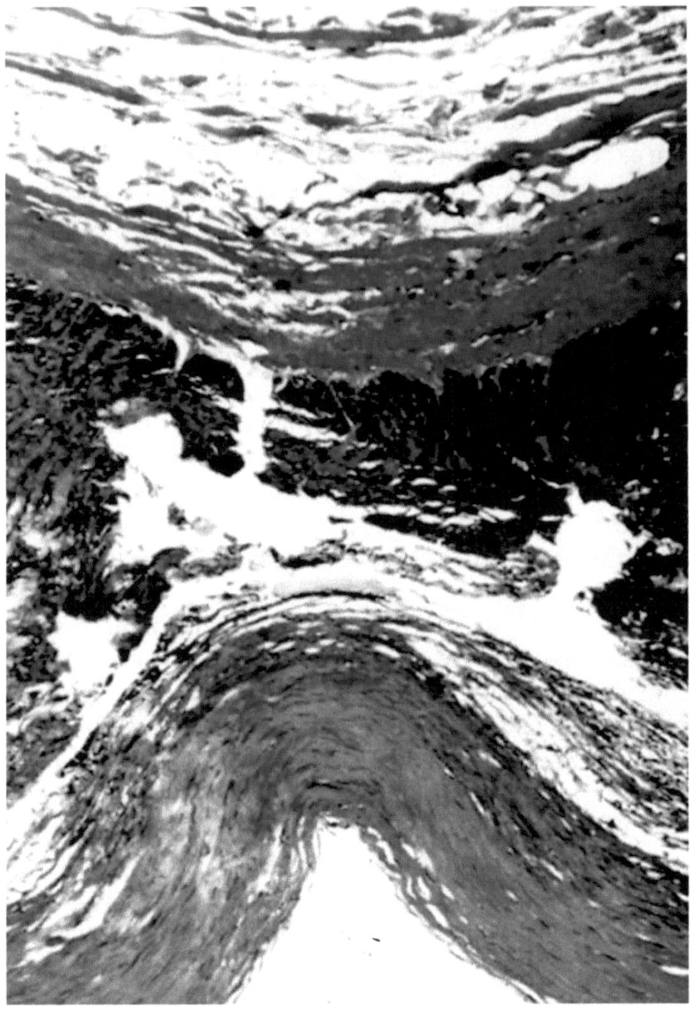

Fig. 2. Histological aspect of a coronary artery after snaring demonstrating lesion of the media layer.

cerebral microembolic signals were analyzed by transcranial Doppler in a randomized clinical trial comparing off-pump vs on-pump revascularization *(12)*. The number of microembolic signals was significant higher in patients operated on with cardiopulmonary support, although there was no significant clinical difference. Another clinical comparative study was performed to evaluate neurological complications. We prospectively examined 81 patients, before and up to 7 d after surgery, to compare the neurological morbidity between on-pump and off-pump procedures. Neurological abnormalities were found in 16 patients operated on-pump and 12 patients in the off-pump cohort. Prolonged coma occurred in one patient who underwent conventional CABG. Permanent stroke occurred in two patients in the on-pump group and one patient in the off-pump cohort. No clinical difference between the two groups was found *(13)*.

To address the inflammatory response associated with bypass grafting, we studied the release of cytokines—tumor necrosis factor-alpha and interleukin-6—as markers of the inflammatory response in patients undergoing conventional coronary revascularization.

Thirty patients were studied; 15 patients received adjunctive methylprednisolone and 15 did not. In this study we demonstrated that the systemic adverse effects caused by inflammatory response after cardiopulmonary bypass were minimized by the use of a corticosteroid *(14)*. We then extrapolated this concept by investigating the effect of avoiding extracorporeal circulation on the release of inflammatory cytokines. Not surprisingly, patients who underwent off-pump CABG demonstrated significantly reduced levels of cytokine release *(15)*.

An important contribution to the developing field of off-pump coronary artery bypass grafting was the introduction by Rivetti et al. *(16)* of a temporary intraluminal shunt that facilitated anastomosis and preserved distal coronary perfusion. We commonly employ this shunt when grafting the right coronary artery, and we believe that it is very important when no backflow can be seen after coronary occlusion.

For many years to follow, skepticism regarding the quality of the anastomosis combined with the natural resistance of surgeons to change routine procedures, rendered us one of a couple of groups in the world persisting with the clinical application of off-pump revascularization.

A landmark event in the field occurred when Benetti proposed a small left thoracotomy to graft left internal thoracic artery to LAD artery *(17)*, a technique that received the often-confusing eponym MIDCAB, for minimally invasive direct coronary artery bypass. This procedure, widely applied and popularized by Calafiore *(18)*, could be considered a natural evolution of the off-pump technique, as it highlighted the minimal-access potential of coronary revascularization.

The initial results with MIDCAB were mixed, and our group published less than optimal early patency rates for left internal thoracic artery to LAD *(19)* anastomoses. Compromising with the minimal access concept, we moved to performing a full sternotomy under a small skin incision. Perhaps the most important legacy of the MIDCAB or LAST (left anterior small thoracotomy) operation, as it is also referred to in the literature, was that it brought attention to cardiac surgeons worldwide that myocardial revascularization could be performed without extracorporeal circulation, much in the same way that Kolessov had done in the past.

Notably, widespread criticism for this procedure soon followed, mainly because of its restricted applicability to patients with single-vessel disease. But this procedure proved that coronary artery bypass performed off-pump through a small incision promoted rapid recovery, avoided blood transfusion, and resulted in fewer postoperative complications, shortened hospital stay, and reduced costs.

Unlike minimally invasive surgery of the abdomen or other body cavities, minimal invasive cardiac surgery has two dimensions: one is avoidance of cardiopulmonary bypass, and the other is limited access. While most agree that the former is of greater physiological importance, the latter seems to be the more attractive to patients.

While full sternotomy allowed the surgeon to reach all coronary branches, heart movement continued to challenge the creation of reliable anastomoses and revascularization of the posterior and lateral walls of the heart. The introduction of mechanical stabilizers as an effective and reproducible means to promote local reduction of heart motion represents perhaps the most important factor in the expansion of beating-heart surgery.

The importance of stabilizers was well documented by Calafiore *(20)*, who demonstrated improved early patency of the left internal thoracic artery and declared a "new era" of cardiac surgery following clinical introduction of the stabilizer. A discussion of the leading stabilizing systems appears later in this book (Chapters 6–8).

Many groups, including ours, adopted the full sternotomy-limited skin incision–mechanical stabilizer approach to off-pump coronary artery bypass with the conviction that two-vessel grafting was as safe and reliable as conventional bypass grafting.

The issue of circumflex artery revascularization, however, remained a major obstacle to complete off-pump revascularization. Exposure of the lateral and posterior walls demanded greater heart mobilization, with more possibilities for hemodynamic instability.

Lima proposed maneuvers for presentation of the marginal branches of the circumflex artery with little hemodynamic instability *(21)*. With several sutures positioned strategically between the inferior vena cava and the left inferior pulmonary vein, the heart can be "verticalized" outside of the chest, creating a true "ectopia cordis."

Some modification in the positioning of the operation table, associated with other maneuvers, allows good exposure of the circumflex branches. The successful application of the "LIMA stitches" and its subsequent modifications allowed complete revascularization and markedly increased the proportion of patients undergoing off-pump bypass grafting.

With this evolution and the introduction by a burgeoning industry of sophisticated enabling stabilizing systems, several groups worldwide have moved toward application of off-pump revascularization to all patients.

We believe that off-pump coronary artery bypass grafting or OPCAB is not a surgical procedure for all patients, and its ubiquitous application should not be seen as a laudable accomplishment. Rather, the technique of beating-heart revascularization should be tailored to the patient's anatomy and needs. In our experience, patients with hypertrophic left ventricles, diffuse atheromatous coronary arteries, and intramyocardial LAD artery are not good candidates for off-pump revascularization.

In almost 20 yr performing coronary artery bypass without extracorporeal circulation in over 3235 patients up to December 2002, we have been rewarded with a 2.8% in-hospital mortality and low morbidity. Following introduction of mechanical stabilizers and techniques for exposure of the circumflex artery branches, our proportion of patients undergoing off-pump revascularization has doubled from 21% to 49%. We expect that in the next few years, as better stabilizers, improved surgical maneuvers, and other technologies such as facilitated anastomotic devices are introduced, our indications will expand.

We believe that myocardial revascularization without cardiopulmonary bypass is a superior treatment for coronary insufficiency and, although, some comparative studies *(22,23)* with low-risk patients do not demonstrate improved clinical outcomes, the real superiority will become more obvious as OPCAB is applied to more patients with severe preoperative comorbidities *(24–26)*. It follows, then, that if OPCAB is a better technique for high-risk patients, it should be a better technique for all patients. While this is our belief, clinical confirmation is needed. The decision to use cardiopulmonary bypass must be individualized, but we do believe that today's coronary surgeon must be able to perform OPCAB and conventional CABG with equal expertise.

REFERENCES

1. Goetz RH, Rohman M, Haller JD, Dee R, Rosenak SS. Internal mammary-coronary anastomosis. A nonsuture method employing tantalum rings. J Thorac Cardiovasc Surg 1961;41:378–386.
2. Kolessov VL. Mammary artery coronary anastomosis as method of treatment for angina pectoris. J Thorac Cardiovasc Surg 1967;54:535–544.
3. Favaloro RG. Saphenous vein autograft replacement of severe segmental coronary artery occlusion technique. Ann Thorac Surg 1968;5:334–339.

4. Trapp WG, Bisarya R. Placement of coronary bypass graft without pump oxygenator. Ann Thorac Surg 1975;19:1–9.
5. Ankeney JL. To use or not to use pump oxygenator in coronary bypass operation. Ann Thorac Surg 1975;19:108–109.
6. Buffolo E, Andrade JCS, Succi JE, et al. Revascularizaçã o direta do miocárdio sem circulaçã o extracorpórea. Descriçã o da técnica e resultados iniciais. Arq Bras Cardiol 1982;38:365–373.
7. Benetti FJ. Direct coronary surgery with saphenous vein bypass without cardiopulmonary bypass or cardiac arrest. J Cardiovasc Surg. 1985;26:217–222.
8. Gerola LR, Moura LAR, Buffolo E, Leão LEV, Soares HC, Gallucci C. Garroteamento da artéria coronária na revascularizaçã o do miocárdio. Relaçã o entre o grau de aterosclerose e a lesão vascular: estudo experimental. Rev Brasil Cir Cardiov 1987;2:64–69.
9. Gerola LR, Moura LAR, Leão LEV, Soares HC, Branco JNR, Buffolo E. Arterial wall damage caused by snaring of the coronary arteries during off-pump revascularization. Heart Surgery Forum 2000;3(2):103–107.
10. Vega H, Leão LEV, Silva LA, et al. Surgical myocardial revascularization without using extracorporeal circulation in patients with acute myocardial infarct treated previously with intravenous streptokinase. Rev Hosp S Paulo 1990;2:75–78.
11. Buffolo E, Summo H, Aguiar LF, Teles CA, Branco JNR. Myocardial revascularization in patients 70 years of age and older without the use of extracorporeal circulation. Am J Geriatr Cardiol 1997;6:6–9.
12. Malheiros SMF, Massao AR, Gabbai AA, et al. Is the number of microembolic signals related to neurologic outcome in coronary bypass surgery? Arc Neuropsychiatr 2001;59:1–5.
13. Malheiros SMF, Brucki SMD, Gabbai AA, et al. Neurological outcome in coronary artery surgery with and without cardiopulmonary bypass. Acta Neurol Scand 1995;92:256–260.
14. Brasil LA, Gomes WJ, Salomão R, Fonseca JHP, Branco JNR, Buffolo E. Uso de corticóide como inhibidor da resposta inflamatoria sistêmica induzida pela circulaçã o extracorpórea. Rev Bras Cir Cardivasc 1999;14(3):254–268.
15. Brasil LA, Gomes WJ, Salomão R, Buffalo E. Inflammatory response after myocardial revascularization with or without cardiopulmonary bypass. Ann Thorac Surg 1998;66:56–59.
16. Rivetti LA, Gandra SMA. Initial experience using an intraluminal shunt during revascularization of the beating heart. Ann Thorac Surg 1997;63:1742–1747.
17. Benetti FJ. Video assisted coronary bypass surgery. J Cardiac Surg 1995;10:620–625.
18. Calafiore AM, Gianmarco GD, Teodori G, et al. Left anterior descending coronary artery grafting via left anterior small thoracotomy without cardiopulmonary bypass. Ann Thorac Surg 1996;61:1658–1665.
19. Buffolo E, Teles C, Aguiar LF, et al. Left anterior small thoracotomy and left anterior descending anastomoses: immediate postoperative analyses. J Am Clin Cardiol 1997;29:716.
20. Calafiore AM, Vitolla G, Mazzei V, Teodori G, Di Gianmarco G, Iovino T, Iaco A. The LAST operation: technique and results before and after stabilization era. Ann Thorac Surg 1998;66:998–1001.
21. Lima RC. Padronizaçã o técnica de revascularizaçã o do miocárdio da artéria circunflexa e seus ramos sem circulaçã o extracorpórea. Tese Doutorado. São Paulo: Universidade Federal de São Paulo/Escola Paulista de Medicina.
22. Vural KM, Tasdemi O, Karagaz H, Emir M, Tarcon O, Bayazit K. Comparison of the early results of coronary artery bypass grafting with and without extracorporeal circulation. Thorac Cardiovasc Surg 1995;43(6):620–625.
23. Kshettry VR, Flavin TF, Emery RW, Nicoloff DM, Arom K, Peterson RJ. Does multivessel off-pump coronary artery bypass reduce postoperative morbidity? Ann Thorac Surg 2000;69:1725–1730.
24. Yokoyama T, Baumgartner FJ, Gheissari A, Capouya ER, Panagiotides GP, Declusion RJ. Off-pump versus on-pump coronary bypass in high-risk subgroups. Ann Thorac Surg 2000;70:1546–1550.
25. Güller M, Kirali K, Toker ME, et al. Different CABG methods in patients with chronic obstructive pulmonary disease. Ann Thorac Surg 2001;71:152–157.
26. Ricci M, Karamanoukian HL, Abraham R, et al. Stroke in octogenarians undergoing coronary artery surgery with and without cardiopulmonary bypass. Ann Thorac Surg 2000;69:1471–1475.

4 Tailoring Minimal Invasive Coronary Bypass to the Patient

Michael A. Borger, MD, PHD
and M. Anno Diegeler, MD, PHD

CONTENTS

Introduction
OPCAB
MIDCAB
Partial Sternotomy CABG
Port-access CABG
Dresden Technique
TECAB
Summary
References

INTRODUCTION

Application of minimally invasive cardiac surgery techniques, in particular coronary bypass, is becoming increasingly widespread. A review of surgical practice in 72 North American hospitals, encompassing 17,000 coronary bypass operations performed in 1999, revealed that 16% of procedures were performed off-pump *(1)*.

While a large number of minimally invasive coronary bypass techniques have been developed, some controversy exists over what actually constitutes "minimally invasive." For the purposes of this chapter we will define minimal invasive coronary bypass as any procedure performed without the aid of cardiopulmonary bypass (CPB) and/or through a minimal access approach (that is, nonmedian sternotomy).

Furthermore, the substantial number of newly developed operations has led to a confusing array of names and acronyms, including OPCAB, MIDCAB, TECAB, and others. Our definition of each of these acronyms will be addressed in their respective subsequent sections. Each operative technique offers certain advantages and disadvantages over the

From: *Contemporary Cardiology: Minimally Invasive Cardiac Surgery, Second Edition*
Edited by: D. J. Goldstein and M. C. Oz © Humana Press Inc., Totowa, NJ

other coronary bypass procedures. One of the most difficult tasks for cardiac surgeons is to determine which operation is appropriate for which patients. The purpose of this chapter is to provide a framework for identifying the optimal surgical technique for specific patient populations—that is, tailoring the coronary bypass operation to the patient's needs.

A few cautionary words are necessary before proceeding. First, it should be stressed that each of the minimal invasive techniques discussed below is associated with a learning curve of skill and knowledge acquisition. Therefore, surgeons must take into account their own level of experience, as well as the experience of their respective institutions, when determining the optimal surgical approach for specific patient populations. Second, individual patient preferences should always be considered when determining the appropriate operation. Patient preferences may become more important over time because of increasing access to medical information through the Internet and patient-to-patient communications. However, we strongly recommend against surgeons performing operations that are clearly beyond their own level of comfort, experience, or knowledge simply to meet patient expectations. Strong patient preferences may therefore require referral to a surgeon or to a center that is experienced with performing the procedure in question. Third, it should be remembered that conventional coronary bypass surgery is always a viable alternative to each of the minimal invasive techniques listed below and is still a kind of "gold standard" for coronary revascularization. Fourth, surgeons should not hesitate to employ conventional coronary bypass in patients who do not meet minimal invasive inclusion criteria. Because the focus of this book is minimal invasive cardiac surgery, however, we will not discuss conventional on-pump coronary bypass in any detail.

OPCAB

For the purpose of this chapter we will define off-pump coronary artery bypass (OPCAB) as coronary revascularization on a beating heart, without the aid of CPB, through a standard median sternotomy. Improved stabilizing devices (see Chapters 6–8) have enabled surgeons to perform beating-heart surgery with greater facility and sense of comfort, and have allowed operating times to become similar to or less than conventional coronary bypass surgery *(2)*.

The main advantage of OPCAB is the avoidance of CPB with all of its documented deleterious effects. Avoiding CPB may lower the risk of neurological complications, renal dysfunction, bleeding, and systemic inflammatory activation (all discussed in more detail below). Another major advantage of OPCAB is the similarity of its operative technique to conventional coronary bypass. The full sternotomy approach allows revascularization of all major coronary territories, an option that is not possible for other minimal invasive techniques using a limited access. Furthermore, rapid institution of CPB is easily achieved, which increases the safety of the procedure, particularly during the learning period.

The main disadvantage of OPCAB is that the complete sternotomy approach increases surgical trauma, increases the risk of postoperative dehiscence and instability, and, most important, increases the risk of wound infection. The approach is therefore not really "minimally invasive," and no benefit can be gained in postoperative patient comfort or time to ambulation.

Another disadvantage is that beating-heart surgery is technically more demanding and may compromise the quality of revascularization, particularly for surgeons with limited experience. However, a number of studies from experienced centers have revealed that OPCAB results in excellent early and intermediate graft patency rates, roughly equivalent to conventional coronary bypass *(3,4)*. Although long-term results are not yet available, there is no foreseeable reason to expect diminished patency rates over time compared to conventional techniques.

The encouraging results for OPCAB have led investigators to try to determine which patient populations are optimal for this technique. Although some surgeons state that OPCAB should be employed in all patients, we do not endorse such a rigid recommendation. Table 1 summarizes our current recommendations for the indications and contraindications for OPCAB coronary revasularization.

Cardiac Indications and Contraindications for OPCAB

The types of cardiac pathology that are suitable and unsuitable for OPCAB surgery are fairly well agreed upon in the literature. OPCAB is indicated for multivessel coronary disease because all territories can be adequately exposed with pericardial stay sutures and stabilizing devices. Hemodynamic compromise may occur, particularly during exposure of the circumflex territory. Exposure of the posterior left ventricle impairs cardiac function by obstructing inflow to the right ventricle and by inducing diastolic dysfunction in the left ventricle. Coronary flow may also become impaired, particularly in the territory of the circumflex artery *(5)*. Furthermore, mitral valve incompetence may increase during cardiac displacement and atrial fibrillation may occur. The majority of these hemodynamic problems are temporary, however, and most can be managed conservatively with monitoring, physiological support, and patience. We have found that measuring left atrial pressure can also be helpful and is easily performed. In addition, atrial pacing at a rate of 90/min often provides further hemodynamic stabilization.

Some types of coronary artery lesions preclude the use of beating-heart surgery. Diffuse coronary artery calcification makes temporary vessel occlusion nearly impossible and therefore OPCAB should be avoided in these patients. A deep intramyocardial left anterior descending coronary artery (LAD) severely complicates the dissection and exposure of this vessel on a beating heart, thereby necessitating conventional coronary bypass under cardioplegic arrest to achieve a reproducible quality of revascularization. Temporary occlusion of a dominant right coronary artery with a noncritical stenosis may cause significant ischemia and arrhythmias *(6)*. A shunt, or a more distally performed occlusion at the posterior interventricular artery, may enable OPCAB to be performed in such patients. Some authors state that severe left main stenosis carries increased risk for OPCAB surgery, but this point is controversial *(7)*.

Other types of cardiac pathology that require increased caution during OPCAB revascularization are severe left ventricular (LV) dysfunction, markedly elevated LV end-diastolic pressure, and moderate to severe mitral regurgitation. Although these patients could benefit the most by avoiding CPB, their hemodynamic management requires experienced cardiac anesthetic and surgical teams. If OPCAB is attempted in these patients, emergency conversion to CPB (so-called crash CPB) should be avoided whenever possible, because the subsequent results are particularly poor. In addition, we recommend against OPCAB surgery in patients with uncontrolled ventricular arrhythmias. Such patients should undergo revascularization using conventional coronary bypass techniques.

Noncardiac Indications and Contraindications for OPCAB

OPCAB plays an important role for patients who are at high risk for complications of CPB (*see* Table 1). Elderly patients may benefit from OPCAB, predominantly by lowering the risk of neurological injury. Elderly age is consistently identified as one of the most important risk factors for stroke during coronary artery bypass grafting (CABG). Ricci et al. compared outcomes in 97 octogenarians undergoing beating-heart surgery to 172 octogenarians having conventional coronary bypass *(8)*. These investigators found a 0% incidence of stroke in OPCAB patients, compared to 9% for conventional patients. In addition, OPCAB may lower the incidence of other complications in elderly patients. Demers and Cartier demonstrated lower rates of atrial fibrillation and transfusion requirements in elderly patients undergoing OPCAB surgery when compared to conventional surgery *(9)*.

Patients with a calcified ascending aorta may benefit the most from OPCAB surgery. Off-pump total arterial revascularization can be performed without aortic cannulation or crossclamping, thereby eliminating the most important cause of embolic stroke during coronary bypass surgery *(10)*. Gaudino et al. compared two techniques for coronary revascularization in 211 patients with diffuse atherosclerosis of the ascending aorta *(11)*. They found that OPCAB resulted in a lower incidence of neurological complications, renal insufficiency, and intensive care unit (ICU) and hospital lengths of stay when compared to revascularization during ventricular fibrillation. Although total arterial revascularization eliminates the need for ascending aortic manipulation, saphenous vein grafts can also be used in patients with a diseased ascending aorta. Newly developed automated devices allow for proximal anastomoses to be constructed between the saphenous vein and the ascending aorta, while avoiding clamping of the ascending aorta.

OPCAB may also be indicated in patients at high risk for postoperative neurological impairment. OPCAB is associated with decreased cerebral microemboli, the predominant cause of postoperative neuropsychological impairment *(12)*. We used transcranial Doppler monitoring to demonstrate that patients undergoing off-pump surgery experienced on average 11 cerebral microemboli during the operation compared to 394 in conventional bypass patients *(13)*. Lowering the number of cerebral microemboli during coronary bypass was directly associated with better postoperative cognitive performance *(12,13)*.

Patients with severe carotid stenosis or a history of previous neurologic injury are particularly high-risk groups for postoperative neurologic sequelae and may benefit substantially from avoiding the systemic inflammatory effects and micro- and macroemboli associated with CPB. Patients with a prior history of stroke or TIA, or possibly degenerative disorders such as Parkinson's, may be optimal candidates for beating-heart surgery. In addition, patients with recent stroke or long-standing hypertension may benefit from a lower risk of cerebral hemorrhage, because lower levels of anticoagulation are required.

Another subpopulation that may benefit from beating-heart surgery is the patient with renal dysfunction. Avoiding CPB appears to lower the risk of perioperative renal ischemia, which is poorly tolerated in patients with preexisting renal impairment. Ascione et al. performed a randomized trial of beating-heart vs conventional surgery in 50 CABG patients *(14)*. These investigators found that OPCAB resulted in better postoperative glomerular filtration rate and renal tubular function than conventional surgery. Improved renal function should decrease the risk of renal failure, a major cause of postoperative morbidity and resource utilization, in patients with preoperative renal insufficiency. This may also be important for insulin-dependent diabetics, even with normal creatinine levels, since post-CPB renal failure is not uncommon in such patients.

OPCAB may play an important role for patients with chronic obstructive pulmonary disease (COPD). Systemic inflammatory activation and capillary leakage during CPB cause postoperative pulmonary edema and markedly impaired pulmonary function. The impaired pulmonary function is temporary and well tolerated by most patients, but may lead to respiratory failure, prolonged intubation, and/or adult respiratory distress syndrome in patients with preexisting COPD. Guler and colleagues prospectively assessed 58 CABG patients with COPD *(15)*. Beating-heart surgery patients (OPCAB and MIDCAB) had better postoperative forced expiratory volumes (FEV_1) than conventional patients. Improved pulmonary function may lead to decreased risk of postoperative respiratory failure, an important cause of prolonged ICU stay.

Finally, OPCAB may be important for patients with a history of bleeding diathesis. Several investigators have demonstrated that OPCAB is associated with improved platelet counts and platelet function, decreased fibrinolysis, and decreased blood loss when compared to conventional surgery. These findings may be important for patients with documented bleeding diathesis or preoperative anemia, as well as in patients who refuse blood transfusions (i.e., Jehovah's Witness patients).

There are very few noncardiac contraindications for OPCAB surgery (Table 1). However, one special circumstance deserves note. Chavanon et al. found that iatrogenic aortic dissection was 50 times more likely to occur during beating-heart surgery than during conventional CABG *(16)*. Iatrogenic dissection was caused by applying a partial occluding aortic crossclamp in patients with a dilated ascending aorta. Although the incidence of aortic dissection was still low in OPCAB patients (1%), this devastating complication should obviously be avoided whenever possible. Because of their experience, these investigators now recommend against using a partial occluding clamp in patients with an ascending aortic diameter greater than 4.0–4.5 cm *(9)*.

MIDCAB

Minimal invasive direct coronary artery bypass (MIDCAB) is another common form of minimal invasive coronary surgery, comprising approx 10% of all beating-heart operations *(2)*. This procedure is discussed in great detail by Dr. Dullum in Chapter 9. For the purpose of this chapter we will define MIDCAB as coronary revascularization through an anterolateral thoracotomy. The procedure entails dissection of the left internal mammary artery (LIMA) with specialized rib retractors through a small (6–8 cm) anterolateral thoracotomy. The LIMA is then anastomosed to the LAD through the thoracotomy incision, using myocardial stabilizers similar to those used for OPCAB. Although MIDCAB can be performed with the assistance of port-access CPB and cardioplegic arrest (see below), beating-heart techniques are employed in the vast majority of cases.

MIDCAB is usually performed for isolated LAD lesions, but radial artery "T" grafts can also be used to bypass favorable diagonal or intermediate branches. A right anterolateral thoracotomy ("right MIDCAB") can be used for patients with isolated proximal RCA lesions. The right internal mammary artery (RIMA) is harvested using the same

Table 1
Current Recommendations for OPCAB

Pathology	*Indications*	*Contraindications*
Cardiac	Multivessel disease	Intramyocardial LAD Diffusely calcified coronaries RCA stenosis < 80% Severe LV dysfunction ↑↑ LVEDP Moderate MR Ventricular arrhythmias
Noncardiac	Elderly age Calcified ascending aorta Neurologic history Renal dysfunction COPD Bleeding diatheses	Dilated ascending aorta

LAD = left anterior descending artery, RCA = right coronary artery, LV = left ventricle, LVEDP = left ventricular end-diastolic pressure, MR = mitral regurgitation, COPD = chronic obstructive pulmonary disease.

technique as for the LIMA and anastomosed to the mid-RCA. In the vast majority of patients, however, the RCA is diseased down to the crux cordis segment. Because the distal branches of the RCA are inaccessible through this limited access, the classical right MIDCAB is rarely performed.

A special type of limited access procedure can be performed through a transabdominal approach (also known as the subxiphoid procedure) *(17)*. This approach is explored by Dr. Benetti in great detail in Chapter 11. The transabdominal approach involves a chevron-shaped incision in the subxiphoid region, followed by harvesting of the right gastroepiploic artery (GEA) and LIMA, if necessary. The GEA is anastomosed to the RCA, or one of its branches, and the LIMA is anastomosed to the LAD. Although transabdominal technique has the benefit of being feasible for multivessel coronary disease, the approach is markedly different than most cardiac operations and therefore is not used by many cardiac surgeons.

Another special type of MIDCAB surgery is the endoscopic coronary artery bypass (ENDOCAB) procedure. ENDOCAB involves endoscopic harvesting of the LIMA (or RIMA) through three small ports, followed by anastomosis of the LIMA to the LAD (or RIMA to the RCA) through a very small (4–5 cm) anterolateral thoracotomy. As with other MIDCAB procedures, ENDOCAB is usually performed on a beating heart, but can also be done with port-access CPB and cardioplegic arrest.

The major advantages of MIDCAB surgery are avoidance of CPB and avoidance of a complete sternotomy. The benefits of surgery without CPB were covered in detail above. The benefits of surgery without a sternotomy are decreased risk of sternal wound infection and decreased time to ambulation. Several investigators, including our group *(18)*, have demonstrated that MIDCAB is associated with lower postoperative pain scores (except in the immediate postoperative period) and better quality of life than conventional coronary bypass surgery. These benefits are particularly notable with recently developed chest retractors that eliminate the need for rib removal or sternocostal disarticulation.

The main concern about MIDCAB surgery, just as for OPCAB, was the quality of coronary anastomoses. Several surgeons have questioned the ability to perform anastomoses on a beating heart through a small thoracotomy. However, increasing evidence has revealed that excellent patency rates can be achieved with the MIDCAB procedure. In one of the largest series to date, we examined graft patency rates in 618 MIDCAB patients *(19)*. Early postoperative angiography, performed in 585 patients, revealed an overall patency rate of 97.4%. Six-month postoperative angiography was performed in 353 patients and revealed an overall patency of 95.8%, increasing to 97.0% for the last year of the study. Significant graft stenosis was present in 4.5% of patients at 6 mo. Several other investigators have confirmed the excellent results achievable with MIDCAB revascularization *(4)*.

One definite disadvantage of MIDCAB is the inability to institute CPB through an anterolateral thoracotomy. If hemodynamic instability is to occur during the operation, patients must be placed on CPB through the femoral vessels or through a separate median sternotomy incision. Fortunately, with proper patient selection, this is a rare occurrence.- Another disadvantage of MIDCAB surgery is the requirement for single-lung ventilation. The lung should be deflated during IMA dissection, thereby necessitating double-lumen endotracheal intubation. Single-lung ventilation may increase anesthesia time and is contraindicated in patients with severe COPD or pulmonary hypertension. The final disadvantage of MIDCAB is the possibility of postoperative lung herniation. The development of new chest retractors has eliminated the need for rib resection or sternocostal disarticulation, reducing the risk of lung herniation.

Cardiac Indications and Contraindications for MIDCAB

Table 2 summarizes our current recommendations for proper patient selection for MIDCAB surgery. As mentioned previously, the predominant cardiac indication for MIDCAB is isolated high-grade LAD disease. In a subset of patients from the above-mentioned study *(19)*, we randomized 200 patients with isolated high-grade LAD stenosis to receive MIDCAB or PTCA. Because of the surgical nature of the MIDCAB procedure, these patients had a slightly higher prevalence of periprocedural adverse events than PTCA patients. However, 6-mo follow-up revealed that MIDCAB patients had significantly less angina, fewer stenoses, and fewer reinterventions than PTCA patients, particularly those with a complex (type B or C) LAD lesion *(19)*. Therefore, MIDCAB may be the procedure of choice for patients with isolated, complex, high-grade disease of the LAD.

MIDCAB can also be attempted in patients with less severe stenosis of the LAD, particularly if a shunt is employed. However, there is an increased risk of temporary ischemia and hemodynamic instability during vessel occlusion in these patients. Patients with exceptionally favorable diagonal or intermediate vessels may also undergo bypass of these vessels with a "T" graft, but this is a relatively uncommon and challenging procedure. We would recommend this technique only in patients with a normal body mass index. MIDCAB is also the option of choice for redo LAD revascularization, provided the LIMA was not used during the previous operation.

Occasionally, a "right MIDCAB" can be used to revascularize isolated RCA disease. However, this is a more technically demanding procedure than conventional MIDCAB, and it results in significantly lower graft patency rates *(4)*. The transabdominal procedure can be used in patients with both LAD and RCA disease, but again this technique is not commonly used. The subxiphoid approach may be the best alternative, however, for patients with isolated RCA disease who have undergone a previous CABG operation, particularly if a patent LIMA to LAD graft is present.

A special indication for MIDCAB surgery is very-high-risk patients with multivessel disease who cannot tolerate CPB. In such patients PTCA and stenting of the RCA and/or circumflex territory is perfromed, followed by MIDCAB revascularization of the LAD. This so-called hybrid procedure has been performed in several centers with satisfactory results *(20)* and is discussed in great detail in Chapter 15. Isolated MIDCAB may also be indicated for patients with LAD disease and "no-option" RCA or circumflex disease. The procedure results in an incomplete revascularization. However, the options for treating the culprit lesion are limited in such patients, and often their angina can be relieved with a MIDCAB alone.

The cardiac contraindications to MIDCAB are similar to those for OPCAB. We strongly recommend against MIDCAB in patients with an intramyocardial or diffusely calcified or diseased LAD. We also recommend against MIDCAB in patients with a small (<1.5 mm) LAD or an occluded LAD that cannot be localized on the angiogram. MIDCAB may also be difficult in patients with severe left ventricular hypertrophy, since the LAD is often notably displaced to the left.

Noncardiac Indications and Contraindications for MIDCAB

Table 2 summarizes the major noncardiac variables to be considered when deciding if a patient is suitable for MIDCAB surgery. In general, MIDCAB patients fall into two groups. One group is comprised of young, low-risk patients with LAD disease that is favorable for MIDCAB revascularization. Such patients would do well with MIDCAB or conventional coronary bypass, but MIDCAB may be a better option because of quicker rehabilitation and better postoperative quality of life. The second MIDCAB group is comprised of very-high-risk patients with isolated LAD disease or multivessel disease that is to be treated with the hybrid procedure. As discussed above, high-risk patients may benefit greatly by avoiding the deleterious effects of CPB. The noncardiac indications for MIDCAB in such patients are essentially the same as for OPCAB (*see* Table 1). Therefore, elderly patients, patients with a calcified ascending aorta, and patients with preoperative renal insufficiency are likely to benefit from MIDCAB surgery if the coronary anatomy is favorable.

The noncardiac contraindications to MIDCAB are severe COPD and severe obesity. As mentioned previously, MIDCAB requires single-lung ventilation and therefore should not be used in patients with an FEV_1 of less than 1.0 L. Severe obesity (body mass index > 35) is also a contraindication to MIDCAB because of the resultant difficulty with surgical exposure. The MIDCAB approach may also be difficult in women with large breasts. A previous laparotomy is a contraindication for patients in whom a transabdominal procedure is being considered

PARTIAL STERNOTOMY CABG

Another minimal invasive coronary bypass operation is the partial sternotomy CABG. In this technique, the lower half of the sternum is divided in the midline up to the third intercostal space. The rest of the procedure is performed using a specialized sternal retractor *(21)*. Alternatively, an "L"- or "T"-shaped sternotomy can be employed *(22)*.

Table 2
Current Recommendations for MIDCAB

Pathology	*Indications*	*Contraindications*
Cardiac	Isolated high-grade (>80%) LAD stenosis Redo LAD bypass (if LIMA not previously used) RCA stenosis ("right MIDCAB" or subxiphoid) Multivessel disease (hybrid procedure)	Intramyocardial LAD Diffusely calcified LAD LAD < 1.5 mm Severe LV dysfunction Ventricular arrhythmias
Noncardiac	Young, active patients Same indications as OPCAB in high-risk patients	Severe COPD (FEV_1 < 1.0 L) Severe obesity (BMI > 35) Previous laparotomy (subxiphoid procedure only)

LAD = left anterior descending artery, LIMA = left internal mammary artery, RCA = right coronary artery, LV = left ventricle, COPD = chronic obstructive pulmonary disease, BMI = body mass index.

The LITA and RITA can be adequately harvested through this incision, or the GEA can be harvested through a small subxiphoid extension. The partial sternotomy CABG allows for beating-heart revascularization of the LAD and RCA territories. Saphenous vein grafts are not used because the ascending aorta is not exposed.

As with the OPCAB and MIDCAB procedures, the main advantage of the partial sternotomy CABG is the avoidance of CPB. The advantages of a partial sternotomy over a complete sternotomy (OPCAB) are a smaller incision (10–12 cm), less traction on the brachial plexus, and lower risk of postoperative sternal dehiscence or infection. The advantages of the partial sternotomy procedure over MIDCAB are the ability to perform double-vessel revascularization, the familiar surgical technique, and the ease of conversion to full sternotomy and CPB.

The main disadvantage of partial sternotomy CABG is prolonged operative times, particularly in the early stages of learning this procedure *(22)*. The difficulties with surgical exposure, as well as the nominal advantages over a complete sternotomy technique, have led most surgeons to choose conventional OPCAB over partial sternotomy CABG.

Table 3 displays our current recommendations for partial sternotomy CABG. The main cardiac indication is double-vessel (LAD and RCA) disease. If the RCA is bypassable in its midsection, then the RITA is employed. If a posterior branch of the RCA needs to be bypassed, then the GEA is used. The cardiac contraindications to partial sternotomy CABG are the same as for OPCAB surgery.

Because partial sternotomy CABG is performed without the use of CPB, the noncardiac indications are the same as for OPCAB. The only noncardiac contraindication, if the GEA is to be used, is a previous laparotomy.

PORT-ACCESS CABG

Port-access CABG refers to coronary revascularization, with CPB support and cardioplegic arrest, through a small anterior thoracotomy *(23)*. The patient is placed on

Table 3
Current Recommendations for Partial Sternotomy CABG

Pathology	*Indications*	*Contraindications*
Cardiac	Double-vessel disease (LAD and RCA)	Same as for OPCAB
Noncardiac	Same as for OPCAB	Previous laparotomy (if GEA is to be used)

LAD = left anterior descending artery, RCA = right coronary artery, GEA = gastroepiploic artery.

CPB through the femoral vessels and an endoaortic balloon is used to separate the coronary and systemic circulations.

The main advantage of port-access CABG is that distal anastomoses are performed on a quiescent, bloodless field through a minimal access incision. In addition, patients with double-vessel disease (LAD and circumflex territory) can be revascularized successfully with this procedure.

There are several disadvantages to port-access CABG. The main disadvantage is the risk of retrograde aortic dissection, particularly in patients with peripheral vascular disease. Port-access CABG is contraindicated in patients with peripheral vascular disease, aortic aneurysmal dilation, or calcification or plaques in the ascending aorta. Aortic regurgitation is another contraindication to this procedure, although retrograde cardioplegia can be employed through a transjugular coronary sinus catheter in such patients. Another major disadvantage of port-access CABG is the risk of endoaortic balloon migration with resultant cerebral ischemia. In addition, the procedure entails prolonged operative and CPB times, and is more expensive than all alternative techniques at the present time.

Multi-institution registries have demonstrated that port-access CABG can be performed in low-risk patients with acceptable results *(23)*. Because of the risks of major complications, however, we do not currently recommend this procedure over MIDCAB (for isolated LAD disease) or OPCAB (for multivessel disease).

DRESDEN TECHNIQUE

Another form of minimal invasive coronary bypass is the Dresden technique *(24)*. For this procedure, an anterolateral thoracotomy is performed in the third intercostal space, with disarticulation of the adjacent sternocostal junctions. The aorta and right atrium are directly cannulated through this incision, and the aorta is occluded with a conventional clamp.

The Dresden technique has the same main advantage as port-access CABG—coronary surgery on an arrested heart—without the major disadvantages of endoaortic balloon migration or retrograde aortic dissection. The presence of peripheral vascular disease is not a limitation for this technique. In addition, the Dresden technique can be used for patients with double-vessel disease, i.e., LAD and high obtuse marginal branches of the circumflex. Endoscopic harvesting of both thoracic arteries can be performed with this approach and may actually enhance the ease of the procedure, particularly if using the recently available da Vinci Telemanipulator system (Intuitve Surgical; Mountain View, CA).

The main disadvantage of the Dresden technique is the limited and unfamiliar access to the heart. The more posterior marginal branches as well as the right coronary artery are difficult to expose. In addition, the third rib is disarticulated from its sternal connection and may cause significant postoperative discomfort. Procedure times are prolonged and technical demands are increased. Perhaps because of these limitations, the Dresden technique is currently performed in few surgical centers.

TECAB

Total endoscopic coronary artery bypass (TECAB) is an experimental procedure currently being examined in a few cardiac surgery centers. LIMA harvesting and coronary revascularization is performed through four very small (1–2 cm) incisions, using robotic techniques *(25,26)*. The procedure was originally performed with port-access CPB support, but concerns about its complications has led to the use of beating-heart techniques.

The main advantage of TECAB is decreased postoperative pain and time to ambulation. The main disadvantages are markedly prolonged operative times, a high rate of conversion to MIDCAB, the need for a specialized surgical team, and increased costs.

TECAB is still an experimental surgical approach and is currently performed in low-risk patients with isolated, high-grade LAD stenoses. The RIMA can also be used for diagonal or intermediate coronary bypass in exceptional patients *(25)*. Contraindications for TECAB are an intramyocardial, diffusely diseased, or noncritically stenosed LAD. Any clinical pulmonary disease, chest deformations, or previous surgery of the left chest are also contraindications to TECAB.

It should be stressed that TECAB should be reserved for centers that are experienced in robotic techniques. Owing to the steep learning curve, this approach should only be performed under a strict scientific protocol. Further developments in endoscopic stabilizers and automated anastomotic devices may increase the feasibility of this procedure in the future.

SUMMARY

The purpose of this chapter was to make current recommendations about which minimal invasive coronary bypass procedure is suitable for which patient groups. The recommendations are likely to change, however, as more data and new enabling technologies become available. As stated earlier, every minimal invasive procedure has its own learning curve of skill and knowledge acquisition. When deciding which technique to use, surgeons must be aware of their own limitations as well as the limitations of their institutions. Standard conventional coronary bypass should always be considered an option.

We currently recommend OPCAB surgery for patients with multivessel coronary disease who are at high risk for complications during CPB. OPCAB should be strongly considered in elderly patients and in patients with ascending aortic atherosclerosis, previous neurological injury, renal impairment, or COPD.

MIDCAB revascularization is the procedure of choice for patients with isolated, high-grade LAD stenosis. Low-risk and high-risk patients may benefit significantly from this procedure.

The partial sternotomy CABG and Dresden technique are other viable minimal invasive operations, but are not commonly performed. The subxiphoid procedure may be particularly helpful for redo CABG patients requiring isolated RCA revascularization.

We currently do not recommend port-access CABG because of the risk of major complications. TECAB is currently an experimental procedure, but may become feasible in the future.

REFERENCES

1. Brown PP, Mack MJ, Simon AW, et al. Comparing clinical outcomes in high-volume and low-volume off-pump coronary bypass operation programs. Ann Thorac Surg 2001;72:S1009–S1015.
2. Mack MJ. Is there a future for minimally invasive cardiac surgery? Eur J Cardiothorac Surg 1999;16:S119–S125.
3. Puskas JD, Thourani VH, Marshall JJ, et al. Clinical outcomes, angiographic patency, and resource utilization in 200 consecutive off-pump coronary bypass patients. Ann Thorac Surg 2001;71:477–484.
4. Stanbridge RDL, Hadjinikolaou LK. Technical adjuncts in beating heart surgery. Comparison of MIDCAB to off-pump sternotomy: a meta-analysis. Eur J Cardiothorac Surg 1999;16:S24–S33.
5. Grundeman PF, Borst C, van Herwaarden JA, Verlaan CW, Jansen EW. Vertical displacement of the beating heart by the octopus tissue stabilizer: influence on coronary flow. Ann Thorac Surg 1998;65:1348–1352.
6. Diegeler A, Matin M, Falk V, et al. Indication and patient selection in minimally invasive and off-pump coronary artery bypass grafting. Eur J Cardiothorac Surg 1999;16:S79–S82.
7. Yeatman M, Caputo M, Ascione R, Ciulli F, Angelini GD. Off-pump coronary artery bypass surgery for critical left main stem disease: safety, efficacy and outcome. Eur J Cardiothorac Surg 2001;19:239–244.
8. Ricci M, Karamanoukian HL, Abraham R, et al. Stroke in octogenarians undergoing coronary artery surgery with and without cardiopulmonary bypass. Ann Thorac Surg 2000;69:1471–1475.
9. Demers P, Cartier R. Multivessel off-pump coronary artery bypass surgery in the elderly. Eur J Cardiothorac Surg 2001;20:908–912.
10. Borger MA, Ivanov J, Weisel RD, Rao V, Peniston CM. Stroke during coronary bypass surgery: principal role of cerebral macroemboli. Eur J Cardiothorac Surg 2001;19:627–632.
11. Gaudino M, Glieca F, Alessandrini F, et al. The unclampable ascending aorta in coronary artery bypass patients: a surgical challenge of increasing frequency. Circulation 2000;102:1497–1452.
12. Borger MA, Peniston CM, Weisel RD, Vasiliou M, Green REA, Feindel CM. Neuropsychological impairment after coronary bypass surgery: effect of gaseous emboli during perfusionist interventions. J Thorac Cardiovasc Surg 2001;121:743–749.
13. Diegeler A, Hirsch R, Schneider F, et al. Neuromonitoring and neurocognitive outcome in off-pump versus conventional coronary bypass operation. Ann Thorac Surg 200;69:1162–1166.
14. Ascione R, Lloyd CT, Underwood MJ, Gomes WJ, Angelini GD. On-pump versus off-pump coronary revascularization: evaluation of renal function. Ann Thorac Surg 1999;68:493–498.
15. Guler M, Kirali K, Toker ME, et al. Different CABG methods in patients with chronic obstructive pulmonary disease. Ann Thorac Surg 2001;71:152–157.
16. Chavanon O, Carrier M, Cartier R, et al. Increased incidence of acute ascending aortic dissection with off-pump aortocoronary bypass surgery? Ann Thorac Surg 2001;71:117–121.
17. Subramanian VA, Patel NU. Transabdominal minimally invasive direct coronary artery bypass grafting (MIDCAB). Eur J Cardiothorac Surg 2000;17:485–487.
18. Diegeler A, Walther T, Metz S, et al. Comparison of MIDCAB versus conventional CABG surgery regarding pain and quality of life. Heart Surg Forum 1999;2:290–295.
19. Diegeler A, Spyrantis N, Matin M, et al. The revival of surgical treatment for isolated proximal high grade LAD lesions by minimally invasive coronary artery bypass grafting. Eur J Cardiothorac Surg 2000;17:501–504.

20. Cohen HA, Zenati M, Smith AJC, et al. Feasibility of combined percutaneous transluminal angioplasty and minimally invasive direct coronary artery bypass in patients with multivessel coronary artery disease. Circulation 1998;98:1048–1050.
21. Niinami H, Takeuchi Y, Ichikawa S, Suda Y. Partial median sternotomy as a minimal access for off-pump coronary artery bypass grafting: feasibility of the lower-end sternal splitting approach. Ann Thorac Surg 2001;72:S1041–S1045.
22. Lichtenberg A, Klima U, Harringer W, Kim PY, Haverich A. Mini-sternotomy for off-pump coronary artery bypass grafting. Ann Thorac Surg 2000;69:1276–1277.
23. Grossi EA, Groh MA, Lefrak EA, et al. Results of a prospective multicenter study on port-access coronary bypass grafting. Ann Thorac Surg 1999;68:1475–1477.
24. Gulielmos V, Brandt M, Dill HM, et al. Coronary artery bypass grafting via median sternotomy or lateral thoracotomy. Eur J Cardiothorac Surg 1999;16:S48–S52.
25. Kappert U, Cichon R, Schneider J, et al. Technique of closed chest coronary artery surgery on the beating heart. Eur J Cardiothorac Surg 2001;20:765–769.
26. Mohr FW, Falk V, Diegeler A, et al. Computer-enhanced "robotic" cardiac surgery: experience in 148 patients. J Thorac Cardiovasc Surg 2001;121:842–853.

5 OPCAB

A Primer on Technique

John D. Puskas, MD, MSc

CONTENTS

INTRODUCTION
PREOPERATIVE EVALUATION
OPERATIVE PROCEDURE
SEQUENCE OF GRAFTING IN OPCAB
CARDIAC DISPLACEMENT AND PRESENTATION OF CORONARY TARGETS
CORONARY STABILIZATION AND GRAFTING
PERFUSION-ASSISTED OPCAB
SUMMARY
REFERENCES

INTRODUCTION

Coronary artery bypass without the use of cardiopulmonary bypass off-pump coronary artery bypass (OPCAB), is gaining popularity due to recent scientific reports showing its safety. OPCAB is performed to avoid the diffuse inflammatory response, multiorgan dysfunction, and neurological complications associated with cardiopulmonary bypass. The authors and others have recently shown excellent graft patency, improved outcomes, and lower costs with OPCAB *(1)*.

Experience with OPCAB over 5 yr has allowed an evolution in surgical technique. Early in the experience, it was common to require inotropic support for hemodynamic instability during OPCAB. Since refining techniques for cardiac positioning and stabilization, use of inotropes is infrequent. With patience and persistence, OPCAB can be performed in the vast majority of coronary revascularization patients. Patients for whom OPCAB may be inappropriate are those in cardiogenic shock, those suffering ischemic

From: *Contemporary Cardiology: Minimally Invasive Cardiac Surgery, Second Edition*
Edited by: D. J. Goldstein and M. C. Oz © Humana Press Inc., Totowa, NJ

arrhythmias, and those with physical conditions that profoundly limit rotation of the heart (pectus excavatum or previous left pneumonectomy). Intramyocardial or unusually small or calcified coronary arteries may be safely bypassed off-pump only with the benefit of considerable experience.

PREOPERATIVE EVALUATION

Coronary revascularization candidates must undergo a complete history and physical exam. If the Allen's test is inconclusive, radial and ulnar artery duplex examinations are performed before radial arteries are harvested. Pulmonary function tests are performed only in patients with severe chronic obstructive pulmonary disease (COPD) or active pulmonary disease. Criteria for preoperative carotid duplex examination include left main disease, peripheral vascular disease, carotid bruits, history of stroke or transient ischemic attack, heavy tobacco use, or age over 65 yr. If significant carotid disease is suggested by duplex examination, then a carotid angiogram is obtained. When > 79% stenosis is present, staged carotid endarterectomy followed by coronary revascularization is performed.

OPERATIVE PROCEDURE

All patients undergoing OPCAB require invasive monitoring during operation. At a minimum, an arterial line and central venous line are required. Significantly depressed left ventricular function mandates a Swan–Ganz catheter. Those patients with severe ventricular dysfunction may benefit from preoperative intra-aortic balloon pump *(2)*. Good communication between the surgeon and the anesthesiologist throughout the procedure is essential. Multiple displacements of the heart during OPCAB subject the patient to repeated hemodynamic changes and require an attentive anesthesiologist throughout the procedure.

The OPCAB procedure differs in many ways from on-pump CABG, but the skin entry and sternotomy are identical. A #10 blade knife is used through the skin and fat, down to fascia. Electrocautery is then utilized only selectively for bleeding and to divide the muscles and fascia at the middle of the sternum. Standard sternotomy is performed with a sternal saw. An upward-lifting Favoloro-type mammary retractor is used to harvest the LIMA and/or the RIMA. This retractor aids in exposure of the arteries and minimizes chest wall trauma. Heparin is given (1.5 mg/kg) with a target ACT > 300 s. Heparin (3000 units) is reinfused every 30 min to maintain an ACT > 300 s. This regimen is prompted by the recognition that heparin metabolism is more rapid in warm OPCAB patients than in those cooled on cardiopulmonary bypass.

After heparin is given, the mammary is divided and a mixture of papaverine and lidocaine is injected into the lumen of the mammary artery and allowed to reside there for 15–30 min. The Medtronic sternal retractor (Octobase™) is placed. This retractor is designed specifically for the Medtronic Octopus III (Medtronic, Minneapolis, MN) stabilizer, which can be secured to any aspect of the retractor.

A wide "T"-shaped pericardiotomy is performed, dividing the pericardium from the diaphragm down towards—but not into—the left and right phrenic nerves. The left and right pericardiophrenic artery and vein branches are carefully clipped and divided to avoid postoperative bleeding. Both pleural spaces are opened widely. Care is taken during the dissection to clip any large vessels encountered and to avoid the phrenic nerves. It is important to divide the diaphragmatic muscle slips that insert on the right side of the xiphoid, to allow elevation of the right hemisternal border, creating space for rightward cardiac displacement. Similarly, excision of a large right-sided pericardial fat pad will provide additional room. Placement of two rolled towels under the right limb of the sternal retractor elevates the right sternal edge, allowing the heart to be repositioned toward the right without compression against the sternum or retractor. One or two heavy pericardial sutures are placed on the left pericardium above the phrenic nerve. It is important to divide the left side of the pericardium off the diaphragm toward the phrenic nerve, so that traction on this left pericardium may assist in rotating and displacing the heart toward the right to visualize the left lateral wall.

The most important traction suture is a deep posterior pericardial suture placed approximately two-thirds of the way between the inferior vena cava and the left pulmonary vein at the point where the pericardium reflects over the left atrium. Care should be taken with placement of this suture to avoid the aorta, esophagus, left lung, and pulmonary veins. The suture is covered with a rubber catheter to prevent trauma to the epicardium. When this suture is retracted toward the patient's feet, it elevates the base of the heart toward the ceiling and lifts the apex vertically with remarkably little change in hemodynamics. When the deep pericardial traction suture is retracted toward the left shoulder, it rotates the heart from left to right. A variety of cotton slings may be applied at the base of this suture to aid in displacing the heart into the right pleural cavity. The slings may be particularly helpful during OPCAB in the setting of cardiomegaly.

All patients undergo epiaortic ultrasound, which may add only 1–2 min to the procedure. Epiaortic ultrasound guides the surgeon in individualized placement of aortic clamps and proximal anastomoses to reduce the risk of embolism of atherosclerotic debris from the ascending aorta. Grade IV or V atherosclerosis of the ascending aorta precludes aortic crossclamping and mandates a change in the site of proximal anastomoses. Other possible sites for proximal anastomoses include the innominate artery, LIMA, and RIMA.

The heart is allowed to roll with gravity into the left or right chest, facilitated by table rotation and traction suture(s) and occasionally a cotton sling. The heart should never be compressed against the sternum or pericardium. The right pericardial traction sutures are released when exposing the left side of the heart and similarly the left traction sutures are released when exposing the right coronary artery. Pericardial sutures on both the right and left sides are never under tension simultaneously when displacing the heart to expose coronary targets. Gentle application of these techniques maintains stable hemodynamics while providing excellent exposure. On rare occasions, bradycardia and cardiomegaly may coexist and the resulting ventricular distention may hinder effective cardiac displacement. Temporary epicardial atrial pacing may significantly reduce cardiac size and improve target vessel exposure during OPCAB in this difficult circumstance.

SEQUENCE OF GRAFTING IN OPCAB

In off-pump coronary surgery, the chosen sequence of grafting is important to maintain hemodynamic stability and avoid critical ischemia. As a general rule, the collateralized vessel(s) are grafted first and then reperfused by performing the proximal anastomosis(es) or unclamping the internal mammary flow or connecting the perfusion-assisted direct coronary artery bypass (PADCAB) apparatus. The last coronary target grafted is the collateralizing vessel(s). This strategy obviates interrupting vital flow from the collateralizing vessel(s) to the collateralized vessels until after the collateralized vessel(s) have been grafted.

Performing the proximal anastomoses first makes estimation of graft length difficult. At times the proximal anastomoses may be performed early in the operative sequence to aid in early reperfusion of a collateralized vessel. If the LIMA → LAD graft must be performed first, it may be necessary to leave a long mammary pedicle to avoid tension on the LIMA anastomosis during subsequent cardiac displacement to expose lateral wall targets.

A preferred sequence of grafting is as follows.

1. Perform the anastomosis to the completely occluded, collaterized vessel(s) first. The collateralizing vessel may then be safely grafted. This strategy will minimize myocardial ischemia.
2. The LIMA → LAD anastomosis should be performed first if the LAD is collateralized or in cases of tight left main stenosis. This anastomosis is performed last when the LAD is the collateralizing vessel.
3. The proximal anastomosis can be performed first or early after the distal anastomosis if the target is a critical, collateralized vessel. This allows simultaneous perfusion during the occlusion of the collateralizing vessel and minimizes overall myocardial ischemia.
4. Beware of the large proximally stenosed right coronary artery. The right coronary artery, particularly if large and dominant, can cause significant problems when occluded during OPCAB. Acute occlusion of a moderately stenotic right coronary artery may lead to severe hemodynamic compromise due to bradycardia. The surgeon must be prepared to use an intracoronary shunt or epicardial pacing to correct bradyarrhythmias promptly.
5. Beware of mitral regurgitation in OPCAB. Prolonged cardiac displacement combined with mitral regurgitation may contribute to a downward hemodynamic spiral. Progressive elevation of pulmonary pressures and increasing regurgitation on TEE may signal impending right heart falure. Ischemic mitral regurgitation should be addressed early in the procedure. This is accomplished by grafting and perfusing the culprit vessel responsible for papillary muscle dysfunction.
6. Finally, graft sequence should be individualized, depending on anatomic patterns of coronary occlusion and collateralization, myocardial contractility, atherosclerosis of the ascending aorta, conduit availability, and graft geometry.

CARDIAC DISPLACEMENT AND PRESENTATION OF CORONARY TARGETS

It is important to understand that the cardiac displacement techniques for exposure of the inferior and lateral vessels are different. The lateral vessels are approached by allowing the base of the heart to descend and rolling the apex of the heart under the right sternal border. As mentioned, the right pleural cavity is opened and the traction sutures on the right pericardium are released. The left-sided traction sutures are pulled up taut on the retractor and the table is rotated sharply to the right to aid in rolling the heart into the right chest. The deep stitch is pulled toward the patient's left shoulder and secured to the drapes. The Octopus III stabilizer (Medtronic, Minneapolis, MN) (*see* Chapter 6) is mounted on the right side of the retractor and its arm reaches across the heart, both aiding in presentation and accomplishing stabilization of the obtuse marginal coronary arteries. A cotton sling may facilitate exposure of the marginal vessel in cases of cardiomegaly.

For the RCA and inferior wall vessels such as the PDA and LV branch or PLOM, the deep stitch is pulled toward the feet and clamped to the drapes. The Octopus III stabilizer is attached to the left limb of the OPCAB sternal retractor ("Octobase," Medtronic,

Minneapolis, MN). The patient is placed in Trendelenburg's position with the bed tilted to the right. The base of the heart is elevated. The apex is oriented vertically.

In contrast to targets on the inferior and lateral walls, the anterior vessels (LAD and diagonals) are exposed with very little manipulation of the heart. The deep stitch is secured to the left drapes and the Octopus III brought onto the heart from the caudal aspect or left limb of the retractor. Care is taken to divide the pericardium to allow the mammary pedicle to fall posteriorly in the apex of the left chest.

CORONARY STABILIZATION AND GRAFTING

The Octopus III is a suction device, not a compression device. It is therefore possible to achieve good tissue capture while applying the device at the mechanical median of the cardiac cycle, rather than vigorously compressing the cardiac chambers. Thus, stabilization is optimized, while mechanical interference with ventricular function is minimized. Once the device is applied, a few seconds may be needed for the heart to recover. If hemodynamics are compromised, the degree of compression should be reduced and the mechanical median of the cardiac cycle should be more clearly identified by releasing the knob of the Octupus arm while maintaining suction. The suction is maintained to avoid losing tissue capture. After the appropriate position for the limb is determined, the Octopus arm is tightened once more. The malleable pods on the Octopus III allow one to spread the epicardium adjacent to the coronary targets, significantly improving visualization of the vessel. The malleable pods may be bent up or down, or in a curve. They may be bent or rotated independent of each other to accommodate irregular epicardial surfaces.

After optimal exposure is obtained, a soft silastic vessel loop (Quest Medical, Allen, TX) is placed around the target vessel for occlusion. The loop is placed proximal to the chosen anastomatic site—never distally. It is wise to avoid entrance into the ventricle and trauma to the epicardial veins with the vessel loops. When this occurs, a superficial epicardial suture will reliably stop bleeding. The vessel loop may be directed out of the surgeon's field of view with the aid of a loose pericardial suture serving as a "pulley."

Once the distal anastomosis is underway, it is critical for the anesthesia team to communicate continuously with the surgical team. Any changes in hemodynamics should be addressed quickly. Bradyarrhythmias may be promptly and easily treated with atrial and/or ventricular pacing. Occlusion of the right coronary artery proximal to the AV nodal artery may cause bradycardia, which responds reliably to epicardial pacing.

The target vessel is opened with a coronary knife and the arterotomy is extended with coronary scissors. The field is kept free of blood by dispersing the retrograde bleeding with a humidified CO_2 blower (DLP, Medtronic, Minneapolis, MN). The mister-blower utilizes warm, humidified, pH-balanced fluid and carbon dioxide to clear the target site of blood and help expose the intima of the coronary artery. It is important to blow on the target only when placing the needle through the tissue, to minimize intimal trauma. (Endothelial injury is discussed at length in Chapter 2.) Good visualization is critical for a precise anastomosis. The intima of both the conduit and coronary artery is visualized with each stitch. Optical magnification (3.5× loups), headlight, and Castro needle drivers are used on all anastomoses. Each distal anastomosis is constructed with 8-0 monofilament suture, to optimize precision, unless severe calcification requires a larger, stronger needle.

An intracoronary (or aortocoronary) shunt may be placed if significant hemodynamic compromise occurs due to ischemia after target vessel occlusion. The shunts (Medtronic, Minneapolis, MN) range in size from 1.5 to 3.0 mm in 0.25-mm increments. These are easily placed and removed. They are used infrequently, but are kept available in the room for all cases. Intracoronary shunts may be particularly helpful with large right coronary arteries (where bradyarrhythmias may occur), intramyocardial vessels (where placement of an occlusive vessel loop may be hazardous), and with critical anatomy (where occlusion of a key collateralizing vessel may be poorly tolerated). The coronary shunt is removed prior to tying the suture on the distal and flow is reestablished. Air is allowed to expel from the anastomosis prior to tying the suture. The conduit should be occluded with an atraumatic bulldog clamp until the proximal anastomosis is performed, in order to prevent retrograde bleeding and loss of coronary perfusion pressure.

At least two corporations have recently introduced cardiac positioning devices (Expose™, Guidant and Starfish™, Medtronic), which use suction to attach to the apex of the heart and can elevate and displace the heart to provide exposure of coronary targets with little hemodynamic compromise. These devices are aids in exposure/presentation and are not designed for coronary stabilization. They are used in conjunction with coronary stabilizers, such as the Octupus III, and may facilitate OPCAB exposure, particularly in cases of cardiomegaly and depressed left ventricular function.

PERFUSION-ASSISTED OPCAB

With experience and gentle application of the principles described above, virtually all coronary vessels can be safely exposed, stabilized, and grafted during OPCAB. However, the cumulative effect of sequential coronary occlusions can lead occasionally to a downward spiral of hemodynamic stability. At times, it may be helpful to provide accessory perfusion to the myocardium while other vessels are occluded. Perfusion-assisted direct coronary artery bypass (PADCAB) allows for direct perfusion of myocardium subtended by a coronary bypass target artery, either during performance of the distal anastomosis, by means of an olive-tipped intracoronary catheter, or after completion of the distal anastomosis, by providing controlled flow down the conduit. Inflow to the circuit and pump is provided by a catheter placed in the ascending aorta or femoral artery. The Quest Medical MPS (Quest Medical, Allen, TX) allows for exact control of coronary perfusion pressure *(3,4)*. Pharmacological additives and temperature control may accentuate its protective effects. The coronary perfusion pressure during PADCAB is independent of systemic pressure. This technique is especially helpful in collateralized targets, as coronary flow may be driven through collaterals to supply adjacent myocardium. It is also possible to measure and document graft patency and flows with the circuit. Multiple grafts may be perfused simultaneously by use of a multilimbed perfusion set. It is important to continue flow through all the grafts simultaneously, when the proximal anastomoses are performed. Each should be disconnected from the multilimb perfusion set separately to perform its proximal anastomosis. PADCAB is used selectively by the authors to minimize regional ischemia and improve myocardial protection in cases of critical coronary anastomosis and profound cardiac dysfunction. Some practitioners use PADCAB routinely, to optimize myocardial perfusion and hemodynamic stability for all OPCAB cases.

Proximal anastomoses to the aorta are performed with an aortic partial occlusion clamp. The systolic pressure is brought down to approx 90–95 mmHg before application of the clamp. Once the clamp is applied, the aortotomies are created with a 4.0-mm aortic punch. The application of the aortic clamp is guided by the results of epiaortic ultrasound scanning as discussed above. Vein graft anastomoses are constructed with 5-0 or 6-0 monofilament suture and arterial grafts with 7-0 monofilament suture. Any graft taken as a "T" off the IMA is anastomosed with 8-0 monofilament. Air is expelled by tying the final suture after removing the cross-clamp. The vein grafts are kept occluded until punctured with a 25-gauge needle to expel air. Arterial grafts are not punctured but are allowed to backbleed prior to cross-clamp removal.

After completion and reperfusion of all grafts, protamine is administered (0.75–1.0 mg/kg) to correct the ACT to approx 150 s. As hemostasis is being achieved, three chest tubes are routinely placed, one in each pleural space and one in the mediastinum. Temporary pacing wires are used only if the patient requires epicardial pacing immediately prior to chest closure.

The chest is closed in standard fashion. Nine sternal wires are used routinely to facilitate a tight sternal closure. Interrupted fascial sutures below the xiphoid ensure a tight fascial closure. The subdermis and skin are closed with running absorbable sutures.

SUMMARY

As with other new techniques, there is a learning curve associated with OPCAB. With persistence and patient attention to detail, this technique can be mastered and performed reproducibly and reliably. OPCAB may show improved outcomes compared with conventional CABG, especially in patients for whom cardiopulmonary bypass has elevated risks. It is therefore important for all cardiac surgeons to be comfortable with this technique.

REFERENCES

1. Puskas JD, Thourani VH, Marshall JJ, et al. Clinical outcomes, angiographic patency, and resource utilization in 200 consecutive off-pump coronary bypass patients. Ann Thorac Surg 2001;71(5):1477–1483; discussion 1483–1484.
2. Murphy DA, Craver JM, Jones EL, et al. Surgical management of acute myocardial ischemia following percutaneous transluminal coronary angioplasty. Role of the intra-aortic balloon pump. J Thorac Cardiovasc Surg 1984;87(3):332–339.
3. Guyton RA, Thourani VH, Puskas JD, et al. Perfusion-assisted direct coronary artery bypass: selective graft perfusion in off-pump cases. Ann Thorac Surg 2000;69(1):171–175.
4. Puskas JD, Vinten-Johansen J, Muraki S, Guyton RA. Myocardial protection for off-pump coronary artery bypass surgery. Semin Thorac Cardiovasc Surg 2001;13(1):82–88.

6 Mechanical Stabilization

The Medtronic Octopus System

Michael Gibson, MD, *Robert B. Beauford,* MD, *and Daniel J. Goldstein,* MD

CONTENTS

Introduction
Development Of The Octopus Tissue Stabilizer
Hemodynamic Changes Encountered With The Octopus Tissue Stabilizer
Histological Changes Associated With The Octopus Tissue Stabilizer
Octopus Off-pump Clinical Experience
Conclusion
References

INTRODUCTION

Worldwide, coronary artery bypass grafting (CABG) using cardiopulmonary bypass (CPB) is performed in over 750,000 patients a year. However, the morbidity associated with extracorporeal circulation and oxygenation is indisputable *(1)*. This fact, combined with developments in enabling technologies and early data suggesting improved coronary surgery outcomes by avoiding extracorporeal circulation *(2,3)*, has led to the resurgence of beating-heart or off-pump coronary artery bypass (OPCAB). The initial skepticism over OPCAB hinged largely on the lack of good mechanical stabilization technology for operating on the beating heart. Currently, several methods of immobilization have been introduced to accomplish this task. Of the proposed mechanical, electrical, and pharmacological stabilization techniques, the mechanical approach has proven to be the most popular. Early experience with OPCAB relied on the use of sutures to

From: *Contemporary Cardiology: Minimally Invasive Cardiac Surgery, Second Edition*
Edited by: D. J. Goldstein and M. C. Oz © Humana Press Inc., Totowa, NJ

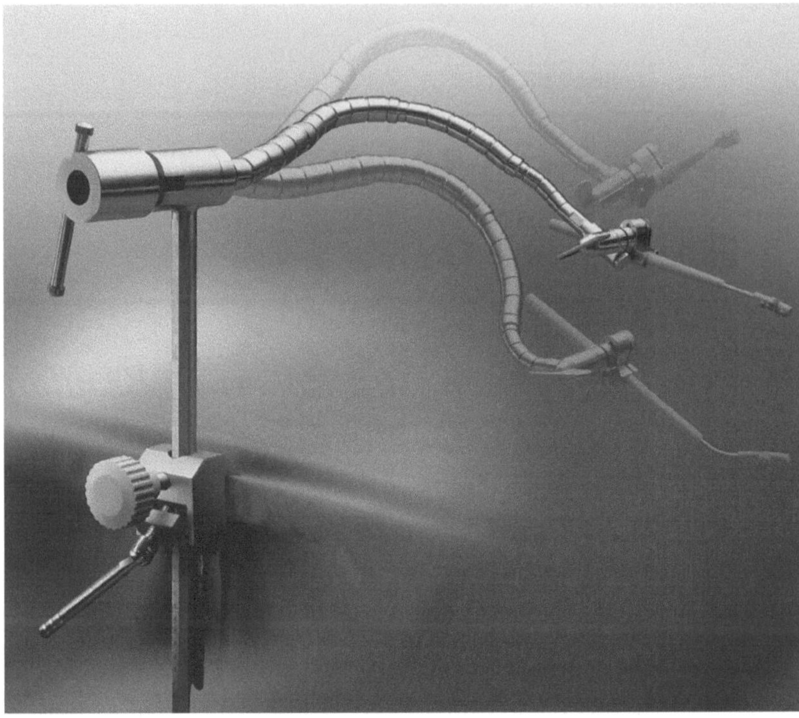

Fig. 1. The Medtronic Octopus 1 tissue stabilizer system. (Courtesy of Medtronic Cardiac Surgery Technologies.)

stabilize the coronary target. At present several suction and pressure systems developed by industry have entered the marketplace. Table 1 details the different mechanical methods.

Borst and colleagues *(4)* at Utrecht University Hospital in The Netherlands pioneered the development of an immobilization device based on the principle of suction. Now known as the Medtronic-Utrecht Octopus® Tissue Stabilization System, it uses a table-mounted mechanical stabilizer combined with suction for epicardial fixation. This device has evolved significantly since its introduction in 1995. This chapter deals with the development of the Octopus, analysis and comparison of the different Octopus prototypes, hemodynamic changes encountered with its use, histological effects of suction, and clinical experience associated with its use. Two of the other leading stabilization systems, the Genzyme OPCAB elite system, and the Guidant OPCAB system are discussed in great detail in Chapters 7 and 8.

DEVELOPMENT OF THE OCTOPUS TISSUE STABILIZER

The evolution of local immobilization devices began in 1994 with the utilization of epicardial stay sutures in the porcine heart. This progressed into an epicardial ring sutured into place. Ultimately, these early attempts at local stabilization proved to be cumbersome and ineffective. Finally, attachment to the epicardium was achieved by suction— and thus the birth of the Medtronic Octopus system. The early system consisted of two prototypes, an "Encircling Octopus," which surrounds the anastomosis circumferentially and the "endo-Octopus," which is placed on either side of the coronary artery.

The first-generation Octopus (**Fig. 1**) involved an adjustable table-mounted clamp with an articulating arm with a "ball-and-sleeve" design and a tissue stabilizer. The tissue

Table 1
Cardiac Muscle Stabilization[a]

	Epicardial stay sutures	*Stay sutures + vessel loops*	*Suction method*	*Pressure/friction technique*
Movement reduction	+/–	+	+++	++
Presentation	+/–	+	++	+/–
Efficacy at all sites	+	+	++	+/–
Stability versus slipping	+	++	++	+/–
Ease of application	+++	+++	+	+/–
Learning curve	–	–	++	+
Potential damage to coronaries	–	+	–	–
Risk of bleeding	–	+	–	–

[a]Adapted (with permission) from ref. *1*, p. 61.

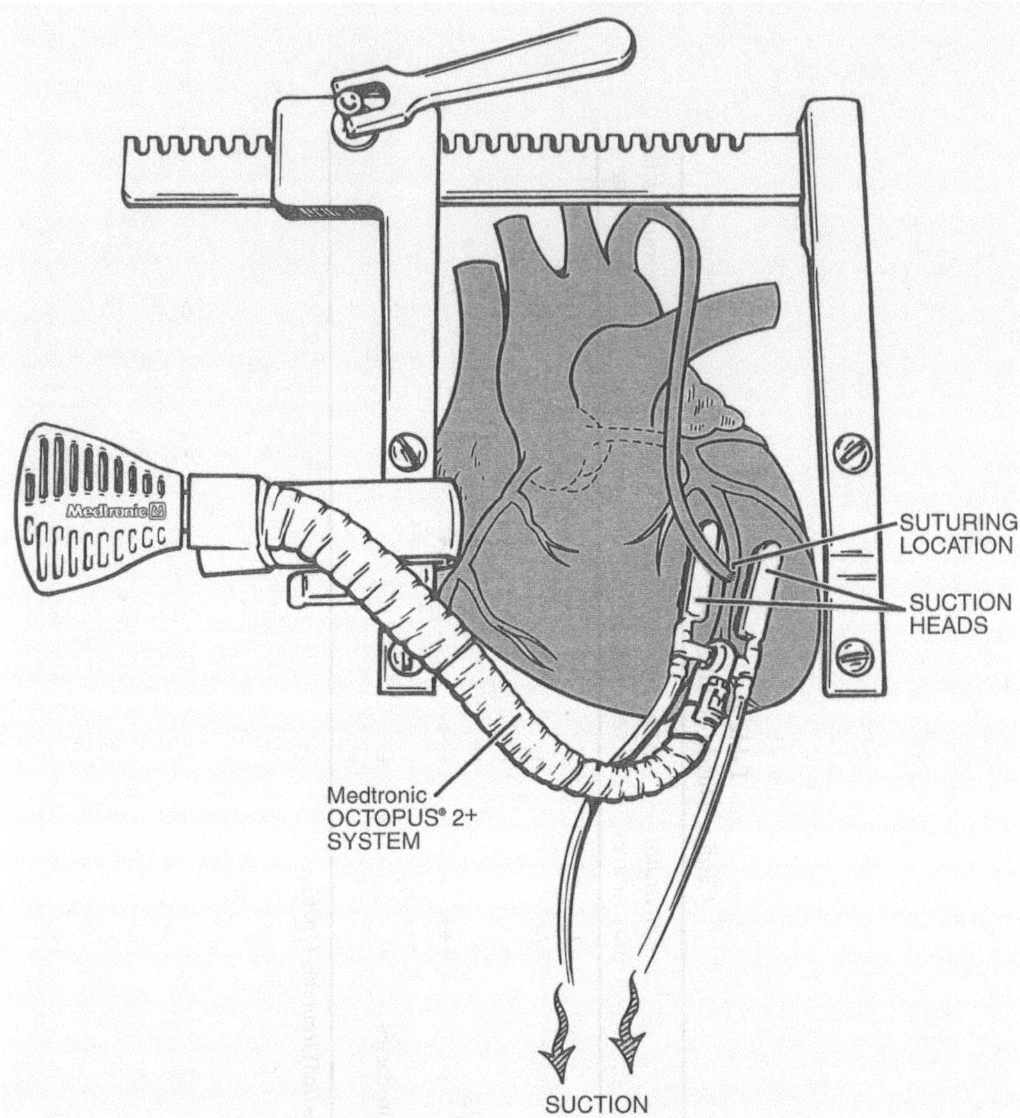

Fig. 2. A pictograph of the Medtronic Octopus 2+ attached to the sternal retractor overlying the heart. (Courtesy of Medtronic Cardiac Surgery Technologies.)

stabilizer had numerous configurations and a malleable arm for positioning. Minimization of motion of the beating heart was considerable. However, there was still some movement in the long axis and difficulty with exposure of the circumflex system. Its bulkiness led to difficulty with manipulation and positioning. These concerns led to the development of the Octopus 2+ tissue stabilizer (**Fig. 2**), which allowed increased motion control at the anastomosis. Additionally, improved multivessel access and mounting was obtained with the four-cup pod stabilizer, a stronger articulating arm, and an improved retractor mount (instead of a table mount). To allow improved ease with coronary anastomosis, the Octopus 2+ LP (low-profile) tissue stabilizer (**Fig. 3**) was developed with a 23% decrease in the pod height.

Additional refinements led to the Octopus 3 (**Fig. 4**), which consists of malleable stabilizer pods to allow better adaptability to patient heart contours. This leads to easier

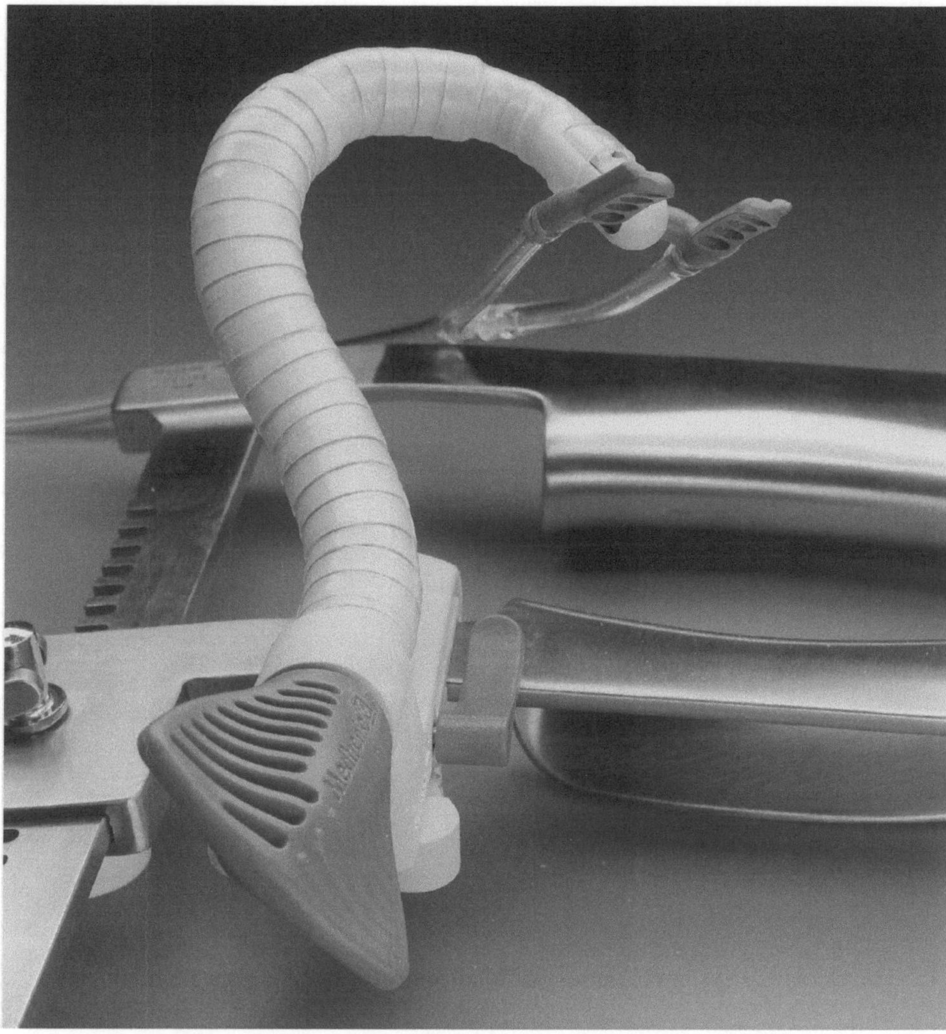

Fig. 3. The Medtronic Octopus 2+ LP tissue stabilizer system. (Courtesy of Medtronic Cardiac Surgery Technologies.)

positioning for exposure of the posterior heart. The Octopus 3 design with its malleable stabilizer pods is manipulated with suction for improved anastomotic site exposure. Table 2 compares and contrasts the different Octopus tissue stabilizer models. As incomplete revascularization in off-pump patients became a growing issue, so did questions about access to the lateral and inferior walls of the heart. This, combined with growing concerns about hemodynamic compromise associated with deep pericardial sutures, led to the develpment of the Octopus Starfish™ heart postitioner (**Fig. 5**) as an adjunct to the Octopus 3 stabilizer. This multiappendage suction device was designed to be connected to the apex of the heart and greatly enhances exposure.

Further developments came with introduction of Octopus System II, which consists of the Octopus 4 stabilizer (**Fig. 6**) and Starfish 2 positioner. Both now have a turret design with 360° movement. This dramatically increases the arm reach and positioning possibilities. Additionally, the devices are less obstructive owing to a smaller "whaletail" for locking the position and a single vacuum line (versus two) on the Octopus 4.

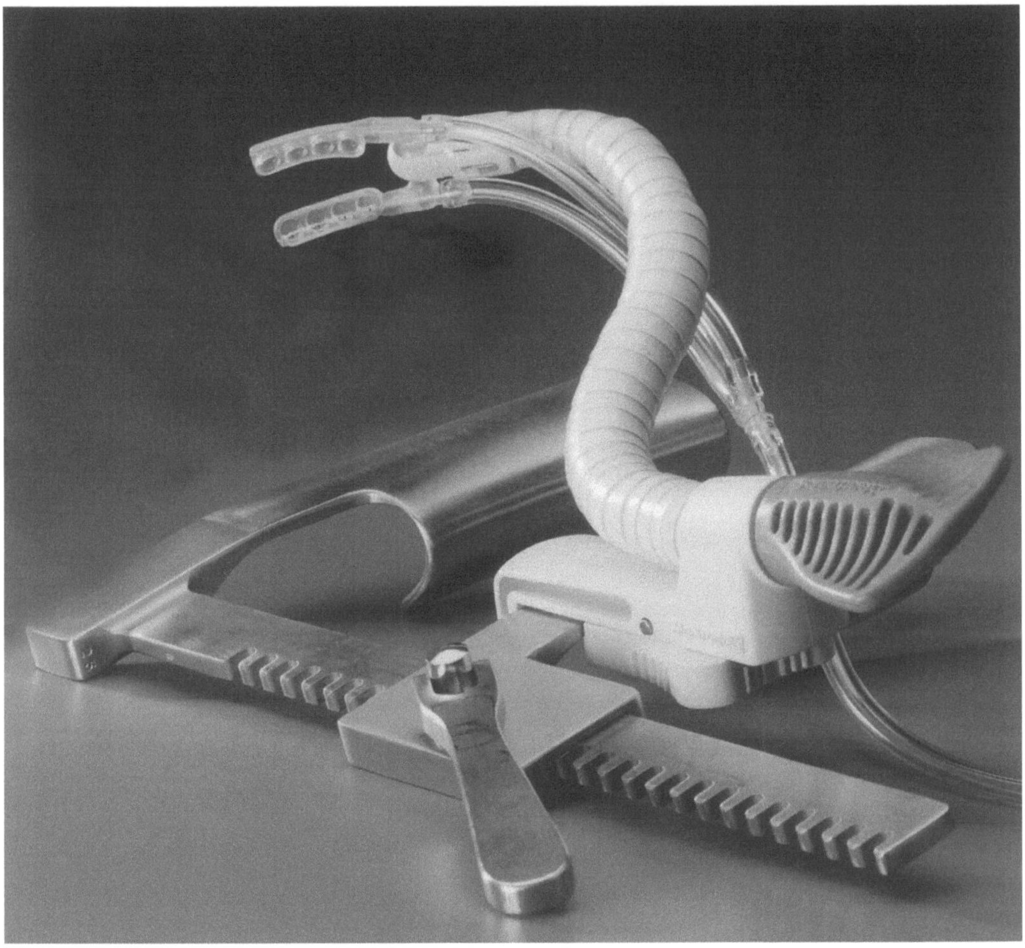

Fig. 4. The Octopus 3 system (Courtesy of Medtronic Cardiac Surgery Technologies.)

HEMODYNAMIC CHANGES ENCOUNTERED WITH THE OCTOPUS TISSUE STABILIZER

As the popularity of off-pump coronary revascularization has grown, more investigations have been carried out to prove its safety. Concerns have arisen regarding difficulty in grafting the circumflex coronary artery territory and posterior surface, maintenance of adequate blood pressure and forward output with cardiac manipulation, and development of myocardial ischemia with cardiac manipulation. These hemodynamic changes, which could potentially lead to the inability to perform OPCAB, have been evaluated using the Octopus Tissue Stabilizer. **Figure 7** and Table 3 demonstrate changes in hemodynamic parameters with various maneuvers. These maneuvers include fixation with the Octopus, vertical displacement of the heart, Trendelenburg 20° positioning, and return to baseline. Hemodynamic changes associated with positioning included decreased stroke volume (SV), increased heart rate (HR), and decreased cardiac output (CO) with vertical displacement. These are thought to be secondary to biventricular pump failure, which improves with Trendelenburg positioning at the expense of augmented left and right ventricular preloads and an increased heart rate *(5)*. Complete inability to obtain hemo-

Table 2
Comparison of Octopus Designs

Octopus Circumflex System	*Movement/stabilization*	*Ease of grafting*	*Anastomotic ease*
1	a. Increased z motion[a] b. Less stable due to long articulating arm	Difficult	Difficult
2+	a. Decreased z motion b. Improved stability	Improved compared to Octopus 1	Improved
2+ LP	a. Decreased z motion b. Improved stability	Improved compared to Octopus 1	Decreased pod height allows increased ease
3	a. Improved contact with the posterior heart b. Increased y motion	Improved compared to Octopus 1	Potentially difficult due to increased y motion

[a]Motion in the z direction relative to the x-y plane.

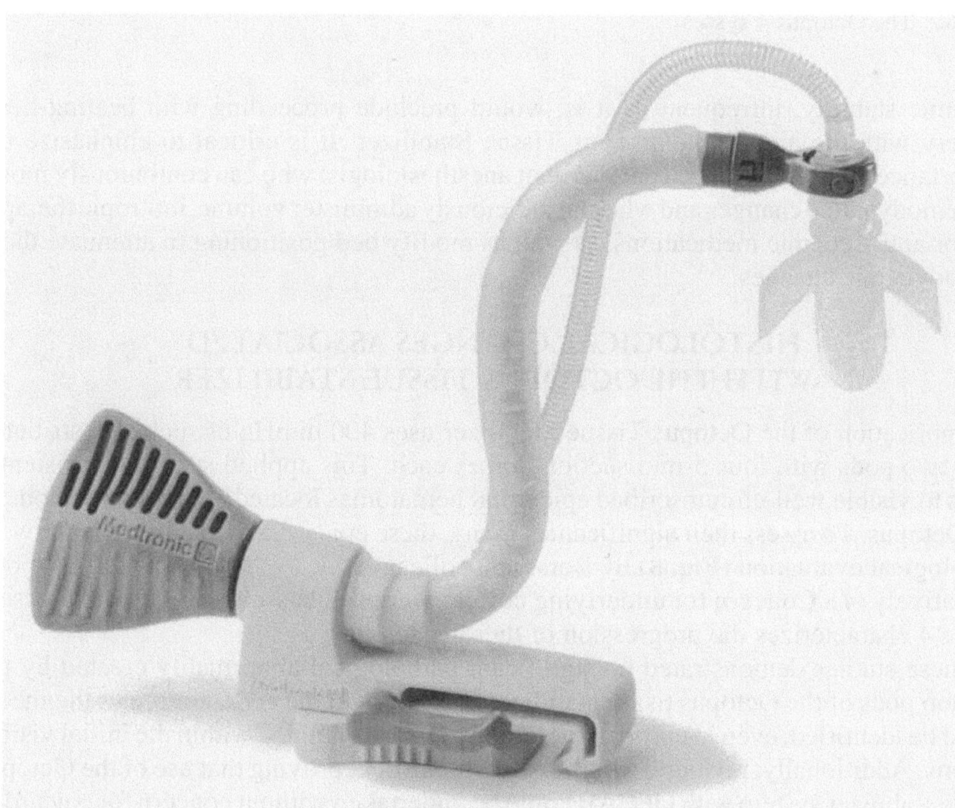

Fig. 5. The Octopus Starfish heart positioner.

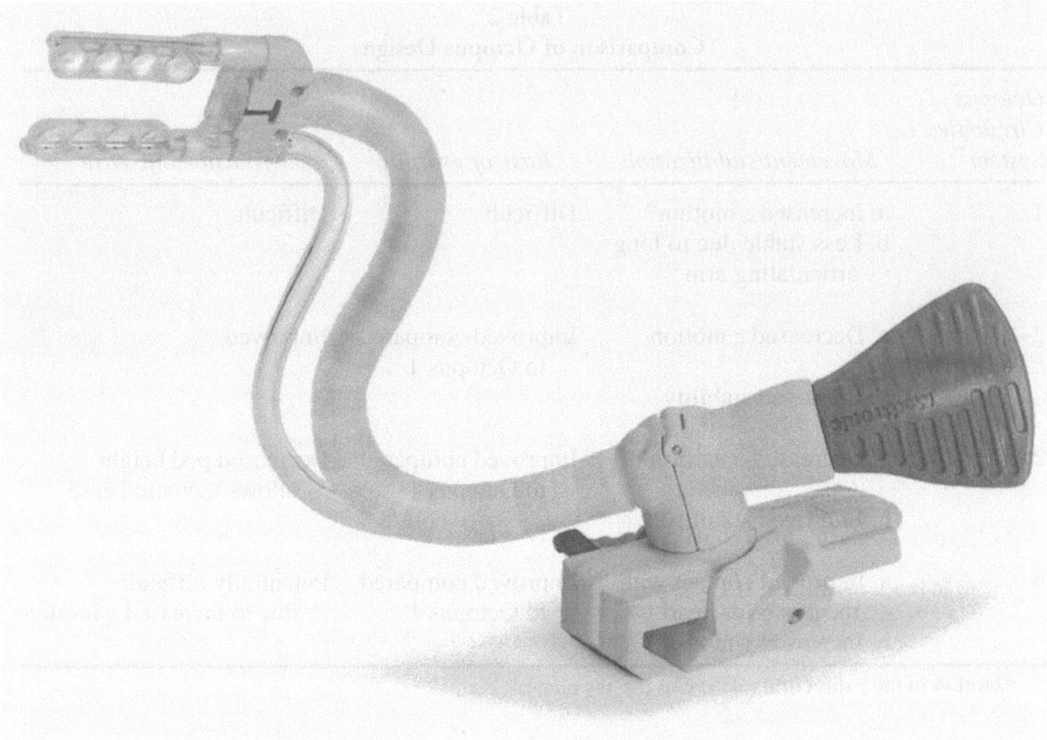

Fig. 6. The Octopus 4 system.

dynamic stability, infrequent as it is, would preclude proceeding with beating-heart surgery with the aid of the Octopus Tissue Stabilizer. It is critical to emphasize the importance of an experienced and vigilant anesthesiologist who can continuously monitor hemodynamic changes and who can judiciously administer volume, inotropic therapy, and/or anti-ischemic medications, as well as modify bed positioning to attenuate these hemodynamic changes.

HISTOLOGICAL CHANGES ASSOCIATED WITH THE OCTOPUS TISSUE STABILIZER

Application of the Octopus Tissue Stabilizer uses 400 mmHg of suction distributed over two pods with four 5-mm suction domes each. This applied suction consistently leads to visible well-circumscribed epicardial hematomas located at the suction pods of the Octopus. To assess their significance, if any, these epicardial hematomas underwent histological evaluation (**Fig. 8**) by Borst and colleagues at 1–4 h, 48 h, and 6 wk postoperatively *(4)*. Concern for underlying coronary arterial vessel injury was addressed. Table 4 characterizes the progression of these lesions.

These studies demonstrated no significant pathological abnormality created by the suction pods of the Octopus tissue stabilizer. No injury to the endothelium or the media could be identified, even in coronary or lymph vessels contained within the initial visible lesions. Additionally, no mural thrombi were identified, proving that use of the Octopus tissue stabilizer system with OPCAB could be undertaken without concern for epicardial injury.OPCAB revealed initial concerns with hemodynamic instability with heart and

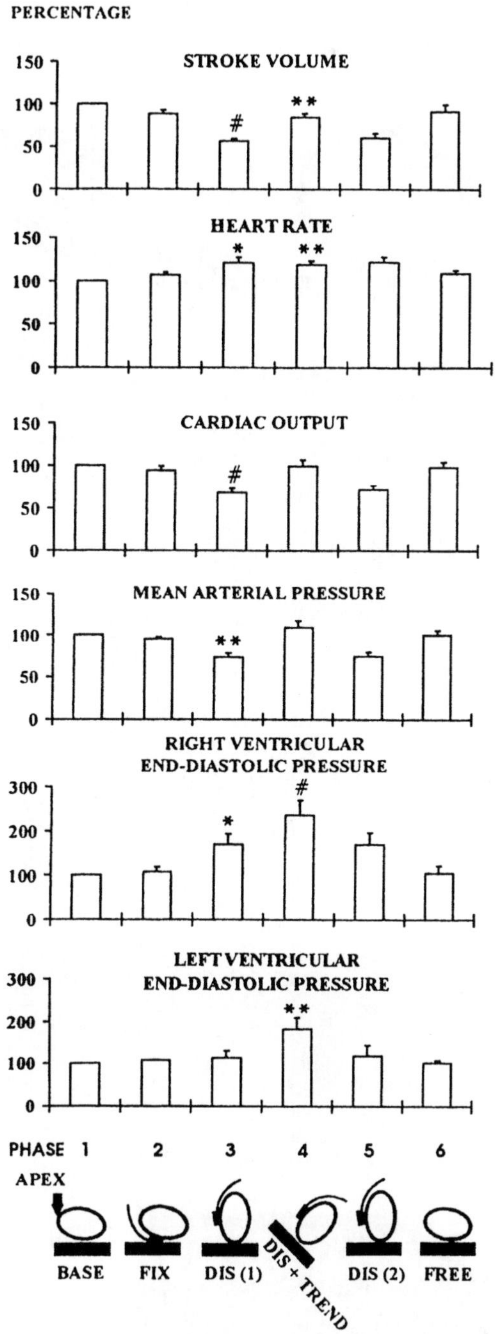

Fig. 7. Relative changes in hemodynamic parameters during vertical displacement of the beating porcine heart by the Utrecht Octopus and the effect of head-down tilt (BASE = pericardial control position; FIX = fixation of the suction tentacles to the posterior cardiac wall; DIS (1) = displacement of the heart by the Octopus; TREND = Trendelenburg maneuver (20° head-down tilt); DIS (2) = retracted heart with table returned to horizontal position and FREE = pericardial position after release of the Octopus. (Statistical comparison with control values: $*p < 0.05$, $**p < 0.01$, $\#p < 0.001$. (Reprinted with permission from the Society of Thoracic Surgeons [Ann Thorac Surg 1997;63:90–91]) *(5)*.

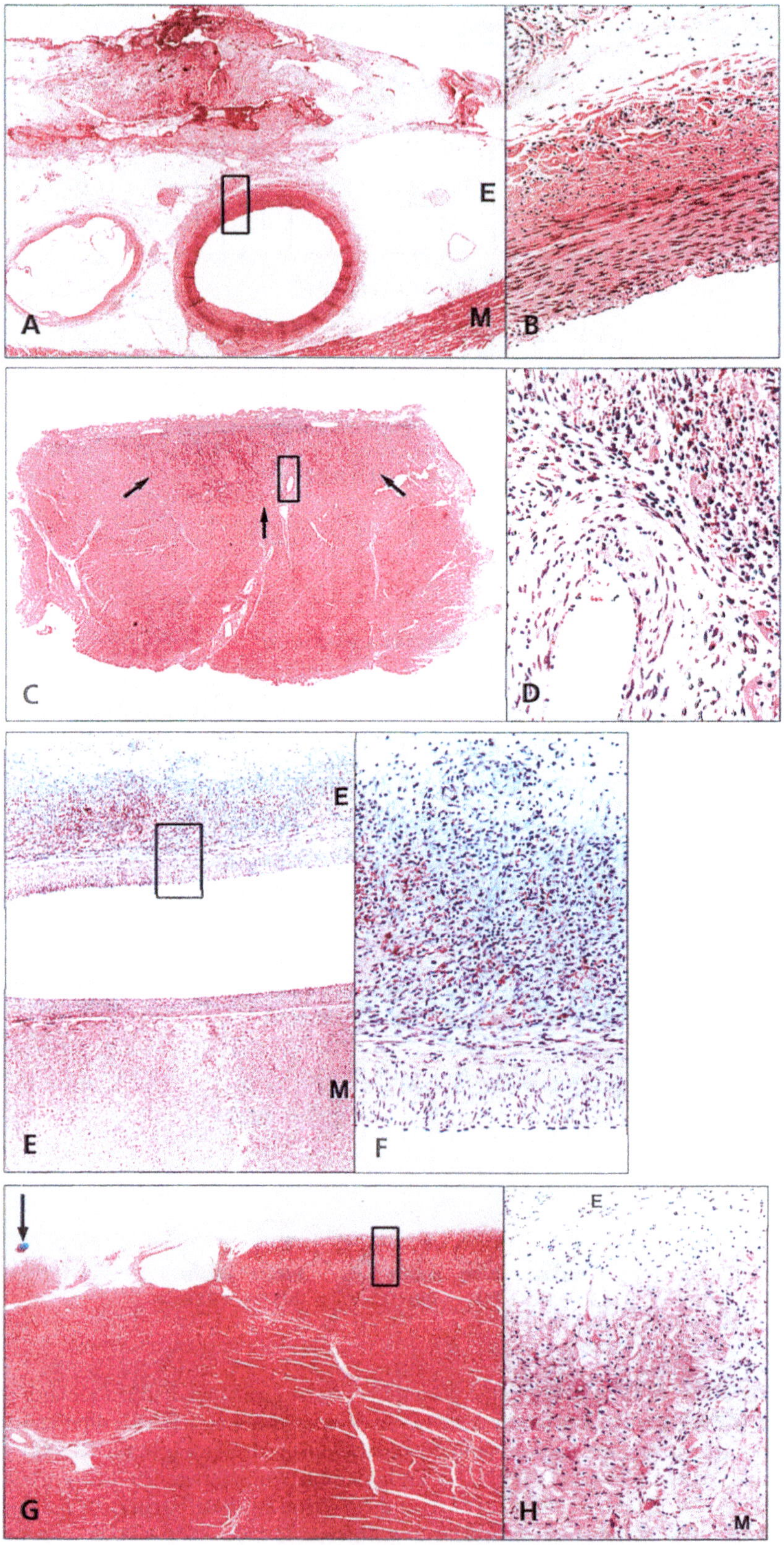

Fig. 8.

Table 3
Changes in Hemodynamic Parameters with Various Maneuvers

Variable[a]	*Basal Values*	*Fixation with Octopus*	*Vertical Displacement*	*Trendelenburg 20-degree Head Down*	*Vertical Displacement*	*Freely Beating Heart*
SV (mL)	75	65	43	62	44	68
HR (bpm)	52	55	62	61	63	57
CO (L/min)	3.8	3.5	2.6	3.7	2.7	3.7
MAP (mmHg)	46	44	34	49	34	45
RVEDP (mmHg)	5	5	8	11	8	5
LVEDP (mmHg)	7	7	7	11	7	7
MRAP (mm Hg)	4	4	5	7	5	4
MLAP (mm Hg)	7	7	8	9	6	7
SVR (dyn s cm^{-5})	931	918	921	931	894	987

Adapted (with permission) from "changes in hemodynamic parameters with various maneuvers," Ann Thorac Surg 1997; 63,S91 (*5*).

[a]SV=stroke volume; HR=heart rate; CO=cardiac output; MAP=mean arterial pressure; RVEDP=right ventricular end-diastolic pressure; LVEDP=left ventricular end-diastolic pressure; MRAP=mean right atrial pressure; MLAP=mean left atrial pressure; SVR=systemic vascular resistance.

Fig. 8. *(facing page)* Histology of suction lesions **(A,B)** Acute suction lesion induced by the encircling Octopus. **(A)** After 45 min of suction on top of the LAD and its concomitant vein. Note the hemorrhage in the upper part of the thick epicardial layer (E) and the absence of mural thrombi in the vessels. M, myocardium. Magnification: 18X. **(B)** Detail of A, showing the intact layers of the arterial wall close to the superficial hemorrhage of the LAD. Magnification 165X. **(C,D)** Suction lesion 48 h after immobilization by the encircling Octopus. **(C)** The arrows point at the edge of the myocardial lesion induced by 22 min of suction at the OM area. Magnification: 18X. **(D)** Detail of C showing intramural coronary artery branch embedded in suction lesion consisting of interstitial hemorrhage and infiltrate. Note the uninjured layers of the arterial wall. The myocytes show a mixed

continued on page 86

Table 4
Progression of Suction Induced Trauma

Post-op	*Visible lesion*	*Hemorrhage*	*Infiltrate*	*Dead myocytes*	*Coronary injury*
1–4 h	+	+	–	–	–
48 h	+	–	+[a]	+[b]	–
6 wk	–	–	–	–	–

[a]Densely cellular fibroblastic tissue consisting of cells with prominent nucleoli and exhibiting mitotic figures.
[b]Few.

OCTOPUS OFF-PUMP CLINICAL EXPERIENCE

To assess the safety and efficacy of this unique stabilization system, we surveyed the largest clinical experiences from the English literature. These results are summarized in Table 5. Van Dijk et al. *(6)* randomized 281 patients to OPCAB and conventional CABG. Their conversion rate was 1.4% and there were no reported device-related complications. They concluded that omitting cardiopulmonary bypass led to reduced cardiac enzyme release, reduced use of blood products, and a slightly shorter hospital stay. They reported that, in selected patients, off-pump CABG is safe and yields a short-term cardiac outcome comparable to that of conventional CABG. Hart et al. *(7)* conducted a retrospective study of all Octopus-supported OPCAB patients by the seven training institutions for the device. The authors studied 1582 patients, of whom 44 (2.8%) were converted to conventional CABG. They point out that only three (0.2%) were converted urgently; the other 41 were converted "electively." The authors ultimately concluded that Octopus-supported OPCAB was a safe procedure with widening applicability. Spooner et al. *(8)* reviewed a 2-yr three-institution experience with the Octopus system involving 456 patients. Conversion to CABG occurred in 13 of 469 patients (2.8%), four of which were secondary to hemodynamic instability. They concluded that the Octopus devices were safely applied with low morbidity. Whitman et al. *(10)* studied the uniform safety of OPCAB using the Octopus system at three institutions among 239 patients. Among the three institutions, 10 patients (4.0%) were converted. They concluded that stabilization with the Octopus system provided predictable, reproducible immobilization with minimal morbidity and decreased costs. Hart *(11)*, in a separate later study, surveyed 230 multivessel Octopus-supported OPCAB patients. Four of these patients (1.7%) were converted to conventional CABG and were subsequently excluded from analysis. Of the remaining 226, Hart pointed out that all regions of the coronary circulation were acces-

continued from page 85

appearance of injured and normal cells. Magnification: 270X. **(E,F)** Suction lesion 48 h after immobilization by the encircling Octopus. **(E)** Longitudinal section through the OM branch shows a patent artery without mural thrombus within the lesion induced by 45 min of suction. E, epicardium. M, myocardium. Magnification: 50X. **(F)** Detail of E, showing interstitial hemorrhage and infiltrate in the epicardium adjacent to the artery. Note the absence of any injury to the arterial wall. Magnification: 165X. **(G,H)** Suction site 6 wk after immobilization by the encircling Octopus. **(G)** Typical example of tissue section at suction site (OM area) identified by intraoperative suture wire (arrow). In spite of 25 min of immobilization, no fibrous tissue was found in the myocardium. Magnification: 18X. **(H)** Detail of G, showing normal myocytes but a fuzzy rather than well-demarcated transition between myocardium (M). (Reproduced with permission from **ref.** *(1)*.

Table 5

Octopus Off-Pump Clinical Experience

Authors	*Van Dijk et al. (6)*	*Hart et al (7)*	*Spooner et al (8)*	*Whitman (10)*	*Hart (11)*[b]
Number of patients	142	1582	456	239	226
Study design	Multicenter randomized prospective trial	Multicenter retrospective review	Multicenter retrospective review	Multicenter retrospective review	retrospective review
Demographics					
Mean age (yr)	61 63.9	NA	62.3	NA	
Mean LVEF	77% nL 23% mod[a]	55.4	NA	56.6	51
% diabetics	9	26.4	NA	26	30.1
Data					
Mean no. of grafts/patient	2.4	2.31	1.9	1.8	2.7
Operating time (h)	4.2NA	NA	NA	NA	
Conversion rate %	7.7	Elective 2.6 / urgent 0.2	Elective 2.6 / urgent 0.2	4.11	.7
Intraoperative IABP %		0.7	0.4	NA	0
Results (%)[d]					
Mortality (2.87)	0	1	0.32	0	0
Post-op MI (1.09)	3.5[c]	1.30.8	0 0.4		
Atrial fib (19.37)	20	14.9	13.3	11	NA
Stroke (1.65)	0.7	0.6	0.2	0	0.4
Renal Failure (3.14)	0	0.9	NA	NA	0.4
Reop for bleeding (2.32)		1.2	1	0.8	0
Follow-up					
Mean follow-up	1 mo	NA	NA	NA	NA
Recurrent angina	NA	NA	NA	NA	NA
Angioplasty	1.4	NA	NA	NA	NA
Reop CABG	0	NA	1.3	NA	NA

[a]Normal left ventricular function reported in 77% patients (109) "moderate left ventricular function" reported in the remaining 23%.
[b]later study done by Hart which included a cohort of new patients.
[c]rate of MI is reported as outcome 1-month after surgery, specific details about the immediate perioperative period was unavailable.
[d]result variables are displayed as a percent with STS benchmarks for all CABG patients in parenthesis.
[e]LVEF=left ventricular ejection fraction; IABP=intraaortic balloon pump; MI=myocardial infarction; fib=fibrillation; CABG=coronary artery bypass graft.

sible. He further concluded that the Octopus system is safe, efficacious, and applicable in a wide range of patients.

Of the represented studies, there were no reported device-related complications. Furthermore, when looking at end points of mortality, atrial fibrillation, stroke, postoperative renal failure, and reoperation for bleeding, OPCAB with the aide of the Octopus compares favorably with published STS benchmarks for *all CABG* patients *(9)*.

CONCLUSION

Myocardial presentation and anastomotic site immobilization remain the most critical factors influencing the accuracy of the off-pump anastomosis. Early clinical use of patient positioning. Most authors acknowledge these perturbations but have shown them to be safely and easily overcome. This requires a dedicated and vigilant anesthesia team, judicious use of inotropes, and continuous echocardiographic and Swan–Ganz monitoring. Other concerns involving mechanical trauma resulting from application of the Medtronic Octopus tissue stabilizer system have been addressed by histopathological examination, which has demonstrated that, even in the presence of visible lesions, there exists no microscopic evidence of trauma to underlying tissue structures or blood vessels. Finally, results of recent publications relating to complications and mortality compare favorably with regard to Society of Thoracic Surgery benchmarks for all CABG patients. In short, OPCAB utilizing the Medtronic Octopus tissue stabilizer system is a safe and efficacious alternative to conventional coronary artery bypass grafting with CPB.

REFERENCES

1. Jansen Erik WL. Towards Minimally Invasive Coronary Artery Bypass Grafting. Utrecht, 1998.
2. Mack MJ. Perspectives on minimally invasive coronary artery surgery. Current assessment and future directions. Int J Cardiol 1997;62(suppl 1):S73–S79
3. Bowles BJ, Lee JD, Dang CR, et al. Coronary artery bypass performed without the use of cardiopulmonary bypass is associated with reduced cerebral microemboli and improved clinical results. Chest 2001;119(1):25–30.
4. Borst C, Jansen EWL, Tulleken CAF, et al. Coronary artery bypass grafting without interruption of native coronary flow using a novel anastomosis site restraining device ('Octopus®'). J Am Coll Cardiol 1996;27:1356–1364.
5. Grundeman PF, Borst C, van Herwaarden JA, et al. Hemodynamic changes during displacement of the beating heart by the utrecht Octopus® method. Ann Thorac Surg 1997;63:S88–S92.
6. van Dijk, Nierich AP, Jansen EWL, et al. Early outcome after off-pump versus on-pump coronary bypass surgery. Circulation 2001;104:1761–1766.
7. Hart JC, Spooner TH, Pym J, et al. A review of 1582 consecutive Octopus® off-pump coronary bypass patients. Ann Thorac Surg 2000;70:1017–1020.
8. Spooner TH, Hart JC, Pym J. A two-year, three institution experience with the Medtronic Octopus®: systematic off-pump surgery. Ann Thorac Surg 1999;68:1478–1481.
9. Society of Thoracic Surgeons National Database Benchmarks 1997 Coronary artery bypass only patients.
10. Whitman GJ, Hart JC, Crestanello JA, Spooner TH. Uniform safety of beating heart surgery using the Octopus® tissue stabilization system. J Card Surg 1999 Sep–Oct;14(5):323–329.
11. Hart JC. Multivessel off-pump coronary bypass with the Octopus® experience in 226 patients. J Card Surg 2000 jul–Aug;15(4):266–272.

7 Mechanical Stabilization Systems

The Genzyme-OPCAB Elite System

William E. Cohn, MD *and Marc Ruel,* MD, MPH

CONTENTS

INTRODUCTION
THE GENZYME-OPCAB ELITE SYMSTEM AND IMMOBILIZER PLATFORM
EXPOSURE OF THE INFERIOR AND LATERAL WALLS
MECHANISM OF ADVERSE HEMODYNAMIC EFFECTS
EXPOSURE TECHNIQUES
CONCLUSION
REFERENCES

INTRODUCTION

Off-pump coronary artery bypass grafting (OPCAB) has been performed since the early years of coronary surgery, with case series documenting its feasibility dating back to the 1970s *(1–4)*. Nevertheless, OPCAB only recently gained widespread acceptance and entered the mainstream of clinical practice, propelled by a greater awareness of the potential morbidity of cardiopulmonary bypass and aortic manipulation.

The introduction of self-retaining coronary stabilizers and the development of techniques for their use are key factors that have led to the recent popularity of OPCAB. When used properly, stabilization systems provide a relatively bloodless and motionless field that allows for the construction of a technically accurate anastomosis. One such system is the Genzyme-OPCAB Elite System (Genzyme Surgical, Fall River, MA), which we have been involved with since its inception.

Although most surgeons can intuitively use stabilizers to accomplish off-pump revascularization of the left anterior descending and diagonal coronary arteries, a more systematic approach is required to successfully graft vessels on the inferior, posterior,

From: *Contemporary Cardiology: Minimally Invasive Cardiac Surgery, Second Edition*
Edited by: D. J. Goldstein and M. C. Oz © Humana Press Inc., Totowa, NJ

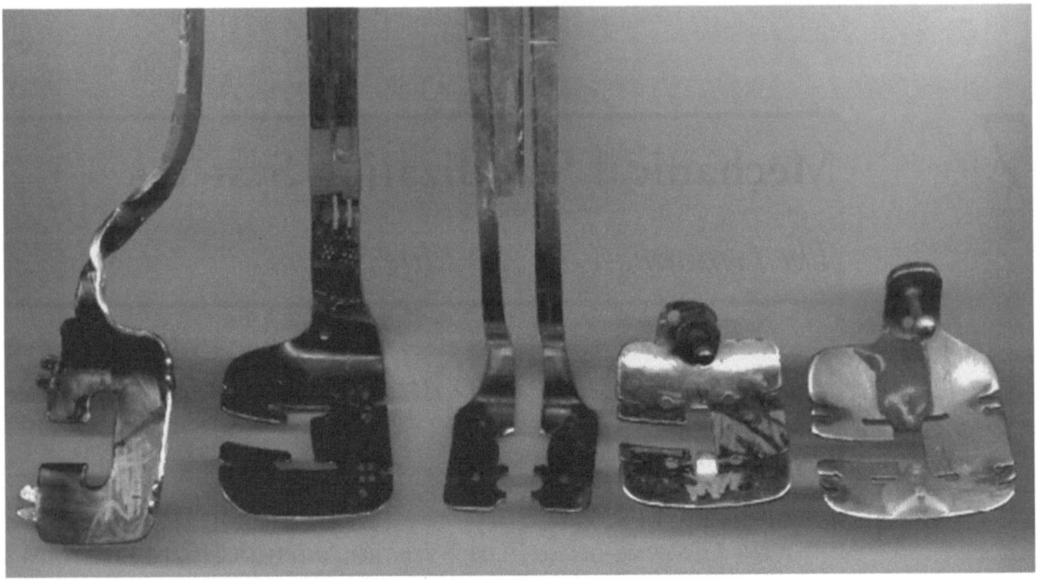

Fig. 1. Five of the 11 early prototypes of the Genzyme stabilizer are shown. Each was fashioned from a soup spoon or ladle. The iteration on the far right most closely resembles the first commercial product.

and lateral walls of the left ventricle. This chapter describes the mechanism of function and detailed instructions for use of the Genzyme system, as well as a number of exposure and stabilization techniques that have contributed to improving the feasibility, safety, and popularity of multivessel OPCAB worldwide.

THE GENZYME-OPCAB ELITE SYSTEM AND IMMOBILIZER PLATFORM

At the heart of the Genzyme Elite OPCAB system is the Immobilizer coronary stabilizer. The Immobilizer utilizes a proprietary mechanism to effect coronary stabilization and local coronary occlusion. This mechanism, called coronary capture, was developed to limit residual motion at the anastomotic site and to minimize physical forces and geometric distortion of the coronary required to achieve hemostasis.

The Immobilizer evolved from fairly humble beginnings. The first 11 prototypes were cut from the bodies of spoons and spatulas purchased at a grocery store not far from Boston's Beth Israel and Deaconess hospitals (**Fig. 1**). Refinements in design resulted in progressive improvement in function. After a number of iterations, the stabilizer was taken from the animal lab to the operating room, where it performed well. After several additional refinements, a licensing agreement was reached between the Beth Israel Hospital and Genzyme Surgical to produce and market the stabilizer. Initially marketed under the name "Cohn Cardiac Stabilizer," it found immediate support in the cardiac surgical community due to the extremely stable operative field it provided. Since its release in January 1998, it has undergone further refinement, evolving into the current Immobilizer platform (**Fig. 2**).

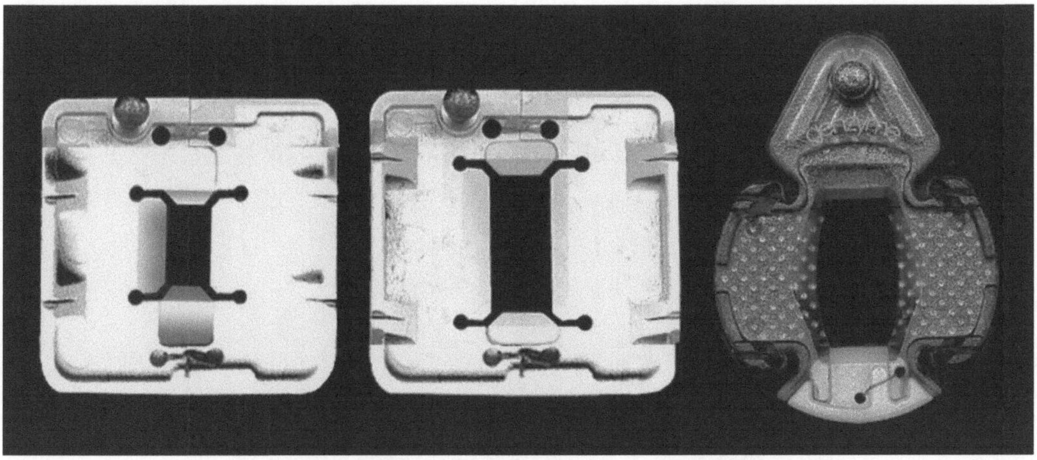

Fig. 2. Three iterations of the commercial stabilizer platform are shown. The Cohn Cardiac Stabilizer on the left provided excellent stability, but the small window was felt to crowd the anastomosis. It was soon followed by the "Large Mouth" Cohn, which provided more room. The current platform, the Immobilizer, eliminates the need to pass the tapes through the center window, allowing for faster setup.

The Immobilizer Platform and Coronary Capture

The Immobilizer is an ovoid plate in the center of which lies a rectangular foramen or window. At the proximal and distal ends of the window are plastic buttresses that project slightly below the plane of the plate. Each buttress is flanked by a pair of cleats that allow a silicone elastic tape to be affixed under tension. At one end of the plate is a detachable segment that facilitates removal of the Immobilizer after graft completion. At the opposite end is a pivot that connects the Immobilizer to the articulating arm (**Fig. 3**).

The coronary capture mechanism integrated into the design of the Immobilizer platform results in compression of the coronary between a single taut segment of silicone elastic tape and a flat plastic surface. As a result, intimate contact is maintained between the epicardial surface and the stabilizer resulting in improved stability. More important, the flattening of the coronary results in gentle coronary occlusion. This method of coronary occlusion is advantageous from several perspectives. As the coronary is compressed between two flat structures, coronary distortion is minimized. Whereas many techniques require circumferential snaring and coronary strangulation to effect occlusion, the biplanar compression effected by the Immobilizer is more analogous to that seen with atraumatic vascular clamps (**Fig. 4**). This is especially important if the coronary segment being snared is diseased, as circumferential snaring of an atherosclerotic vessel is more likely to result in plaque rupture and vascular injury (**Fig. 5**). Biplanar compression may result in less distortion of posterior or hemicircumferential plaque. Furthermore, because the silicone elastic tapes are pulled to the sides, only a small fraction of the tape tension, that portion that is perpendicular to the stabilizer, is transmitted to the coronary, decreasing the risk of coronary injury (**Fig. 6**).

Many find that the capture technology utilized by the Genzyme Immobilizer, when used correctly, provides improved anastomotic site stability. This is due in part to the fact

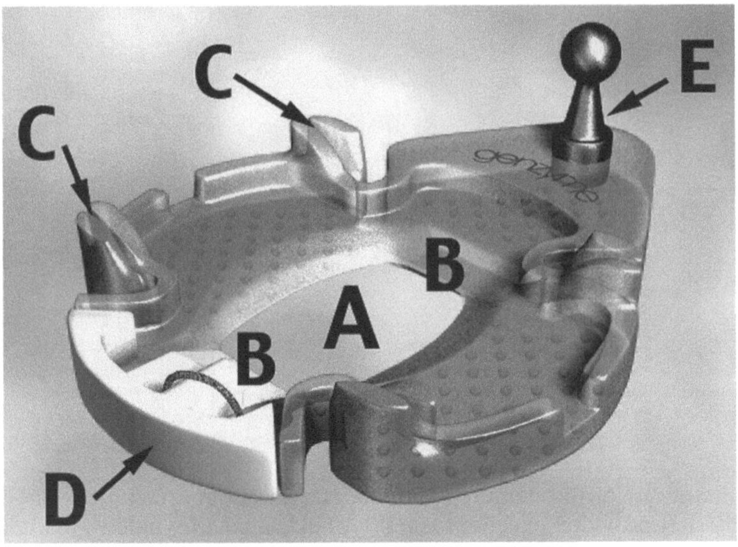

Fig. 3. The five key features of the Immobilizer Platform are (**A**) the anastomotic window, (**B**) the proximal and distal buttresses, (**C**) the paired flanking tape cleats, (**D**) the detachable segment, and (**E**) the metal pivot.

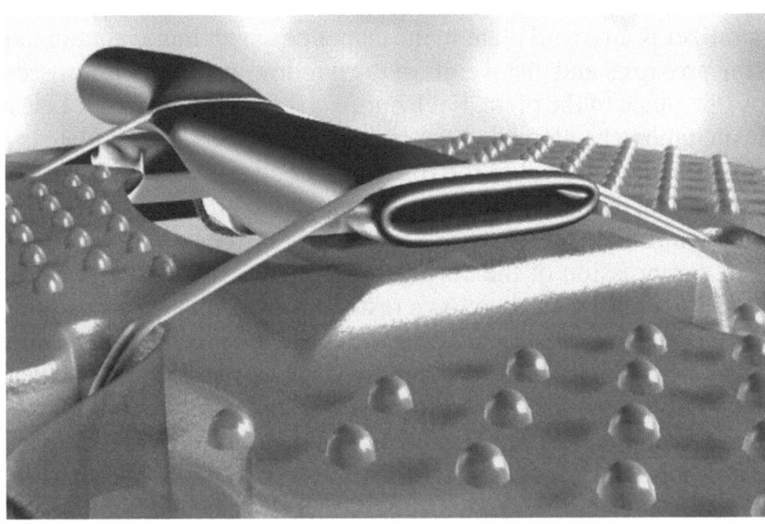

Fig. 4. When using the Immobilizer, the coronary is occluded by biplanar compression between the flat undersurface of the plastic buttress and a straight segment of silicone elastic tape.

that the Immobilizer stabilizes the coronary segment directly, rather than indirectly by stabilizing the adjacent epicardium. It is well recognized by OPCAB surgeons that excessive downward pressure on the heart surface paradoxically compromises rather than improves stability. The upward force created by the silicone elastic tapes ensures intimate contact between the textured bottom surface of the Immobilizer and the epicardium, despite the use of nominal downward pressure. This allows stability to be optimized and prevents stabilizer slippage during grafting.

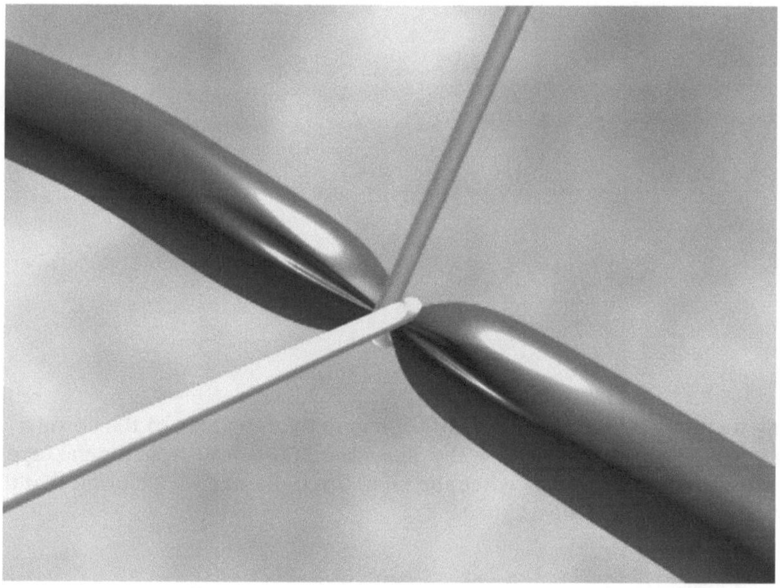

Fig. 5. Circumferential strangulation has the potential to injure delicate coronary arteries, especially if applied to a diseased vessel segment.

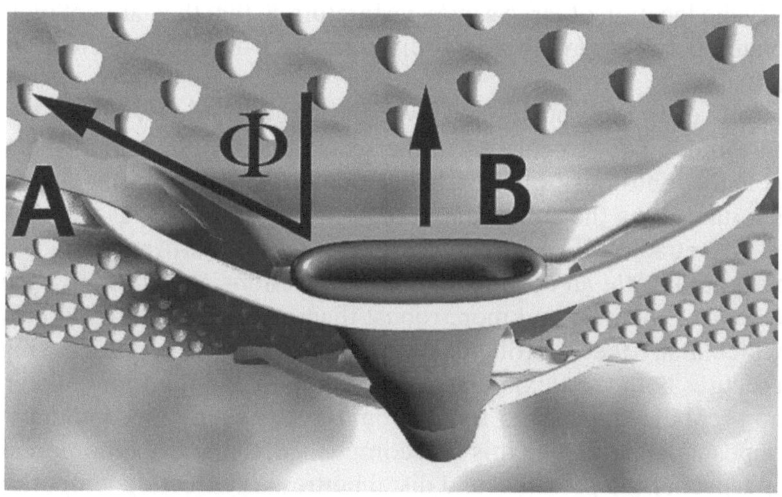

Fig. 6. A simple vector analysis illustrates that only a fraction of the tape tension **A** is transmitted to the coronary artery through the normal vector **B**. The maximum tape tension A is limited by the tape cleat, which will hold only 2 N.

Immobilizer Use

Prior to positioning the Immobilizer, silicone elastic tapes are placed deep to the target coronary artery approx 2.0 cm apart and as perpendicular as possible with respect to the long axis of the vessel. Accurate spacing is essential to achieve good hemostasis (**Fig. 7**). Although the needle on the tapes is intentionally blunt, care is taken to avoid injury to septal perforators and coronary veins and to ensure that the tapes pass deep to the artery.

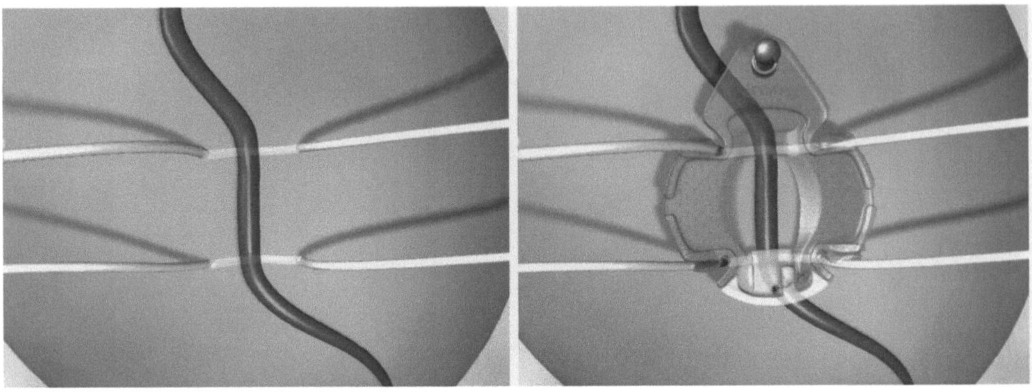

Fig. 7. Placing the tapes symmetrically with respect to the long axis of the coronary is essential so that the target site remains centered in the anastomotic window. Spacing the tapes 2 cm apart facilitates occlusion of the coronary when the tapes are tightened by ensuring that the tapes and proximal and distal buttresses are aligned.

Creating a defect in the epicardium prior to passing the needle allows passage with less force and greater tactile sense, minimizing the risk of vascular injury. If resistance is encountered during this maneuver, the needle is withdrawn and redirected until a resistance-free path is identified. A careful review of the preoperative cineangiogram allows one to identify the location of large septal perforators so that they are not included in the segment isolated between proximal and distal tapes, which can result in troublesome backbleeding.

The Immobilizer is then positioned over the target coronary artery such that the intended anastomotic site is centered in the rectangular window, and the articulating green arm is locked into position. The base of the articulating arm locks securely to a metal rail that runs along the entire length of both sternal blades, as well as the rack of the Elite OPCAB retractor. Like other systems, the stabilizer arm and retractor have been designed to accommodate an infinite number of positions and configurations (**Fig. 8**). The Elite retractor is heavier and more robust than most other commercially available retractors, which many feel contributes to the stability of the system. A single locking mechanism secures both the flexible arm configuration and the Immobilizer pivot.

After the Immobilizer is locked in position, the tapes are placed under tension and wedged in opposing cleats. Once this is accomplished, the artery is compressed against the posterior aspect of the proximal and distal buttresses, effecting temporary coronary occlusion and isolation, as described above.

The decision of whether to use a single proximal tape or proximal and distal flanking tapes is complex and is in part determined by the surgeon's preference. Generally, completely occluded vessels that fill by distal collaterals are more likely to have brisk backbleeding if only a proximal tape is used. Similarly, the rich septal collaterals between the LAD and PDA vessels generally make flanking tapes a good idea. Furthermore, it should be noted that often stability is improved with flanking tapes cleated under tension. As some surgeons prefer not to manipulate the coronary distal to the anastomotic site unless necessary, however, a good rule of thumb is to place flanking tapes, and cleat one or both only as needed for hemostasis.

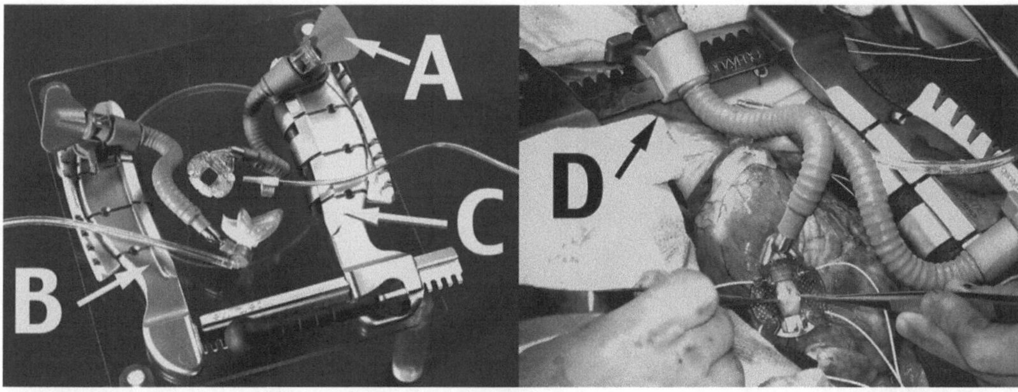

Fig. 8. The articulating flexible arm and the Immobilizer pivot are locked securely in position by tightening a single mechanism. The flexible arm can be attached to either blade of the retractor **A**, **B** as well as to the rack **C**.

The Immobilizer Platform and Intracoronary Shunts

In the early evolution of OPCAB, placement of intracoronary shunts was felt to be a necessary step to avoid ischemia and hemodynamic instability while the distal anastomosis was being constructed. With increased experience, there has been a trend away from shunting, as it has been shown to be superfluous in the overwhelming majority of grafts. Nevertheless, there remain occasional situations where shunting may be prudent. These include the large dominant RCA with a moderate stenosis that must be grafted proximal to the origin of the PDA branch, the LAD with moderate stenosis that must be grafted in the proximal half of the vessel, and any situation where a large coronary with moderate stenosis must be grafted prior to revascularization of an adjacent collateral dependent territory. Although intracoronary shunts can be readily employed with the Genzyme Immobilizer, in this setting we prefer the use of aortocoronary shunts. Aortocoronary shunts consist of an arterial source catheter, generally a no. 5 French cannula inserted in the ascending aorta, hooked by large-bore iv tubing to a silicone olive-tipped coronary catheter. The Immobilizer is positioned as described earlier, but only a proximal tape is used. The appropriately sized olive-tipped catheter is inserted into the distal coronary lumen providing flow. Although there is a moderate amount of line resistance in this arrangement, the blood delivered to the coronary distal to the anastomotic site is much greater than that seen with traditional intracoronary shunts, which convey the already compromised proximal flow through a resistive tube. As aortocoronary shunts are linear rather than "T"-shaped, and extend only down the distal vessel, they are easier to remove after completion of the anastomosis (**Fig. 9**).

EXPOSURE OF THE INFERIOR AND LATERAL WALLS FOR PERFORMING MULTIVESSEL OPCAB

Clearly, one of the most important developments in the evolution of multivessel OPCAB has been the techniques for exposing branches of the circumflex and right coronary arteries on a beating heart. Understanding the mechanisms of hemodynamic compromise during manipulation of the heart is essential in learning to perform OPCAB.

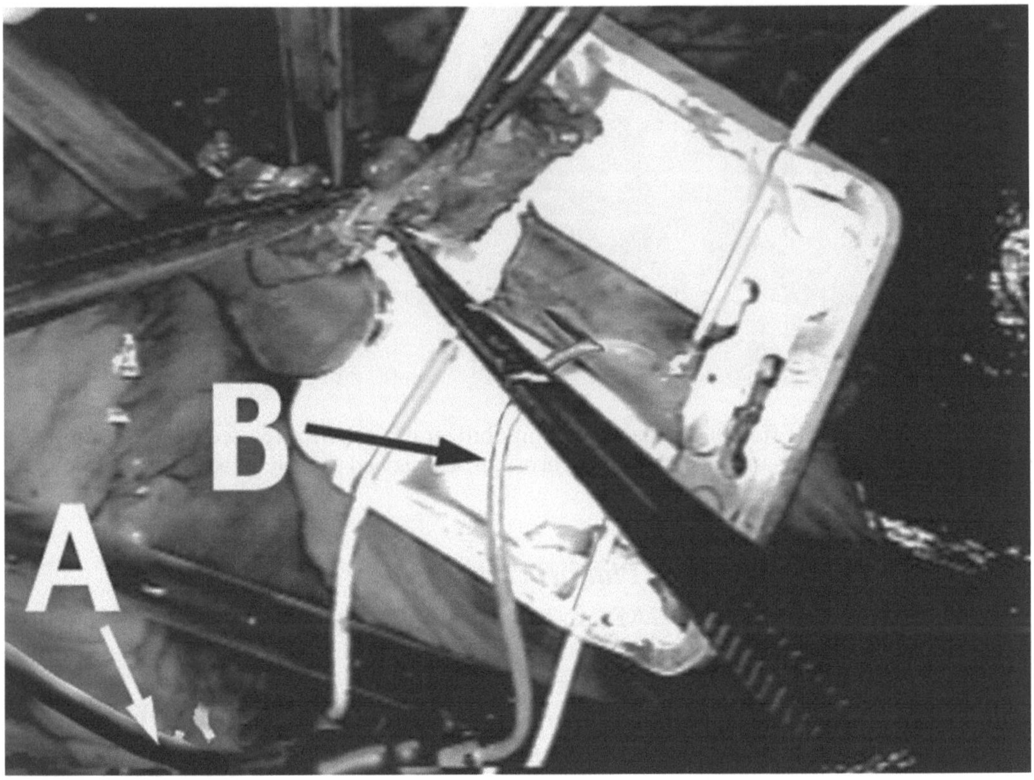

Fig. 9. A short segment of plastic tubing **A** conveys arterial blood from a no. 5 French cannula placed in the ascending aorta through a Nylon olive-tipped cannula **B** to the distal LAD.

These mechanisms are stabilizer-independent, and can be seen with pressure-type and epicardial suction-type stabilizers, as well as with the Genzyme Immobilizer.

MECHANISMS OF ADVERSE HEMODYNAMIC EFFECTS

Left ventricular compression, right ventricular compression, and coronary insufficiency are responsible for the majority of adverse hemodynamic effects resulting from exposure and stabilization of the heart during OPCAB *(5–7)*. These mechanisms are reviewed below.

Left Ventricle

The application of pressure with the coronary stabilizer during exposure of the circumflex system constrains the lateral wall of the left ventricle, leading to diastolic dysfunction and decreased left ventricular end-diastolic volume (LVEPV), stroke volume, and cardiac output *(7)*. Although volume loading and Trendelenburg positioning can attenuate these effects by elevating left ventricular filling pressures, these measures may also exacerbate intraoperative third-space fluid sequestration. The use of short-acting α-adrenergic agents can help in maintaining perfusion pressure in this setting, but may be associated with an increased risk of perioperative mesenteric ischemia *(8)*. Furthermore, mitral regurgitation can also occur during exposure of the lateral wall, possibly related to deformation of subvalvular structures in combination with coronary insufficiency. Exposure techniques that minimize or eliminate left ventricular deformation during OPCAB are therefore desirable.

Right Ventricle

Exposure of the lateral wall of the left ventricle displaces the heart toward the right, resulting in right ventricular compression against the pericardium and right hemisternum. The relatively low pressure in the right ventricle makes it particularly vulnerable to deformation and to reduction in right ventricular end-diastolic volume (RVEDV) *(6,9)*, with decreased right ventricular stroke volume leading to poor left ventricular filling and a drop in cardiac output. Volume loading and Trendelenburg positioning can only partially compensate for this effect, and the recourse to intraoperative right ventricular assist devices has been proposed as palliation for right ventricular compromise *(10,11)*; preferable, however, are exposure techniques that minimize right ventricular deformation and render the use of these costly devices unnecessary.

Coronary Insufficiency

Decompensated coronary disease, coronary snaring, and reduced cardiac output during heart manipulation can also lead to hemodynamic instability, which is best prevented by planning a revascularization strategy that minimizes myocardial ischemia and by using exposure techniques that maintain coronary perfusion pressure at all times. Useful axioms include the revascularization of occluded or severely stenosed coronary arteries first, the construction of proximal anastomoses after each distal anastomosis that involves a free graft, the availability of temporary pacing during snaring of a moderately stenosed right coronary artery, the constant optimization of afterload and coronary perfusion pressure by the anesthesiologist, and the selective use of intracoronary shunts, aortocoronary shunts, or assisted coronary perfusion devices such as the PADCAB™ system *(12)*. The use of an intra-aortic balloon pump can also prove useful in select cases *(13)*.

EXPOSURE TECHNIQUES

Depending on the size and shape of the heart and the dimensions of the chest cavity, visualization of the proximal obtuse marginal and posterolateral branches of the circumflex system may be obstructed by the left hemisternum. Although intuitive attempts at improving exposure may involve displacing the coronary stabilizer's arm toward the right (thereby increasing its application pressure), this maneuver usually leads to hemodynamic problems as well as paradoxically poor stabilization. Maximized access and stability at the anastomotic site with minimal compromise of cardiac performance is most readily achieved when the stabilizer is applied with little or no pressure; thus, coronary stabilizers should be used only to stabilize the anastomotic field rather than assist at retracting the heart. Exposure is best obtained with maneuvers such as the use of deep pericardial sutures, right pleurotomy and pericardiotomy, right hemisternal elevation, and apical suction devices, each of which is described below.

Deep Pericardial Sutures

One of the most important advances in exposure techniques for OPCAB has been the use of deep pericardial sutures. These sutures, when placed under tension, create a ridge

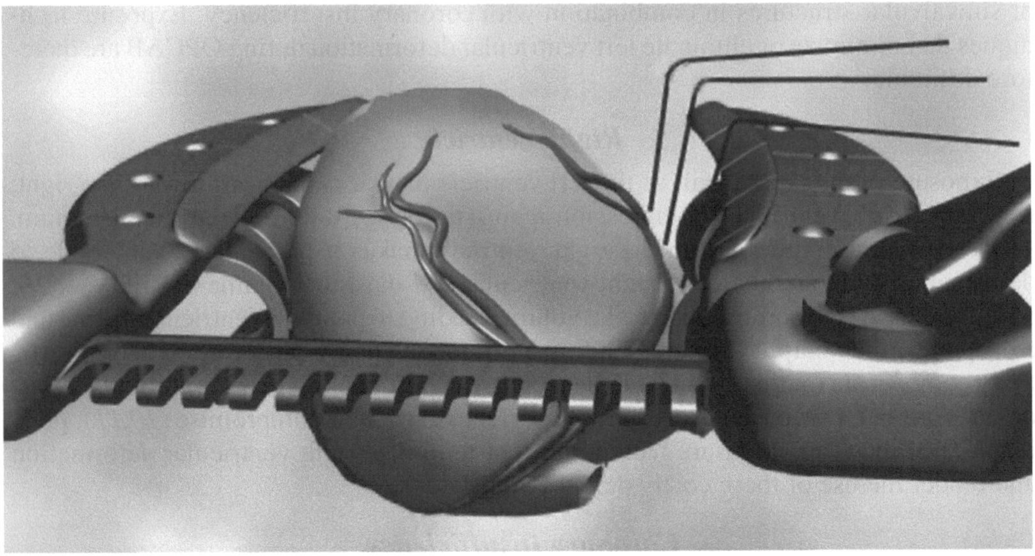

Fig. 10. Placement of deep pericardial sutures results in rotation of the heart to an "apex up" orientation. Often the heart protrudes above the plane of the chest wall in this position.

of pericardium that supports the base of the lateral left ventricle adjacent to the atrioventricular groove and allows the heart to be rotated rightward to assume an "apex-up" position (**Fig. 10**). In this subluxed position, the apex of the heart points toward the ceiling and protrudes through the sternotomy incision, often in a plane above that of the sternal retractor. This generally allows for adequate exposure of the lateral and inferior aspects of the left ventricle before applying the coronary stabilizer.

Placement of deep pericardial sutures may vary between surgeons and according to the patient's anatomy. Generally, one or two 2-0 silk sutures are placed in the pericardium posterior to the left phrenic nerve immediately anterior to one or both left pulmonary veins. Two additional sutures are placed deep in the oblique sinus behind the left atrium, and to the left and posterior to the inferior vena cava (**Fig. 11**). Care must be taken when placing these sutures to avoid injury to underlying structures such as the esophagus and lung *(14)*. The suture in the oblique sinus is particularly important to obtain good exposure of the lateral wall near the base of the heart. One commonly used technique, called the "stockinet," consists of placing a single deep pericardial suture in this location to secure the midpoint of a 50-cm gauze strip deep in the oblique sinus. Subsequent traction on the two ends of the strip can then be adjusted to optimize exposure of different surfaces of the heart.

Regardless of the technique used, deep pericardial traction sutures generally allow for presentation of the lateral, inferior, and even posterior wall of the heart with little change in left ventricular geometry or LVEDV, providing adequate access for multivessel grafting while maintaining hemodynamic stability. In some patients, however, additional maneuvers such as those outlined below are necessary to accomplish this aim effectively.

Right Pleurotomy and Pericardiotomy

Right pleurotomy and right vertical pericardiotomy constitute helpful technical adjuncts in patients with difficult lateral wall exposure. Human pericardium is quite

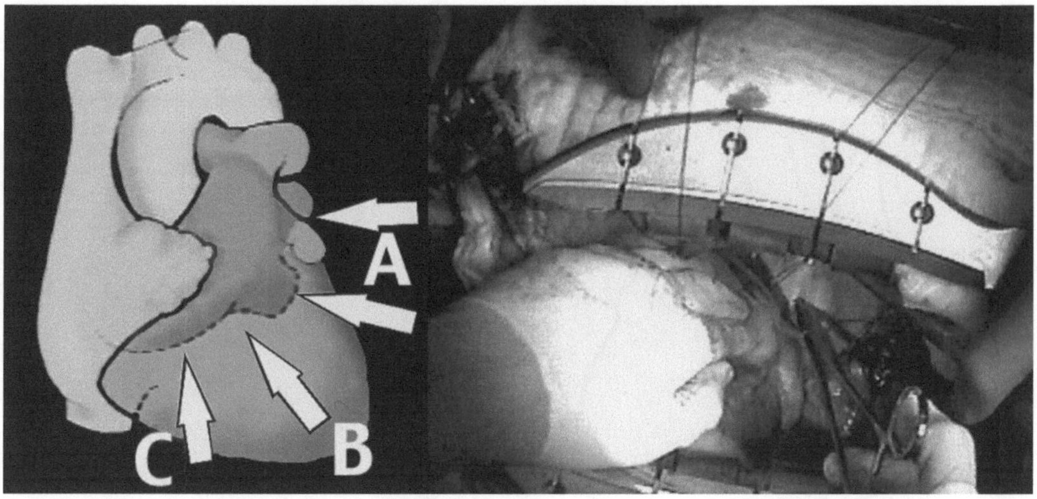

Fig. 11. Deep pericardial sutures are placed posterior to the left phrenic nerve adjacent to the left upper and lower pulmonary veins **A**, behind the left atrium **B**, and posterior and to the left of the inferior vena cava **C**. The operative photo shows the heart being lifted and rotated to the right to allow suture placement.

flexible but very inelastic. This inelasticity accounts for the profound hemodynamic effects caused by acute tamponade from a relatively small volume of intrapericardial fluid. As such, the posterior pericardium, right lateral pericardium, and diaphragmatic pericardium therefore constitute a fixed-volume cusp or pocket. It is into this pocket that the right ventricle is compressed during extreme rightward rotation of the heart. By opening the right pleura widely and incising the pericardium, the pocket is vented, allowing the heart to herniate into the right pleural space while maintaining RVEDV.

Right lateral pericardiotomy can be performed with a right vertical incision extending from the cut edge of the initial anterior pericardiotomy, 2 cm cephalad and parallel to the diaphragm, down to the level of the inferior vena cava with care taken at avoiding injury to the right phrenic nerve (**Fig. 12**). The 2-cm rim of pericardium on the diaphragm facilitates closure of the pericardiotomy once grafting is complete. In some circumstances, one may also benefit from removing the right pericardiophrenic fat pad, which can be quite large, and decreasing tidal volume to provide additional room for the easily deformed right ventricle. Caution should be taken when measuring right-sided grafts, as closure of the lateral pericardial incision may affect their lie.

Many surgeons skilled in the OPCAB procedure avoid right pleurotomy and lateral pericardiotomy on the contention that incising the lateral pericardium and entering an additional body cavity is inconsistent with the objective of decreased invasiveness. While many cases can indeed be performed successfully without it, this maneuver facilitates the reproducible performance of a precise anastomosis during multivessel OPCAB. Furthermore, right pleurotomy does not leave a scar, nor is it associated with significant morbidity or additional length of stay after coronary surgery.

Right Hemi-Sternal Elevation

Asymmetric right hemisternal elevation can further improve lateral wall exposure when used in conjunction with the techniques described above. Once the right lateral

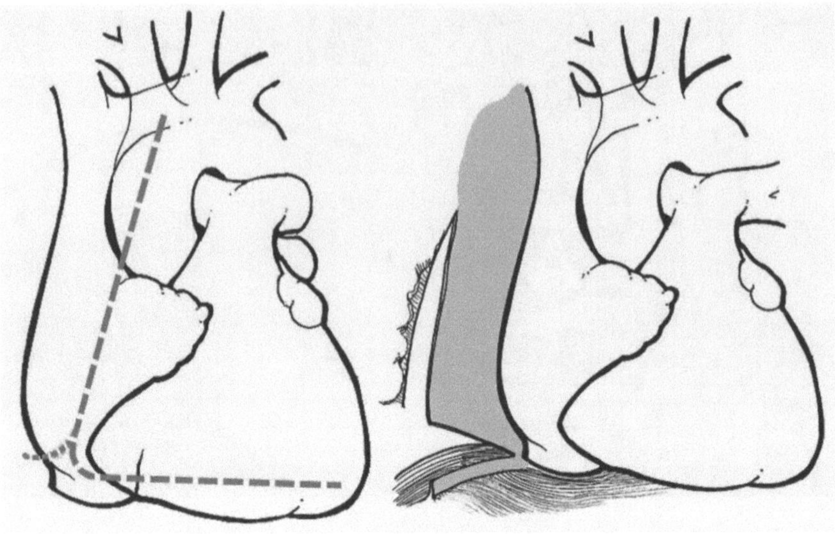

Fig. 12. The pericardial incision is made along the dotted lines shown. The drawing on the right shows the resulting vertical incision in the right lateral pericardium and the widely opened right pleural space.

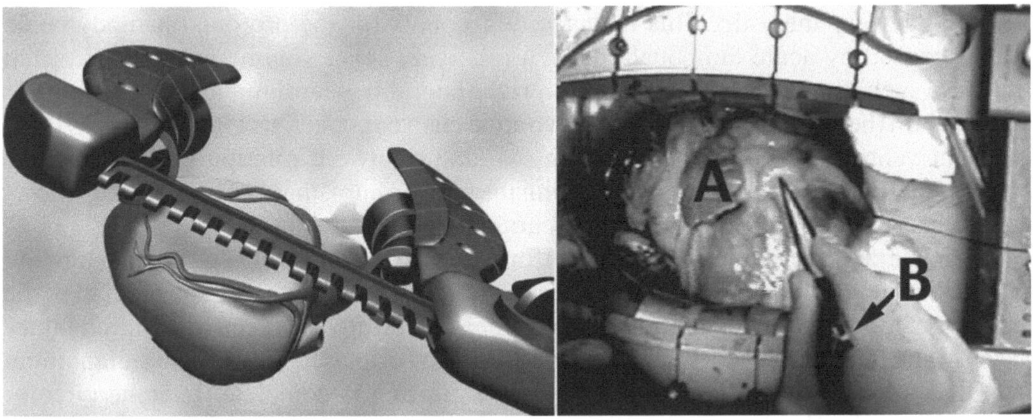

Fig. 13. After creating a right vertical pericardiotomy, opening the right pleural space, and elevating the right sternum, the heart can be readily rotated. The operative photo on the right shows the lateral wall exposure that results. The tip of the forceps is on the proximal aspect of the obtuse marginal branch, where it emerges from the fat in the atrioventricular groove. The left atrial appendage **A** is in the center of the operative field, whereas the apex of the heart **B** is under the right hemisternum.

pericardium and right pleura are incised, it is often the right half of the sternum and right blade of the retractor that limits rightward displacement of the subluxed apex of the heart. By elevating these structures, the apex can clear the posterior aspect of the chest wall. This allows the entire heart to rotate into the right pleural space with little change in left and right ventricular geometry or end-diastolic volume (**Fig. 13**). As a result of these maneuvers, the proximal obtuse marginal and posterolateral branches are brought toward the center of the operative field and into the surgeon's view.

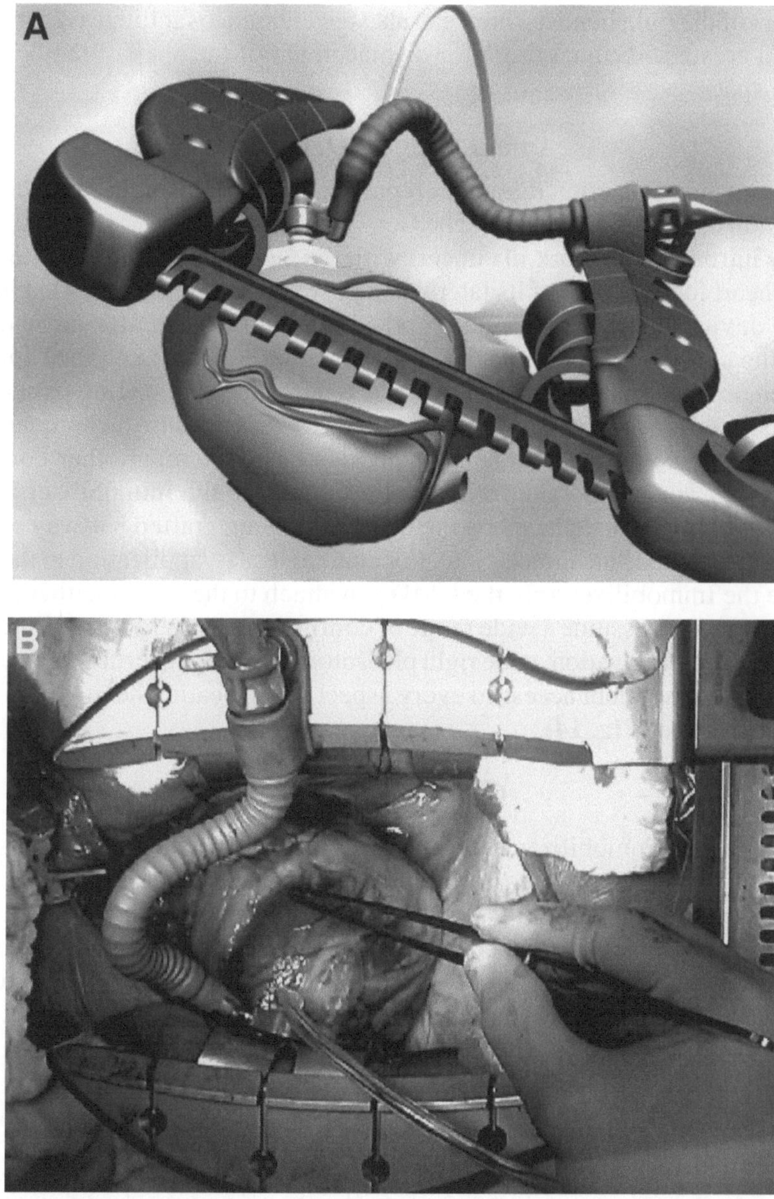

Fig. 14. The HMD (Heart Manipulation Device) when used in conjunction with other maneuvers described, provides quick and reliable access to every aspect of the heart with little compromise in hemodynamic stability.

Right hemisternal elevation is best accomplished if carried out as the sternotomy incision is being performed. By applying anterior traction on the right chest wall when the retractor is first spread, costal microfractures that inevitably form during sternal opening will occur predominantly in the right-sided ribs. The resulting increase in flexibility of the right chest wall will subsequently prevent the need for exaggerated tilting of the sternal retractor, which is often required to overcome the left chest wall's tendency to rise after left internal mammary artery harvest. The diaphragmatic insertion on the inferior aspect of the right hemisternum can also be released to facilitate right hemisternal elevation and create additional room for displacement of the apex of the heart into the right pleural space.

Apical Suction Devices

Self-retaining apical suction retractors represent a welcome addition to the operative armamentarium of OPCAB surgeons. The Genzyme HMD (Heart Manipulation Device) was recently introduced to work in concert with the Genzyme-OPCAB Elite System to position the heart for exposure of its lateral and posterior aspects (**Fig. 14**). Although the use of these devices involves supplemental expenses, the easy affixation of the suction cup to the cardiac apex or adjacent inferior or lateral wall and the rapid locking into a chosen position make them an attractive adjunct for challenging patients. Apical suction can be used alone or in conjunction with the other exposure techniques described above. The HMD suction head is smaller and lower profile than other commercially available devices, and can be placed in close proximity to the Immobilizer platform. It is often most effective when placed on the heart wall being grafted halfway between the apex of the heart and the anastomotic site. For smaller hearts, application to the apex may suffice. Like the Immobilizer arm, the HMD can attach to the rack or either blade of the Elite retractor, and can assume a wide range of configurations. When used in conjunction with right hemisternal elevation, wide right pleurotomy, and right vertical pericardiotomy, the HMD provides excellent access to every aspect of the beating heart with little hemodynamic compromise (**Fig. 14**).

CONCLUSION

Introduction of the Immobilizer, recent changes in the stabilizer arm, and most recently, introduction of the Genzyme Heart Manipulation Device, have resulted in continued improvement in the Genzyme-OPCAB Elite System from both performance and ease-of-use perspectives. It is likely that continued improvements in tools and exposure techniques over the next several years will make multivessel OPCAB an increasingly attractive approach for the next generation of cardiothoracic surgeons.

REFERENCES

1. Ankeney JL. To use or not to use the pump oxygenator in coronary bypass operations. Ann Thorac Surg 1975;19:108–109.
2. Trapp WJ, Bisarya R. Placement of coronary artery bypass graft without pump oxygenator. Ann Thorac Surg 1975;19:1–9.
3. Benetti FG, Naselli G, Wood M, Geffner L. Direct myocardial revascularization without extracorporeal circulation: experience in 700 patients. Chest 1991;100:312–316.
4. Buffolo E, Andrade JCS, Branco JNR, Aguiar LF, Teles CA, Gomes WJ. Coronary artery bypass grafting without cardiopulmonary bypass. Ann Thorac Surg 1992;61:63–66.
5. Nierich AP, Diephuis J, Jansen EW, Borst C, Knape JT. Heart displacement during off-pump CABG: how well is it tolerated? Ann Thorac Surg 2000;70(2):466–472.
6. Mathison M, Edgerton JR, Horswell JL, Akin JJ, Mack MJ. Analysis of hemodynamic changes during beating heart surgical procedures. Ann Thorac Surg 2000;70(4):1355–1360; discussion 1360–1361.
7. Biswas S, Clements F, Diodato L, Hughes GC, Landolfo K. Changes in systolic and diastolic function during multivessel off-pump coronary bypass grafting. Eur J Cardiothorac Surg 2001;20(5):913–917.
8. Reilly PM, Wilkins KB, Fuh KC, Haglund U, Bulkley GB. The mesenteric hemodynamic response to circulatory shock: an overview. Shock 2001;15(5):329–343.

9. Grundeman PF, Borst C, Verlaan CW, Meijburg H, Moues CM, Jansen EW. Exposure of circumflex branches in the tilted, beating porcine heart: echocardiographic evidence of right ventricular deformation and the effect of right or left heart bypass. J Thorac Cardiovasc Surg 1999;118(2):316–323.
10. Lima LE, Jatene F, Buffolo E, et al. A multicenter initial clinical experience with right heart support and beating heart coronary surgery. Heart Surg Forum 2001;4(1):60–64.
11. Sharony R, Autschbach R, Porat E, et al. Right heart support during off-pump coronary artery bypass surgery—a multi-center study. Heart Surg Forum 2002;5(1):13–16.
12. Guyton RA, Thourani VH, Puskas JD, et al. Perfusion-assisted direct coronary artery bypass: selective graft perfusion in off-pump cases. Ann Thorac Surg 2000;69(1):171–175.
13. Kim KB, Lim C, Ahn H, Yang JK. Intraaortic balloon pump therapy facilitates posterior vessel off-pump coronary artery bypass grafting in high-risk patients. Ann Thorac Surg 2001;71(6):1964–1968.
14. Zamvar V, Deglurkar I, Abdullah F, Khan NU. Bleeding from the lung surface: a unique complication of off-pump CABG operation. Heart Surg Forum 2001;4(2):172–173.

8 Mechanical Stabilization Systems

The Guidant OPCAB System

Marc W. Connolly, MD
and Valavanur A. Subramanian, MD

CONTENTS

INTRODUCTION
GOAL OF OPCAB SURGERY
TECHNICAL CONSIDERATIONS AND STRATEGIES
INSTITUTIONAL OPCAB EXPERIENCE
CONCLUSION
REFERENCES

INTRODUCTION

In January 1997, the Guidant Corporation Cardiac Surgery Group introduced the first widely used beating-heart stabilizer system for MIDCAB procedures. From the experience gained since these initial MIDCAB procedures *(1,2)*, the Access MV OPCAB System™ was introduced in 1998 for multivessel, sternotomy off-pump CABG, leading to greater surgeon acceptance of the OPCAB procedure and to the development of further enabling technologies and devices. Introduced in 2000, the latest Guidant OPCAB System (Axius™ Stabilizer and *Xpose*™ Apical Positioning Device) has greatly assisted the surgeon in providing improved hemodynamic stability and access to lateral wall circumflex vessels—increasing the overall comfort level of the surgeon.

Presently, at Lenox Hill Hospital, 98% of all CABG procedures are performed off-pump, with the 1–2% on-pump cases performed for deep intramyocardial left anterior descending vessels and severe diffuse distal disease requiring extensive endarterectomies. This chapter outlines our OPCAB operative technique with the use of Guidant Axius Stabilizer with the *Xpose* Apical Positioning Device System, and briefly, discuss our OPCAB hospital outcomes.

From: *Contemporary Cardiology: Minimally Invasive Cardiac Surgery, Second Edition*
Edited by: D. J. Goldstein and M. C. Oz © Humana Press Inc., Totowa, NJ

GOAL OF OPCAB SURGERY

The primary goal of OPCAB is to obtain complete revascularization using standard anastomotic techniques to all critically stenosed coronary arteries without the use of cardiopulmonary bypass (CPB). To avoid the use of CPB and its potential adverse perioperative complications, hemodynamic stability needs to be maintained and coronary ischemia avoided or minimized throughout the entire procedure. A consistent, well-planned operative strategy is implemented to achieve this goal.

TECHNICAL CONSIDERATIONS AND STRATEGIES

Cardiac Anesthesia

All patients are monitored intraoperatively with arterial line pressure, Swan–Ganz catheter with mixed venous oximetry, central body temperature, foley urimetry, and transesophageal echocardiography.

Intravenous neosynephrine and nitroglycerin are most commonly used for pharmacological support. Occasionally, Primacor (Sanofi–Synthelabo) is used in patients with poor left ventricular function, elevated pulmonary pressures, and/or hemodynamically compromising acute ischemia. Rarely, levophed and IABP are used to support hemodynamics.

Coronary Artery Anatomy

Coronary artery anatomy strategies have been discussed in detail previously *(3)*. To avoid intraoperative ischemia, the sequence of grafting, coronary shunting, and perfusion of completed bypass grafts by performing proximals first or with the use of perfusion cannulae should be well thought out before skin incision. An individual patient's coronary anatomy and lesions, left ventricular function, and regional wall motion abnormalities should be taken into preoperative consideration when planning a patient's intraoperative strategy to avoid ischemia and hemodynamic compromise, leading to conversion to cardiopulmonary bypass support.

Sternotomy and Pericardiotomy

The skin incision is made from two to three finger breadths below the sternal notch to the inferior tip of the xiphoid. Sternotomy is performed in usual fashion. The Guidant OPCAB retractor is placed and the sternum is opened, manually elevating the right side to increase room for placement of the right ventricle during positioning for lateral wall exposure.

The pericardium is incised with electrocautery completely along the diaphragm, then superiorly with the superior mediastinal fat pad to the innominate vein. The right pericardium is further loosened by incising its diaphragmatic attachments toward the vena cava, carefully avoiding the phrenic nerve. Also, the pericardial attachment along the right ascending aorta near the innominate artery is incised to increase laxity of the right pericardium. Having a loose, movable right pericardium is critical to avoid right ventricular compression and hemodynamic instability when performing lateral and posterior wall coronary artery anastomoses. Infrequently, the right pleura is opened further to increase the space under the right sternum to displace the right heart during positioning.

Pericardial sutures are placed only along the anterior edge of the left side, never on the right. Pulling up on these left pericardial sutures can usually expose the left anterior descending without having to place deep pericardial sutures or use the *Xpose*.

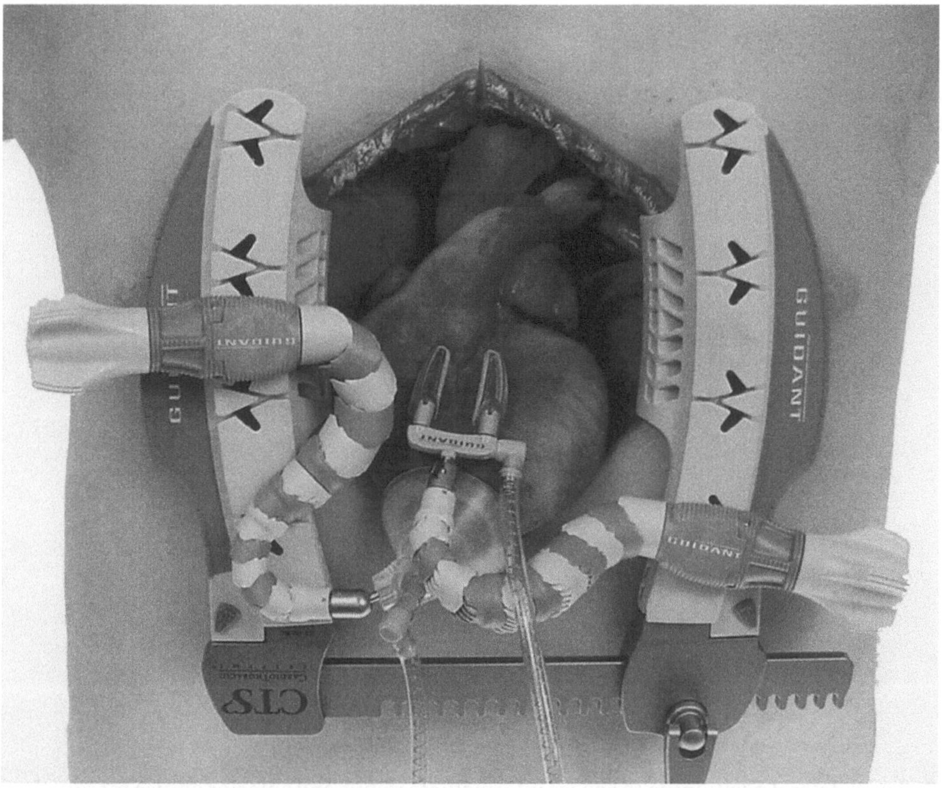

Fig. 1. Anterior positioning with *Xpose* apical device and LAD stabilization with Axius suction foot. (Used by permission of Guidant Corporation, Santa Clara, CA.)

The Guidant OPCAB retractor provides excellent mediastinal exposure. The retractor's curved sternal blades pull the heart anteriorly toward the surgeon as the sternum is opened. The numerous suture guides along both sides provide for placement of silastic tapes, coronary artery traction sutures, and pericardial sutures, thus avoiding unnecessary clamps. A deep large blade retractor is also available for obese patients.

Heart Displacement

The *Xpose* Apical Positioning Device has greatly improved exposure to all vessels while maintaining hemodynamic stability. The *Xpose* Apical suction device provides excellent access to the anterior (**Fig. 1**), anterolateral (**Fig. 2**), lateral (**Fig. 3**), posterior (**Fig. 4**), and inferior vessels (**Figs. 5** and **6**). In large hearts, the suction cup can even be placed on the lateral apical wall to gain access to circumflex vessels near the AV groove, or on the right ventricle to expose the left anterior descending or distal right coronary artery.

The most important aspect of heart positioning and displacement is to prevent compression and decreased filling of the right ventricle. Elongating the heart by pulling out and upward with the *Xpose* improves right ventricular and left ventricular preload and function during displacement. As discussed previously, a loose right-sided pericardium or opening into the right pleural space helps avoid right ventricular compression and hemodynamic deterioration.

In over 600 cases using *Xpose*, we have not experienced any avulsion of the epicardium, but bruising or an epicardial "hickey" is common without adverse sequelae. Dullum

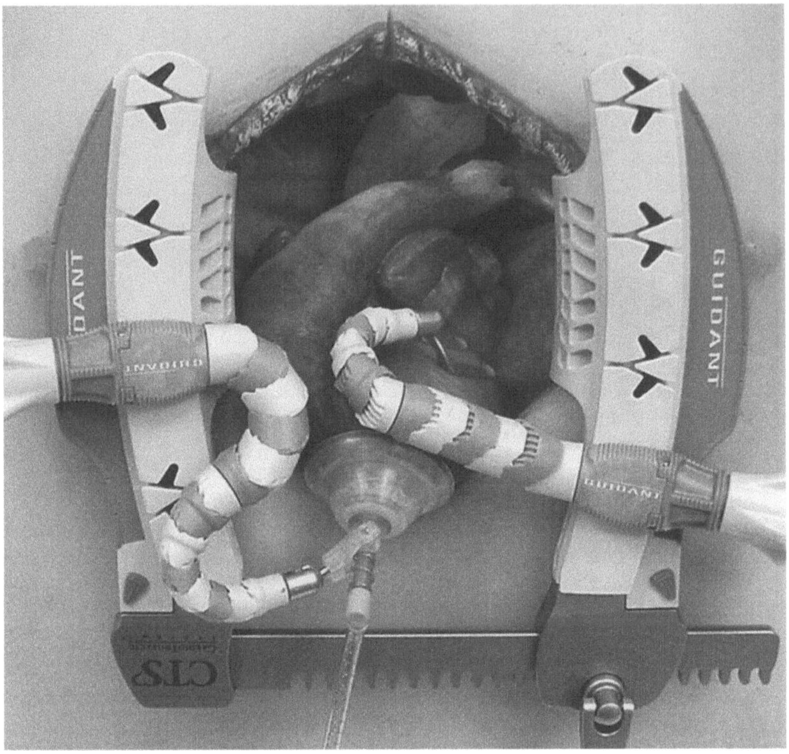

Fig. 2. Anterolateral positioning to access intermediate ramus and anterior obtuse marginal vessels with antegrade placement of mechanical Axius stabilizer. (Used by permission of Guidant Corporation, Santa Clara, CA.)

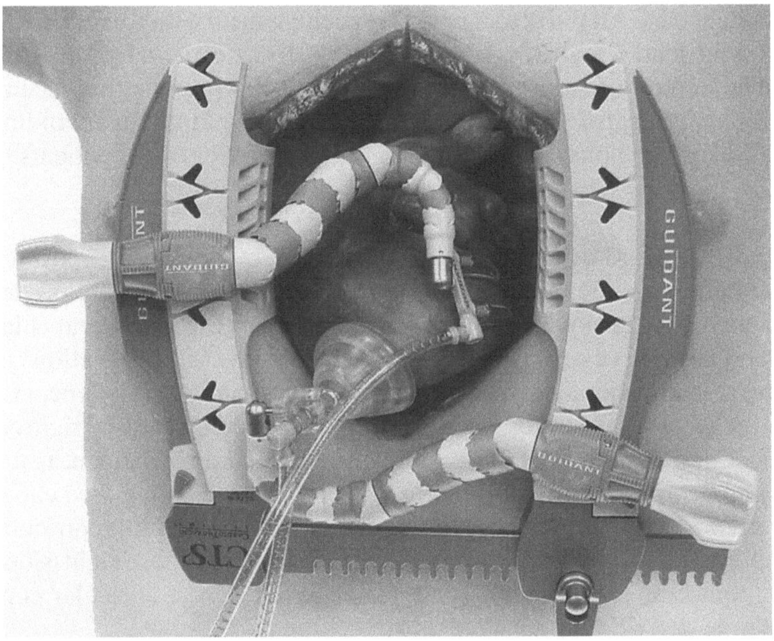

Fig. 3. Lateral exposure of circumflex vessels using *Xpose* apical device with antegrade placement of Axius suction stabilizer. (Used by permission of Guidant Corporation, Santa Clara, CA.)

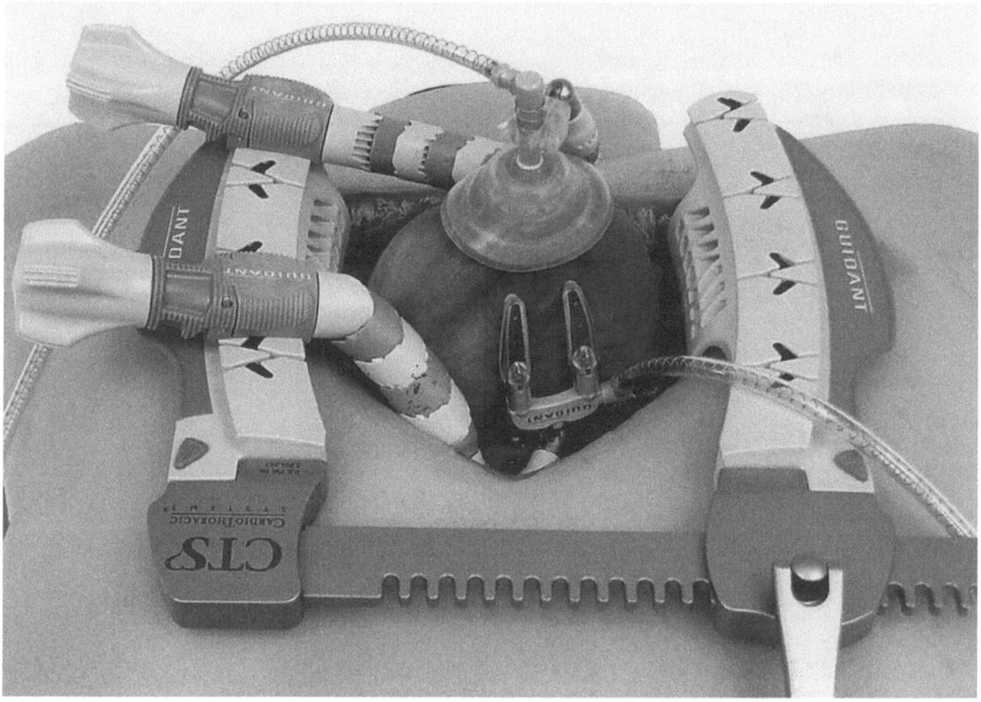

Fig. 4. Posterior exposure to posterior lateral ascending or posterior obtuse marginal vessels using *Xpose* apical position device and Axius suction stabilizer. Notice apex of heart pulled anteriorly and cephalad. (Used by permission of Guidant Corporation, Santa Clara, CA.)

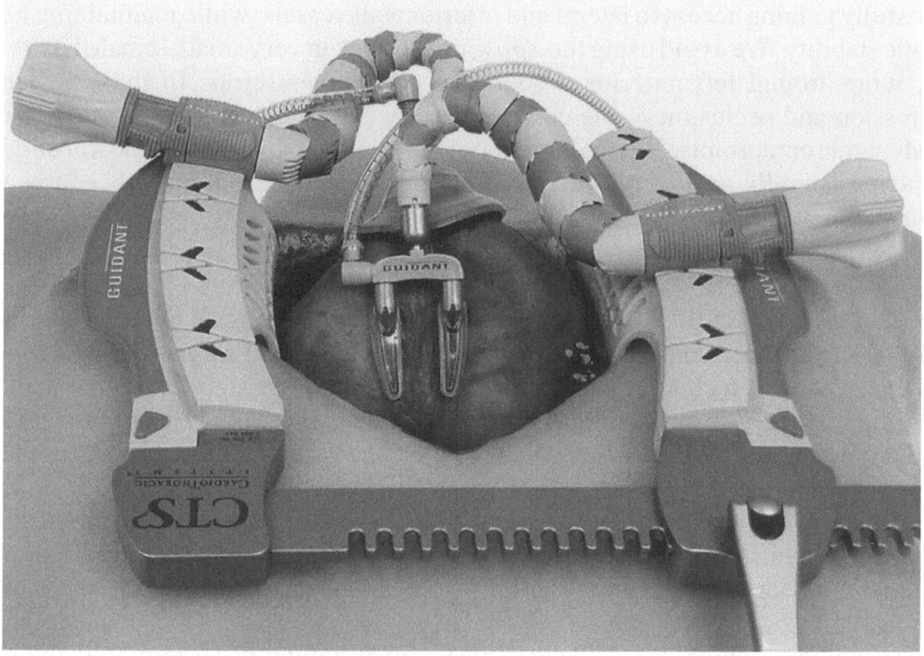

Fig. 5. Inferior exposure of posterior descending artery with *Xpose* apical device and retrograde placement of Axius suction stabilizer. Apex of heart pulled anterior and cephalad. (Used by permission of Guidant Corporation, Santa Clara, CA.)

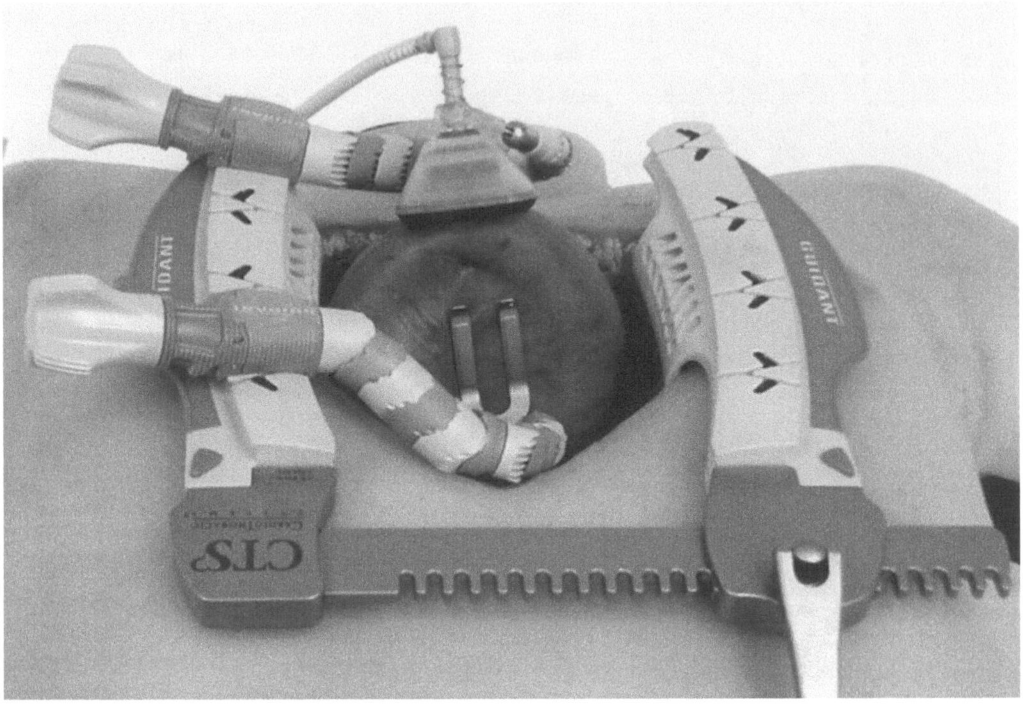

Fig. 6. Inferior exposure with *Xpose* apical device and antegrade placement of Axius mechanical stabilizing foot. (Used by permission of Guidant Corporation, Santa Clara, CA.)

and Resano *(4)* describe their initial experience with the *Xpose* in five case reports, successfully gaining access to lateral and inferior wall vessels, while maintaining hemodynamic stability. We avoid using the *Xpose* on the apex in very small, female hearts with large, wrap-around left anterior descending coronary arteries. In these instances, compression and occlusion of the coronary artery can occur, producing ischemia and hemodynamic compromise. In two patients where this was experienced, the *Xpose* devise was moved laterally away from the left anterior descending and the procedures were completed uneventfully.

Vessel Stabilization

The Guidant Axius Off-Pump System has various stabilizing technologies available to suit the particular needs and comfort level of the individual surgeon. The Axius stabilizing arm has link technology for accurate placement of the stabilizing foot without a protruding stabilizing arm extending above the sternal plane. The Axius stabilizer can be placed anywhere on the OPCAB retractor to gain access to the desired coronary artery and is available in two types: suction (**Fig. 1**) or mechanical (**Fig. 2**). The foot can be placed retrograde (**Fig. 5**) or antegrade (**Fig. 6**) to the vessel, depending on the surgeon's preference. An earlier-generation Access Ultima™ Stabilizing System with an offset mechanical foot and curved fluted shaft is also available, and is still preferred by some surgeons.

We encourage surgeons to try all available Guidant stabilizing systems with the *Xpose* Apical Positioner for the various vessel exposures to find what system provides him or her the best access and stabilization with consistent hemodynamic stability. The melding of an individual surgeon with specific available technology produces a comfort level for consistent, reproducible results.

Proximal Anastomosis

Proximal anastomoses in a deep chest with a hyperdynamic heart that produces movement of the aorta can be more difficult than distal anastomoses. To prevent loss of aortic vascular control with the partial occlusion clamp and potential aortic complications, great care should be taken when performing the proximal anastomoses.

The adventitial layer between the aorta and main pulmonary artery is widely separated to allow for proper placement of the partial occlusion clamp. The anesthesiologist is asked to maintain the systolic arterial pressure between 90 and 110 mmHg before placement of the partial occlusion clamp. If the aorta and partial occlusion clamp are moving too much for proper suture placement, a supporting towel, lap pad, or the hand of the assistant can stabilize the clamp while suturing. The aortic clamp is gently removed after completion of proximal anastomoses.

Proximal anastomoses can be performed before distals to reperfuse coronary beds as coronary anastomoses are completed to prevent ischemia. Proximal anastomotic devices may also be used in diseased ascending aortas, thereby avoiding partial clamping.

LENOX HILL OPCAB EXPERIENCE

Beginning in May 1999, Lenox Hill Hospital began a dedicated OPCAB program. All eligible multivessel CABG patients underwent unselected, intention-to-treat OPCAB procedures. Our experience gained from the use of the Access Ultima OPCAB System (Guidant, Santa Clara, CA), made available in May 1999, provided a comfort level and confidence in approaching our CABG patients in this intention-to-treat model. The development of the Axius and *Xpose* systems has assisted in decreasing our conversion rate to cardiopulmonary bypass.

Betweem April 1998 and January 2002, over 1300 patients underwent multivessel full sternotomy OPCAB procedures. The mean number of grafts was 3.22. Conversion to CPB occurred in 3.1% of patients over the entire series, improved to 1.4% in the last 6 mo. The most common etiology of conversion to CPB was hemodynamic ischemic deterioration and presence of deep intramyocardial left anterior descending arteries.

A retrospectively comparison to conventional CABG performed in previous years at our institution demonstrated that OPCAB patients had a significantly less overall perioperative complication rate (10% vs 18%, $p < 0.0001$), deep sternal infection (1.4% vs 3.2%, $p < 0.02$), reoperation for bleeding (2.2% vs 6.3%, $p < 0.0001$), hospital mortality (1.6% vs 3.4%), and stroke rate (1.1% vs 3.1%, $p < 0.004$). Length of stay was also significantly decreased (6.1 d vs 7.2 d, $p < 0.01$). The perioperative myocardial infarction rate was similar in both groups (0.8% OPCAB vs 1.1% conventional).

CONCLUSION

With over 1300 OPCAB and 500 MIDCAB procedures performed at Lenox Hill, the Guidant Off-Pump Vessel Stabilizing Systems have enabled us to perform presently over 98% of our CABG procedures without cardiopulmonary bypass. Hemodynamic stability and excellent vessel stabilization can be achieved in the majority of multivessel OPCAB patients, allowing for proper anastomotic suture placement and achievement of complete revascularization.

Further development in enabling off-pump technologies are needed to obtain even greater access and stabilization to deep proximal obtuse marginal circumflex vessels and to prevent conversion to cardiopulmonary bypass. As technology develops, greater surgeon acceptance will increase and CABG patient outcomes will improve. Anastomotic devices will most likely play an important part in this future development.

REFERENCES

1. Subramanian V, Sani G, Benetti F, et al. Minimally invasive coronary artery bypass surgery: a multicenter report of preliminary clinical experience. Circulation 1995;92(suppl):645.
2. Calafiore A, DiGiammarco G, Teodori G, et al. Left anterior descending coronary artery grafting via left anterior thoractomy without cardiopulmonary bypass. Ann Thorac Surg 1996;61:1658–1665.
3. Connolly M, Subramanian V, Patel N. Multivessel coronary artery bypass grafting without cardiopulmonary bypass. Op Tech Thoracic 2000;5:166–175.
4. Dullum M, Resano F. *Xpose*™: A new device that provides reproducible and easy access for multivessel beating heart bypass grafts. Heart Surg Forum 2000;3(2):113–118.

9 The MIDCAB Operation

Mercedes K. C. Dullum, MD
and Albert J. Pfister, MD

CONTENTS

Definition
History
Indications And Contraindications
Surgical Technique
Postoperative Results
References

DEFINITION

For purposes of this discussion, a minimally invasive direct coronary artery bypass (MIDCAB) is considered to be any surgical coronary revascularization performed on the beating heart ("off-pump") through an incision other than a median sternotomy.

HISTORY

Interestingly, the initial attempts at surgical myocardial revascularization were performed on the beating heart via a thoracotomy. Vineberg *(1)* in 1946 implanted the internal mammary artery directly into the cardiac muscle. In 1967, Kolessov *(2)* reported direct coronary revascularization of the LAD and obtuse marginal via a thoracotomy without cardiopulmonary bypass. Sabiston *(3)* is often credited with performing the first coronary artery bypass graft of a saphenous vein graft to the right coronary artery via a median sternotomy. The ease of this incision and the excellent exposure that it afforded quickly made median sternotomy the incision of choice for coronary revascularization. Other surgeons including Favaloro, Garrett, Trapp, Bysana, and Ankeny *(4–7)* continued to demonstrate the safety of off-pump coronary bypass.

The improvements in cardiopulmonary bypass technology combined with the safety and efficacy of cardioplegia in the 1960s changed the approach to coronary bypass. The

From: *Contemporary Cardiology: Minimally Invasive Cardiac Surgery, Second Edition*
Edited by: D. J. Goldstein and M. C. Oz © Humana Press Inc., Totowa, NJ

ability to perform distal anastomoses in a bloodless field on a motionless target dramatically increased the reproducibility of coronary artery bypass grafting (CABG). Coronary bypass via median sternotomy done on cardiopulmonary bypass with cardioplegic arrest became (and some would argue still is) the gold standard for coronary revascularization.

In the 1980s, Benetti *(8)* in Argentina began a resurgence of off-pump coronary surgery, reporting his early experiences in 1985 and performing his first left anterior thoracotomy for CABG in 1988. He reported the results of his series in 1990 *(9)*. Pfister *(10)* in 1992 demonstrated the safety of off-pump bypass surgery (most via median sternotomy) in the United States. MIDCAB was introduced to the United States in 1994, and in 1995 Subramanian and colleagues *(11)* reported the first MIDCAB multicenter study of over 150 patients.

Following these early reports, great momentum and enthusiasm for learning and performing MIDCABs ensued. After this early expansion in the late 1990s, interest in the procedure reached a plateau for several reasons: (1) the limited applicability, because the procedure was used only for single-vessel bypass; (2) the steep learning curve required to become skillful at the operation; (3) the development of off-pump multivessel bypass techniques via median sternotomy; and (4) improved percutaneous therapies.

INDICATIONS AND CONTRAINDICATIONS

The surgeon's decision to perform the MIDCAB procedure should depend on his or her belief that it is the procedure of choice to produce the best clinical outcome for the patient. The procedure should be tailored to the patient and not vice versa.

Several patient populations can be considered for MIDCAB approaches. First are patients with isolated LAD and/or diagonal lesions. These usually represent restenosis following transcatheter therapy or patients with complex lesions not suitable for percutaneous revascularization. Second are patients with more than single-vessel disease and a contraindication to sternotomy in whom the non-LAD lesion is to be treated percutaneously, a so-called hybrid approach *(12,13)* (see Chapter 15). Third is the group of patients who can be adequately revascularized via a nonsternotomy approach and who have a high risk of complications resulting from cardiopulmonary bypass. These would include patients with a recent or high risk for stroke, uncontrolled diabetes, renal insufficiency, hematological disorders, advanced age, lung disease, calcified ascending aortas, redos, and patients whose religious conviction preclude transfusion. Finally, patient preference must be considered, for example, those patients who wish to return to manual labor or strenuous physical activity earlier. MIDCAB is an excellent alternative in patients who require a redo CABG to the LAD only, whether the LIMA has been used previously or not. In the latter case a "homegrown LIMA" can be made using a radial artery or segment of saphenous vein with proximal inflow via the axillary artery *(14–16)* (as will be explained below). A MIDCAB via a posterolateral thoracotomy can be performed on patients who are redos with patent LIMA to LAD and who require grafting of the lateral wall *(17)*.

Contraindications for this procedure are based on a variety of anatomical, technical, and clinical considerations. We consider the MIDCAB operation (via anterior thoracotomy) to be a single-vessel bypass to the LAD. Initially, our group attempted to perform multivessel bypass via an anterior thoracotomy, but found that it was less painful for the patient and more expeditious to perform multivessel bypass through a median sternotomy. Therefore, we consider multivessel disease to be a relative contraindication for MIDCAB.

Patients with deep chest walls or breasts too large to accommodate the instruments for access, and those with small, deeply intramyocardial and/or calcified target vessels should also be considered unsuitable candidates for MIDCAB. Patients with pulmonary insufficiency who are unable to tolerate single-lung ventilation may represent a relative contraindication to MIDCAB. While it is possible to perform the operation with both lungs being ventilated, it can be tedious and time-consuming. Chronic obstructive pulmonary disease (COPD) by itself is not a contraindication to MIDCAB. Interestingly, COPD frequently makes it easier to harvest the LIMA and to access the heart, since the COPD enlarges the anterior–posterior dimension of the chest cavity. The ideal first patient for MIDCAB has the following characteristics: single-vessel coronary artery disease represented by total occlusion of the LAD with good collaterals; a 2 mm or greater diameter distal vessel that is epicardial and not calcified; normal ventricular function; a thin chest wall; and mild to moderate COPD. We believe that patients with decompensated heart failure or recalcitrant arrhythmias represent contraindications to MIDCAB. Clearly, access is much better through a sternotomy in these situations. Finally, conversion from a MIDCAB approach to a sternotomy, either on or off bypass, is rare, but not unheard of. Situations that require conversion from a thoracotomy approach include patients with an inaccessible LAD (deeply intramyocardial, or technically difficult to graft on the beating heart), inadequate conduit, uncontrolled arrhythmias, or hemodynamic compromise.

SURGICAL TECHNIQUE

Different variations of the MIDCAB procedure are used, depending on the patient's specific need for revascularization. These various approaches include: (1) the left anterior thoracotomy performed through the fourth or fifth intercostal space (standard MIDCAB); (2) the xiphoid approach performed through the xiphisternum; (3) the left anterior thoracotomy combined with an infraclavicular incision for axillary artery inflow; (4) the endoscopic approach; (5) the posterior lateral thoracotomy, particularly in redo patients and those who need circumflex grafting only; and (6) the transabdominal approach as described by Subramanian *(18)*. Regardless of approach, it is of utmost importance to have an anesthesiologist who is proficient with anesthesia for off-pump surgery and can maintain a comfortable, safe working environment for the surgeon. Each of these approaches will be discussed separately.

Left Anterior Thoracotomy

The patient is positioned supine on the table. In our experience, we initially elevated the left chest with a rolled sheet, but have now abandoned this, as with current instrumentation it is easier to harvest the left internal mammary artery. External defibrillator pads are placed, particularly in redo patients. The positioning of these pads should allow for a sternotomy access. Routine coronary artery bypass graft prepping and draping is performed with exposure of the entire left the chest laterally over to the axilla. A 6- to 10-cm incision is made over the fourth intercostal space (ICS) (**Fig. 1**). This incision is usually just below the nipple, but may be placed above in asthenic men. The incision is started two fingerbreadths lateral to the midline. In women, performing the incision

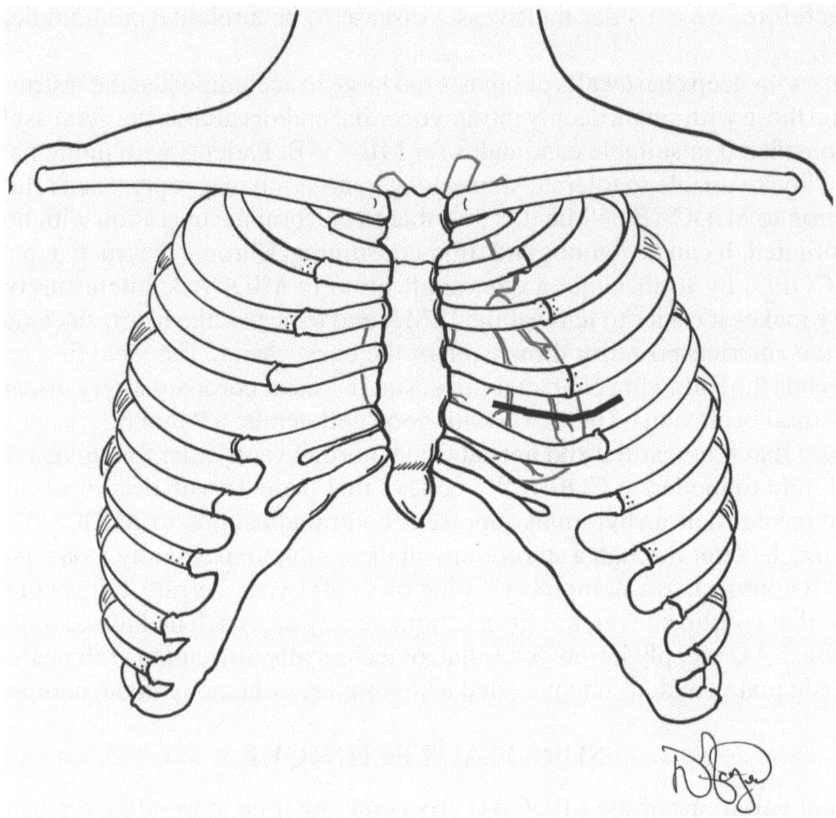

Fig. 1. The incision is performed at the fourth intercostal space, below the nipple.

1–2 cm below the inframammary crease allows for better healing, as there is not constant friction and maceration at the incision site. The pleural space is entered and the LIMA retractor (Guidant Corporation, Cupertino, CA) is inserted. A double-lumen endotracheal tube or bronchial blocker is used to collapse the ipsilateral lung; however, if necessary, the lung can be packed out of the way with warm lap packs. Care is taken to mobilize any pleural or cardiac adhesions (particularly in redos) prior to insertion and opening of the retractor, to prevent inadvertent damage to these organs. Dissection of the internal mammary artery under direct vision is the same as through the sternotomy except that it is from a mirror-image lateral location. Identification of the internal mammary artery medially is important prior to extensive dissection or traction, due to the possibility of injuring it before the pedicle has been mobilized. The endothoracic fascia is scored and mobilized. The collateral branches to the intercostal vessels are identified, clipped, and divided with electrocautery or scissors. The harmonic scalpel can also be used for the dissection. Mobilizing a short length of the LIMA pedicle without too much traction is important at the beginning of the dissection to prevent avulsion of the branches. The LIMA should be mobilized proximally to the subclavian vein and distally to one intercostal space below the incision (**Fig. 2**). A LIMA pedicle length of approx 15–17 cm is required for a tension-free anastomosis. The highest intercostal branch of the LIMA should be clipped and divided to prevent coronary steal. This phenomenon has seldom been seen in our experience; however, if identified in the postoperative period, the inter-

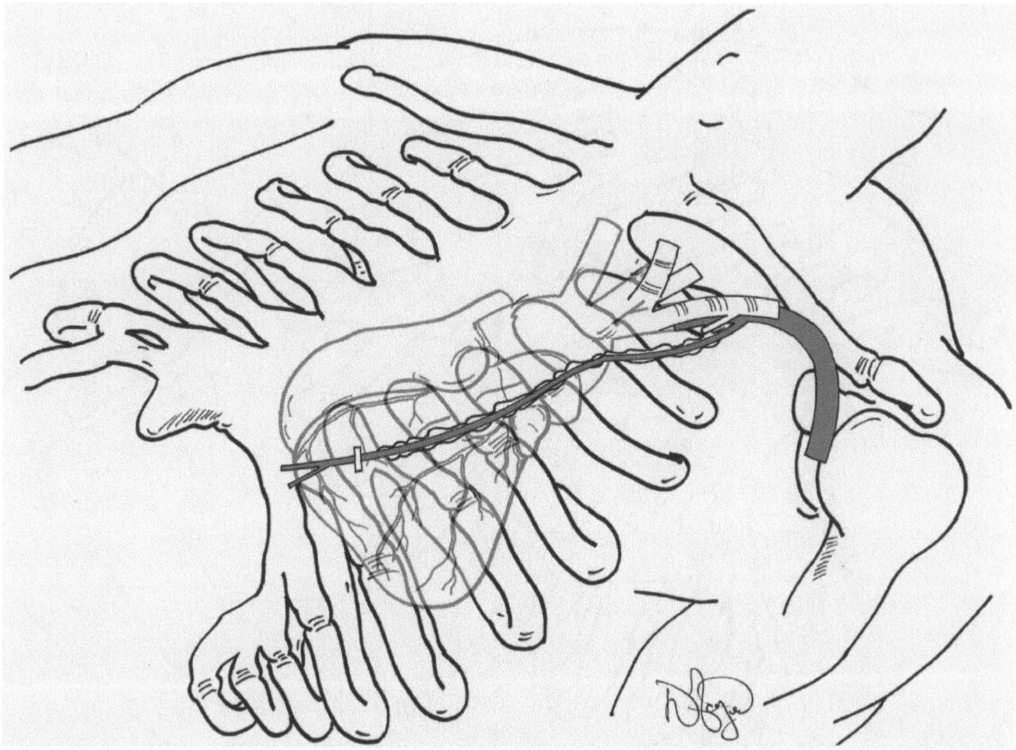

Fig. 2. The endothoracic fascia is incised and the LIMA dissected. The pedicle is freed proximally to the subclavian vein and to one intercostal space distal to the incision.

costal branch can be embolized percutaneously. The distal end of the internal mammary artery is freed and can be clipped after heparin has been administered. To prevent damage to the LIMA, we prefer harvesting the internal mammary artery as a pedicled rather than a skeletonized graft. Identification of the LAD can be performed prior to the LIMA dissection by opening the pericardium before starting the dissection. The pericardium is opened over the pulmonary artery and should be dissected distally to the apex and proximally to the mediastinal tissue. It is important to have studied the angiogram carefully so that the diagonal branches can be used as landmarks to locate the LAD and prevent inadvertently grafting the wrong vessel. The LAD can usually be identified as it emerges lateral to the pulmonary artery and courses medially to the apex. It behooves the surgeon to take a few moments to identify the LAD correctly, as ventricular enlargement or adhesions can alter the cardiac position and rotate the LAD out of view. Tension on the pericardium allows the surgeon to reposition the heart and bring the LAD into the surgical site. We currently use the Guidant MIDCAB system with separate retractors for the LIMA harvest and anastomosis. The LIMA retractor should be opened slowly, as this reduces the risk of rib fracture and pain. Once the LIMA has been harvested, the patient is systemically heparinized (3 mg/kg) and the LIMA is divided distally and prepared for grafting. Pericardial traction sutures are placed pulling the upper ones toward the left shoulder and the lower ones laterally, as this rotates the heart into the midline of the incision. The compression stabilizer is placed and the immobility of the graft site and presence of stable hemodynamics are confirmed prior to proceeding. Proximal occlusion

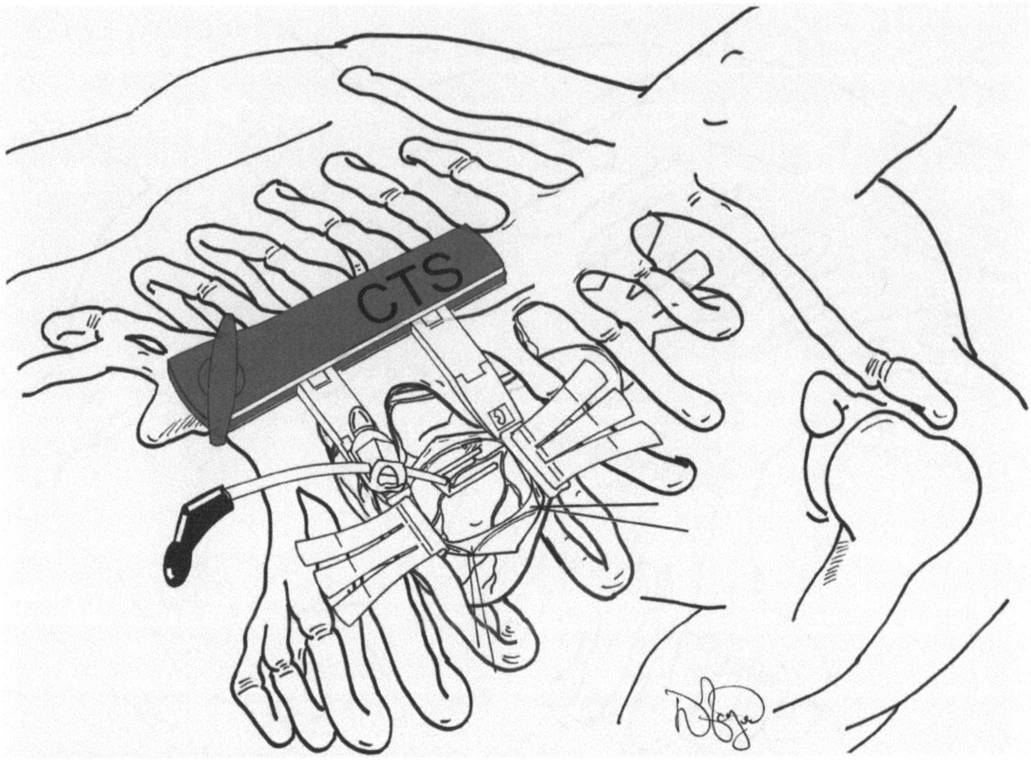

Fig. 3. The anastomosis is performed with local stabilization and proximal occlusion. A shunt can be used if necessary. The LAD is rotated into view with pericardial sutures.

of the LAD is obtained by passing a pledgeted silastic tape around the vessel (**Fig. 3**). If deemed necessary, a shunt may be placed. Preischemic conditioning is not routinely performed, but the anesthesiologist is notified prior to occlusion of the vessel. The LAD is then opened and the anastomosis is performed with running 7 or 8 prolene. The use of anastomotic clips may facilitate creation of this anastomosis. Once the anastomosis is completed, the LAD and LIMA should be flushed prior to tying the last suture or placing the last clip. We recommend tacking the LIMA pedicle to the epicardium. The pedicle should be attached medially to the mediastinal tissue without tension. It is necessary to reexpand the lung under direct vision to ensure that the lung rises over and not under the LIMA pedicle, so as to prevent the risk of avulsion of the pedicle. The heparin is fully reversed with protamine. Once hemostasis is adequate, the mediastinal fat pad is brought back over to cover the anastomosis. One Blake drain is placed in the left pleural space. Local anesthetic block in the intercostal spaces is performed with marcaine. The incision is closed in the usual fashion, first with pericostal sutures and then completing the other layers of tissue.

Left Anterior Thoracotomy with Axillary Artery Inflow

In patients in whom the LIMA cannot be used, i.e., in which the LIMA has been damaged in the harvest, or in redo patients with a previously used and occluded LIMA, or for LIMAs that have sustained radiation damage, a radial artery or saphenous vein can be used with axillary artery inflow. In these patients, once the LAD is identified and found

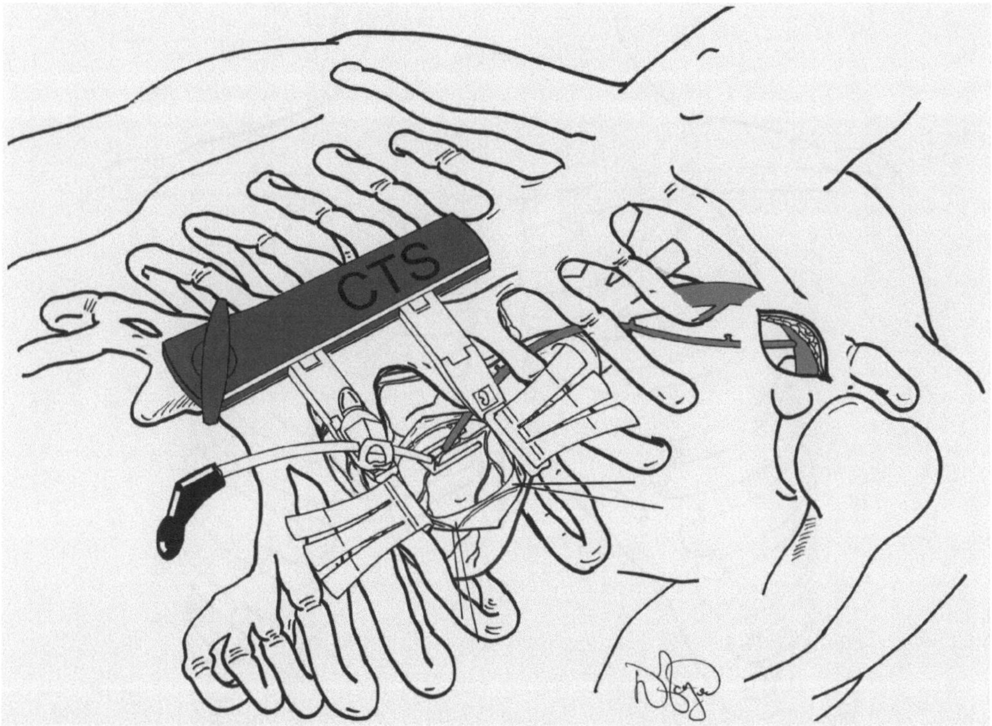

Fig. 4. The axillary artery is accessed through an infraclavicular incision. Once the proximal end of the graft is anastomosed to the axillary artery, it is tunneled in to the chest along the mediastinum to the LAD.

to be graftable, a segment of radial artery or saphenous vein is harvested. The axillary artery is then accessed through an infraclavicular incision. The proximal end of the conduit is then sewn to the axillary artery, then brought into the chest through the pectoral fascia in the first or second intercostal space. The conduit is then brought to the LAD with care to tack it to the mediastinal tissue to prevent avulsion from the lung (**Fig. 4**). The rest of the operation follows as described above for the left anterior thoracotomy.

T MIDCAB or H Graft

A variation of the left anterior thoracotomy MIDCAB known as the (T MIDCAB) or the (H Graft) has been described by Cohn, Caulson, and Wolfe *(19–21)*. In these cases, a limited anterior thoracotomy is performed and a short length of the LIMA is exposed. A segment of radial artery graft is then anastomosed between the LIMA and LAD. This allows for limited dissection, specifically in high-risk patients or those in whom dissection is difficult. Favorable results have been reported with this technique, but it is important to ligate the LIMA distally to prevent coronary steal.

Xiphoid MIDCAB

Calafiore has further validated the "standard " MIDCAB approach with the results of his limited-access small thoracotomy (LAST) operation *(22)*. It is important to note that patients have experienced more early postoperative pain than originally expected. Alternatively, another variation of the original MIDCAB is one in which a xiphoid approach

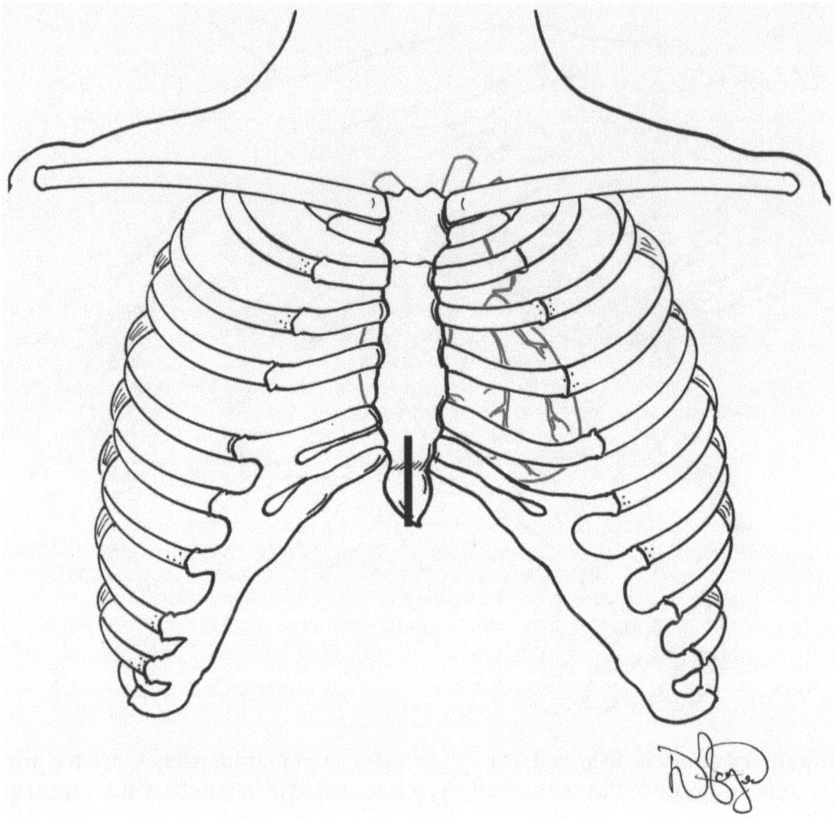

Fig. 5. A 7- to 8-cm incision is made over the xiphoid.

is taken to the distal LIMA and LAD *(23,24)*. The xiphoid MIDCAB appears to be a simpler, less painful approach than that through a left anterior thoracotomy.

A vertical midline 6- to 8-cm skin incision is made over the xiphoid (**Fig. 5**). The xiphoid process is then divided and the incision is extended into the lower sternum for one or two interspaces if necessary. A Rultract® mammary artery retractor is used to elevate the left side of the costal margin and the distal LIMA is identified. All efforts are made to leave the pleura intact during the dissection. The LIMA is harvested at a level proximal to the third to fourth interspace (**Fig. 6**). Heparin (10,000 units) is administered and the mammary artery is divided distally and prepared for grafting.

The pericardium is then opened and the edges retracted with sutures. These sutures allow the heart to be elevated and rotated medially with the assistance of a saline-filled glove placed in the pericardial well (**Fig. 7**). The LAD is then stabilized with a mechanical stabilizer and an arteriotomy is performed. Proximal occlusion may be obtained by the use of a pledgeted silastic tape surrounding the proximal LAD, or, alternatively, an appropriately sized intracoronary shunt is used to allow distal perfusion during the anastomosis (**Fig. 8**). Distal coronary occlusion is never used. A bloodless field is maintained with the use of a CO_2 blower. The LIMA-to-LAD anastomosis is performed with running 7-0 Prolene® and the pedicle is tacked to the epicardium (**Fig. 9**). The ventricle is then allowed to fall back into the pericardial well, and a trough is cut in the pericardium to

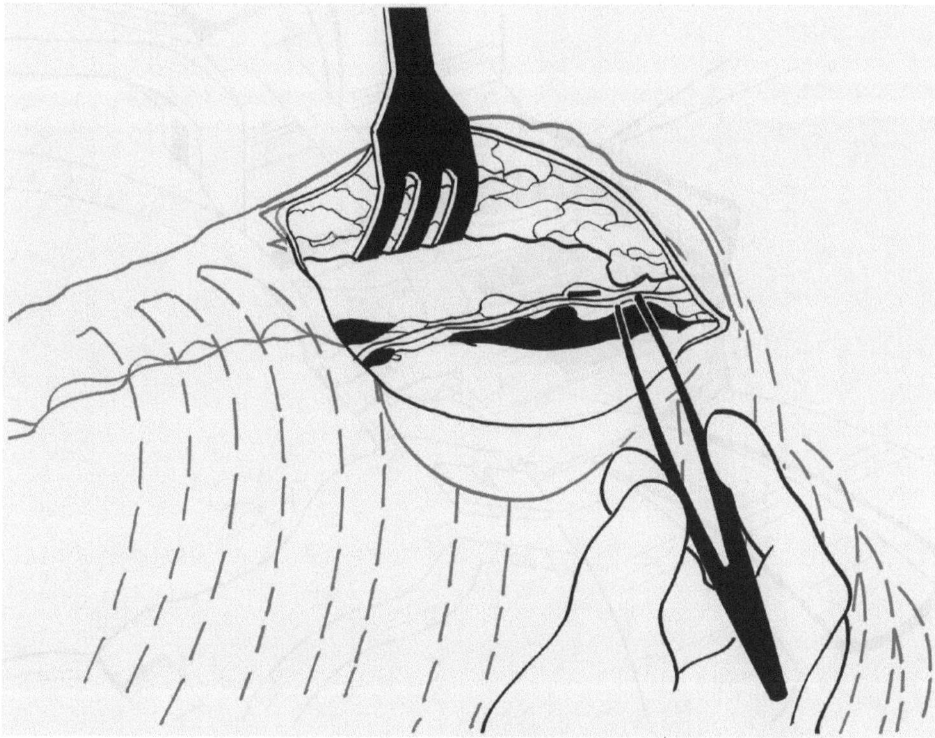

Fig. 6. The LIMA is harvested proximally to the third or fourth ICS.

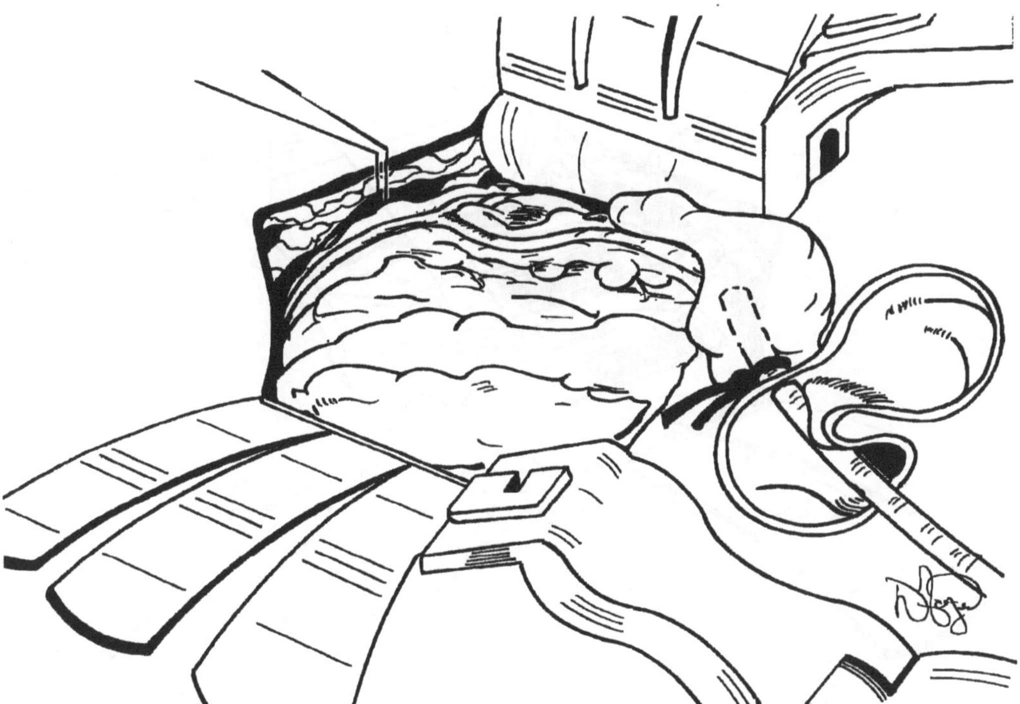

Fig. 7. The LAD is brought into view with the glove and pericardial sutures.

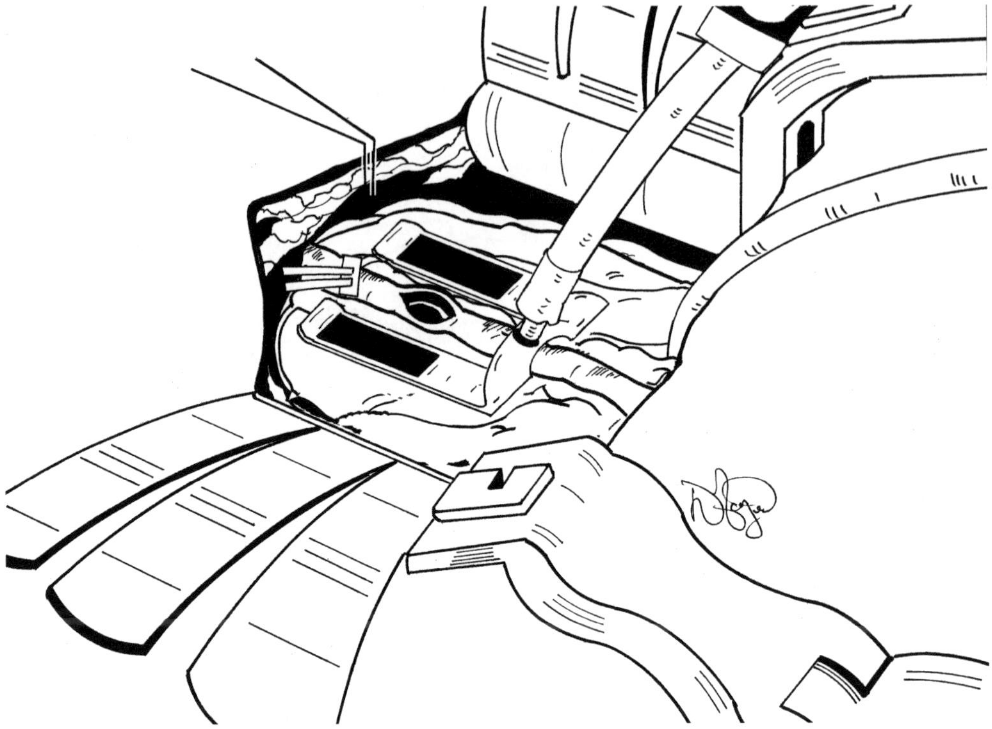

Fig. 8. The vessel is stabilized for the anastomosis.

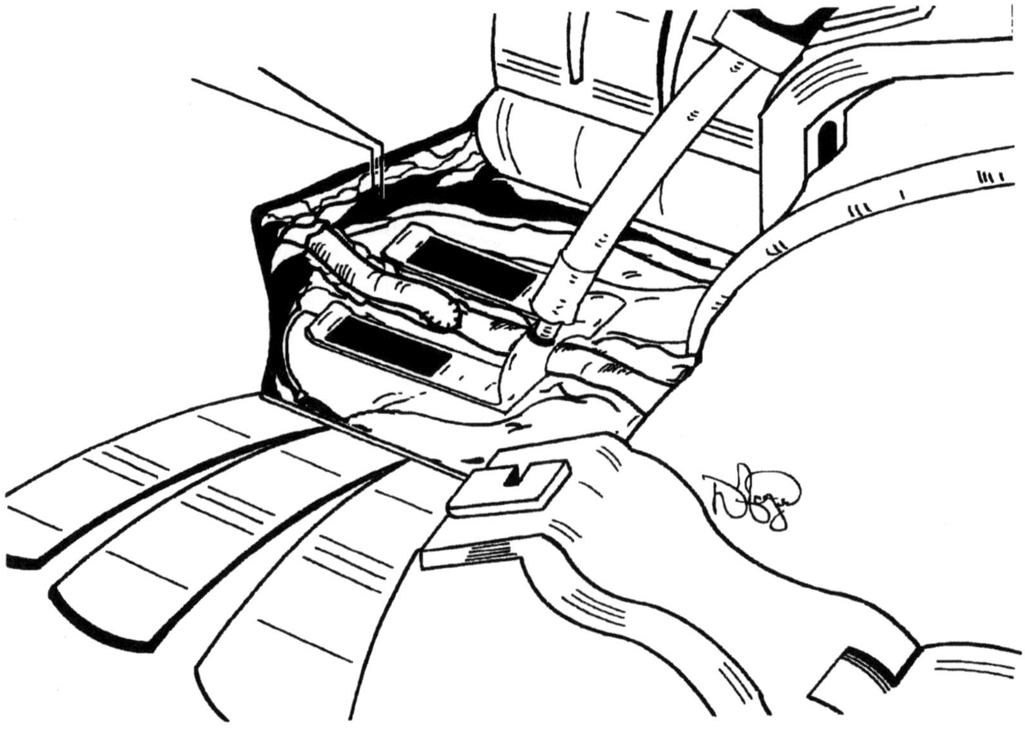

Fig. 9. Completed xiphoid MIDCAB anastomosis.

prevent kinking of the LIMA pedicle. A small soft drain is then placed in the pericardial well extending into the pleura (if it is open). Patients are usually extubated in the operating room and are kept in the intensive care unit overnight.

In a recent report of xiphoid MIDCAB *(24)*, 10 patients underwent LIMA to LAD grafting by this approach. Mean age was 73 yr (range 52–86). There were no reops, and most patients had multiple comorbidities with Parsonnet scores ranging from 3 to 41.5 *(25)*. Three patients underwent hybrid percutaneous intervention on the first postoperative day. Postoperative length of stay ranged from 3 d to 29 d, with the older and hybrid patients requiring longer stays. There were no deaths, but 2 of the hybrid patients had major complications resulting in a prolonged hospital stay. The first had pericardial tamponade and low cardiac output after receiving heparin on the first postoperative day for the placement of an intracoronary stent. This complication required reexploration and drainage. After the initial experience with this patient who suffered delayed tamponade, a soft drain was left in the pericardial well until the day after percutaneous revascularization in all subsequent hybrid patients. The second patient also had bleeding and low cardiac output after percutaneous intervention, requiring placement of an intra-aortic balloon pump.

Postoperative angiograms in the hybrid patients showed that the LIMA-to-LAD anastomoses were patent. Transthoracic Doppler evaluation was done in three nonhybrid patients and showed good diastolic augmentation, suggesting anastomotic patency. In this initial group of patients reported there were no mortalities and the postoperative complications were not compounded by the xiphoid incision.

Xiphoid MIDCAB is a safe and effective approach for grafting the LIMA to the LAD. The proximity of the distal LAD and distal LIMA to the left costal margin makes the anatomy favorable for this approach. By avoiding chest wall incisions and intercostal retraction, pain is lessened. We believe that the xiphoid approach to isolated LIMA-to-LAD anastomosis deserves further pursuit with controlled studies, comparing the morbidity and mortality from this procedure to alternative approaches for hybrid or isolated surgical revascularization.

Left Posterior Lateral Thoracotomy MIDCAB

The left lateral thoracotomy is the best approach when grafting vessels of the circumflex system *(18)*. It is a safe approach in redos, especially with patent LIMAs. The patient should be positioned to allow for femoral cannulation if necessary. External defibrillation pads should also be placed prior to starting the procedure, and the radial artery or saphenous vein conduits may need to be harvested before placing the patient in the right lateral decubitus position. A 10-cm thoracotomy is performed and the left lung is freed, mobilizing all adhesions and releasing the inferior pulmonary ligament up to the pulmonary vein. The circumflex vessel can be identified once the pericardium is opened, and can frequently be found by following the previous graft down to the target coronary vessel. The conduit can then be anastomosed to the descending thoracic aorta after heparinization. One note of caution with this proximal anastomosis is that there may be significant atherosclerotic disease in the descending aorta, which could affect the inflow. Proximal occlusion of the coronary artery is then obtained and the distal anastomosis can be performed. The compression stabilizers work best for this approach. Usually a shorter length of conduit will be needed for grafting the circumflex system through a left posterolateral thoracotomy rather than through a median sternotomy. The graft should be brought underneath the pulmonary ligament and measured prior to grafting, being careful

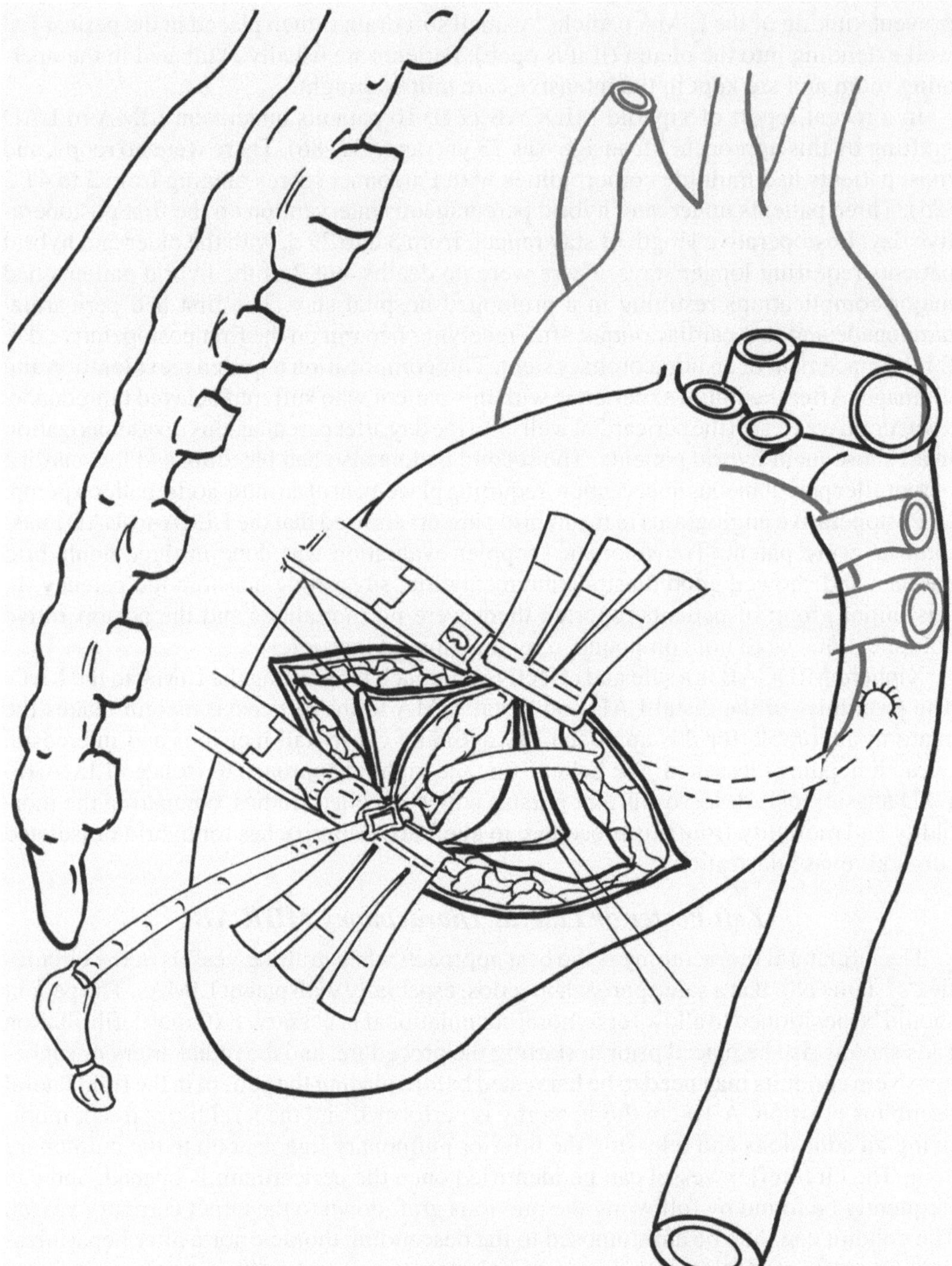

Fig. 10. The proximal end of the graft is attached to the descending thoracic aorta. The conduit is the passed below the inferior pulmonary ligament and anastomosed to the coronary artery. (Courtesy of Guidant Corporation, modification of original illustration by Michael Morejohn.)

to prevent kinking once the lung is reexpanded (**Fig. 10**). A pleural drainage tube is placed and then the chest closed in the usual fashion.

Endoscopic MIDCAB

Mack reported on the early use of thoracoscopically assisted coronary artery surgery for harvesting of the LIMA *(26)*. Other reports described thoracoscopically harvesting both LIMAs and then performing bilateral anterior small thoracotomy incisions for grafting the LAD and RCA systems *(27)*. The use of video assistance for minimally invasive coronary bypass has enjoyed great success as shown by Wolf *(28)*, and has advanced at many centers with excellent results.

This field has now progressed to robotic assistance, "RAVECAB," as described by Boyd in Ontario *(29,30)*, and TECAB, performed by Diegler's group in Germany *(31,32)*. Closed-chest totally endoscopic coronary bypass is no longer a fantasy and has now evolved into a reality with good early results *(33,34)*. Endoscopic and robotic surgery are described in detail in other chapters of this book.

POSTOPERATIVE RESULTS

Pain management and the development of multivessel beating-heart surgery have restricted the growth of conventional MIDCAB. The use of thoracic blocks, epidurals, and intrathecal morphine has not had the beneficial results expected in MIDCAB surgery, and many patients still experience early pain. However, these patients usually recover more quickly than sternotomy patients and are able to resume regular activities sooner. The majority of patients who have MIDCABs are extubated in the operating room or soon after in the intensive care unit. Early and late clinical outcomes have been excellent, and the angiographic results in these patients have shown durable patency. Calafiore *(35)* reported on 540 patients who were scheduled to undergo LIMA to LAD using his left anterior small thoracotomy (LAST) approach. In 5.2% of the patients, the LAST operation could not be performed for technical reasons. Thirty-day results included blood transfusions in 3.3%, reoperation for bleeding in 1.9%, atrial fibrillation in 9%; pericarditis in 1.2%, and delayed chest wound healing 2.9%. There was a 30-d 1% mortality and 1.2% late mortality. A total of 26 patients (5.1%) required reoperation, 3.5% within 30 d, and 1.6% later than 30 days. Three patients required repeat angioplasty, one patient within 30 d after the MIDCAB and two thereafter. Calafiore found that with increasing experience and improved instrumentation, the incidence of reoperation after his initial group decreased in his last 100 patients. Reoperation was required in one patient due to conduit occlusion. Mack and Magovern reported on a group of 103 patients undergoing MIDCAB operations from December 1996 through December 1997 *(36)*. Most of these patients (97%) underwent angiography, with 99% patency and 91% with Fitz-Gibbons grade A patency *(37)*. There were two operative noncardiac deaths, and in both patients patent grafts were documented. Three patients who underwent intraoperative angiography had graphs revised with improved flow. Incidence of reoperation for bleeding, stroke, and atrial fibrillation were 3.9%, 9%, and 1.7%, respectively. Interestingly, early angiography after MIDCAB has demonstrated that early stenosis (not occlusion) often resolves within 6–10 mo on angiographic follow-up. A recent report by Diegler and his group *(38)* showed early and 6-mo patency rates of the LIMA-to-LAD anastomosis of 97% and 95%, respectively, with a 3% reintervention rate. Mehran et al. *(39)* reported on our single-center experience with MIDCABs in 274 patients. The mortality was lower in the latter 174 patients than in the initial 100; however, this was not statistically significant. There was a 4% occurrence of major adverse cardiac events in the initial group and 1% in the last group. At 1 yr, the reintervention rate was approximately 2.9% and the actuarial survival rate was 98% in both groups. In the year after surgery, none of the patients who had angiographic follow-up in the study showed a restenosis of the arterial bypass conduit.

Undoubtedly, there is a learning curve associated with the MIDCAB operation. Despite this, it has been shown that this procedure can be performed with excellent clinical results and, in an effort to tailor the bypass operation to our patients, MIDCAB should be part of the armamentarium of every coronary surgeon.

REFERENCES

1. Vineberg AM. Development of anastomosis between coronary vessels and transplanted mammary artery. Med Assoc J 1954;71:594.
2. Kolessov VI. Mammary artery-coronary anastomosis as method of treatment for angina pectoris. J Thorac Cardiovasc Surg 1967;54:535–544.
3. Sabiston DC. The coronary circulation. Johns Hopkins Med J 1974:314.
4. Ankeny JL. To use or not to use the pump oxygenator in coronary bypass operations. Ann Thorac Surg 1975;19:108–109.
5. Favoloro RG, et al. Current status of coronary artery bypass graft (CABG) surgery. Semin Thorac Cardiovasc Surg 1994;6:67–71.
6. Garrett HE, Dennid EW, DeBakey ME. Aorto-coronary bypass with saphenous vein graft:seven year follow up. JAMA 1973;223:792–794.
7. Trapp WG, Bisarya R. Replacement of coronary artery bypass graft without pump oxygenator. Ann Thorac Surg 1975;19:1–8.
8. Benetti FJ. Direct coronary surgery with saphenous vein bypass without either cardiopulmonary bypass or cardiac arrest. J Cardiovasc Surg 1985;26:217–222.
9. Benetti FJ, Nasellli G, Wood M, Geffner L. Direct myocardial revascularization without extracorporeal circulation. Experience in 700 patients. Chest 1991;100:312–316.
10. Pfister AJ, Zaki MS, Garcia JM, et al. Coronary artery bypass without cardiopulmonary bypass. Ann Thorac Surg 1992;54:1085–1091.
11. Subramanian VA, Sani G, Benetti FJ, Calafiore AM. Minimally invasive coronary bypass surgery: a multicenter report of preliminary clinical experience. Circulation 1995(suppl 8);92:S1645.
12. Cohen HA, Zenati M. Integrated coronary revascularization J Invasive Cardiol 1999;11(3):184–191.
13. Farahat F, Depuydt F, VanPraet F, et al. Hybrid cardiac revascularization using a totally closed-chest robotic technology and a percutaneous transluminal coronary dilatation. Heart Surg Forum 2000;9403.
14. Bonatti J, Coulson A, Bakhshay S, Posch L, Sloan T. The subclavian and axillary arteries as inflow vessels for coronary artery bypass grafts—combined experience from three cardiac centers. Heart Surg Forum 2000;741718.
15. Flege JB, Wolf RK, Minimally invasive axillary—coronary artery bypass. Heart Surg Forum 2000;3(3):238–240.
16. Shabb B, Khalil I. Minimally invasive axillary–LAD saphenous vein bypass. Heart Surg Forum 1999;2(3):254–255.
17. Baumgartner FJ, Gheissari A, Panagiotides GP, et al. Off-pump obtuse marginal grafting with local stabilization: thoracotomy approach. Ann Thorac Surg 1999(Sep);68(3):946–948.
18. Subramanian VA, Patel NU. Transabdominal minimally invasive direct coronary artery bypass grafting (MIDCAB). Eur J Cardiothorac Surg 2000;17(4):485–487.
19. Cohn W, Suen H, Weintraub R, Johnson R. The "H" graft: an alternative approach for performing minimally invasive direct coronary artery bypass. J Thorac Cardiovasc Surg 1998;115:148–151.
20. Coulson A, Bakshay S. The "T-MIDCAB" procedure. Use of extension grafts from the undisturbed LIMA in high risk patients. Heart Surg Forum 1998;1(1):54–59.

21. Miyaji K, Wolf R, Flege J. Minimally invasive direct coronary artery bypass using H graft for pleural symphysis. Ann Thorac Surg 1999;68(1):234–235.
22. Calafiore AM, DeGiammarco GD, Teodori G, et al. Left anterior descending coronary artery grafting via left anterior small thoracotomy without cardiopulmonary bypass. Ann Thorac Surg 1996;61: 1658–1665.
23. Benetti F. Minimally invasive coronary surgery (the xyphoid approach). Eur J Cardiothorac Surg 1999;16(suppl 12):S10–S11.
24. Dullum M, , Block J, Benetti F, et al. Xiphoid MIDCAB: report of the technique and experience with a less invasive MIDCAB. Heart Surg Forum 1999;2(1):77–81.
25. Parsonnet V, Dean D, Bernstein AD. A method of uniform stratification of risk for evaluating the results of surgery in acquired adult heart disease. Circulation 1989;79:(suppl 1):I3–I12.
26. Mack M, Acuff T, Yong P, Jett G, Carter D. Minimally invasive thoracoscopically assisted coronary artery bypass surgery. Eur J Cardiothorac Surg 1997;12(1):20–24.
27. Watanabe G, Misaki T, Kotoh K, Yamashita A, Ueyama K. Bilateral thoracoscopic minimally invasive direct coronary artery bypass grafting using internal thoracic arteries. Ann Thorac Surg 1998;65(6):1673–1675.
28. Kagami M, Wolf R, Flege J. Surgical results of video-assisted minimally invasive direct coronary artery bypass. Ann Thorac Surg 1998;67:1018–1021.
29. Boyd W, Kiaii B, Novick R, et al. RAVECAB: improving outcome in off-pump minimal access surgery with robotic assistance and video enhancement. Can J Surg 2001;44(1):45–50.
30. Kiaii B, Boyd W, Rayman R, et al. Robot-assisted computer enhanced closed-chest coronary surgery: preliminary experience using a harmonic scalpel (R) and Zeus (TM). Heart Surg Forum 2000;3(3):194–197.
31. Falk V, Diegler A, Walther T, et al. Total endoscopic computer enhanced coronary artery bypass grafting. Eur J Cardiothorac Surg 2000;17(1):38–45.
32. Falk V, Diegler A, Walther T, et al. Total endoscopic off-pump coronary artery bypass grafting. Heart Surg Forum 2000;3 (1):29–31.
33. Kappert U, Schneider J, Cichon R, et al. Closed chest totally endoscopic coronary artery bypass surgery: fantasy or reality? Curr Card Rep 2000;2(6):558–563.
34. Kappert U, Schneider J, Cichon R, et al. Robotic coronary artery surgery—the evolution of a new minimally invasive approach in coronary artery surgery. Thorac Cardiovasc Surg 2000;48(4):193–197.
35. Calafiore A, Contini M, et al. Minimally invasive coronary artery bypass grafting on the beating heart: the European experience. In: Oz MC, Goldstein DJ, eds. Minimally Invasive Cardiac Surgery. Totowa, NJ: Humana Press, 1999:110–113.
36. Mack M, Magovern J, Acuff T, et al Results of graft patency by immediate angiography in minimally invasive coronary artery surgery. Ann Thorac Surg 1999;68(1):383–390.
37. FitzGibbon G, Kafka H, Leach A, et al. Coronary artery bypass graft fate and patient outcome: angiographic follow-up of 5,065 grafts related to survival and reoperation in 1,388 patients during 25 years. J Am Coll Cardiol 1996;28:616–626.
38. Diegler A, Matin M, Falk V, et al. Coronary bypass grafting without cardiopulmonary bypass: technical considerations, clinical results, and follow-up. Thorac Cardiovasc Surg 1999;47(1):14–18.
39. Mehran R, Dangas G, Stamou SC, et al. One-year clinical outcome after minimally invasive direct coronary artery bypass. Circulation 2000;102:2799–2802.

10 Minimally Invasive Coronary Artery Bypass Grafting on the Beating Heart

The European Experience

Antonio M. Calafiore, MD,
Michele Di Mauro, MD, *Alessandro Pardini*, MD,
Antonio Bivona, MD,
and Stefano D'Alessandro, MD

CONTENTS

INTRODUCTION
LEFT ANTERIOR SMALL THORACOTOMY (LAST OPERATION)
MEDIAN STERNOTOMY
DISCUSSION
REFERENCES

INTRODUCTION

The prospect of grafting the internal mammary artery (IMA) to the left anterior descending (LAD) artery via a thoracotomy without the aid of cardiopulmonary bypass (CPB) was first explored by Kolessov in 1967 *(1)*, and further applied by Favaloro *(2)*, Garrett *(3)*, Trapp *(4)*, and others. The early wave of enthusiasm for this technique soon wavered with the widespread availability of CPB and cardioplegia, which allowed for a motionless and bloodless operative field. The unequivocal and widespread success of conventional coronary artery bypass grafting (CABG) limited the use of unsupported bypass grafting. Two developments in the early 1990s revived the technique of myocardial revascularization without CPB: (1) the emergence of minimally invasive technology applicable to the chest, and (2) the promising results of "pumpless" bypass grafting reported by a number of authors *(5–7)*.

In our opinion, the definition of minimally invasive cardiac surgery encompasses all approaches that avoid cardiopulmonary bypass, regardless of mode of surgical access

From: *Contemporary Cardiology: Minimally Invasive Cardiac Surgery, Second Edition*
Edited by: D. J. Goldstein and M. C. Oz © Humana Press Inc., Totowa, NJ

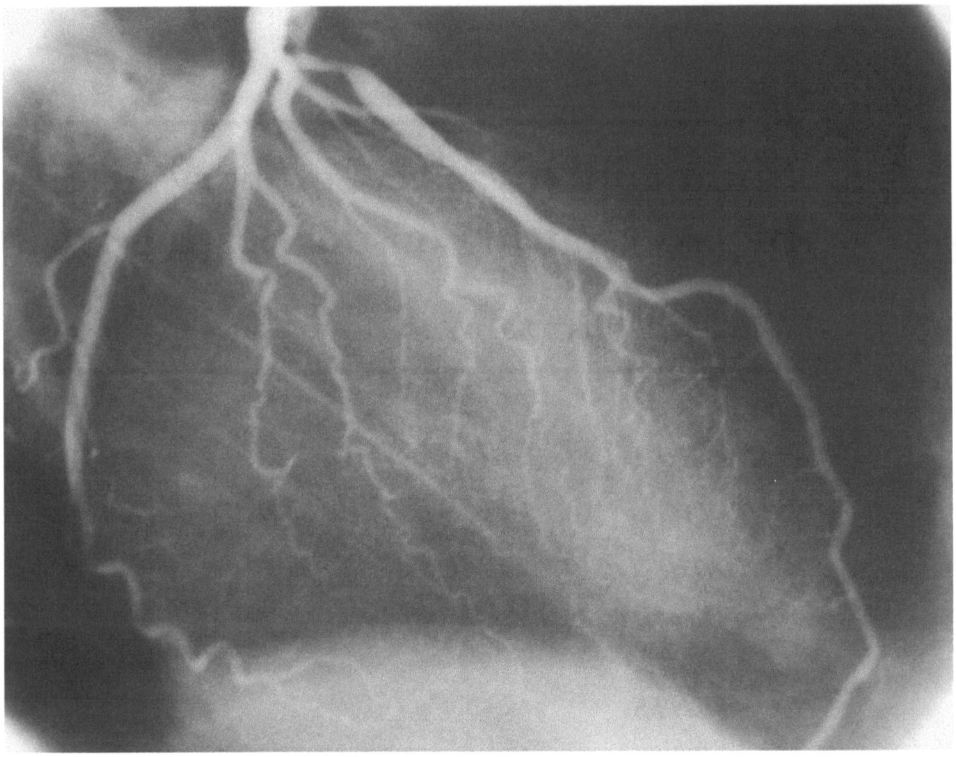

Fig. 1. Angiographic demonstration of an intramyocardial LAD. This constitutes a contraindication to off-pump grafting.

(i.e., full sternotomy, thoracotomy, etc.). In this chapter, we report our experience with myocardial revascularization without CPB utlilizing two different approaches: (1) the left anterior small thoracotomy and (2) the median sternotomy.

LEFT ANTERIOR SMALL THORACOTOMY (LAST OPERATION)

The promising clinical reports of minimally invasive coronary artery bypass grafting (MICABG) demonstrating excellent early patency, low morbidity and mortality, and shortened hospital stays stimulated a worldwide interest in these techniques. Our group popularized MICABG through a left anterior small thoracotomy, coining the term the "LAST" operation *(8)*.

Surgical Indications

Candidates for the LAST operation include patients with isolated LAD disease in whom a percutaneous transluminal coronary angioplasty (PTCA) was unsuccessful, impossible (occluded LAD), or contraindicated (proximal and/or complex stenoses). Patients with two-vessel disease (right coronary or circumflex plus LAD) in which the non-LAD vessel is occluded and recanalized or with a mild stenosis or stenosis that could be dilated are also considered. In addition, patients with multivessel disease in which the lesion in the other vessels can be addressed percutaneously (hybrid approach explored elsewhere in this book) are suitable candidates. Finally, patients for whom extracorporeal circulation is deemed a high-risk undertaking, including patients with malignancies, renal failure, generalized vasculopathy, coagulation disorders, and advanced age, are also considered.

Contraindications to the LAST operation are limited to anatomic considerations and are strictly related to the impossibility of performing the left internal mammary artery (LIMA) to left anterior descending artery (LAD) anastomosis because of an unsuitable or unreachable LAD. In some patients, unfavorable conditions can be detected preoperatively. Presence of left subclavian stenosis or occlusion precludes the LAST operation because it can result in a coronary steal syndrome *(9,10)*. An intramyocardial vessel, often discernible at angiography (**Fig. 1**), is also an absolute contraindication. The latter is best diagnosed on angiographic oblique right anterior projections in which the vessel is seen to progress downward and then, after a few centimeters, turn upward (toward the epicardium). An LAD of <1.5 mm or a calcified LAD preclude this approach. Exquisite attention must be given to the area 2–4 cm distal to the second diagonal branch because this is the usual anastomotic site. We rely on the evaluation of different angiographic projections to show the internal size of the distal LAD, the quality of its walls, and its position relative to the epicardial surface. In the majority of cases, however, the final decision to proceed or not with the LAST approach is made at operation.

Surgical Technique

After establishing hemodynamic monitoring, general endotracheal anesthesia with a single-lumen endotracheal tube is instituted. Early in our experienee, we relied on the use of double-lumen endotracheal tubes to optimize left-sided exposure. With increased experience, we have abandoned its routine use.

In our most recent experience, anesthesia was induced with fentanyl (2 µg/kg) and propofol (2.0–2.5 mg/kg) and was maintained with fentanyl in bolus (0.8 µg/kg) and propofol (0.4–1.2 µg/kg) in continuous infusion. Muscular relaxation was obtained with atracurium besilatum. During the closure of the chest, the infusion of propofol was reduced and then stopped, to achieve a rapid awakening of the patient and, if possible, his or her disconnection from mechanical ventilation. As soon as the chest was closed, a continuous infusion of agents (90 mg/24 h ketoralac, 10 mg/24 h metoclopramide, and 200 mg/24 h tramadol) was started for at least 24 h.

Access to the heart is obtained via LAST in the fourth or fifth intercostal space, depending on angiographic criteria. The pleural cavity is entered, the ribs are retracted, and the pericardium is incised parallel to the sternum. The LAD is inspected and the feasibility of the operation is considered. In the presence of any contraindication (as described above), the chest is closed and median sternotomy is performed. In the first part of our experience the LIMA was harvested for a short length (4–5 cm), usually extending from the superior intercostal space to the level of the inferior rib. In our early experience, if the LAD lay excessively lateral, the inferior epigastric artery was used to prolong the LAD in an end-to-end fashion (**Fig. 2**). Occasionally, a saphenous vein graft would be used to achieve the necessary length (**Fig. 3**). This technique has been reported previously *(11)*. Since April 1997, the availability of better instruments has allowed us to procure a longer segment of the LAD. Indeed, the IMA Access Retractor (CardioThoracic Systems, Cupertino, CA) has allowed extended IMA dissection to the level of the bifurcation inferiorly and first rib superiorly. Following systemic heparinization (1 mg/kg), 3 mL of papaverine (1 mg/mL) are injected into the LIMA, and the vessel is clipped distally *(11)*.

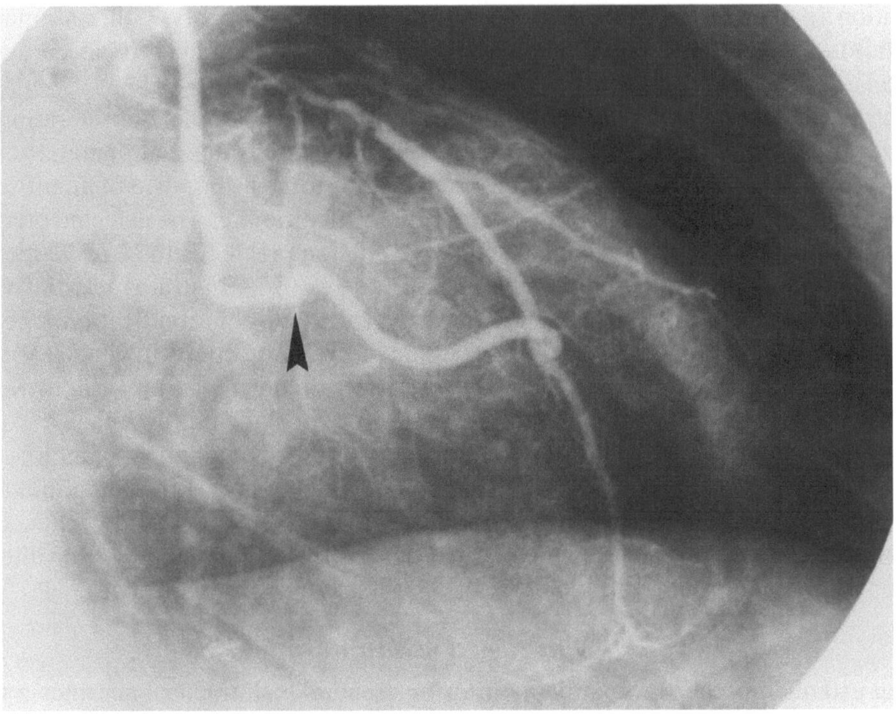

Fig. 2. The inferior epigastric artery is anastomosed end to end to the LIMA to allow grafting of an abnormally lateral LAD.

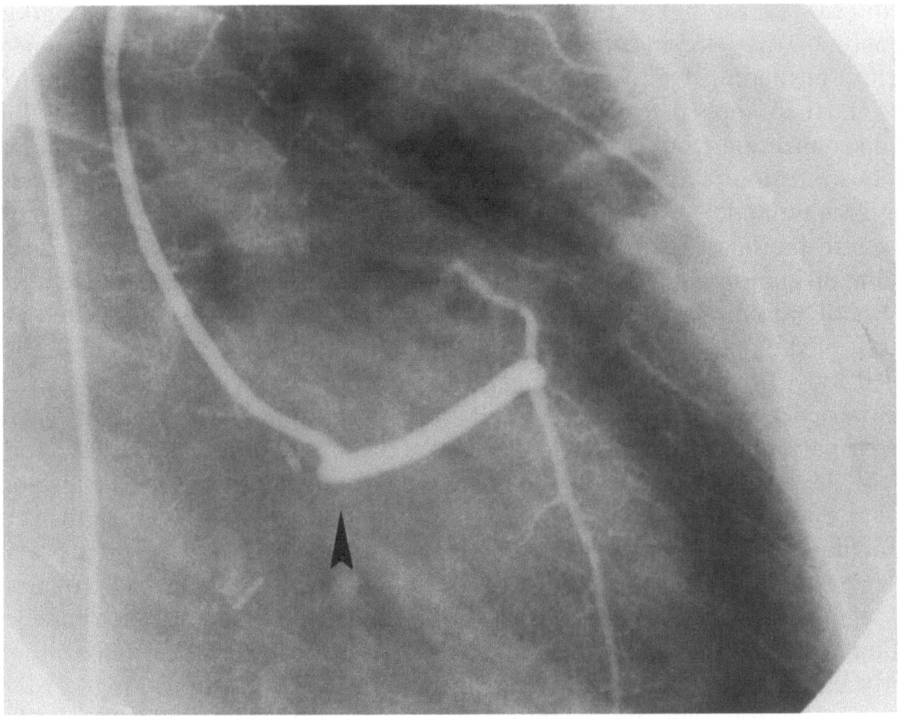

Fig. 3. Use of an interposition saphenous vein graft to achieve LIMA-LAD grafting in a laterally placed LAD.

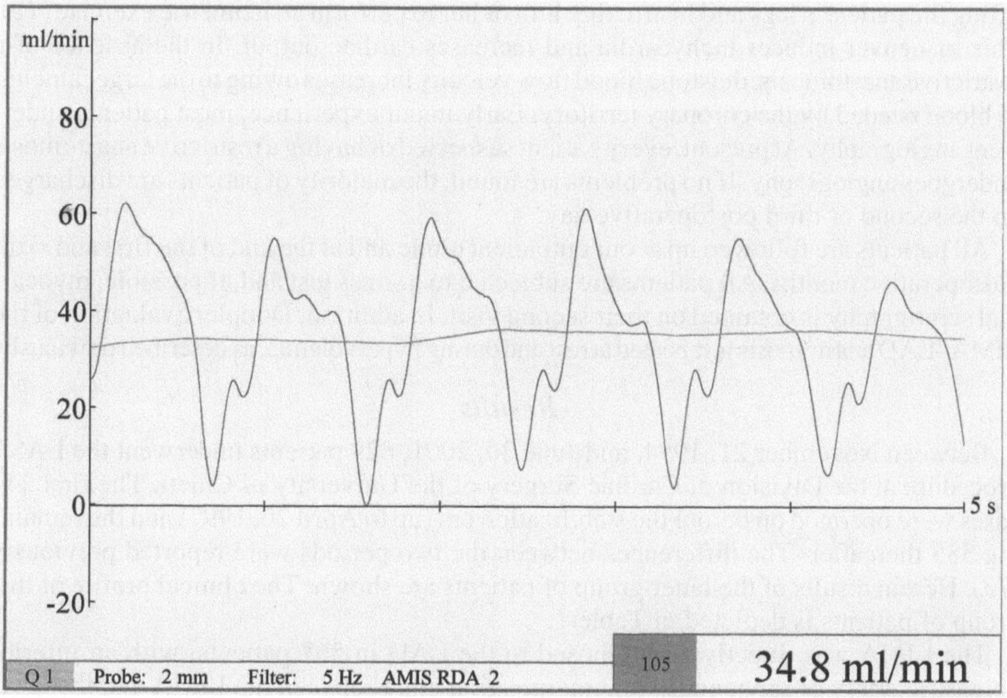

Fig. 4. Flow meter: mean flow and the shape of the curve.

The LAD is then occluded proximally and distally using a 4-0 Prolene suture with a 25-mm needle, snared on a small piece of silicone tubing, to avoid direct compression of the coronary artery. A stabilizer with two feet connected to the retractor is positioned parallel to the LAD and pushed down gently. This maneuver minimizes the effect of the beating heart on the operative field, making the LAD virtually motionless. No preconditioning of the distal LAD territory is performed.

The distal LIMA is prepared in the usual fashion. The anastomotic site of the LAD is dissected and incised with a scalpel for a distance of 4–5 mm. The anastomosis is created using two running sutures of 8-0 Prolene. The anastomosis is created by "parachuting" the stitches at the heel and apex, and the anastomosis is completed by running the Prolene sutures in standard vascular fashion. The LIMA and LAD are unclamped and meticulous hemostasis is obtained. The flow inside the graft is then measured with a flowmeter (Transonic, Ithaca, NY, USA, and Medi-Stim, Oslo, Norway) evaluating both the mean flow and the shape of the curve (**Fig. 4**).

During the first part of our experience, we routinely reversed the heparin with a 1:1 dose of protamine, but we have abandoned heparin reversal more recently. A thoracotomy tube is positioned in the chest along with a small catheter, which is used to infuse analgesics. The wound is closed in the usual manner.

Postoperative Course

The patient is extubated in the operating room, or shortly after arrival at the intensive care unit. Routine blood samples, electrocardiogram, and chest roentgenogram are obtained. After a few hours of observation, the patient is transferred to the ward. The chest tube and pleural catheter are removed on the morning of the first postoperative day. Evaluation of LIMA flow is repeated at rest and after acutely induced hypervolemia, by lifting the patient's legs and instructing him or her to perform an isometric exercise *(12)*. This maneuver induces tachycardia and increases cardiac output. In the absence of a restrictive anastomosis, diastolic blood flow velocity increases owing to the larger amount of blood needed by the coronary territory. Early in our experience, most patients underwent angiography. At present, every patient suspected of having a restrictive anastomosis undergoes angiography. If no problems are found, the majority of patients are discharged on the second or third postoperative day.

All patients are followed up at our outpatient clinic and at the end of the first and sixth postoperative months. All patients are subjected to a stress test and, if possible, myocardial scintigraphy is obtained on their second visit. In addition, Doppler evaluation of the LIMA–LAD anastomosis is repeated at rest and during hypervolemia, as described previously.

Results

Between November 21, 1994, and June 30, 2001, 829 patients underwent the LAST procedure at the Division of Cardiac Surgery of the University of Chieti. The first 244 cases were operated on before the stabilization era (up to April 20, 1997) and the remaining 585 thereafter. The differences between the two periods were reported previously *(13)*. Herein results of the latter group of patients are shown. The clinical profile of this group of patients is depicted in Table 1.

The LIMA was directly anastomosed to the LAD in 562 patients, with an inferior epigastric artery or saphenous vein interposition graft between the LIMA and the LAD in 18 patients. In two patients the LIMA was used to graft a diagonal branch; in four redo cases, a saphenous vein was used from axillary artery to LAD, and in two patients a radial artery was used as a bridge from the *in situ* LIMA to the LAD. Mean occlusion time was 17.2 ± 6.2 min, distal anastomotic time was 9.5 ± 8.1 min, and mean operation time was 2.0 ± 0.6 h. Postoperative data are displayed in Table 2. All patients had Doppler flow evaluation, at rest or during Azoulay maneuver, angiography, or both. Globally, the patency rate was 99.1% and the incidence of perfect anastomosis was 98.1%.

Among the 585 patients who underwent the LAST procedure, early and late mortality were 2.9% and 1.9%, respectively. Early deaths were due to cardiac causes in four cases (sudden death due to infero-lateral myocardial infarction with widely patent graft at necropsy in two cases; low output syndrome, preoperatively present and not reversed by the graft, widely patent at necropsy; cardiac tamponade in a patient who had a successful stent placement on the right coronary artery 3 d after the LAST procedure), and not cardiac-related in two cases (cerebral hemorrhage, abdominal complication).

Late deaths were cardiac in six instances (three sudden deaths and two acute myocardial infarction) and not cardiac-related in five cases (one cerebrovascular accident, three malignancies, and one car accident).

Eight patients (1.4%) were reoperated on, due to conduit occlusion (seven) or anastomotic malfunction (one). All patients underwent an uneventful reoperation, via median sternotomy. Nine patients (1.5%) required percutaneous intervention, four due to progression of LAD disease progression, and five on another coronary territory.

At a mean follow-up of 38.5 ± 15.1 mo, 569 patients (97.3%) are alive and asymptomatic with or without medical treatment; 554 patients (94.7%) are alive, asymptomatic, and without a repeated surgical or cardiological intervention on the LAD.

Five-year survival and event-free survival were 96.1 ± 1.0 and 93.2 ± 1.2, respectively (**Fig. 5**).

With increasing experience and new instruments, angiographic results are improving. We reported recently our early angiographic results. In a series of 190 patients, patency

Table 1
Clinical Profile of 585 Patients Undergoing the LAST Operation

Age	
Mean	62 ± 10 yr
Range	32–88
≥ 75 yr	56 (10.8%)
Female	74 (12.6%)
Urgent	75 (12.8%)
Single-LAD disease	295 (50.4%)
EF (%)	
Mean	61 ± 12
Range	15–90
≤ 35%	13 (2.2%)
Diabetes	101 (17.3%)
Previous MI	262 (44.8%)
Redo	34 (5.8%)
Other comorbidities[a]	126 (21.5%)

[a]Age ≥ 75, malignancy, coagulopathy, HIV, diffuse cerebrovascular disease, chronic renal failure.

Table 2
Postoperative Data for 585 Patients Undergoing LAST Operation

Extubation by 2 h	495 (84.6%)
Reop for bleeding	17 (2.9%)
Transfusion	22 (3.8%)
ICU length of stay (h)	6.6 ± 8.3
Stroke	0
Perioperative MI	2 (0.3%)
Atrial fibrillation	50 (8.3%)
Postoperative length of stay (d)	3.1 ± 1.2
Discharged by postop day	187 (32%)

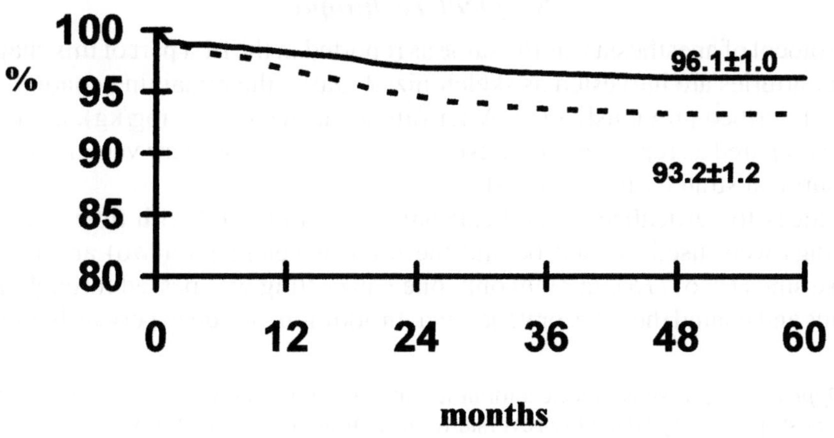

Fig. 5. Five-year survival and event-free survival (LAST operation).

rate was 98.9% and perfect patency rate was 97.4 *(14)*. After a mean follow-up of 11.1 ± 9.5 mo, patency rate and perfect patency rate were 94.4% (34/36) and 91.7% (33/36), respectively.

An unexpected finding occurred during our experience. Six patients with anastomotic or conduit anomalies on postoperative evaluation showed reversal to normal anatomy after a mean period of 94 ± 56 d from the first angiography (**Fig. 6A,B**). We feel this is due to adventitial hematomas or clots that resolve with time. At present, decisions to reoperate on the basis of an imperfect angiographic appearance of the anastomosis or of the conduit are delayed for 2 mo, at which time the angiography is repeated *(8)*.

MEDIAN STERNOTOMY

Between January 1995 and May 20, 1997, only patients with favorable anatomy were considered for off-pump coronary bypass grafting. However, among them, the procedure was performed only in patients with high risk factors for institution of cardiopulmonary bypass (CPB), as marginal branch or posterior descending artery grafting was difficult and cumbersome. The remaining patients had only grafts to the LAD, diagonal branches, or right coronary artery proximal to the crux. During this period, only 129 patients were operated on without CPB (13.3% of the patients operated on with median sternotomy), with 2 conversions to CPB (1.6%).

In May 1997, we introduced a technique for heart verticalization that allowed exposure of the lateral and inferior walls *(15)*. Thereafter, the incidence of patients operated on without CPB rose through June 30, 2001, to 50% (1134/2268, with 54 conversions or 4.8%).

Clinical and angiographic election criteria utilized in this group of patients included: (1) the coronary vessels had to be epicardial, with an internal size diameter >1.2 mm and with no calcifications at the level of the anastomotic site; (2) the marginal branches had to be long, with a uniform internal size up to the midportion of the vessel, as this is often the anastomotic site; (3) electric stability had to be present, as the risk of severe ventricular arrhythmias during manipulation is high; (4) while ejection fraction *per se* was not a contraindication for beating-heart revascularization, an enlarged heart can make the exposure of the lateral wall difficult; (5) need for multiple sequential grafts was considered a contraindication up to the end of December 1997, as we concentrated our attention in obtaining a good end-to-side anastomosis. Since January 1998, sequential grafts have been routinely performed without CPB if necessary.

Surgical Technique

The protocol of anesthesia was the same as reported in the first part of this chapter. The mammary arteries are harvested as skeletonized grafts; the remaining conduits are harvested as described previously *(12)*. After full heparinization (3 mg/kg), all the arterial grafts are prepared as reported previously *(11)*.The target coronary vessels are explored and the surgical strategy is confirmed.

Techniques to verticalize of the heart have been modified with time. At first, four gauze slings were used, passed behind the inferior vena cava (two) and through the transverse sinus (two) *(15)*. In 1999 only one gauze sling was passed through the transverse sinus and behind the inferior vena cava. In addition, one deep pericardial suture was

---

Fig. 6. (*Opposite page*) Anastomotic anomalies, at first angiography on postoperative day 2 (**A**), and 4 mo postoperatively (**B**). Note reversal to normal-appearing anatomy.

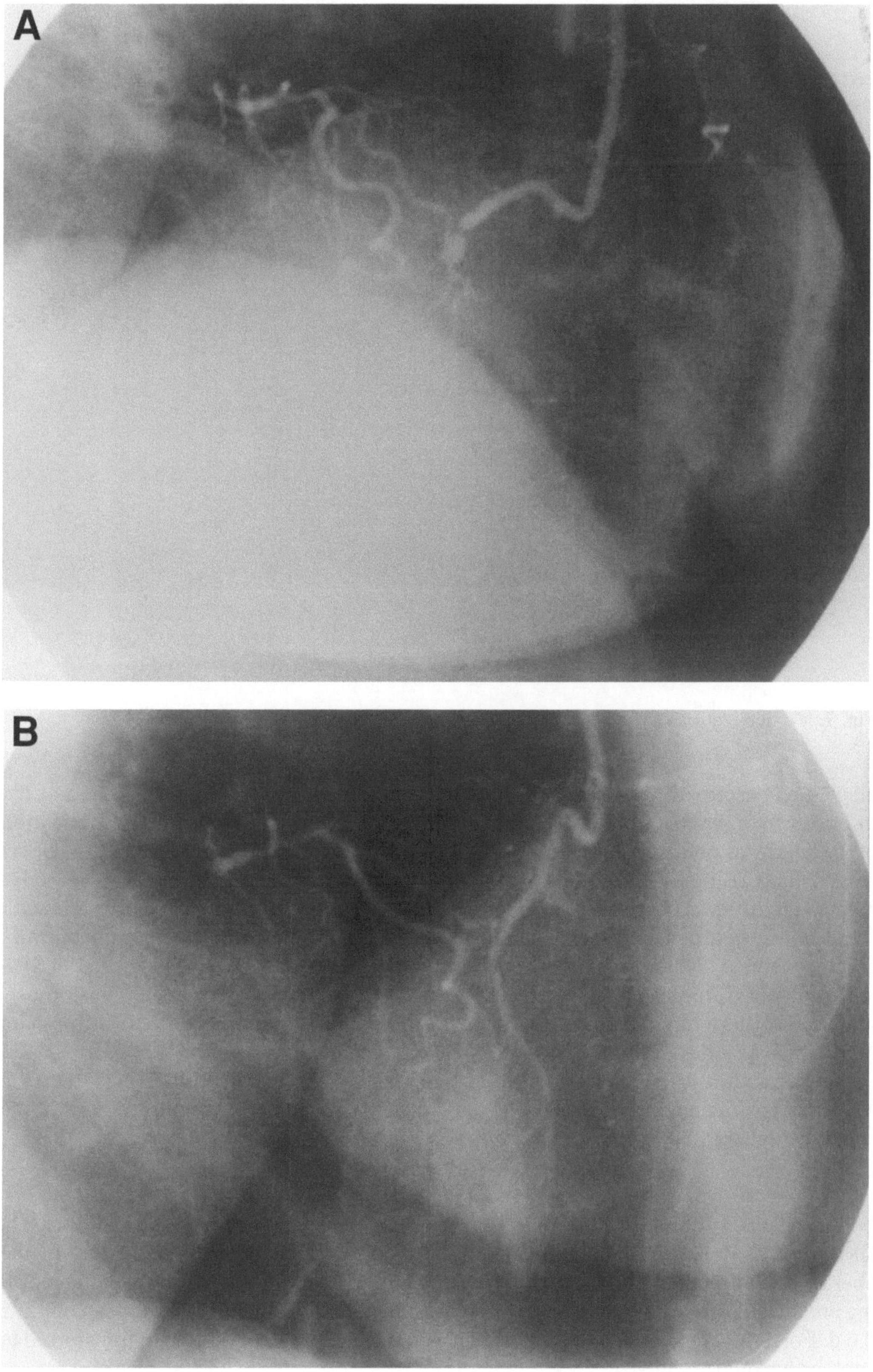
A
B

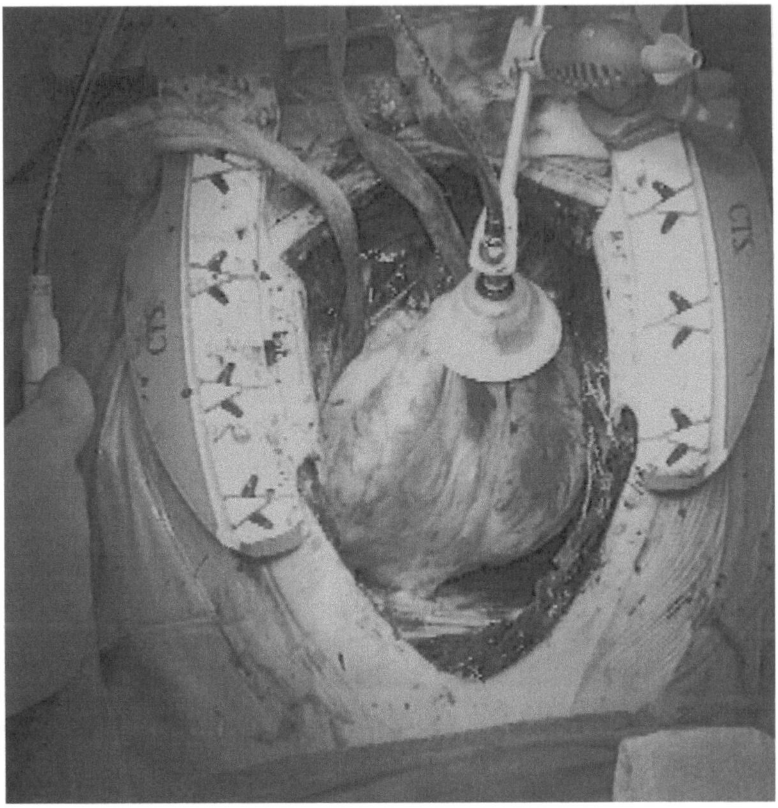

Fig. 7. Verticalization of the heart as obtained with the Xpose.

placed, as described by Lima *(16)*, between the left inferior pulmonary vein and the inferior vena cava, with a third sling in the same place. More recently, the verticalization of the heart was obtained with the Xpose™ (Guidant Corporation, Cupertino, CA, USA) (**Fig. 7**) and a single Lima stitch with a single additional sling, if necessary. Hemodynamic stability was obtained with Trendelenburg position, addition of volume and with small boluses of a vasopressor when needed (metaraminol or diluted norepinephrine), and mechanical stabilization was obtained with CTS stabilizers (Acces Ultima™ System, Guidant Corporation, Cupertino, CA, USA) *(17)*. At the end of every anastomosis the flow in the graft is measured using a flow meter (Cardiomed, Medi-Stim Oslo, Norway; Transonic System, Ithaca, NY, USA).

Blood lost during the procedure is reinfused in the patient using a cell saver (DIDECO, Mirandola, Modena, Italy). Protamine is reversed 0.5:1 and the wound is closed in the usual fashion.

Postoperative Course

All patients were admitted to the ICU, where they remained for a mean of 13.7 ± 17.8 h. Globally, 41.3% of the patients were discharged from the ICU the same day of the operation. This percentage rises to 66.7% if only the procedures performed in the morning are considered. The patients were discharged from the hospital after a mean of 4.2 ± 2.6 d. Forty-seven percent were sent directly home and the remaining wre transferred to another hospital.

Table 3
Comparison of Pre- and Intraoperative Data Among Patients Undergoing Coronary Revascularization with and Without CPB Support

	Off-Pump CABG	*Conventional CABG*	*p Value*
n	1134	1134	
Age (yr)	65 ± 10	64 ± 10	ns
Age ≥ 75 yr	160 (14.1%)	166 (14.6%)	ns
Female	210 (18.5%)	212 (18.7%)	ns
LVEF (%)	58 ± 13.5	56 ± 13.6	< 0.001
LVEF ≤ 35%	70 (6.2%)	75 (6.6%)	ns
Urgent operation	259 (22.8%)	251 (22.1%)	ns
Diabetes	250 (22%)	284 (25%)	ns
Left main disease	135 (11.9%)	134 (11.8%)	ns
Redo	19 (1.7%)	87 (7.7%) < 0.01	
Anastomoses/patient	2.4 ± 0.8	3 ± 1	< 0.001
Sequential grafts	217	574	< 0.001
Carotid surgery	24 (2.1%)	24 (2.1%)	ns

Table 4
Comparison of Clinical Outcomes Between OPCAB (*n* = 1134) and Conventional CABG) *n* = 1134) Patients

	Off-Pump CABG	*Conventional CABG*	*p Value*
	1134	1134	
Conversion to CPB	53 (4.8%)	NA	
Mortality	17 (1.5%)	37 (3.3%)	0.005
Inotrope use >24 h	32 (2.8%)	69 (6.1%)	0.002
Perioperative MI	10 (0.9%)	33 (2.9%)	<0.001
CK-MB peak (IU/L)	25 ± 42	48 ± 82	<0.001
Stroke	9 (0.8%)	13 (1.1%)	ns
Bleeding mL/24 h	399 ± 431	435 ± 409	0.041
Transfusion	263 (23.2%)	388 (34.2%)	<0.001
Atrial fibrillation	117 (10.3%)	135 (11.9%)	ns
Early major events	59 (5.2%)	110 (9.7%)	<0.001

Results

Between January 1995 and July 2001, 1263 patients underwent myocardial revascularization on a beating heart via a median sternotomy at our institution. Up to May 20, 1997, patients were strictly selected, lacking any technique for heart verticalization. In 129 patients, 211 distal anastomoses were performed (1.7 ± 0.7/patient). Among them, only 12 were performed on the lateral wall and 5 on the inferior wall.

Following introduction and application of verticalization techniques, selection criteria were relaxed and more patients were operated upon without CPB.

From May 21, 1997 to June 30, 2001, 1134 patients (50% of patients operated on via a median sternotomy in this period) had myocardial revascularization on a beating heart without CPB. Comparative data with patients operated on with CPB in the same time frame are listed in Tables 3 and 4.

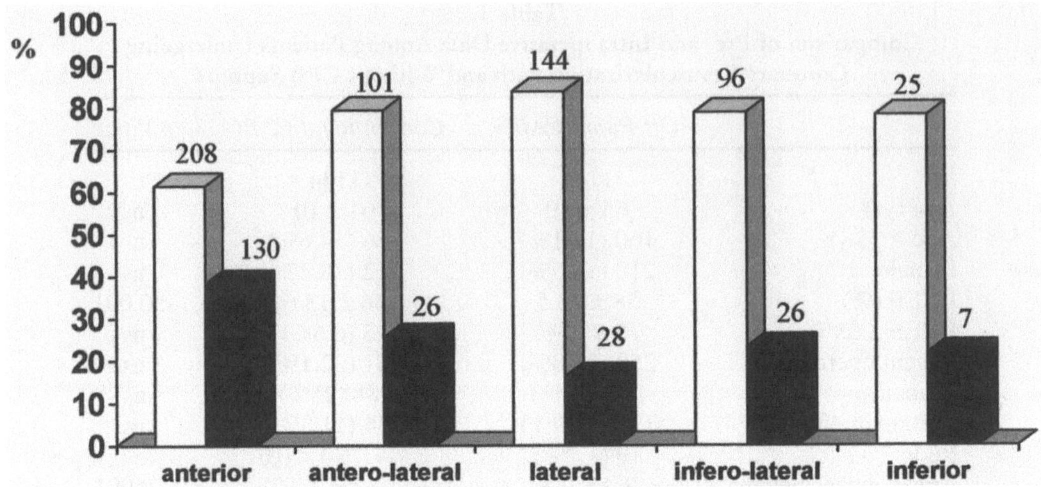

Fig. 8. Sequential grafts according to target territories. White bars depict conventional bypass patients and dark bars represent beating-heart revascularization patients.

Patients in the off-pump group had a higher ejection fraction, a lower incidence of redo, and fewer anastomoses per patient, with less sequential grafting (**Fig. 8**). However, both groups had the same expected risk according to EuroSCORE, 3.6 vs 3.7 (p = ns).

Mortality was lower in the off-pump group, as was the incidence of acute myocardial infarction, need for inotropes, and need for transfusion. Incidence of cerebrovascular accidents and atrial fibrillation was similar in both groups.

After a mean follow up of 12.7 ± 11.7 mo, 20 patients who underwent myocardial revascularization without CPB died, 10 due to cardiac causes (2 due to heart failure, 2 due to acute myocardial infarction, and 6 sudden deaths) and 10 due to other causes (3 due to cerebrovascular accident, 1 due to sepsis, 2 after abdominal aneurysm surgery, 2 due to malignancy, 1 from intestinal ischemia, and 1 from respiratory failure associated with pulmonary fibrosis).

In the conventional cardiopulmonary bypass group, nine patients died after a mean follow-up of 4.0 ± 3.0 months. Six deaths were due to cardiac causes.

After a mean of 7.0 ± 3.4 mo, seven off-pump recipients needed a repeat coronary intervention. Of these, five required repeat bypass grafting (two graft failures, three with progression of the disease) and two underwent percutaneous interventions (2 graft failures). After a mean of 13.5 ± 10.3 mo, two patients operated on with conventional CPB required reop CABG for graft failure. Four-year survival for the off-pump and conventional groups was 96.0 ± 0.6 and 97.1 ± 0.5, respectively (p = ns) (**Fig. 9**). Event-free survival was 96.3 ± 0.6 for patients who had beating-heart revascularization and 95.7 ± 0.6 for patients operated on with CPB support (p = ns) (**Fig. 10**).

Early angiographic results, shown in a previous report *(18)*, were similar to those obtained with CPB support. A high patency rate (98.2%) of marginal branch grafts is a very important issue, as lateral wall grafting is a major problem in myocardial revascularization without CPB.

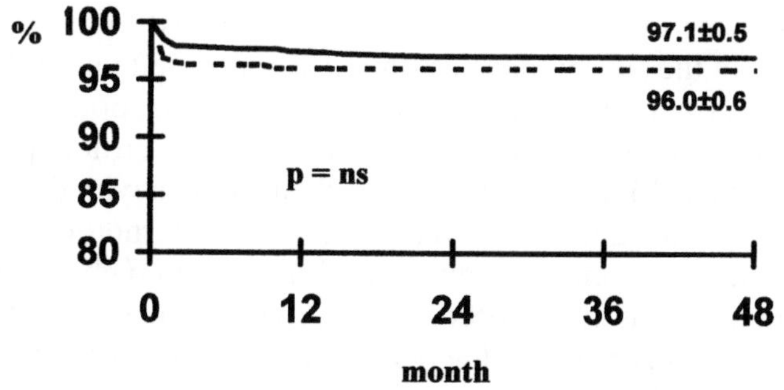

Fig. 9. Four-year survival of patients undergoing OPCAB (dashed line) and conventional CABG (solid line).

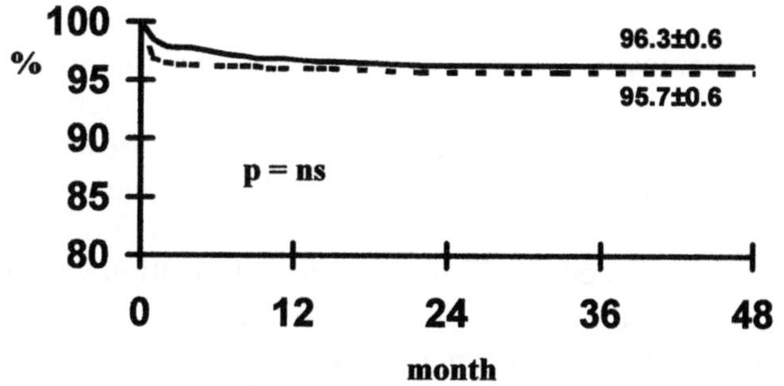

Fig. 10. Four-year event-free survival for patients undergoing beating-heart revascularization (solid line) and conventional CPB-supported bypass grafting (dashed line).

DISCUSSION

Myocardial revascularization without CPB is an accepted surgical strategy. Its benefit becomes evident in patients for whom CPB may have potential complications, as in the elderly or in patients with severe preoperative organ dysfunction.

The benefit of the LAST operation in particular is obvious during the early psotoperative recovery. These patients have short lengths of stay and faster return to social activities. The use of a LAST approach vs percutaneous interventions in patients with single-vessel disease is an interesting question. The ability to offer a LIMA-to-LAD anastomosis with very high early and midterm patency, the most important factor for long-term survival *(19)*, and with a safe, minimally invasive operation offers significant advantages over coronary artery stenting.

Despite this, stenting of the proximal LAD remains the first treatment for these lesions. However, application of coronary artery stenting to patients with type C lesions is associated with high failure rates and worse midterm outcomes than MIDCAB *(20)*. Even if the new coated-stent technology confirms a low risk of restenosis, the LAST operation is a well-standardized operation with good early and long-term results and remains a valid surgical option for single LAD disease.

One of the criticisms to the LAST operation was related to the possibility of flow competition if some of the side branches of the LIMA were left undivided. Indeed, some anecdotal reports *(21)* where single cases of ligature or embolization of huge side branches of the internal mammary artery to reverse ischemia in the LAD territory have been reported.

The concept that the LIMA can only be partially harvested with the minithoracotomy LAST approach is not true. During conventional median sternotomy, the LIMA is harvested up to the subclavian vein. The most proximal side branch is the first intercostal artery, the same branch that is divided during LIMA harvesting via a LAST approach. The very first part of the LIMA is never harvested, and lies the costolateral branch in this portion and some other subclavian artery branches. It is important to note that in 30% of the cases, these branches have a common origin with the LIMA *(22,23)*. If the flow competition between the side branches of the LIMA and the LAD were a clinical problem, it would have been present in all instances of myocardial revascularization regardless of approach.

Moreover, the physiology of coronary circulation is such that the nutritive flow happens mainly during diastole, whereas in the muscular territories the nutritive flow is mainly systolic *(24,25)*. An undivided side branch could cause flow competition, but only if it is addressed to a territory perfused during diastole, as the lungs, but this situation is very rare.

When multiple grafts are needed, off-pump revascularization via median sternotomy is the approach of choice. Although myocardial revascularization without CPB was the initial approach in the early era of coronary surgery *(1,25)*, the advent of safe CPB and cardioplegic arrest limited the interest in a technique that was more technically demanding. In fact, even though several groups continued to perform such a procedure *(5,6,26)*, the surgical technique was far from being well established and grafting the lateral wall was rarely done *(27)*.

In recent years, a new way of performing the operation was developed. The introduction of stabilizers and different techniques to verticalize the heart *(15,16,28–30)* were striking improvements that modified the feasibility of the procedure. The hemodynamic changes during the verticalization, when present *(31)*, are small enought to have no effect on the surgical outcome *(32)*.

Although some studies showed that, in patients in whom CPB was not used, there was significant reduction of the inflammatory response *(33)*, improvement in neurocognitive outcome *(34)*, and no increase in extracerebral water *(35)* in comparison with patients operated on with CPB; primary end points (mortality, CVA, and acute myocardial infarction incidence) were never reported to be lower in off-pump recipients.

In our recent report, we were able to demonstrate with the aid of stepwise logistic regression that CPB is an independent variable for early death, perioperative myocardial infarction, and early major events (the composite of death, low output syndrome, perioperative AMI, cerebrovascular accident, acute renal failure, acute respiratory failure, and acute abdominal complication) (Table 5) *(17)*. We believe that, if myocardial revascularization can be done without CPB, patients will experience lower morbidity and mortality.

Lack of angiographic studies in patients who underwent coronary surgery on a beating heart had led surgeons to question the safety and efficacy of the operation. Our angiographic studies demonstrated satisfying patency rate; even if some loss of patency occurs during the first year related to perioperative technical inadequacies, it holds true for every coronary anastomosis independent of the surgical technique *(18)*.

Table 5
Stepwise Logistic Regression Analysis of Risk Factors for Untoward Clinical Outcomes

	Early Death		*Stroke*		*Early MI*		*EME*[d]	
Risk Factor	*OR (95% CI)*	*p Value*	*OR (95% CI)*	*p Value*	*OR (95% CI)*	*p Value*	*OR (95% CI)*	*p Value*
Age ≥ 75 yr	—	—	—	—	2.2 (1.0–5.0)	0.0465	—	—
AMI[a] > 24 h	18.7 (2.8–123.7)	0.002	31.8 (2.7–365)	0.0055	—	—	18 (3.0–108)	0.0016
Chronic renal failure[b]	—	—	—	—	—	—	2.9 (1.4–6.4)	0.0058
Diabetes	2.2 (1.1–4.2)	0.016	—	—	—	—	—	—
LVEF ≤ 35%	2.9 (1.3–6.5)	0.011	9.3 (3.2–27.1)	<0.00001	3.0 (1.2–7.3)	0.017	3.5 (2.1-5.90)	0.0001
Heart failure	4.0 (1.5–10.4)	0.005	—	—	6.7 (2.4–18.7)	0.0003	3.4 (1.7–6.90)	0.0006
Preop IABP[c]	21.9 (2.2–222.4)	0.009	—	—	17.2 (1.5–192.1)	0.0208	—	—
Left main disease	—	—	3.9 (1.3–11.8)	0.0151	—	—	—	—
Unstable angina	—	—	—	—	2.8 (1.4–5.6)	0.0049	2.0 (1.4–3.0)	0.0002
Ventricular arrhythmia	—	—	—	—	—	—	2.9 (1.3–6.8)	0.013
Cardiopulmonary bypass	2.2 (1.1–4.3)	0.022	—	—	2.5 (1.2–5.2)	0.0185	1.8 (1.2–2.6)	0.0034
Carotid endarterectomy	—	—	9.0 (1.9–43.7)	0.006	—	—	—	—

[a]Acute myocardial infarction.
[b]Defined as serum creatinine ≥ 2.0 mg/dL.
[c]Intra-aortic balloon pump.
[d]Early major events (composite of death, low-output syndrome, acute myocardial infarction, cerebrovascular accident, acute respiratory dailure, acute renal failure, abdominal complication).

Myocardial revascularization without CPB is a surgical strategy that, in selected cases, can have satisfying early and midterm results. Selection of patients, in our experience, is the key to the success of the procedure. Tailoring the strategy to the patient will improve the already excellent outcomes currently achieved with coronary bypass grafting.

REFERENCES

1. Kolessov VI. Mammary artery-coronary artery anastomosis as method of treatment for angina pectoris. J Thorac Cardiovasc Surg 1967;54:535–544.
2. Favaloro RG. Saphenous vein autograft replacement of severe segmental coronary artery occlusion. Ann Thorac Surg 1968;5:334–339.
3. Garrett HE, Dennid EW, DeBakey ME. Aortocoronary bypass with saphenous vein graft. Seven year follow-up. JAMA 1973;223:792–794.
4. Trapp WG, Bisarya R. Placement of coronary artery bypass graft without pump oxygenator. Ann Thorac Surg 1975;19:1–9.
5. Benetti FJ, Naselli G, Wood M, Geffner L. Direct myocardial revascularization without extracorporeal circulation: experience in 700 patients. Chest 1991;100:312–316.
6. Buffolo E, de Andrade CS, Branco JN, Teles CA, Aguilar LF, Gomes WJ. Coronary artery bypass grafting without cardiopulmonary bypass. Ann Thorac Surg 1996;61:63–66.
7. Moshkovitz Y, Lusky A, Mohr R. Coronary artery bypass without cardiopulmonary bypass: analysis of short-term and mid-term outcomes in 220 patients. J Thorac Cardiovasc Surg 1995;1(10):979–987.
8. Calafiore AM, Di Giammarco G, Teodori G, et al. Left anterior descending coronary artery grafting via left anterior small thoracotomy without cardiopulmonary bypass. Ann Thorac Surg 1996;671: 1658–1665.
9. Bryan FC, Allen RC, Lumsden AB. Coronary-subclavian steal syndrome: report of five cases. Ann Vasc Surg 1995;9(1):115–122.
10. Breall JA, Grossman W, Stillman IE, Gianturco LE, Kim D. Atherectomy of the subclavian artery for patients with symptomatic coronary-subclavian steal syndrome. J Am Coll Cardiol 1993;21(7): 1564–1567.
11. Calafiore AM, Di Giammarco G, Luciani N, et al. Composite arterial conduits for a wider myocardial revascularization. Ann Thorac Surg 1994;58:185–190.
12. Calafiore AM, Teodori G, Di Giammarco G, et al. Minimally invasive coronary artery bypass grafting on a beating heart. Ann Thorac Surg 1997;63:S72–S75.
13. Calafiore AM, Vitolla G, Mazzei V, et al. The LAST Operation: techniques and results before and after the stabilization era. Ann Thorac Surg 1998;66:998–1001.
14. Calafiore AM, Di Giammarco G, Teodori G, et al. Midterm results after minimally invasive coronary surgery (LAST operation). J Thorac Cardiovasc Surg 1998;115:763–771.
15. Calafiore AM, Di Giammarco G, Teodori G, Mazzei V, Vitolla G. Recent advances in multivessel coronary grafting without cardiopulmonary bypass. Heart Surg Forum 1998; 33589.
16. Lima R Revascularizacion a o da artèria circunflexa sem auxilio da CEC. In: XII encontro dos discipulos do dr. EJ Zerbini, Curitiba, 1995. Sessao de videos. Curitiba, Parana, Sociedade dos discipulos do dr. EJ Zerbini Outtubro de 1995: 6.b.
17. Calafiore AM, Di Mauro M, Contini M, et al. Myocardial revascularization with and without cardiopulmonary bypass in multivessel disease. Impact of the strategy on early outcome. Ann Thorac Surg 2001;72:456–463.
18. Calafiore AM, Teodori G, Di Giammarco G, et al. Multiple arterial conduits without cardiopulmonary bypass. Early angiographic results. Ann Thorac Surg 1999;67:450–456.
19. Loop FD. Internal thoracic artery grafts—biologically better coronary arteries. N Engl J Med 1996;334:263–265.
20. Mariani MA, Boonstra PW, Grandjean JG, et al. Minimally invasive coronary artery bypass grafting versus coronary angioplasty for isolated type C stenosis of left anterior descending artery. J Thorac Cardiovasc Surg 1997;114:434–439.
21. Hartz RS, Heuser RR. Embolization of IMA side branches for post CABG ischemia. Ann Thorac Surg 1997;63:1765–1766.
22. Henriquez-Pino JA, Gomes WJ, Prates JC , Buffolo E. Surgical anatomy of the internal thoracic artery. Ann Thorac Surg 1997;64:1041–1045.

23. Calafiore AM, Contini M, Iacò AL, et al. Angiographic anatomy of the left internal mammary artery. Ann Thorac Surg 1999;68:1636–1639.
24. Kern MJ, Bach RG, Donohue TJ, et al. Role of large pectoralis branch artery in flow through a patent left internal mammary artery conduit. Cathet Cardiovasc Diagn 1995;34:240–244.
25. Favaloro RG, Effler DB, Groves LK, Sheldon WC, Sones FM. Direct myocardial revascularization by saphenous vein graft. Present operative technique and indications. Ann Thorac Surg 1970;10:97–111.
26. Ankeney JL. To use or not to use the pump oxigenator in coronary bypass operation. Ann Thorac Surg 1975;19:108–109.
27. Tasdemir O, Vural KM, Karagoz H, Bayazit K. Coronary artery bypass grafting on the beating heart without the use of the extracorporeal circulation: review of 2052 cases. J Thorac Cardiovasc Surg 1998;116:68–73.
28. Spooner TH, Dyrud TE, Monson BK, Dixon GE, Robinson LD. Coronary artery bypass on the beating heart with the Octopus: a North American experience. Ann Thorac Surg 1998;66:1032–1035.
29. Angelini GD, Lucchetti V. An inexpensive method of heart stabilization during coronary artery operation without cardiopulmonary bypass. Ann Thorac Surg 1998;1477–1478.
30. Bergsland J, Karamanoukian HL, Soltosky PR, Salerno TA. "Single suture" for circumflex exposure in off pump coronary artery bypass grafting. Ann Thorac Surg 1999;67:1653–1658.
31. Mathison M, Edgerton JR, Horswell JL, Akin JJ, Mack MJ. Analisys of haemodynamic changes during beating heart surgical procedures. Ann Thorac Surg 2000;70:1355–1361.
32. Nierich AP, Diephuis J, Jansen EWL, Borst C, Knape JTA. Heart displacement during off pump CABG: how well is it tolerated?. Ann Thorac Surg 2000;70:466–472.
33. Ascione R, Lloyd CT, Underwood MJ, Lotto AA, Pitsis AA, Angelini GD. Inflammatory response after coronary revascularization with or without cardiopulmonary bypass. Ann Thorac Surg 2000;69: 1198–1204.
34. Diegeler A, Hirsch R, Schneider F, et al. Neuromonitoring and and neurocognitive outcome in off pump versus conventional coronary bypass operation. Ann Thorac Surg 2000;69:1162–1166.
35. Anderson RE, Li TQ, Hindmarsh T, Settergren G, Vaage J. Increased extracellular brain water after coronary artery bypass grafting is avoided by off-pump surgery. J Cardiothorac Vasc Anesth 1999;13:698–702.

11 Minimally Invasive Coronary Artery Bypass Grafting

The South American Experience

Federico J. Benetti MD, PHD
and Maximo Guida MD

CONTENTS

INTRODUCTION
MINIMALLY INVASIVE CORONARY SURGERY
SURGICAL TECHNIQUE
MATERIALS AND METHODS
RESULTS
DISCUSSION
REFERENCES

INTRODUCTION

It is widely accepted that the single most important development in cardiac surgery was the introduction and refinement of extracorporeal circulation via cardiopulmonary bypass (CPB). The ensuing advances in cardioplegia and myocardial protection provided a motionless and bloodless field for accurate reparative surgery and improved event-free survival for patients undergoing a variety of cardiac procedures. Further advances in myocardial protection along with developments in percutaneous catheter-based intervention fostered a decade of debate regarding the definitive treatment for ischemic coronary artery disease.

Prior to the introduction of percutaneous transluminal coronary angioplasty (PTCA), coronary artery bypass grafting (CABG), rather than an initial strategy of medical therapy, resulted in longer survival and better quality of life in specific subgroups of patients with multivessel disease *(1–3)*. With the introduction of PTCA in 1977, the use of less invasive

From: *Contemporary Cardiology: Minimally Invasive Cardiac Surgery, Second Edition*
Edited by: D. J. Goldstein and M. C. Oz © Humana Press Inc., Totowa, NJ

methods for coronary revascularization rapidly expanded *(4)*. The well-publicized and much-quoted BARI trial, in which patients with multivessel disease were randomized to CABG or PTCA, concluded that there was no statistically significant difference in late survival between the two treatment strategies. Of note, however, the rate of repeat percutaneous intervention or subsequent revascularization was 42% in the PTCA group vs 3% in the CABG group. Indeed, 31% of the patients initially randomized to PTCA ultimately underwent CABG procedure anyway. Of great interest was the finding that the subset of patients with treated diabetes who underwent CABG was found to have a significant survival advantage over those receiving PTCA *(5)*.

The fact that the left internal mammary artery (LIMA) connected to the left anterior descending artery (LAD) is the single most powerful predictor of long-term survival has not been refuted even in cardiology circles *(6)*. In fact, despite the advances in catheter-based treatment methods, proximal and diffuse LAD disease still remain problematic and continue to have restenosis or reintervention rates much higher than bypass grafting of this vessel *(7)*. The advantages of PTCA include decreased trauma, shorter hospital stay and recovery, and, though somewhat debatable, lower costs. It is clear that patients are often willing to take the less invasive option despite being educated to the risks for restenosis and reintervention rates in order to avoid anesthesia, sternotomy, and cardiopulmonary bypass *(8)*.

As reviewed elsewhere in this book, the earliest coronary operations were done without the use of the extracorporeal circulation *(9–16)*. These initial experiences were largely ignored after the advent of precise, reproducible, bloodless, and motionless heart surgery; despite this, these pioneering experiences demonstrated the feasibility of beating-heart revascularization.

The era of cardiopulmonary bypass coronary surgery flourished and results continued to improve. However, it became increasingly obvious that extracorporeal circulation has deleterious effects in all body systems *(17–26)*.

MINIMALLY INVASIVE CORONARY SURGERY

Benetti *(27,28)* and Buffolo *(29)* repopularized beating-heart coronary revascularization (OPCAB) by expanding the technique, addressing lesions of the circumflex system, and applying it to diverse clinical scenarios. Experimentation with several surgical access approaches (other than full sternotomy) were used, including left anterolateral, posterolateral, and right anterolateral thoracotomies as well as partial sternotomy. Thoracoscopy was used for the first time to dissect the LIMA without opening the pleural cavity. The LIMA was then anastomosed to the LAD through a small left anterior thoracotomy in 1994 *(30–32)*, marking the era of the minimal-access cardiac surgery, and the eponym MIDCAB (minimally invasive direct coronary artery bypass) was coined.

A new series of technological developments allowed widespread application of the MIDCAB technique *(33–36)* as detailed in Chapter 9. A prospective multicenter study evaluating MIDCAB vs conventional bypass grafting demonstrated equivalent LIMA to LAD patency rates *(37)*. Today, coronary surgery in the beating heart (OPCAB and/or MIDCAB) is routine in many hospitals around the world, confirming the advantages of these procedures *(38,39)*.

In 1997 we began to examine the possibility of ambulatory coronary surgery. The approach was based on access via a xiphoid (or lower sternotomy) approach. Using three-dimensional visualization, the LIMA was harvested and anastomosed to the LAD

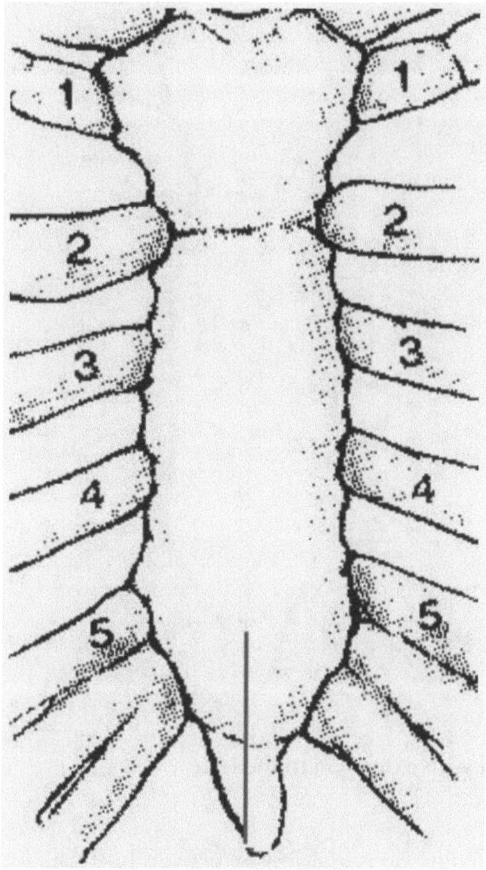

Fig. 1. Lower midsternal incision for the xiphoid approach.

(40–42). Important advantages of this approach include reduced postoperative pain and preservation of intact pleural cavities, increasing the possibility of early discharge *(43,44)*.

We have now applied current technology through a lower sternotomy approach for multivessel revascularization in several patients with the aim of discharging them within 24 h of operation *(40–42)*. The following paragraphs describe our technique and results with ambulatory coronary surgery.

SURGICAL TECHNIQUE

The original technique was developed in 1997 *(40–42)*. Currently, we do not use the videoscope routinely and we always extend the sternal incision to the left, right, or both to fit the retractor adequately (**Figs. 1–3**). Preoperative measurements with the cardioscan are very helpful to evaluate the internal mammary artery diameter and presence of collaterals. It is also very important to measure the distance to potential anastomotic sites, as it will dictate the length of mammary needed to reach the target comfortably (**Figs. 4** and **5**). Following lower sternal incision, a mammary retractor (Favaloro type) is used to dissect one or both mammary arteries (**Fig. 6**). Additional conduits are harvested and anastomosed to the LIMA if necessary (**Fig. 7**). Care is taken not to enter either pleural cavity. When the LIMA is the only conduit needed, we harvest approx 7 cm of length. We

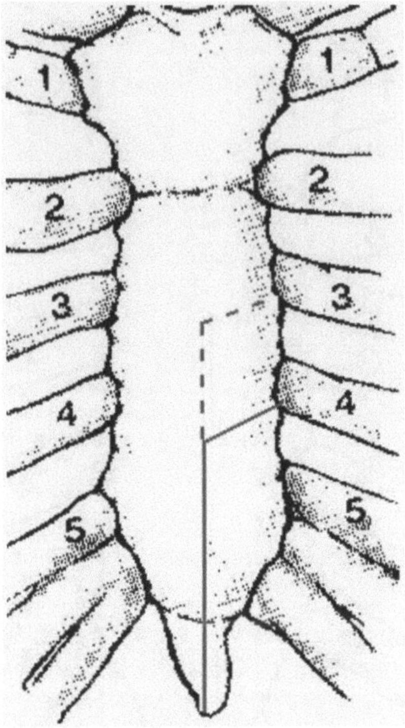

Fig. 2. Midsternal incision with extension to the left.

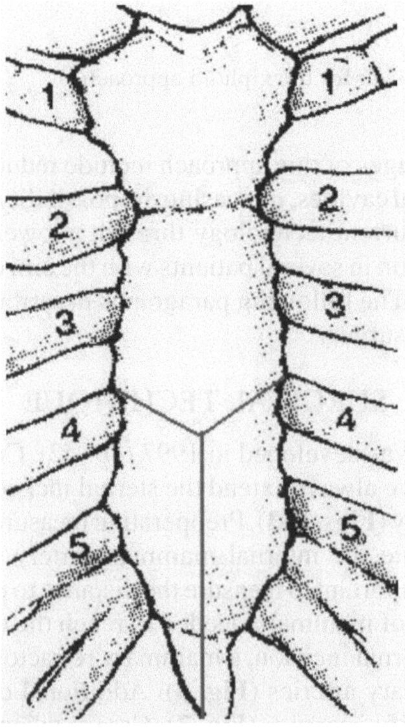

Fig. 3. Midsternal incision with bilateral extensions.

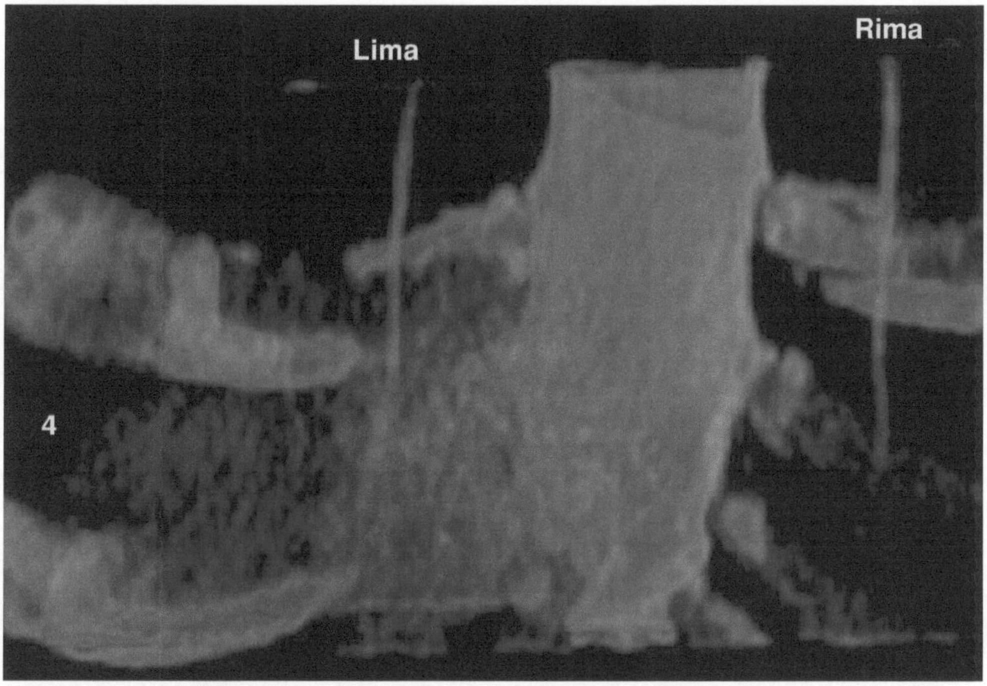

Fig. 4. Preoperative Cardioscan demonstrating the internal mammary arteries.

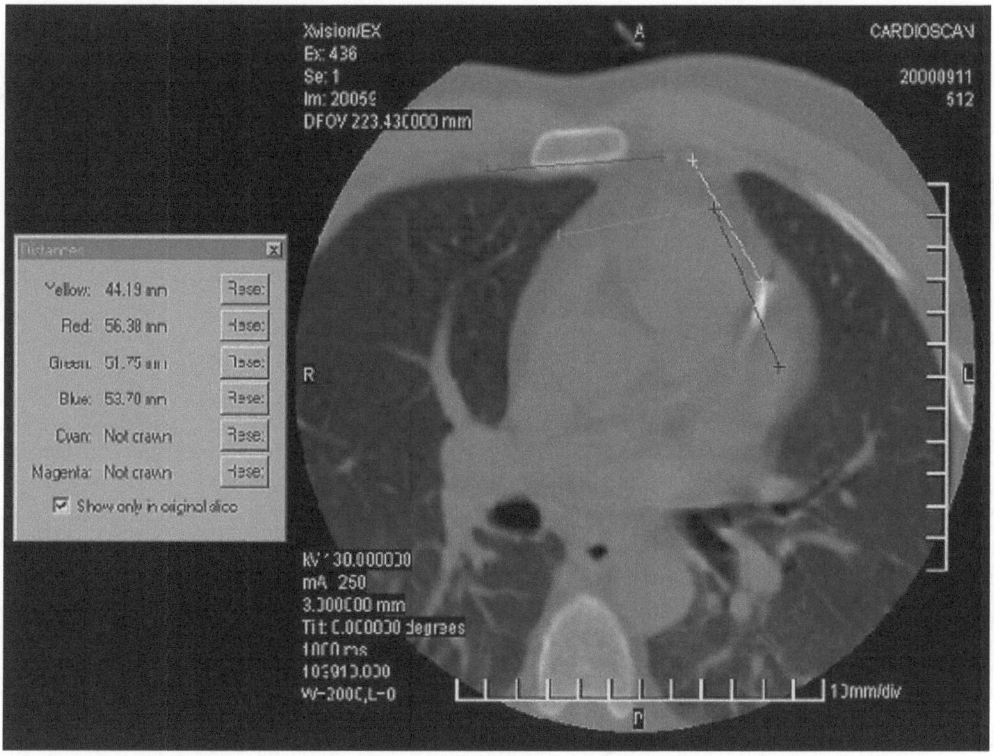

Fig. 5. Preoperative measurements with the Cardioscan system.

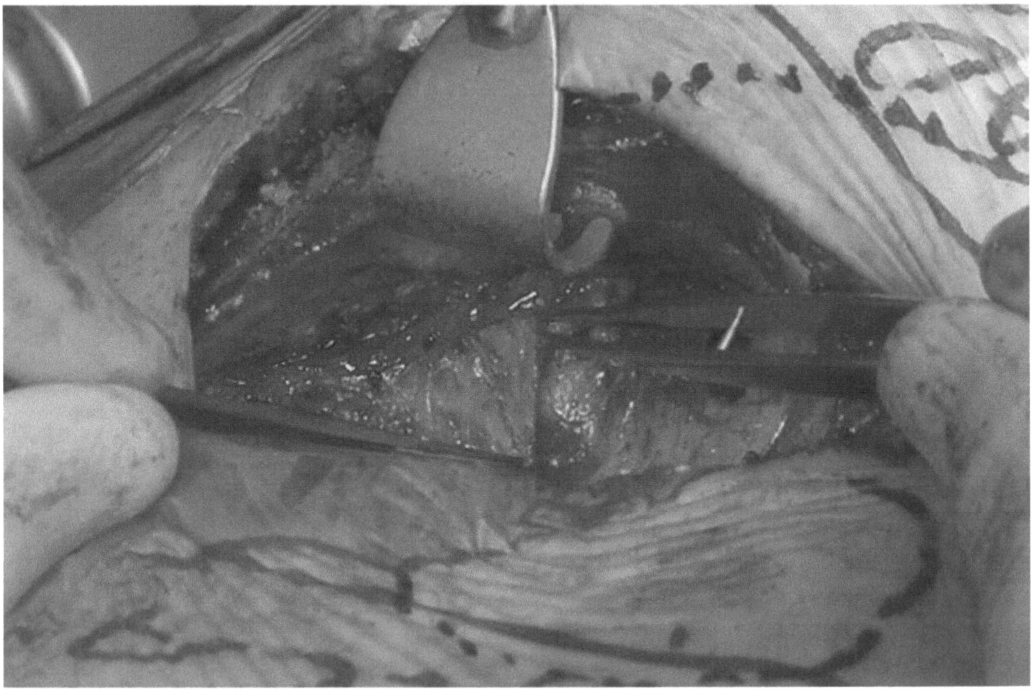

Fig. 6. Dissection of the mammary artery.

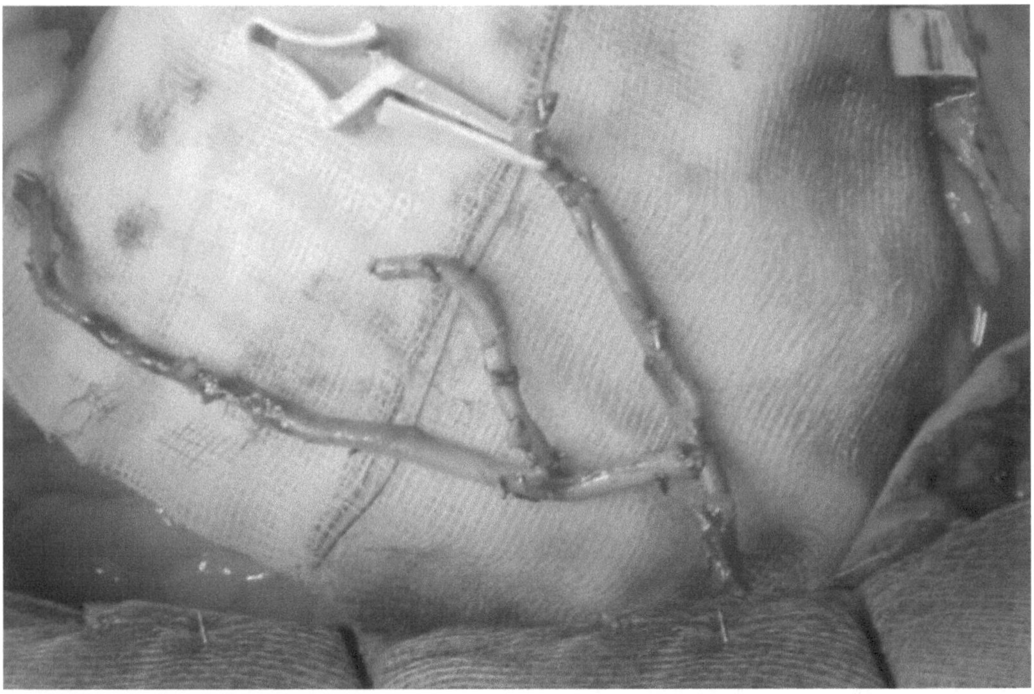

Fig. 7. Conduits used to create the y-grafts from the LIMA.

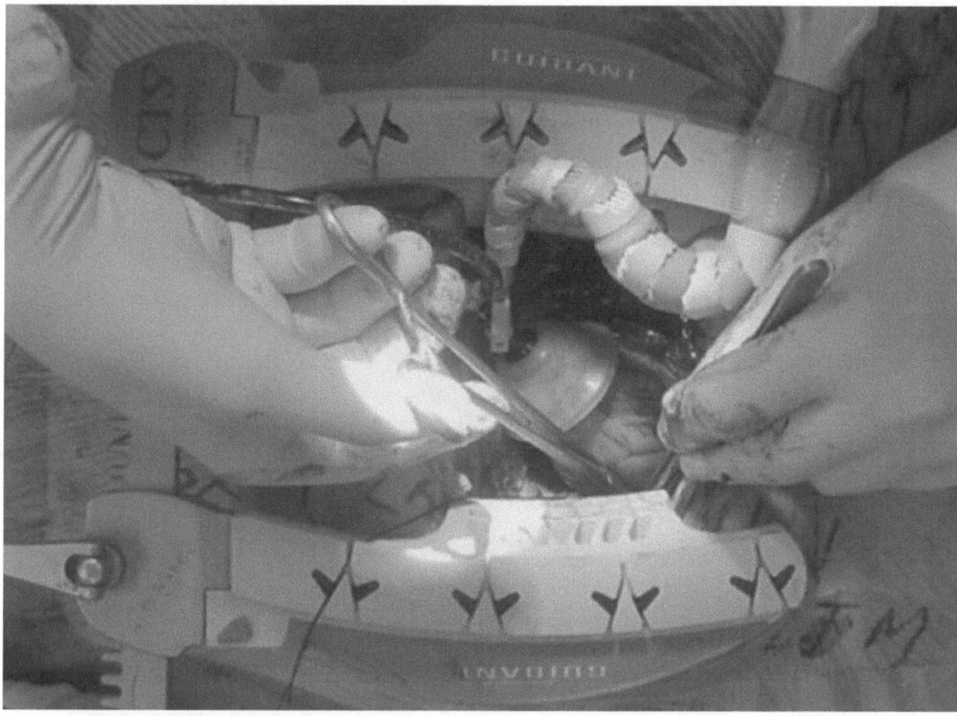

Fig. 8. Use of the *Xpose* apical system.

do not believe the steal phenomenon is clinically relevant and hence we do not bother clipping LIMA branches. It is critical to measure the exact distance between the mammary and the potential site in the LAD with the heart in a normal position to avoid any kinking or angulation, particularly at the level of the sternum. Because the mammary is attached to a fixed point, we take these measurements after the pericardium has been opened and with the retractor in place.

The pericardium is opened to the left of the pulmonary artery and toward the left ventricular apex and a flap is created to the right. A stitch is then placed in the left edge of the pericardium. We position the Xpose™ Apical Positioning Device (**Fig. 8**), trying to minimize cardiac manipulation to avoid atrial fibrillation *(30)*. We routinely use the Guidant stabilization system to perform the anastomosis (**Fig. 9**). Upon completion of the anastomosis, and after satisfactory hemostasis has been achieved, drains are carefully placed to avoid any damage to the conduits.

After closing the sternum with one to three wires, we infiltrate all intercostals spaces and the path of the drainage with local anesthesia to enhance the chance of early extubation.

MATERIALS AND METHODS

Between October 1997 and June 2001, 85 patients were operated through the xiphoid (lower sternotomy). Among this group of patients, 15 (12 men, 3 women) with a mean age of 65 yr (range 45–78) were discharged within 24 h after the operation, although some of the patients stayed for a few more hours in the facilities for practical reasons *(42)*.

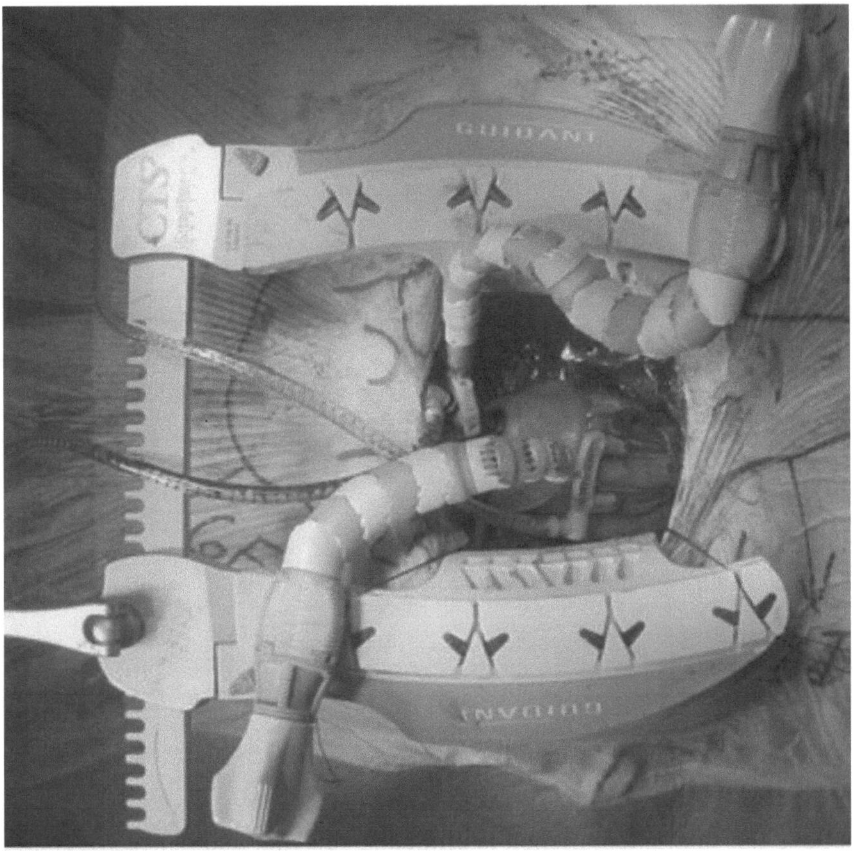

Fig. 9. Use of stabilizer to perform the anastomoses.

RESULTS

Operative mortality was 1% (one patient). Conversion to complete sternotomy occurred in one patient (1%) and Q-wave perioperative infarction occurred in one (1%) patient. In all 16 patients who consented to postoperative angiography, the patency rate was 100%. In the 15 ambulatory patients the mortality was 0% and the perioperative infarction 0%. The postoperatative follow-up ranged between 12 and 44 mo, with an average of 22 mo. All patients were asymptomatic. Five patients have had stress thallium testing, which has demonstrated no active ischemia.

DISCUSSION

Coronary bypass surgery without CPB in the beating heart via different incisions is a proven and reproducible technique *(38–42)* that has the distinct advantages of avoiding the morbidity associated with extracorporeal circulation *(8,17,26)*.

In our mind, the goal of the MIDCAB operation *(31)* was to perform coronary surgery in an ambulatory fashion, based on the time-proven concept that the left internal mammary connected to the LAD is the best long-term treatment for lesions of this artery.

We soon realized that the thoracotomy incision required for the MIDCAB approach created two obstacles to early discharge: significant postoperative pain and invasion of the left pleura. The former often mandates the use of intravenous narcotics, while the latter requires chest tube placement, serial radiographs, and removal of the chest tube, with concerns about pneumothoraces and pleural effusions. In view of these limitations, we refocused our approach to the xiphoid approach. This strategy avoids pleural entry and is associated with much lesser and more treatable postoperative pain, which together permit the application of coronary bypass grafting to the ambulatory setting. We are now focusing on developing newer methodologies and instrumentation to expand this approach to multivessel grafting. We envision that, as technological improvements are made, multivessel coronary bypass grafting on the beating heart, with multiple arterial conduits, will be feasible via a small incision and permit ambulatory or very early hospital discharge with results that mimic those currently obtained by conventional full sternotomy.

REFERENCES

1. Jones R, Kesler K, Phillips H, et al. Long-term survival benefits of coronary artery bypass grafting and percutaneous transluminal angioplasty in patients with coronary artery disease. J. Thorac Cardiovasc Surg 1996;111:1013–1025.
2. Jones EL, Craver JM, Guyton RA, et al. Importance of complete revascularization in performance of the coronary bypass operation. Am J Cardiol 1983;51:7–12.
3. Califf RM, Mark DB. Percutaneous intervention, surgery and medical therapy: a perspective from the Duke databank for cardiovascular diseases. Semin Thorac Cardiovasc Surg 1994;6:120–128.
4. King SB III, Lembo NJ, Weintraub WS, et al. Emory angioplasty versus surgery trial (EAST): design, recruitment and baseline description of patients. Am J Cardiol 1995;75:42C–59C.
5. Feit F, Brooks MM, Sopko G, et al. Long-term clinical outcome in the Bypass Angioplasty Revascularization Investigation Registry: comparison with the randomized trial. BARI Investigators. Circulation 2000;101:2795–2802.
6. Loop FD, Internal thoracic artery grafts: biologically better coronary arteries. N Engl J Med 1996;334:263–265.
7. Fischman DL, Lenon MB, Baim DS, et al. A randomized comparison of coronary-stent placement and balloon angioplasty in the treatment of coronary artery disease. N Engl J Med 1994;331:496–501.
8. Roach GW, Kanchuger M, Mangano CM, et al. Adverse cerebral outcomes after coronary bypass surgery. N Engl J Med 1996;335:1857–1863.
9. Vineberg AM. Development of anastomosis between coronary vessels and transplanted mammary artery. Med Assoc J 1954;71:594.
10. Westaby S, Benetti FJ. Less invasive coronary surgery: consensus from the Oxford meeting. Ann Thorac Surg 1996;62:924–931.
11. Goetz RH, Rohman M, Haller JD, et al. Internal mammary-coronary anastomosis: a moisture method employing tantalum rings. J Thorac Cardiovasc Surg 1961;41:378–386.
12. Sabiston DC. The coronary circulation. Johns Hopkins Med J 1974;134:314–329.
13. Kolessov, VI. Mammary artery-coronary artery anastomosis as method of treatment for angina pectoris. J Thorac Cardiovasc Surg 1967;54:535–544.
14. Ankeney JL. To use or not to use the pump oxygenation in coronary bypass operation. Ann Thorac Surg 1975;19:108–109.
15. Garret HE, Dennis EW, DeBakey Me. Aortocoronary bypass with saphenous vein graft. Seven-year follow-up. JAMA 1973;223:792–794.
16. Trapp WG, Bisarya R. Placement of coronary artery bypass graft without pump oxygenator. Ann Thorac Surg 1975;19:1–8.
17. Westby S, Johnson P, Parry AJ, et al. Serum S100 protein: a potential marker for cerebral events during cardiopulmonary bypass. Ann Thorac Surg 1996;61:88–92.
18. Robin ED, McCaurley RF, Notkin H. Long- term cognitive abnormalities associated with cardiopulmonary bypass (CPB) and the Babel effect. Chest 1994;106:278–281.
19. Murkin JM, Martzke JS, Buchan AM, et al. A randomized study of the influence of perfusion technique and pH management strategy in 316 patients undergoing coronary artery bypass surgery. II. Neurologic and cognitive outcomes. J Thorac Cardiovasc Surg 1995;110:349–362.

20. Hiberman M, Derby GC, Spenser RJ, Stinson EB. Sequential path physiological changes characterizing the progression from renal dysfunction to acute failure following cardiac operation. J Thorac Surg 1980;79:838–844.
21. Zenardo G, Michielon P, Paccagnella A, et al. Acute renal failure in the patient undergoing cardiac operation: prevalence, mortality rate an main risk factors. J Thorac Cardiovasc Surg 1994;107: 1489–1495.
22. Corwin HL Sprague SM, DeLaria GA, Norusis MJ. Acute renal failure associated with cardiac operations. J Thorac Cardiovasc Surg 1989;98:1107–1112.
23. Butler J, Rocker GM, Westby S. Inflammatory response to cardiopulmonary bypass. Ann Thorac Surg 1993;55:552–559.
24. Gailiunas P Jr, Chawla R, Lazarus JM, et al. Acute renal failure following cardiac operations. J Thorac Cardiovasc Surg 1980;79:241–243.
25. Bhat JG, Gluck MC, Lowenstein J, et al. Renal failure after heart surgery. Ann Intern Med 1976;84: 677–682.
26. Emunds L H Why cardiopulmonary bypass make patients sick. Strategies to control the blood-synthetic surface interface. Adv Card Surg 1996;6:88–92.
27. Benetti FJ. Cirugía cardiaca a sin CEC o parada cardiaca. Rev de la Federación Argentina de Cardiología 1980;8:3.
28. Benetti FJ. Direct coronary surgery with saphenous vein bypass without either cardiopulmonary bypass or cardiac arrest. J Cardiovasc Surg 1985;26:217–222.
29. Buffolo E, Andrade JC, Succi J, Leao LE, Gallucci C. Direct myocardial revascularization without cardiopulmonary bypass. Thorac Cardiovasc Surg 1985;33:26–29.
30. Benetti FJ, et al. Uso de la toracoscopía en cirugía coronaria para disección de la arteria mamaria interna. Prensa Medica Argentina 1994;81:877–879.
31. Benetti FJ, Ballester C. Use of thoracoscophy and minimal thoracotomy in mammary to coronary bypass to left anterior descending artery, without extracorporeal circulation. J Cardiovasc Surg 1995;36:159–161
32. Benetti FJ, et al. Coronary revascularization with arterial conduits via a small thoracotomy and assisted by thoracoscopy, although without cardiopulmonary bypass. Coronary Revasc 1995;4(1):22–24.
33. Benett FJ. Method for Coronary Artery Bypass. US Patent 5,888,247.
34. Benetti FJ, et al. Access Platform for Internal Mammary Dissection. US Patent 5,730,757.
35. Benetti FJ, et al. Surgical Method for Stabilizing the Beating Heart During Coronary Bypass Surgery. US Patent 5,894,843.
36. Benetti FJ, et al. Surgical Devices for Imposing a Negative Pressure to Fix the Position of Cardiac Tissue During Surgery. US Patent 5,727,569.
37. Meharan R. Long-term patency of LIMA-LAD beating heart anastomosis (POEM) trial The 6th annual Cardiothoracic Techniques & Technologies meeting 2000. January 27–29, 2000. Bal Harbour, FL.
38. Mitchell J, et al. Elimination of cardiopulmonary bypass improves early survival in multivessel coronary artery bypass patients. Society of Thoracic Surgeons, 2001 (Jan), New Orleans, LA, USA.
39. Benetti FJ. Minimally invasive coronary surgery. Seventieth Scientific Sessions of the American Heart Association, Orlando, FL, USA, 1997 (Nov).
40. Benetti FJ. Minimally invasive coronary surgery (the xiphoid approach). Eur J Cardiothorac Surg 1999;16(suppl 2):S10–S11.
41. Guida M, Torrealba C, Rivera J, et al. CTT meeting, New Orleans, LA, USA, 2001.
42. Subramanian VA, Sani G, Benetti FJ, Calafiore A. Minimally invasive coronary bypass surgery: a multicenter-report of preliminary clinical experience. Circulation 1995;92(8):I-645.
43. Diegeler A, et al Minimally invasive coronary bypass experience. Eur J Cardiothorac Surg 2000; 17:501–504.
44. Benetti FJ. Cirugía coronaria directa sin circulación extracorporeal. Buenos Aires: Ed Akadia, 1993.

12 Reoperative Off-Pump CABG

Valavanur A. Subramanian, MD,
James D. Fonger, MD,
and Nilesh U. Patel, MD

CONTENTS

INTRODUCTION
INDICATION FOR PREOPERATIVE PLANNING
PREOPERATIVE PLANNING FOR REOPERATION
ANESTHESIA AND INTRAOPERATIVE MONITORING
SURGICAL TECHNIQUE
OPERATIVE APPROACHES
INSTITUTIONAL EXPERIENCE
REFERENCES

INTRODUCTION

Coronary reoperations continue to play an increasing role in the practice of coronary bypass surgery *(1,2)*. At present, approx 10% of isolated coronary revascularization operations in the United States are reoperations *(3)*. Operative mortality and morbidity are increased for patients undergoing reoperative or redo coronary artery bypass grafting (CABG), with an operative mortality in most series of reoperations three to five times that of primary CABG *(1,2,4–6)*.

Reoperative procedures have several technical obstacles that differentiate them from primary procedures. These problems include: (1) difficulties with sternal reentry, with potential for cardiac and conduit injury during dissection when the surgical plane is obscured by dense adhesions and normal anatomical landmarks are obliterated; (2) availability of conduit; (3) management of patent vein grafts with severe atherosclerosis; (4) myocardial protection in situations where there are complex routes of myocardial perfusion, depending on the status of the native coronary circulation and the patency of the vein or internal mammary artery (IMA) grafts.

From: *Contemporary Cardiology: Minimally Invasive Cardiac Surgery, Second Edition*
Edited by: D. J. Goldstein and M. C. Oz © Humana Press Inc., Totowa, NJ

Alternative strategies currently used include different techniques for sternal reentry, strict avoidance of graft manipulation to minimize the risk of graft atheroembolism, and numerous modifications of myocardial protection, including performing coronary artery bypass grafting without cardiopulmonary bypass through the standard sternal reentry approach *(7–10)*.

Since 1994, alternative nonsternal, minimal-access off-pump approaches (i.e., left anterior thoracotomy, subxyphoid, short lateral thoracotomy, and transabdominal) have been increasingly used in reoperation either alone or in combination *(11–14)*.

INDICATION FOR REOPERATION

Some indications for coronary reoperation are clear and are based on clinical evidence, while other indications must be based on logic. Clear indications include:

1. The presence of late stenosis (≥50%) in vein grafts supplying the LAD or large circumflex and/or right coronary systems that supply viable myocardium.
2. Patients with left main or triple vessel disease and abnormal left ventricular function, or a large LAD coronary artery with a proximal stenosis and multivessel disease who do not have any patent grafts. These indications are based on data from the randomized trials of primary coronary bypass surgery *(15,16)*, and meta-analysis of those data.
3. For patients with severe disabling angina and previous bypass surgery, coronary reoperation is one option that can be considered for the purpose of relieving symptoms *(17)*.

Noninvasive testing can also add information to the anatomic data. When patients exhibit a decrease in left ventricular function associated with stress testing, that situation predicts a worse outcome without surgery, an observation that can aid in decision making.

PREOPERATIVE PLANNING FOR REOPERATION

Since most reoperative candidates have had symptomatic atherosclerosis for at least a decade, they often have far advanced diffuse coronary and noncoronary atherosclerosis. Routine preoperative or intraoperative echocardiography is used to detect the presence of severe ascending and descending aortic atherosclerosis, a problem that may alter strategies for grafts and graft inflow. Preoperative computed tomography (CT) scan of the chest in addition to TEE in patients requiring circumflex CABG to evaluate the descending aorta as a site for proximal anastomosis is helpful. Patients with carotid bruits undergo preoperative noninvasive screening tests for carotid stenosis for possible staged or combined carotid endarterectomy.

Limited availability of bypass conduits is a common problem during reoperation, particularly if the patient has had multiple previous operations. The availability of lower extremity veins with preoperative venous Doppler studies of the greater and lesser saphenous vein systems can be helpful. The surgeon needs to be aware of previous abdominal procedures that may have made the inferior epigastric arteries or the right gastroepiploic artery unusable. If radial artery grafts are a possibility, Doppler studies can demonstrate the integrity of the collateral arterial supply to the hand. The presence of patent inferior epigastric arteries can also be documented noninvasively. If conduits are extremely limited, it is also wise to perform a preoperative angiogram of the internal mammary arteries to make certain they are not atherosclerotic and were not damaged during the previous sternal closure. Lastly, while not ideal, cryopreserved veins are commercially available for use.

ANESTHESIA AND INTRAOPERATIVE MONITORING

Routine hemodynamic monitoring includes a radial artery (sometimes femoral artery) line and a continuous mixed venous oxygen saturation pulmonary artery catheter. After routine double-lumen endotracheal tube placement, a transesophageal echocardiographic probe is inserted. External defibrillator pads (R_2 stat<i> *padz*™, Zoll, Inc., Burlington, MA) are routinely placed prior to skin prepping. Cardiopulmonary bypass machine is always available in the room but not primed.

SURGICAL TECHNIQUE

After exposure of the target coronary vessels by a variety of incisions and operative exposure techniques described below, the patient is routinely heparnized before the local coronary occlusion. The dose of intravenous heparin consists of a bolus intravenous administration of 10,000 IU to keep the activated clotting time (ACT) within a range of 300–350 s. ACT is repeatedly measured every 20–30 min in multivessel grafting prior to each coronary occlusion to make sure that it is in the 300–350-s range, and additional bolus of heparin is given if it is required. This is important in off-pump surgery since there is a hypercoagulable tendency in some patients as the length of the operation increases.

For coronary stabilization, both mechanical stabilizer and epicardial radial sutures on either side of the coronary target site are used routinely. CTS (Cardio Thoracic Systems, Cupertino, CA) MIDCAB Stabilizer platform for anterior thoracotomy and CTS Ultima™ Offset Stabilizer are used routinely in our institution in all other incisional approaches. Local coronary occlusion of a short segment of the artery (2 cm) is obtained with silastic sutures on a blunt needle encircling the entire artery, epicardial fat, and veins placed both proximal and distal to the anastomotic site.

A blower device (Axius™ CO_2 blower, Guidant Corp., Cupertino, CA) is used to keep the field clear of blood and incised edges of the coronary artery separated during the anastomosis. Use of intracoronary shunt is not routine, and contingent on the size of the target and the severity of anatomical obstruction. More frequently, the shunt is used if the size of the coronary artery is $\geq$2 mm and the degree of coronary artery obstruction is < 75%. Coronary anastomosis is performed using 7-0 or 8-0 continuous Prolene suture. Heparin is routinely neutralized with protamine at the end of anastomosis. No intravenous antiarrhythmics are given routinely. If the coronary artery is <2 mm, diffusely diseased, and calcified, and if the patient has a patent intracoronary stent, clopidogrel (Bristol Myers Squibb, New York, NY) is administered via nasogastric tube prior to the coronary artery occlusion and postoperatively and continued daily for 4 wk. Patients are usually extubated either in the operating room before transfer to the intensive care unit (ICU) or within 1–2 h after arrival in the ICU.

Strategies for perioperative pain control included intercostal nerve block (0.5% bupivacaine), epidermal catheter, and, recently, intercostal nerve protectors and intercostal cryoanalgesia. Discomfort due to rib retraction in thoracotomy approaches usually subsides within 2 d compared to the sternotomy approaches. This discomfort during the initial recovery period has been dramatically reduced with the use of new disposable intercostal nerve protectors (Deflector™, ViaMedics, White Bear Lake, MN) and application of cryoanalgesia (Cryohit, Galil Medical, Israel) to the neighboring intercostal nerves before closure. Cryoanalgesia technique results in temporary damage to the nerve's myelin sheath without significant damage to the underlying nerve axon. Interrupting the myelin sheath stops the transmission of pain stimuli, and the sheath regenerates quickly

(2–3 wk) without incident. Leaving the axon intact minimizes the nerve axon regeneration and the chance of developing a subsequent painful neuroma. The pain control with this method extends over 2–3 wk postoperatively.

OPERATIVE APPROACHES

Standard Resternotomy

Standard resternotomy is ideal for patients with no prior patent anterior (i.e., LIMA→LAD, SVG→RCA) grafts and who need multivessel grafting.

Sternal Reentry

To perform the median sternotomy, the skin and subcutaneous tissues are divided sharply, the sternal wires are exposed and cut anterior to the sternum but are not removed. While an assistant elevates both costal margins with retractors, an oscillating saw is used to divide the sternum. The position of the wires posterior to the sternum helps to avoid damage to the underlying structures.

Mediastinal Dissection

Once the sternum is reopened, the two sides of the sternum are dissected away from the underlying structures. On the right side, the pleura usually can be entered safely, and this is also possible on the left side unless a patent ITA graft is present. Complete dissection of the cardiac structures and old bypass grafts is not needed at this time. It is safest to enter the right and left pleural spaces by dissection along the diaphragm, because at that level only a right coronary graft is exposed to possible injury. Once entry into the left pleural space is accomplished at the level of the diaphragm, the mediastinal structures, including a patent left ITA, can be separated from the chest wall by dissection proceeding superiorly.

Exposure of Lateral and Inferior Wall During Resternotomy

The following technique greatly facilitates a good exposure for performance of coronary anastomosis to circumflex branches and distal right coronary artery branches.

1. Limiting the posterior pericardial dissection to anterior to the A-V groove. Posterior pericardial sutures are placed at the junction of the pericardium with its attachment to the A-V groove.
2. Opening of the right pleura widely with dissection of right ventricle and right atrium. This allows the heart to fall into the right pleural cavity during exposure of the posterior wall of the left ventricle.
3. Liberal use of the new apical suction cup device (Xpose Access Device™, Guidant/CTS, Cupertino, CA) (**Fig. 1**) to elongate and pull the heart out of the mediastinal cavity.
4. Division of the attachments of the diaphragm to the anterior costal margin bilaterally. This maneuver creates more space in the chest to move around the heart freely.
5. Placing the sternal retractor from the suprasternal notch down. Then the handle of the retractor is no longer in the way during operation on the inferior and posterior surface of the heart.
6. Partial vertical dissection of central tendon of the diaphragm posteriorly and downward traction on the diaphragm with heavy traction sutures fixed to the abdominal wall. This naturally moves the posterior part of the heart to the right and out of the pericardial cavity.
7. Trendelenburg position.

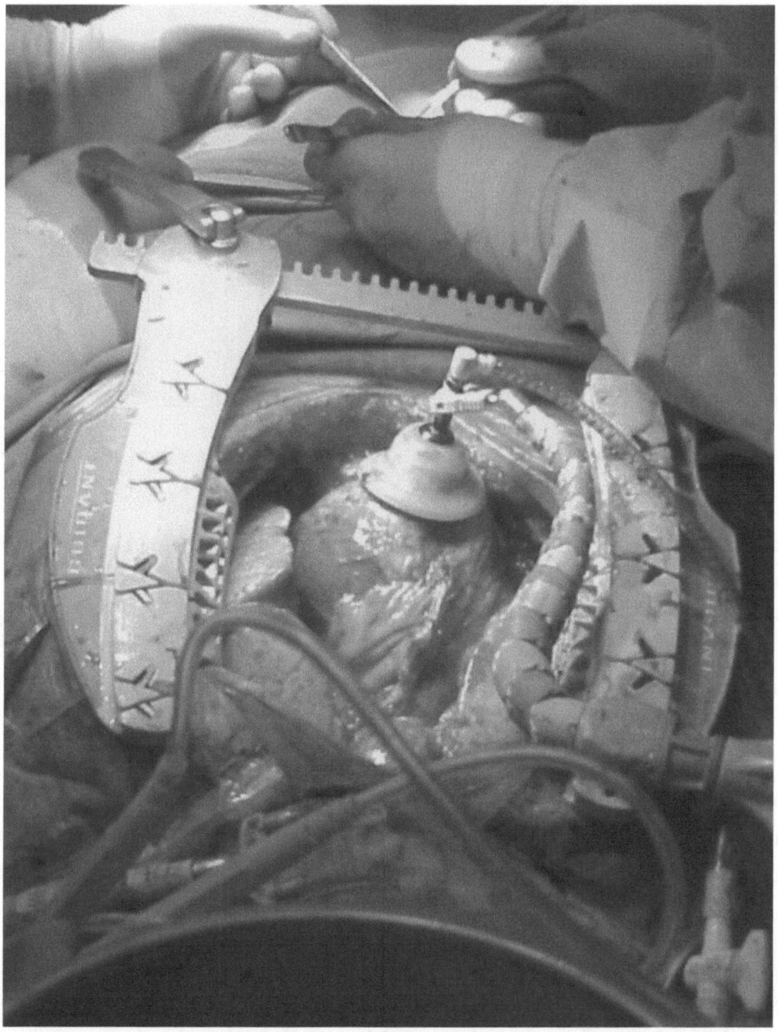

Fig. 1. Use of the Xpose™ apical device to facilitate posterior exposure.

These steps provide an excellent exposure for all the branches of circumflex artery and posterior descending branch of the right coronary artery.

Routine skeletonization of the internal mammary artery (right or left) grafts, use of composite radial artery grafts, and increasing use of the right gastroepiploic artery have made it possible to use multiple arterial grafting in most of the reoperative procedures.

With bilateral mammary artery use in reoperative patients, the radial artery composite grafts are performed end to end to the right mammary artery to revascularize the circumflex branches. The RIMA composite graft is frequently routed anterior to the aorta. Sequential anastomoses are used liberally.

If saphenous vein grafts (SVG) are used in reoperation, the proximal anastomosis is performed to the old hood of the proximal vein graft. Recently, St. Jude Symmetry™ Aortic Proximal Connector (St. Jude Medical, St. Paul, MN) has been used frequently to avoid any clamping of the aorta.

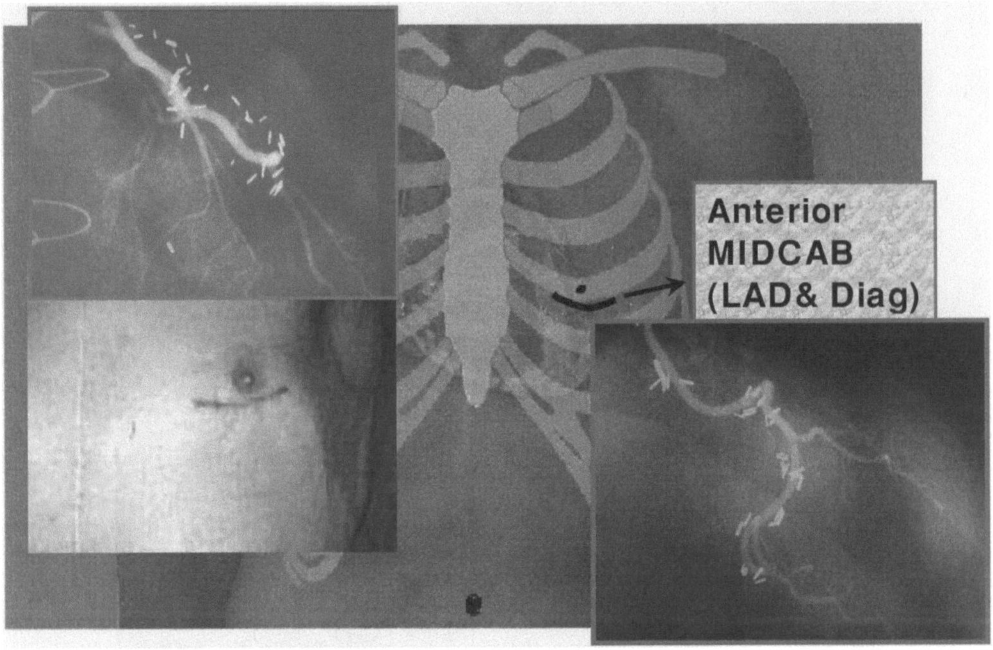

Fig. 2. Classical anterior MIDCAB approach. Angiogram (sequential LIMA to LAD and diagonal arteries) and size of incision are depicted.

For patients who need single or double bypass, minimally invasive direct coronary artery bypass (MIDCAB) approaches through anterior minithoracotomy, short lateral thoracotomy, transabdominal incision, and subxyphoid ministernotomy are used.

Anterior MIDCAB

Anterior MIDCAB is most frequently used for LAD and diagonal revascularization in patients with closed or compromized prior SVG graft to the LAD. Patient is placed in a left semianterolateral decubitus position with a roll under the left scapula. An 8-cm incision over the fourth left intercostal space, with two-thirds of the incision medial and one-third lateral to the nipple is made (**Fig. 2**). The pleura is routinely entered. The left lung is collapsed and the ventilation continues with single right lung ventilation. Routine use of a reusable IMA access retractor system (Thoralift, U.S. Surgical, Norwalk, CT) (**Fig. 3**) creates a wide visual tunnel for exposure of the entire LIMA, allowing its mobilization up to its origin under direct vision. This retractor has several different length blades adaptable to different shapes of the chest. Moreover, by reversing the retractor to the lower chest, the LIMA can be mobilized to its bifurcation at the sixth intercostal space, thus allowing routine sequential anastomoses to the LAD, diagonal and marginal (**Fig. 2**).

In reoperative patients, there is very little endothoracic fascial scarring on the left lateral side of the LIMA pedicle, which makes routine skeletonization of the LIMA easier than in the sternal approach.

Preparation of the LIMA

Prior to the division of the LIMA at the sixth intercostal space, 5000 U of intravenous heparin are given. The LIMA graft is prepared with separate intraluminal injection of verapamil (5 mg in 30 cc of heparnized saline—4 cc injection) and papaverine hydrochlo-

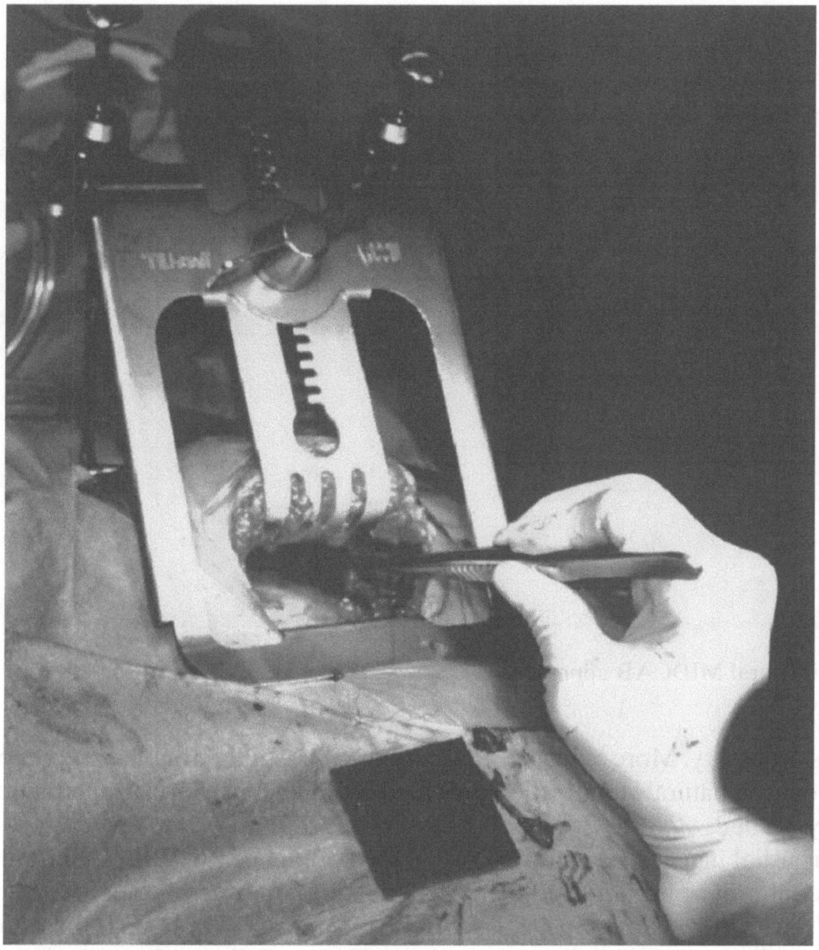

Fig. 3. Thoralift MIDCAB retractor.

ride. Injections are administered without clamping the IMA graft, and no hydrostatic dilatation is used. The distal end of the IMA graft is clipped and allowed to auto-dilate while the coronary artery target site is prepared. This technique for preparation of the IMA graft has been used at our institution over the past decade and has been shown to eliminate any IMA spasm in more than 2000 patients undergoing multiple arterial bypass grafting. Indeed, the arterial conduits are quite large by the time the coronary anastomosis is ready to be performed.

In situations when composite T- or Y-grafting from the LIMA is chosen for grafting of diagonal or ramus intermedius branches through this operative approach (**Fig. 4**), it is essential to construct these anastomoses to the LIMA prior to creation of the LIMA–LAD anastomosis for proper assessment of the length of these grafts.

Exposure of the LAD and Its Branches

After the LIMA is prepared, the IMA retractor system is replaced by the CTS MIDCAB stabilizer platform. Exposure of the target coronary artery (LAD) is easy in reoperation since one can feel the old graft through the pericardium, which easily leads one to the coronary artery just distal to the old anastomotic site. No extensive intrapericardial dis-

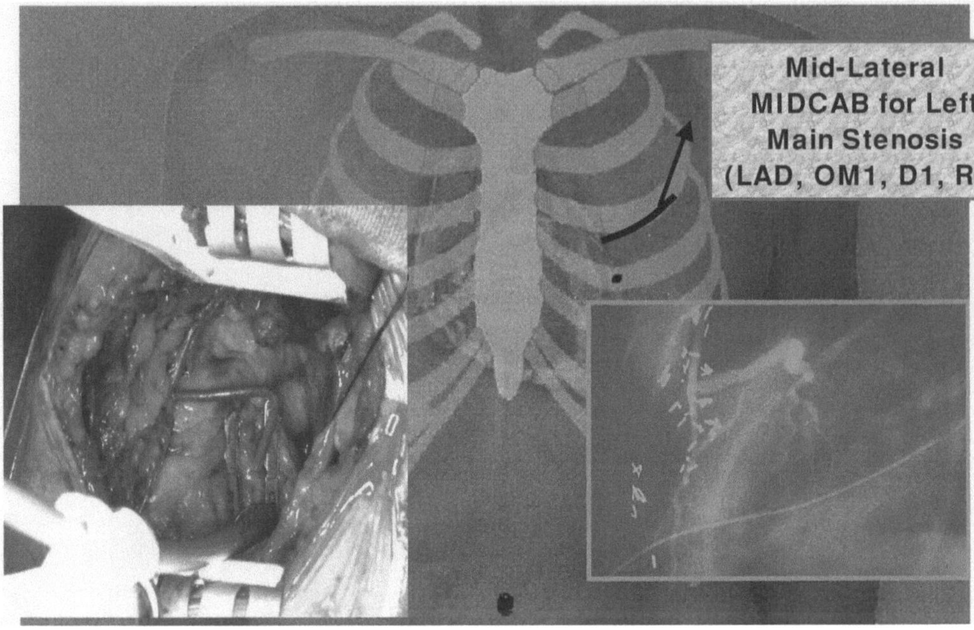

Fig. 4. Midlateral MIDCAB approach.

section is necessary. More extensive dissection will result in troublesome venous bleeding and reduced natural stabilization provided by adhesions. Pericardial traction sutures are rarely needed.

A pericardial incision is made anterior to the phrenic nerve. With an intramyocardial LAD, the intramyocardial tunnel is incised to expose the vessel after antegrade stabilization of the heart with a mechanical stabilizer is achieved. The LAD is then "unearthed" by using two lateral epicardial sutures with tiny Teflon pledgets placed on the sides of the intramyocardial tunnel. In patients with a prior closed IMA graft to LAD, the right gastroepiploic artery graft is harvested via a small upper laparotomy incision and brought through the diaphragm into the left chest to be anastomosed to the LAD.

Subclavian MIDCAB

Subclavian MIDCAB consists of using the radial artery or saphenous vein graft arising from the left axillary artery to graft the LAD or diagonal and ramus intermedius targets (**Fig. 5**). This approach is excellent for patients with prior patent IMA who need diagonal and/or ramus grafts and also in patients with prior occluded IMA who need grafting of the LAD and its branches.

The anterior thoracotomy incision is made again over the left fourth intercostal space, but placed lateral to the nipple to expose the LAD, diagonal and ramus intermedius branches. It is essential to free the adhesions of the medial aspect of the left upper lobe from the apex down to the left hilum, to make sure the graft lies along the medial surface of the hilum to avoid kinking. The coronary target site is exposed as in the anterior MIDCAB. A separate incision is made in intraclavicular fossa one to two fingerbreadths below the left clavicle. The left axillary artery is identified after separating the pectoralis major and pectoralis minor muscle fibers (sometimes division of pectoralis minor muscle).

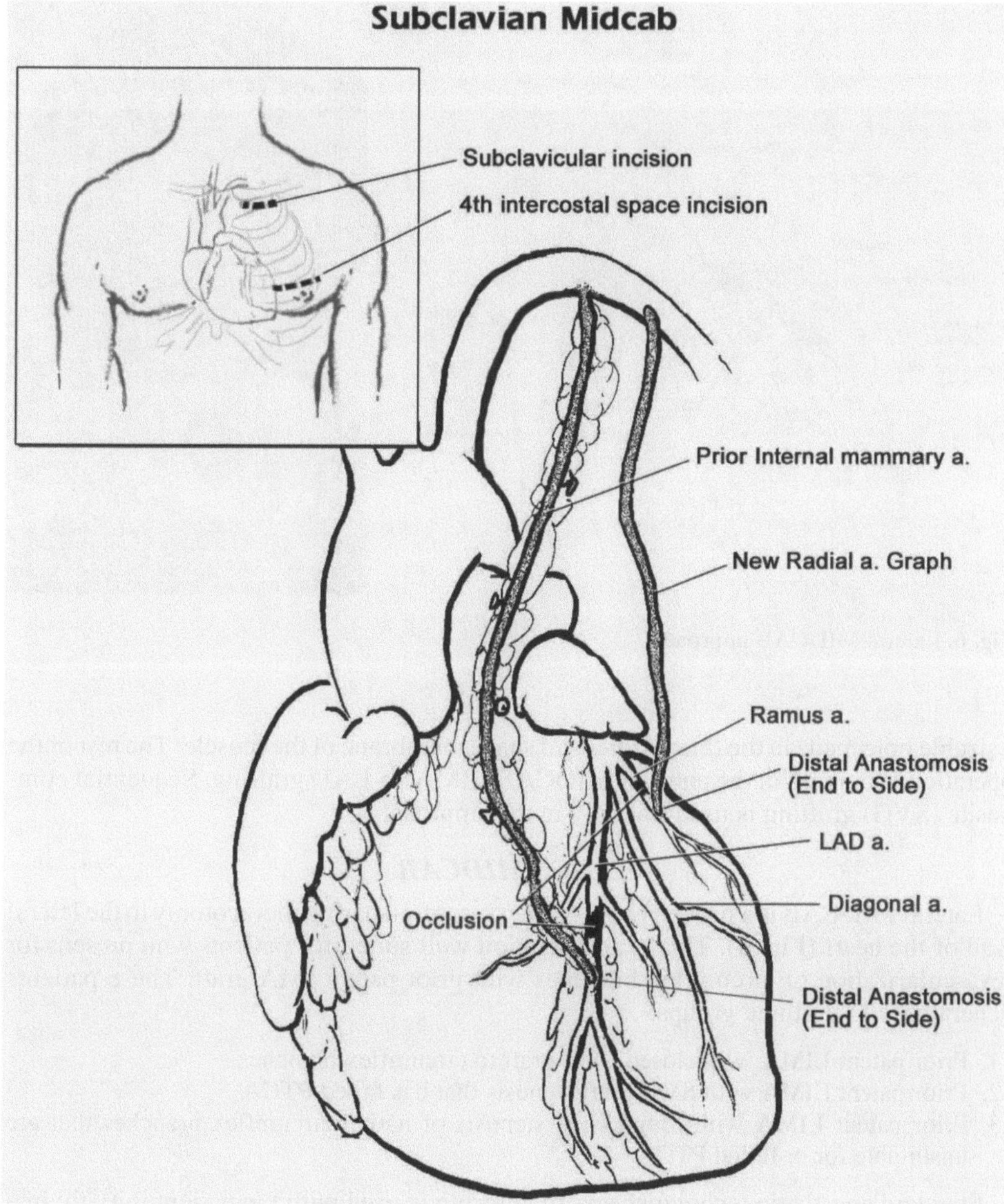

Fig. 5. Subclavian MIDCAB approach.

After division and retraction of these muscles, the clavipectoral fascia is identified and incised. The axillary vein is identified. The axillary artery is inferior to the vein and in most instances the axillary vein has to be retracted away. Heparin is given intravenously (5000 U) and the axillary artery is clamped proximally and distally. A vertical incision from anterior to posterior is made in the inferior aspect of the axillary artery.

The anastomosis of radial artery or SVG graft is performed as a T-graft with the heel of the graft placed posteriorly and inferiorly. The graft is brought in the left chest through

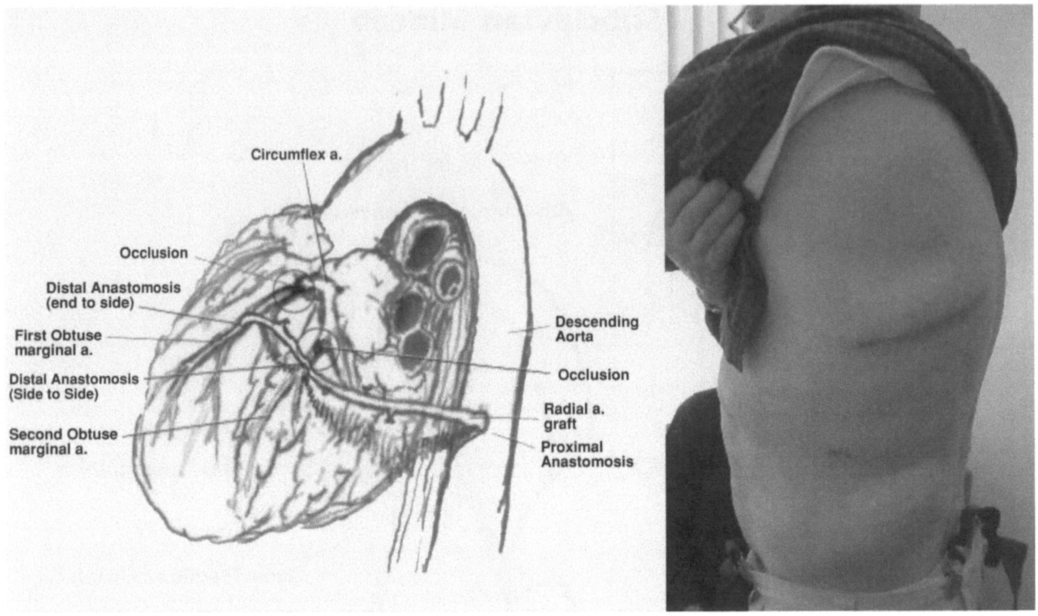

Fig. 6. Lateral MIDCAB approach.

a sizable hole made in the third intercostal space membrane of the muscle. The rest of the operation is done as in the anterior MIDCAB LIMA-to-LAD grafting. Sequential composite (SVG) grafting is used liberally in this approach.

Lateral MIDCAB

Lateral MIDCAB is a limited (3-in.-) access sternal-sparing thoracotomy to the lateral wall of the heart (**Fig. 6**). This is an operation well suited for patients who present for revascularization of circumflex branches with prior patent IMA graft. These patients generally fall into three groups:

1. Prior patent LIMA with closed SVG graft to circumflex branches
2. Prior patent LIMA with SVG graft stenosis that has failed PTCA
3. Prior patent LIMA with progressive stenosis of native circumflex branches that are unsuitable for or failed PTCA

Standard anesthetic techniques and monitoring is used with the patient initially in a supine position. Double-lumen endotracheal intubation is routinely used. Radial artery and SVGs are harvested by endoscopic technique, the grafts are prepared, and the incision is closed. The patient is then turned to the right lateral decubitus standard left posterolateral thoracotomy position. The pelvis and legs are externally rotated (45%) for any emergent access to femoral vessels (i.e., IABP, CPB.) The 3-in. skin incision is made two fingerbreadths below the tip of the scapula, with two-thirds of the incision anterior and one-third posterior to the scapula. Extension of this incision anteriorly is required if grafting of the anterior ramus intermedius branches is necessary in addition to the marginal branches. Posterior extension is required rarely except in instances when the preoperative graft inflow site is determined to be in the proximal left subclavian or proximal descending thoracic aorta and the aortic arch. Most commonly, for grafting of the first and second marginal branches of the circumflex, the fifth intercostal space is entered. The left lung is deflated. In patients with prior multiple operations (more than one coronary reoperation), there may be extensive adhesions between the lung and the chest wall. In these patients, the ribs are retracted and lifted up with a table-mounted IMA retractor hook (Rultract) and sharp dissection of the lung from the chest wall is performed under direct vision, just enough to get a small Finnochieto chest retractor placed in the fifth intercostal space. Further dissection is completed within the chest.

The fourth intercostal space is entered for grafting of the ramus intermedius and the sixth for grafting of the posterolateral and left posterior descending coronary artery branches from the circumflex system. Marsupialization of the serratus anterior and latissimus dorsi muscle with heavy retraction sutures placed through the muscle and brought to the skin and anchored well above and below the skin incision is routine and improves the operative exposure, allowing maximal working space within the chest cavity with the chest retractor in place. Excision of small portions of the posterior part of the fifth and sixth ribs is optional, and occasionally the entire rib is excised. At our institution we have routinely used the CTS Ultima™ Offset Stabilizer, which has excellent retractor blades and gives maximum exposure. This retractor is placed with its handle in the medial aspect of the incision. With the lung clamp retracting the left lower lobe, the inferior pulmonary ligament is incised with cautery, the left lower lobe is dissected from the anterior surface of the distal descending thoracic aorta, and the anteromedial portion of the left lower lobe is dissected away from the pericardium up to the left hilum until the left pulmonary vein becomes visible. In most instances, the lung adhesions to the pericardium are loose and thin and easily dissected away. In patients with prior multiple reoperations with dense adhesions, only the anteromedial surface of the left lower lobe is dissected away from the pericardium and the lateral aspect of the left lower lobe is dissected from the descending thoracic aorta. In this situation the graft is then routed through a small hole in the adhesion between the left lower lobe and the anterior surface of the descending thoracic aorta to be brought to the coronary artery target site. Once the left lower lobe is liberated, this part of the lobe is then packed superiorly into the apex of the thorax with laparotomy gauze pads, thereby providing uninterrupted exposure to the entire surface of the heart posteriorly (**Fig. 7**). The diaphragm is pulled downward with heavy traction sutures placed over the dome of the diaphragm, pulled through the skin at the seventh intercostal space in the anterior axillary line, and tied over a small rubber bolster. Any long nerve retractor hook available in any operating room or the Heartport retractor hook is ideal for this maneuver. This operative maneuver increases the exposure to the posterolateral branch and the left posterior descending coronary artery branch from the circumflex. The pericardium is palpated to locate the old vein grafts when present. In general, the pericardium is opened posterior to the phrenic nerve for grafting of all the circumflex branches except for the ramus intermedius branch, which is exposed via pericardial incision made anterior to the phrenic nerve. Limited dissection of the pericardium is all that is needed to locate the target vessel, usually tracing the old grafts to its anastomotic site. More extensive dissection results in troublesome venous bleeding and reduces the natural stabilization provided by the adhesions. Dissections are rarely carried out anteriorly, and the left internal mammary artery graft is usually not encountered in this operation. After identifying the target vessel, the attention is usually turned to the proximal anastomosis. Advantages of performing the proximal anastomosis first include more accurate measurements and routing of the distended graft conduit, the opportunity to flush atherosclerotic debris from the graft before the completion of the distal anastomosis, and immediate

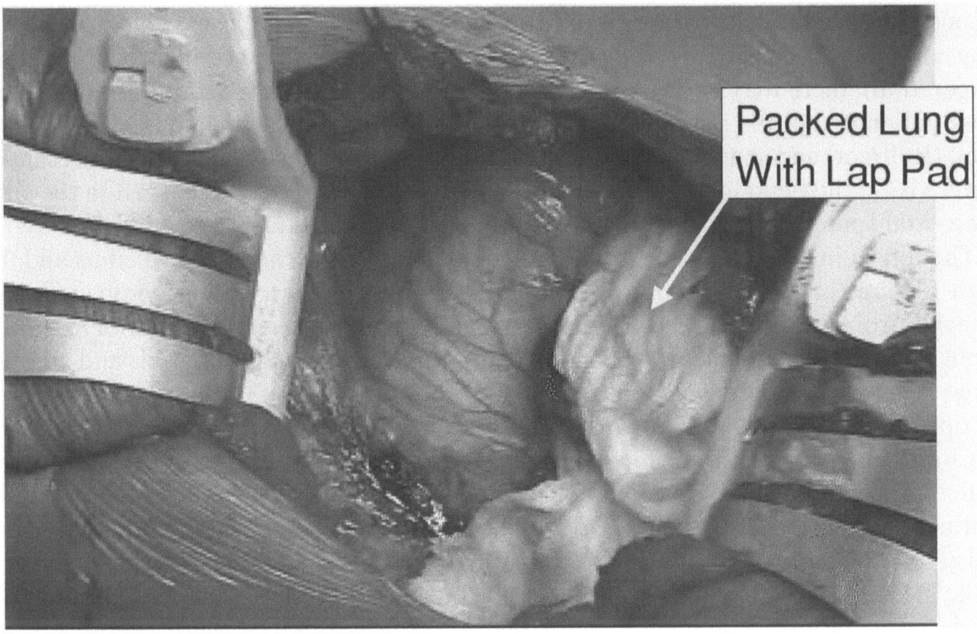

Fig. 7. Exposure of the pericardium on MIDCAB approach.

establishment of flow upon the completion of distal anastomosis. The descending thoracic aorta is assessed below the hilum further by transesophageal or epiaortic echocardiography. Frequently, the proximal anastomosis is performed in the distal descending thoracic aorta midway between the lung hilum and the diaphragm. The heel of the anastomosis is placed proximally, with the toe pointing toward the diaphragm. The proximal anastomosis is completed with the aid of a specially made side-biting clamp on the descending thoracic aorta. This clamp (Scanlan, Inc., St. Paul, MN) has a long handle with a short jaw and is ideally suited for a lateral MIDCAB because of the deep position of the descending thoracic aorta in this approach (**Fig. 8**). The handle of the clamp stays well away from the chest wall and the anastomosis proceeds uninterruptedly with continuous 6-0 Prolene sutures. Recently, a St. Jude Symmetry™ Aortic Connector (St. Jude Medical, St. Paul, MN) has been frequently used for nonclamp technique and is especially useful in this operation due to the deep position of the descending thoracic aorta. If the descending thoracic aorta is atherosclerotic, and there is not a suitable site to be obtained for inflow, the left subclavian artery is used as an inflow. To expose the left subclavian artery, posterior extension of the skin incision is necessary. The proximal portion of this vessel is dissected circumferentially, a side-biting clamp is placed on the artery, or the vessel is occluded with vessel loops. In patients with a patent LIMA graft, a 5-min test occlusion of the subclavian artery is undertaken before opening the artery. During the test occlusion, if there are no electrocardiographic or hemodynamic signs of ischemia, the artery is opened and the proximal graft anastomosis is completed with 6-0 Prolene sutures. If the test occlusion is not tolerated, alternative sites for graft inflow in the aortic arch or in the proximal descending thoracic aorta are chosen. If the arch and the proximal descending thoracic aorta are also heavily atherosclerotic, the left lateral thoracodorsal artery or the left axillary artery have been used for inflow without changing the position of the patient. The lateral thoracodorsal artery is exposed by making a vertical anterior

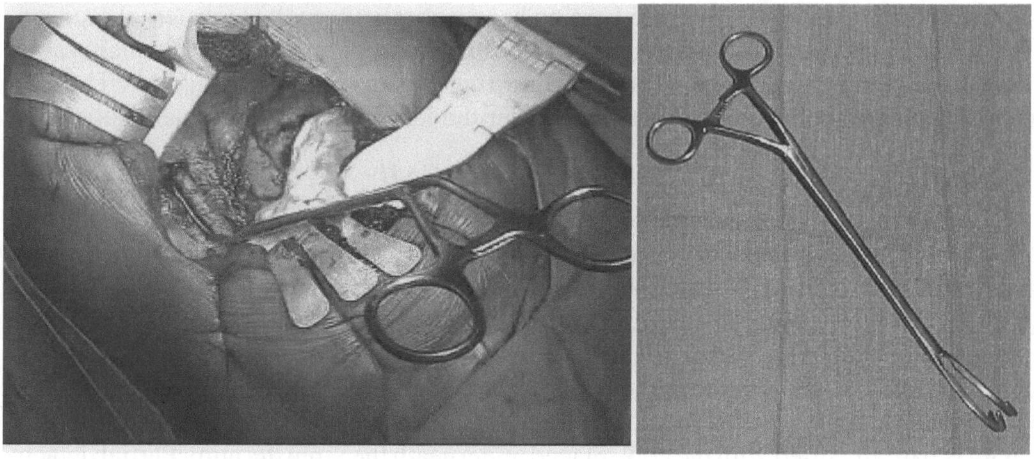

Fig. 8. Aortic clamping in midlateral MIDCAB.

incision in front of the anterior border of the latissimus dorsi and the left thoracodorsal artery. The nerve and vein are identified and carefully separated. End-to-end anastomosis of the graft to the left thoracodorsal artery is performed using fine 7-0 Prolene sutures, and this composite graft is then dropped through a sizable hole in the third intercostal membrane in the anterior axillary line and routed in the major fissure between the upper and the lower lobe of the left lung anterior to the hilum to be anastomosed to the target vessel of the circumflex system. The left axillary artery is approached via an incision posterior to the anterior axillary fold. The axillary artery and vein are identified and anastomosis of the graft to the axillary artery is performed; the graft is then dropped through the third intercostal membrane, coming anterior to the left hilum to be anastomosed to the circumflex branch. In this instance, it is important to mobilize the left upper lobe of the lung from the anterior medial surface of the pericardium, the aortic arch, and the subclavian artery to make the graft lie in a gentle straight route without any kinking. Distal coronary artery anastomosis is completed in a standard fashion running 7-0 polypropylene sutures. The use of intracoronary shunts is optional; the orientation of the graft in most instances is in antegrade fashion with the heel of the anastomosis placed proximally and the toe distally in the coronary artery target site. Occasionally, when the descending thoracic aorta is atherosclerotic and only the lower part of descending aorta is found to be a good inflow site, then anastomosis of the coronary artery target site is performed in retrograde fashion, utilizing the toe pointing toward the proximal and the heel pointing to the distal end of the coronary target site. In all instances the graft has to be tacked very gently over the surrounding tissues to form a nice gentle curve, and the lung is usually inflated after the completion of the anastomosis to assess the final position of the graft. Sequential anastomoses are liberally used in this operation for multivessel grafting.

A recently popularized variation of the lateral MIDCAB is the sternal sparing Thoracab approach *(18)*. The left thoracotomy incision for a Thoracab is longer (4 in.), higher on the chest wall, and more anterior. The proximal source for graft inflow is the ascending aorta with either a side-biting clamp or now a facilitated anastomotic connector. All the native coronary arteries can be visualized and grafted on a beating heart, including the harvesting of the LIMA with grafting to the LAD. With innovative apical suction cup-like devices, the heart can be rotated through this small incision to expose the inferior surface for multivessel CABG on a beating heart entirely through a nonsternal incision. The thoracab approach is being used more often and is particularly good when multivessel beating-heart grafting involves extensive grafting of sites on the lateral wall. The skin incision can also be placed cosmetically under the left breast fold in female patients.

Subxiphoid MIDCAB

The subxiphoid MIDCAB operative approach is ideally suited for grafting of the mid and distal RCA prior to the crux and the proximal part of posterior descending coronary artery with a high origin from the RCA. The right gastroepiploic artery is used as a graft (**Fig. 9**). With the patient in supine position, a vertical incision (3 in.) is made from the xiphisternum to midway between the umbilicus and the sternum (**Fig. 9**). The linea alba is incised and a small V-shaped piece of the xiphisternum is excised. A table-mounted IMA retractor (Rultract) with hooks is placed on the left side of the table and the thoracic cavity is partially lifted with the hook placed underneath the xiphisternum. Partial detachment of the costal attachment of the diaphragm on both sides gives exposure to the mid-right coronary artery and the inferior surface of the right ventricle. Downward sutures on the diaphragm tied to the abdominal wall further increase the exposure. The peritoneum is entered and the gastroepiploic artery is harvested as a pedicle, using a Harmonic scalpel. A vertical incision of the central part of the diaphragm is made and the gastro-epiploic artery is brought over the diaphragm into the mediastinal cavity. A mechanical stabilizer (CTS Ultima™ Stabilizer) is placed vertically to expose the target vessel for coronary artery anastomosis. The stabilizer is used with the handle placed from either the superior or inferior aspect of the incision and the coronary artery is stabilized. The anastomosis is then made in a standard fashion, again using 7-0 Prolene sutures. In a large heart with increased anteroposterior dimension with difficulty in exposure of the distal coronary artery target, the incision needs to be extended into the lower part of the sternum with lateral division of the sternum into the right fifth intercostal space. The distal right coronary artery and posterolateral branch are difficult to access in most instances in this approach.

Transabdominal MIDCAB

Transabdominal MIDCAB is a newer minimally invasive direct coronary artery by-pass operation specifically designed to achieve single and multivessel coronary revascularization in patients including those with distal disease and "full metal jacket" syndrome following prior PTCA in the LAD and RCA, reoperative coronary surgery, and to perform simultaneous bypass via a single incision to the left anterior descending and the right coronary artery and its branches. Our preliminary anatomic observations indicated the following:

1. The rectus abdominus muscle has the strongest downward pull on the lower part of the sternum, so if it is divided the lower sternum can be lifted up farther than the usual position by retractors.
2. When the rib cage is elevated during normal respiration, the lower rib projects directly forward so that the sternum also moves away from the spine, increasing the anteroposterior diameter of the chest by 20%.
3. By dividing the rectus muscle bilaterally and allowing the costal arch to be lifted anteriorly and dividing both costal attachments of the diaphragm, the entire abdominal viscera fall posteriorly, thus increasing the operative exposure and the operative angle to about 60° from the vertical midline of the abdominal incision.

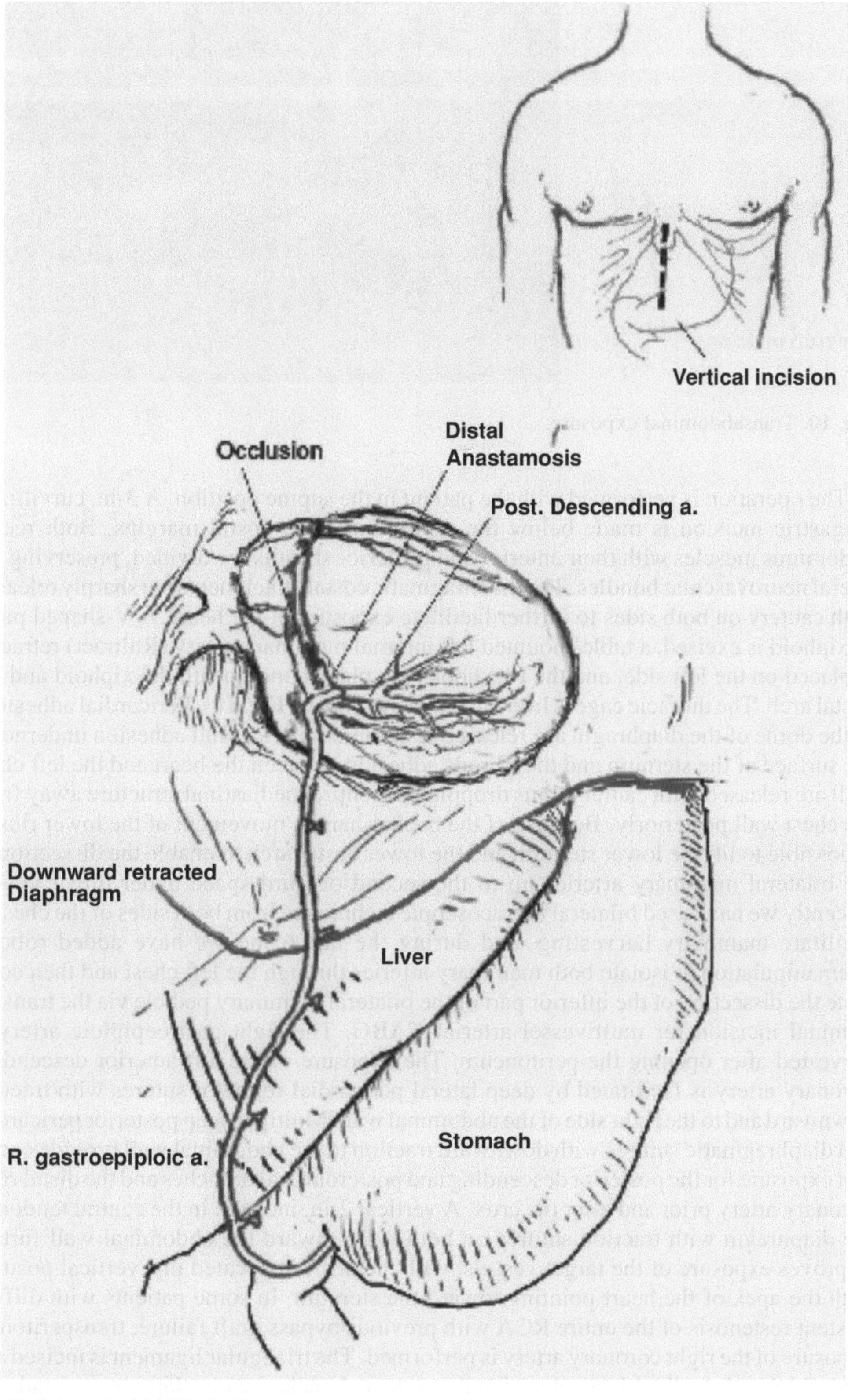

Fig. 9. Subxyphoid MIDCAB approach.

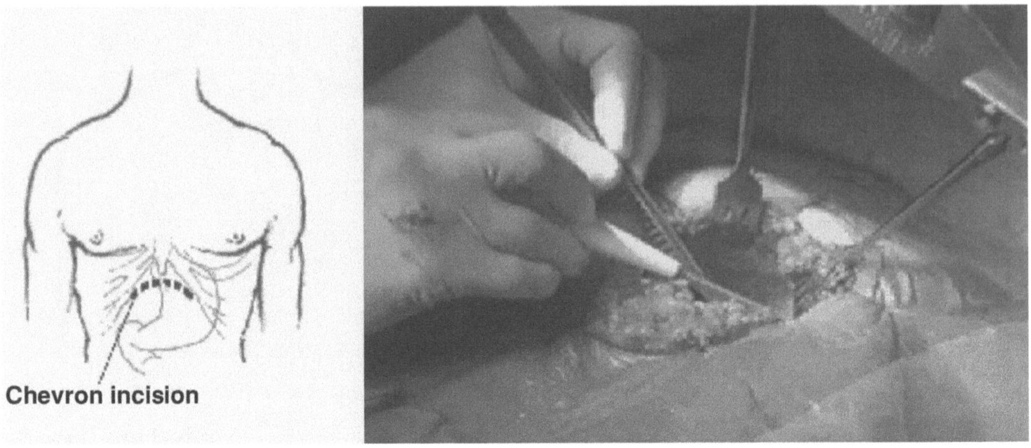

Fig. 10. Transabdominal exposure.

The operation is performed with the patient in the supine position. A 3-in. curvilinear epigastric incision is made below the xiphoid and the costal margins. Both rectus abdominus muscles with their anterior and posterior sheaths are divided, preserving the lateral neurovascular bundles. The diaphragmatic costal attachments are sharply released with cautery on both sides to further facilitate exposure of the heart. A V-shaped piece of xiphoid is excised, a table-mounted left internal mammary artery (Rultract) retractor is placed on the left side, and the two hooks are placed underneath the xiphoid and the costal arch. The thoracic cage is lifted to expose the heart (**Fig. 10**). Pericardial adhesions to the dome of the diaphragm are released. The sternal pericardial adhesion underneath the surface of the sternum and the fibrous adhesion between the heart and the left chest wall are released with cautery, thus dropping the entire mediastinal structure away from the chest wall posteriorly. Because of the bucket-handle movement of the lower ribs, it is possible to lift the lower sternum and the lower costal arch to enable the dissection of the bilateral mammary arteries up to the second or third space under direct vision. Recently we have used bilateral thoracoscopic techniques from both sides of the chest to facilitate mammary harvesting, and during the last 6 mo we have added robotic telemanipulation to isolate both mammary arteries through the left chest and then complete the dissection of the inferior part of the bilateral mammary pedicle via the transabdominal incision for multivessel arterial CABG. The right gastroepiploic artery is harvested after opening the peritoneum. The exposure of the left anterior descending coronary artery is facilitated by deep lateral pericardial retractor sutures with traction downward and to the right side of the abdominal wall. Multiple deep posterior pericardial and diaphragmatic sutures with downward traction to the abdominal wall provide excellent exposure for the posterior descending and posterolateral branches and the distal right coronary artery prior and after the crux. A vertical 2-in. incision in the central tendon of the diaphragm with traction sutures on both sides toward the abdominal wall further improves exposure of the target vessels, with the heart dislocated in a vertical position with the apex of the heart pointing toward the sternum. In some patients with diffuse in-stent restenosis of the entire RCA with previous bypass graft failure, transperitoneal exposure of the right coronary artery is performed. The triangular ligament is incised and the left lobe of the liver is displaced to the right and packed with a laparotomy pad, and then a transverse diaphragmatic incision is made. The stent is palpated and the incision

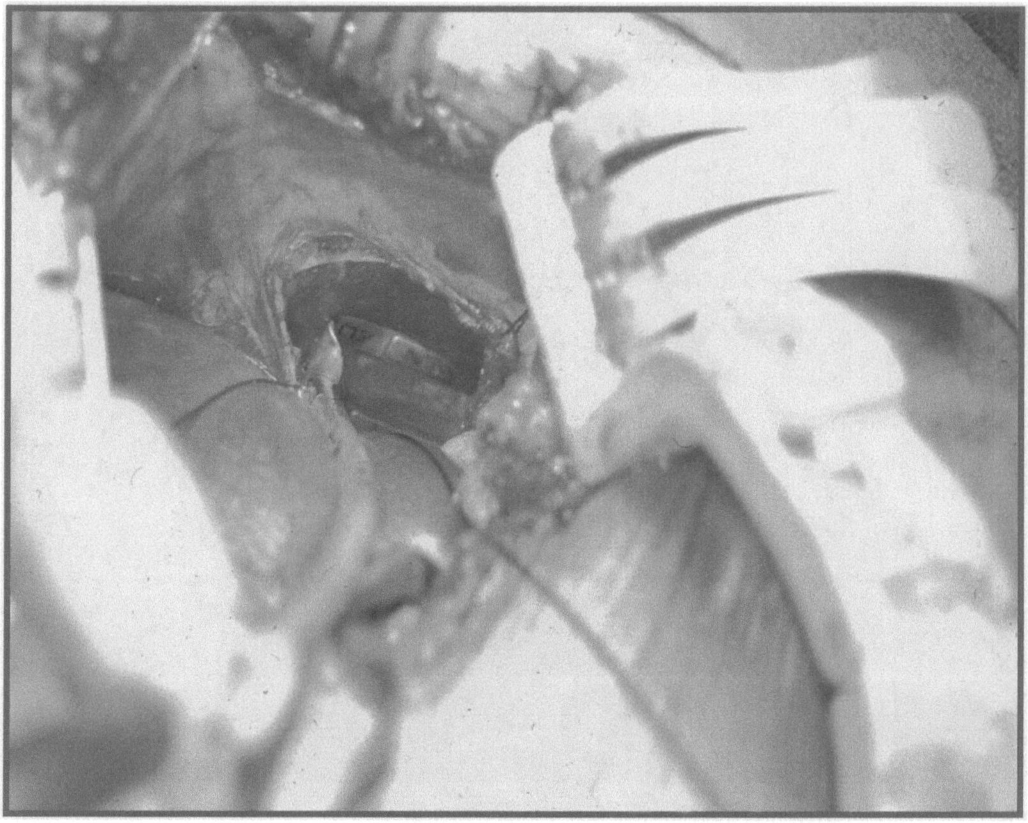

Fig. 11. Transdiaphragmatic incision with stabilization in place.

is then carried out over the coronary artery target site beyond the limit of the stent (**Fig. 11**). The CTS OPCAB retractor is placed either vertically or transversely and the incision is spread. The stabilizer is always placed on the left side and on the inferior part of the retractor. Coronary artery anastomosis is performed in a standard fashion as described in the surgical techniques section. The pleural cavity is rarely entered in these patients, and a small pericardial Blake drainage tube is placed in the posterior part of the mediastinum over the diaphragm, brought through the skin at the lateral aspect of the incision. The incision is closed in layers and the patient is extubated intraoperatively or within the first hour in the ICU. The postoperative invasive monitoring lines are removed within 6 h, and ambulation starts within 24 h. Most patients stay in the hospital for 1–2 d prior to discharge (**Fig. 12**). In addition to the use of bilateral mammary and right gastroepiploic arteries, composite grafting with saphenous vein graft or radial artery conduit anastomosed to the arterial pedicled grafts are sometimes necessary.

RESULTS OF REOPERATIVE OFF-PUMP CABG AT LENOX HILL HOSPITAL

Between April 1994 and December 2001, 499 patients underwent reoperative CABG at our institution. This represents 12.5% of all isolated coronary reoperations during this period. One hundred of these patients had their CABG done on-pump, while the remaining 399 patients had off-pump surgery. Since April 1999, intent to treat all isolated CABG

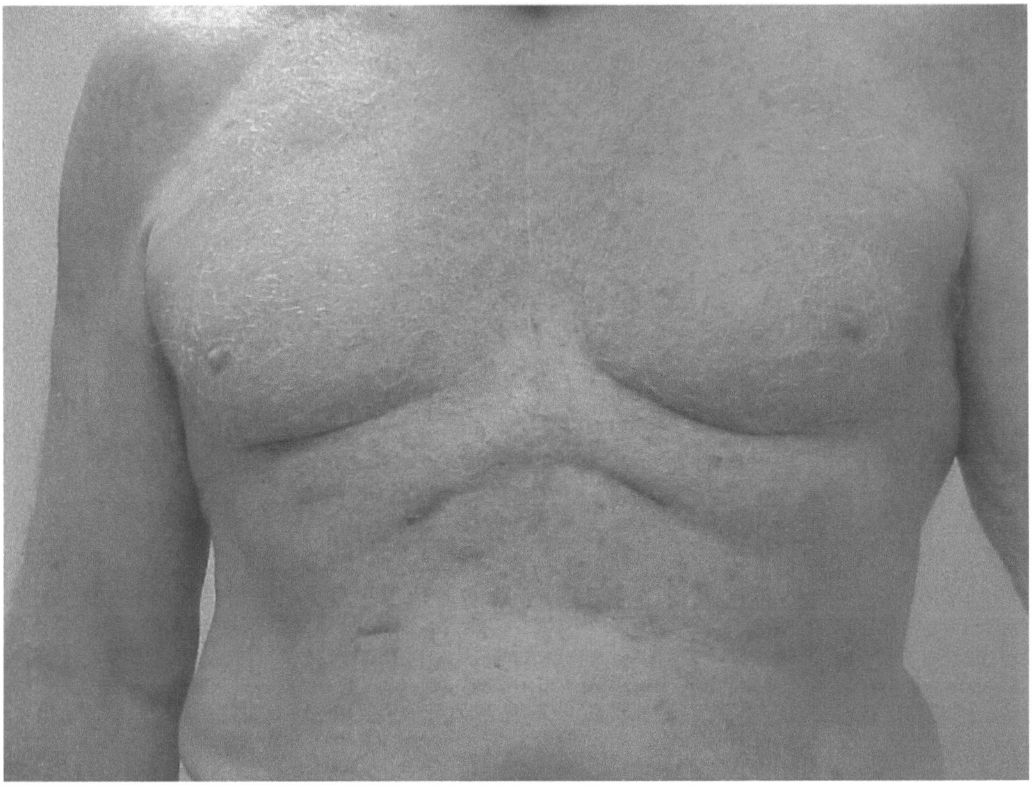

Fig. 12. Postoperative transabdominal MIDCAB incision.

(primary of reoperative) patients with an off-pump approach was initiated at our institution. No reoperative CABGs have been performed on-pump since that time. Of the total 399 off-pump cases, 346 (87%) were performed via nonsternotomy, minimal-access approaches. During the last 18 mo, rare patients have had sternotomy reoperative OPCAB.

The demographics of patient population who had reoperative off-pump CABG via MIDCAB and CABG are shown in Table 1. With experience in minimal access off-pump surgery, the percentage of patients receiving double grafts has increased to 25%. The lowest risk-adjusted mortality is seen in the MIDCAB group, which is better than most series reported on pump reoperative CABG. Postoperative complications and morbidity have also significantly decreased with reoperative off-pump CABG. Strikingly, stroke is practically eliminated with off-pump approaches, especially in view of the high preoperative risk factors associated with this patient population.

The beneficial effect of off-pump approaches is seen even in subgroups including various MIDCAB approaches (Tables 2–4). Of note is the increased percentage of patients receiving double grafts (29.3%) and the absence of stroke in transabdominal and lateral MIDCAB. With increased use of LIMA-to-LAD grafting in the last decade and a half and the continued deterioration of SVG grafts to the circumflex, there has been aggressive use of stenting and PTCA procedures for these patients. Unfortunately the results of SVG graft intervention by PTCA or stenting have been dismal. These patients with prior patent LIMA are frequently referred for reoperative CABG. Most of them need one or two grafts to the circumflex branches in the setting of a patent LIMA and with several occluded vein grafts to other regions of the heart. Hemodynamical stability may depend on the integrity

Table 1
Demographics and Outcomes Among 346 Patients Undergoing Reoperative MIDCAB Approaches (1994–2001)

Preoperative demographics		
Peripheral vascular disease	194	56.1
Multiple previous MI	71	20.5
History of CHF	207	59.8
COPD	41	11.8
Extensively calcified aorta	46	13.3
LVEF ≤ 30	92	26.6
Postoperative complications		
None	316	91.3
Stroke	2	0.6
Q-wave MI	0	0
Deep sternal wound infection	0	0
Renal failure	1	0.3
Risk-adjusted operative mortality		0.76
Number of grafts		
Single	260	75.1
Double	79	22.8
Triple	7	2
Grafts/patient	1.33	

Table 2
Demographics and Outcomes Among 167 Patients Undergoing Reoperative Anterior MIDCAB (1994–2001)

Preoperative demographics		
Peripheral vascular disease	109	65.3
Multiple previous MI	28	16.8
History of CHF	85	50.9
COPD	22	13.2
Extensively calcified aorta	17	10.2
LVEF ≤	52	31.1
Postoperative complications		
None	144	86.2
Stroke	2	1.2
Q-wave MI	0	0
Deep sternal wound infection	0	0
Renal failure	1	0.6
Risk-adjusted operative mortality		0.88
Number of grafts		
Single	126	75.4
Double	37	22.2
Triple	4	2.4
Grafts/patients	1.21	

of the LIMA during reoperative dissection. Even with careful transsternal approach for reoperative grafting in experienced institutions, others have documented that the LIMA is still damaged 5% of the time. When this happens, operative mortality rises threefold,

Table 3
Demographics and Outcomes Among 75 Patients Undergoing Reoperative Transabdominal MIDCAB (1998–2001)

Preoperative demographics		
Peripheral vascular disease	39	52
Multiple previous MI	15	20
Hypertension	51	68
History of CHF	45	60
COPD	9	12
Extensively calcified aorta	13	17.3
LVEF ≤ 30	18	24
Postoperative complications		
None	66	88
Stroke	0	0
Q-wave MI	0	0
Deep sternal wound infection	0	0
Renal failure	0	0
Risk-adjusted operative mortality		0.61
Number of grafts		
Single	52	69.3
Double	22	29.3
Triple	1	1.3
Grafts/patient	1.3	

Table 4
Demographics and Outcomes Among 114 Patients Undergoing Reoperative Lateral MIDCAB (1996–2001)

Preoperative demographics		
Peripheral vascular disease	46	40.4
Multiple previous MI	28	24.6
History of CHF	77	67.5
COPD	10	8.8
Extensively calcified aorta	16	14
LVEF ≤ 30	22	19.3
Postoperative complications		
None	106	93
Stroke	0	0
Q-wave MI	0	0
Deep sternal wound infection	0	0
Renal failure	0	0
Risk-adjusted operative mortality		0.55
Number of grafts		
Single	82	71.9
Double	30	26.3
Triple	2	1.8
Grafts/patient	1.31	

from the expected 3% to 9%. When a limited-access approach, such as lateral MIDCAB, is used, the patent graft is not disturbed and the operative mortality is reduced to 0.5% as shown by our experience.

Multivessel coronary artery disease after prior CABG may present with more than one ischemic myocardial region that cannot be fully addressed via a single limited-access incision. To resolve this, we have been increasingly using two separate minimal-access incisions to address both regions. In some instances we have operated at two different times separated by 1–2 mo with different access approaches.

The experience with evolving facilitated anastomotic technology will further enhance the utility of minimal reoperative CABG. The St. Jude Symmetry™ Aortic Connector (St. Jude Medical, St. Paul, MN) in lateral MIDCAB has already simplified this operation. Novel magnetic connectors *(19)* are being evaluated for distal coronary arterial anastomosis in clinical trials in Europe (*see* Chapter 30). These devices combined with limited-access incisions and robotic assistance, we believe, will pave the way for outpatient reoperative CABG.

REFERENCES

1. Loop FD, Lytle BW, Cosgrove DM, et al. Influence of the internal-mammary-artery graft on 10-year survival and other cardiac events. N Engl J Med 1986;314:1–6.
2. Cameron A, Kemp HG Jr, Green GE. Bypass surgery with the internal mammary artery graft: 15 year follow-up. Circulation 1986;74(suppl III):III-30-6.
3. Lytle BW. Coronary reoperations. In Franco KL, Verrier ED, eds. Advanced Therapy in Cardiac Surgery. B. C. Decker, 1999;84–99.
4. Rosengart TK. Risk analysis of primary versus reoperative coronary artery bypass grafting. Ann Thorac Surg 1993;56:S74–S77.
5. He GW, Acuff TE, Ryan WH, et al. Determinants of operative mortality in reoperative coronary artery bypass grafting. J Thorac Cardiovasc Surg 1995;110:971–978.
6. Loop FD, Lytle BW, Cosgrove DM, et al. Reoperation for coronary atherosclerosis: changing practice in 2509 consecutive patients. Ann Surg 1990;212:378–386.
7. Fanning WJ, Kakos GS, Williams TE Jr. Reoperative coronary artery bypass grafting without cardiopulmonary bypass. Ann Thorac Surg 1993;55:586–589.
8. Mohr R, Moshkovitz Y, Gurevitch J, Benetti FJ. Reoperative coronary artery bypass without cardiopulmonary bypass. Ann Thorac Surg 1997;63(suppl 6):S40–S43.
9. Bergsland J, Hasnain S, Lajos TZ, Salerno TA. Elimination of cardiopulmonary bypass: a prime goal in reoperative coronary artery bypass surgery. Eur J Cardiothorac Surg 1998;14:59–63.
10. Pfister AJ, Zaki S, Garcia JM, et al. Coronary artery bypass without cardiopulmonary bypass. Ann Thorac Surg 1992;54:1085–1092.
11. Subramanian VA. Clinical experience with minimally invasive reoperative coronary bypass surgery. Eur J Cardiothorac Surg 1996;10:1058–1063.
12. Grandjean JG, Mariani MA, Ebels T. Coronary reoperation via small laparotomy using right gastroepiploic artery without cardiopulmonary bypass. Ann Thorac Surg 1996;61:1853–1855.
13. Fonger JD, Doty JR, Sussman MS, Salomon NW. Lateral MIDCAB grafting via limited posterior thoracotomy. Eur J Cardiothorac Surg 1997;12:399–405.
14. Subramanian VA, Patel NU. Transabdominal minimally invasive direct coronary artery bypass grafting (MIDCAB). Eur J Cardiothorac Surg 2000;17(4):485–487.
15. Varnauskas E, the European Coronary Study Group. Twelve-year follow-up of survival in the randomized European Coronary Surgery Study. N Engl J Med 1988;319:332.
16. CASS Principle Investigators, et al. Myocardial infarction and mortality in the Coronary Artery Surgery Study (CASS) randomized trial. N Engl J Med 1984;310:750.
17. Yusuf S, Zucker D, Peduzzi P, et al. Effect of coronary bypass surgery on survival: overview of 10 year results from randomized trials by The Coronary Artery Bypass Graft Surgery Trialists Collaboration. Lancet 1994;344:563–570.
18. Srivastava SP, Kirit NP, Tummala P, et al. Thoracab: an innovative approach to total revascularization without cardiopulmonary bypass and median sternotomy—Srivastava approach. A report of first 160 consecutive cases. Heart Surgery Forum 2001;4(suppl 2):S80.
19. Subramanian VA. Overview of magnetic technology used to facilitate proximal and distal anastomoses. Presented at Euro-College on ATCS: The Key to Advanced Techniques in Cardiac Surgery, Sep 15, 2001, Lisbon, Portugal.

13 Perioperative Evaluation of Graft Patency in OPCAB

Vinod H. Thourani, MD
and John D. Puskas, MD, MSc

Contents

Introduction
Introperative Graft Assessment
Postoperative Graft Assessment
Future Technologies to Evaluate Postoperative Graft Patency
Summary
References

INTRODUCTION

With presently available instrumentation, off-pump coronary artery bypass (OPCAB) grafting via a median sternotomy can now be performed for lesions in virtually any coronary artery with a high degree of patient safety and surgeon comfort. Recent reports have documented excellent short-term outcomes for patients undergoing OPCAB *(1,2)*. Despite multiple clinical studies evaluating clinical outcomes, there remains a paucity of literature evaluating the patency of grafts constructed by OPCAB techniques. Although the introduction of epicardial stabilizers has improved the accuracy with which distal anastomoses on the beating heart can be constructed, there has been concern that the technical difficulties of performing OPCAB could possibly increase the risk of technical anastomotic failure *(3)*. This chapter reviews both the intraoperative and postoperative methods and outcomes of anastomotic evaluation for patients undergoing off-pump coronary artery surgery.

From: *Contemporary Cardiology: Minimally Invasive Cardiac Surgery, Second Edition*
Edited by: D. J. Goldstein and M. C. Oz © Humana Press Inc., Totowa, NJ

INTRAOPERATIVE GRAFT ASSESSMENT

Intraoperative assessment of graft patency has not been commonly performed after conventional coronary artery bypass surgery. Most cardiac surgeons have relied on simple clinical signs (e.g., electrographic tracings or hemodynamic stability) or manual palpation (e.g., fingertips or direct probing) to make a diagnosis of coronary graft occlusion. With the increasing sophistication and popularity of OPCAB, together with the introduction and improvement in tools to measure intraoperative coronary graft flow, there has been a revived interest in documenting graft patency. While angiography remains the definitive test of graft patency, it is time-consuming, often requires cardiology assistance, and is not without risk. A rapid, safe test of graft patency that can be easily performed by the operating surgeon has been sought.

Initially, electromagnetic devices were used to measure the intensity of the electromagnetic field generated by electrically charged red blood cells flowing within the vessels *(4)*. The intensity of the electromagnetic field generated was used to calculate the actual blood flow. However, this technology has been abandoned due to the numerous sources of potential error. These flow measurements were often difficult to obtain, required perfect placement of probes, and necessitated careful calibration of instruments. Finally, the measured values are influenced by the hematocrit and the thickness of the vessel wall *(5)*. Generally, ultrasound technology—Doppler and transit time flow measurement (TTFM)—has replaced electromagnetic techniques *(5–7)*.

Transit Time Flow Measurement

Although the first transit time flow meter was described in 1962 *(8)*, it was not until 1983 that the first flow meter became commercially available. The flow probe consists of two small piezoelectric crystals, one upstream and one downstream, mounted on the same side of the vessel. Opposite the crystal is a small metallic reflector. Each crystal produces a wide pulsed ultrasound beam covering the entire vessel width. The area of the transducers and the distance the beam has to travel between the two transducers are known and are used to calculate the flow of blood through the graft. The probe is connected to a computer and the necessary time for an ultrasound beam, emitted from the upstream crystal to arrive at the downstream crystal after being reflected, and for a signal from the downstream crystal to reach the upstream crystal is measured. Because ultrasound travels faster if transmitted in the same direction as flow, a small time difference between the two beams is calculated as the transit time of flow (TTF). Thus, the blood flow in the graft is proportional to the transit time. All calculations are made automatically by the flow meter and are displayed as milliliters per minute. The level of acoustical coupling is expressed by a color-coded square and as a percentage of the optimal contact. Measurements are not dependent on the angle between the vessel and the probe. Measurements are also independent of the hematocrit level, heart rate, and thickness of the vessel wall. Flow curves, together with flow and pulsatile index (PI) values, are displayed in real time on a video screen.

The PI is a good indicator of the blood flow pattern and, consequently, of the quality of the anastomosis. This number is obtained by dividing the difference between the maximum and minimum flow by the value of the mean flow. The optimum PI should be between 1 and 5; the higher the number, the more suggestive of anastomotic imperfections *(9,10)*. D'Ancano and colleagues suggest revision of any distal coronary anastomosis with a measured intraoperative pulsatile index ≥ 5 *(9,10)*.

The ability of TTFM to detect less than critical stenosis has not been clearly defined. Another limit of TTFM is the lack of standard or nominal curves and flow values for different types of grafts and revascularized vessels. Interpretation of flow curves and TTFM findings is still empirical and dependent on the surgeon's personal experience. Jaber et al. *(11)* reported that differences in flow tracing morphology were virtually indistinguishable from fully patent to moderately stenotic anastomoses. Moreover, grafts with up to 75% stenosis still had predominantly diastolic flow, and only grafts with greater than 75% stenosis exhibited significantly reduced diastolic flow in a canine model.

In order to improve the objectivity of TTFM in detecting significant differences between mild-to-moderate and more severe stenosis, Koening et al. *(12)* have utilized magnitude and phase-component spectral analysis. Furthermore, Cerrito et al. *(13)* designed a neural network to represent an "acceptable" anastomosis of less than 50% stenosis, or an anastomosis that "should be redone" with a stenosis greater than 50%. The future for clinical application of neural network analysis will require a database of graft flow measurements correlated to varying degrees of anastomotic stenosis, validated by angiography. In humans, Salerno and Bergsland have suggested that flow patterns, PI values, flow values, and clinical findings (e.g., electrocardiographic tracing, hemodynamic values) should always be evaluated simultaneously with TTFM to complement important clinical decisions.

Since 1996, Salerno and Bergsland have consistently utilized this technology in patients undergoing OPCAB and have reported on their extensive experience *(6,10,14–17)*. In a series of articles on off-pump coronary surgery, they reported 161 patients undergoing a total of 323 distal anastomoses *(15)*. All completed grafts were tested intraoperatively with TTFM, and the decision to accept or revise any individual graft was based on a decision nomogram using key values readily available from the TTFM output. They noted that 32 grafts (10%) were surgically revised based on unsatisfactory flow curves, the pulsatile index (PI), or both. All revised grafts were found to have a significant technical error, such as an intimal flap, thrombus, conduit kinking, or dissection. In a follow-up study by the same group, the authors *(16)* reported on 464 patients undergoing a total of 1002 flow assessments. A total of 57 grafts (6%) of the distal grafts required revision. The authors *(14)* have eloquently summarized their clinical recommendations in the following seven dictums:

1. Flow must be measured with and without proximal occlusion. A graft obstructed at the toe may show perfectly normal flow if there is significant outflow in the proximal direction.
2. The diastolic flow pattern must be evaluated, as the graft may be compromized with relatively high mean flow. Correspondingly, a graft can be normal with low mean flow.
3. When in doubt, reevaluation of TTFM at a higher blood pressure and/or through an intraoperative pharmacological stress test should be performed with nitroglycerin, papaverine, or adenosine.
4. The presence of air bubbles in the graft may simulate organic obstruction. If this is suspected, the graft should be de-aired.
5. When a malfunctioning graft is diagnosed, it should be immediately revised to prevent ischemia and hemodynamic problems during the remaining procedure.
6. Measurement of the graft flow should be repeated after heparin reversal.

7. Final graft verification should be done just before chest closure, since grafts that are too short or too long may kink on chest closure.

A limited number of studies have determined the validity of the intraoperative transit time flow measurements of grafts in coronary bypass grafting by correlating TTFM with intraoperative or postoperative quantitative angiography. In a small series of 35 patients (28 patients underwent conventional "on-pump" CABG and 7 underwent OPCAB) having 82 distal anastomoses, Takami et al. *(18)* noted that intraoperative flow measurement reflected precisely the short-term (14 ± 5 d) postoperative angiographic quality of the distal anastomoses. They note that the calculations based on the fast Fourier transformation (FFT) of the flow curve allowed distinction of patent from nonpatent grafts. A FFT ratio (the ratio of powers of the fundamental frequency and its first harmonic) greater than 1.0 corresponded with patent grafts (stenosis less than 20%) and those with FFT ratio less than 1.0 corresponded with nonpatent grafts. They conclude that power spectral analysis of the TTFM flow waveform using FFT is useful for intraoperative prediction of anastomotic patency *(19)*.

In contrast, Hol and colleages *(20)* studied 72 patients (21 patients underwent conventional "on-pump" CABG and 51 underwent OPCAB) undergoing 124 grafts. All patients underwent intraoperative TTFM, followed by coronary angiogram in the operating room after chest closure while the patients were under general anesthesia. Follow-up angiography of both grafts and the native coronary arteries was carried out at 3 mo in all cases. Forty-eight grafts were assessed by an additional angiography at 12 mo. The authors concluded that blood flow measurements (mean flow, PI, and waveform) performed intraoperatively could not identify significant stenoses in arterial or vein grafts and were not predictive of long-term graft patency. Furthermore, they believe that blood flow measurements should be interpreted cautiously and viewed as additional evidence to other indicators of graft dysfunction.

Even if interpretation of TTFM findings is still based on personal experience and empirical values, many researchers are focusing their attention on trying to develop nominal TTFM curves and objective mathematical values to improve the applicability of this technology. At the present time, TTFM remains the most popular modality among an armamentarium of intraoperative techniques used to assess OPCAB graft patency.

Doppler Ultrasound

Pulse-wave Doppler ultrasound is another technique commonly employed to assess intraoperative coronary artery graft patency. The ultrasound pencil probe (generally 5–20 MHz) is acoustically coupled to the vessel by a small amount of sterile gel. Sharp dissection is not necessary to measure flow in most conduits. The parameters commonly determined by the pulsed Doppler are flow (L/min), velocity (cm/s), and internal diameter (mm) of the vessel. Furthermore, a total resistance of the graft and coronary bed, along with a pulsatility index (PI) can also be calculated. Although a variety of investigators have evaluated the use of Doppler ultrasound as a tool of flow assessment in patients undergoing on-pump conventional coronary artery bypass grafting *(4,21–26)*, only a few have investigated this tool in OPCAB patients *(27–30)*.

Dr. Chitwood's group *(27)* reported the use of simple continuous-wave Doppler flow assessment of the LIMA graft with concurrent intraoperative angiography via the radial artery in 50 consecutive patients. They used a nonquantitative and subjective methodology for analysis of the Doppler flow signal. Flow was graded as 0 = no flow, 1+ = poor or questionable signal, and 2+ = satisfactory flow with diastolic augmentation. To avoid mistaking retrograde for antegrade flow, assessment was made with a proximal tourniquet still in place. They demonstrated a 75% sensitivity of the Doppler ultrasound in detecting actual problems and 94% specificity. Despite the advent of more sophisticated duplex ultrasound technology, the authors contend that all noninvasive testing may be subject to technical problems with equipment, user error, and subjective interpretation.

More recently, Magovern and his associates *(28)* studied intraoperative color pulsed-Doppler flow methods of graft analysis in 35 patients undergoing elective left internal mammary artery (LIMA) anastomosis to the left anterior descending (LAD) coronary artery via OPCAB. In addition, immediate graft patency was determined with intraoperative angiography using selective injection of the left internal mammary artery from a femoral approach. A normal Doppler study was defined as a diastolic predominant flow pattern with a pan-diastolic flow velocity of greater than 15 cm/s. There was immediate perfect patency with brisk flow in 32 patients (91%), all confirmed by intraoperative angiograms. All patients with abnormal angiograms also had abnormal Doppler flow. In this study, the three patients with imperfect anastomosis were revised. Interestingly, none of these patients demonstrated echocardiographic evidence of ischemia, hemodynamic instability, or any obvious abnormality of the graft. At 2 yr follow-up, all surviving patients were without angina, and 97% were free from reintervention on the LAD. The authors conclude that color pulsed-Doppler analysis was 100% accurate for confirming graft patency and for detecting failed grafts intraoperatively.

Calafiore et al. *(29,30)* have reported that the pulsed-Doppler flow velocity performed perioperatively at rest and after the adjunctive Azoulay maneuver (which transiently augments venous return and increases cardiac output and graft flow) is a reliable technique to follow up patients who undergo OPCAB. They described 100 patients who underwent early postoperative Doppler flow velocity assessment and coronary angiography. They concluded that normal grafts show an increase in diastolic flow velocity whereas stenotic grafts do not. These results were confirmed by angiography.

In general, Doppler flow measurements are not as familiar to cardiac surgeons as angiograms, but they provide useful information and avoid the risks of contrast dye and catheter-related injury. Doppler technology may be expeditiously utilized by experienced OPCAB surgeons wishing to document the patency of distal coronary anastomoses.

Intraoperative Angiography

Angiography is considered the "gold standard" for assessment of anastomotic quality. However, angiography is not readily available in most operating rooms and is invasive, costly, and time-consuming. It has therefore been utilized sparingly in the intraoperative assessment of graft patency during OPCAB *(27,31–37)*.

Chitwood and his colleagues reported that, with some experience, cardiac surgeons can perform intraoperative LIMA arteriography via the left radial artery in 10–15 min *(31)*. The LAD–LIMA patency was visualized under direct fluoroscopy in a series of 20 patients without complications. Intervention based on angiography was required in three patients (15%), two of whom had received sequential LIMA anastomoses. Mild LIMA or LAD spasm was a common finding, which generally resolved after a second contrast injection. The authors felt that intraoperative arteriography offered several advantages over routine postoperative cardiac catheterization prior to hospital discharge: (1) the results were obtained immediately and interventions performed prior to the patient leaving the operating suite; (2) same-day catheterization requiring transfer of the patient from the operating room to a catheterization lab was eliminated; and (3) the cost to the patient for a postoperative coronary catheterization was reduced.

In a follow-up study, Chitwood *(27)* compared the use of continuous-wave Doppler flow assessment of the LIMA graft with concurrent intraoperative surgeon-performed angiography via a radial artery technique in 50 consecutive patients. They suggested that intraoperative arteriographic assessment of grafts be performed (1) in any patient with equivocal Doppler flow signals; (2) in any patient with severely diseased native coronary vessels; (3) in all sequential or complex anastomotic cases; and (4) in any case in which the surgeon is not entirely satisfied with the anastomosis. Furthermore, they noted that intraoperative angiography may be helpful to a surgeon early in the OPCAB learning curve.

Other Techniques for Intraoperative Graft Assessment

Takayama reported that intraoperative coronary angiography using fluorescein in 29 consecutive cases had sufficient resolution only to demonstrate whether an anastomotic stenosis was critical and whether the distribution of graft flow was normal *(38)*. Intraoperative fluorescein angiography provided the cardiac surgeon with insufficient objective data to adequately assess the quality of coronary anastomoses and to make decisions regarding graft revision. However, since this technique does not require selective catheterization of coronary arteries, it is easy to perform.

Thermal coronary angiography (TCA), or infrared thermography, is a noninvasive method that requires no catheter, contrast medium, radiation, or interference with the surgical procedure *(39–42)*. Yet it is similar to angiography in that it gives visual representation of grafts and coronaries arteries. Falk and colleagues *(42)* used this method in 370 on-pump coronary artery bypass patients and successfully documented patency rates for saphenous vein grafts (90.6%) and LIMA grafts (96.2%). However, owing to anatomical reasons, certain coronary arteries could not be visualized and thermal imaging was compromised by excessive epicardial fat pads *(42)*. More recently, Suma et al. *(37)* used thermal coronary artery imaging with a newer-generation infrared camera (IRIS III) in 12 normothermic OPCAB patients undergoing 18 distal anastomoses. One LIMA graft (5.6%) was shown to be closed and was revised. All grafts were restudied by conventional catheter angiography postoperatively, and all were patent. In this small cohort of patients, these authors showed that intraoperative noninvasive coronary imaging with a highly sensitive infrared camera had adequate resolution to detect graft closure, but this technique still offers inadequate resolution to assess coronary anastomoses qualitatively.

At present no alternative method provides the same information and resolution as angiography. Nonetheless, only a small minority of surgeons perform routine intraoperative angiography, owing to technical and logistical concerns. It is foreseeable that a new, less invasive, and equally informative technique of graft assessment might become a widely accepted tool for intraoperative assessment of anastomoses performed during OPCAB, but none presently exists.

POSTOPERATIVE GRAFT ASSESSMENT

Although there is an extensive body of literature containing the results of postoperative angiographic patency rates in conventional coronary artery bypass grafting, only a limited number of series contain information on postoperative angiographic findings following OPCAB.

Results of Early (< 1 mo) Angiography After OPCAB

Schaff and his colleagues *(43)* from the Mayo Clinic studied 15 of 16 patients with angiography immediately following minimally invasive direct coronary artery bypass grafting (MIDCAB). Three patients (20%) required reexploration, and one patient (7%) required reconstruction of the distal anastomosis.

Subramanian et al. *(44)* have shown that mechanical stabilizers can profoundly impact angiographic patency rate. In an off-pump series of 199 patients, 111 patients had postoperative angiographic evaluation and were divided into two groups. In 44 patients MIDCAB operations were performed prior to April 1996, utilizing β-blockers and calcium-channel blockers and intermittent transient cardiac standstill accomplished with 5- to 10-mg intravenous boluses of adenosine. In 67 patients, MIDCAB was performed after April 1996, using a mechanical stabilizer. Early overall graft patency (less than 36 h postoperatively) was 93% (103 of 111 patients). They found that the patency rate for the patients in which MIDCAB was performed with a mechanical stabilizer was significantly improved compared to those performed without a mechanical stabilizer (97% vs 86%, respectively, $p = 0.028$).

Similarly, Cartier and his colleagues in Montreal *(45)* evaluated the quality of LIMA anastomosis to the LAD in 20 patients who underwent beating-heart coronary bypass surgery without stabilization and 14 patients who had OPCAB with a stabilization device. Eight patients in whom the anastomoses were performed without stabilization (8/20, 40%) had stenoses of more than 50%. There was only one stenosis (7%) of more than 50% of coronary luminal diameter among the patients in whom the operation was performed with a stabilizer ($p = 0.02$). In a multi-institutional study, Mack et al. *(46)* reported intraoperative (38 patients) or immediate postoperative (62 patients) angiographic evaluation in 100 of 103 patients undergoing LIMA to LAD by MIDCAB. They found angiographic graft patency of 99%, with Grade A graft patency (no stenosis greater than 50%) being 91%. A total of three grafts (8%) were revised in the operating room; one patient (2%) underwent reoperation and three more (5%) underwent PTCA. Similarly, in a small series of 25 patients, Gill et al. *(47)* completed angiographic follow-up in all patients within 4–6 h postoperatively and noted a 97.5% (28 of 29 grafts) overall patency rate.

At our institution, one surgeon (J.D.P.) routinely performed early postoperative angiography for all OPCAB patients who would consent since November 1996 *(1,2,48)*. A recent review of 378 consecutive patients at Emory University before September 2000 revealed that 287 patients (76%) underwent postoperative cardiac catheterization prior to hospital discharge *(49)*. The average number of distal anastomoses was 2.8 ± 1.1. The angiograms were reviewed by a panel of three cardiologists, and quantitative measurements were performed on all grafts and target vessels.

Postoperative graft angiography was performed within 3 d in 95% of the 287 patients. A total of 737 conduits and 785 distal anastomoses were evaluated. The majority of conduits utilized were the reverse saphenous vein graft and internal mammary graft (Table 1). A variety of target vessels were grafted in this series and are listed in Table 2. At cardiac catheterization, 728 of 737 grafts (98.8%) were patent utilizing the Fitzgibbon classification (Table 3). Eight of 423 saphenous vein grafts were occluded, one of 278 IMA grafts was occluded, and no radial grafts were occluded. There were no differences in patency rates of grafts supplying different regions of the heart (Table 4).

At a mean interval of 15 mo (range 2–42 mo), 90% follow-up was obtained in this population of OPCAB patients. There were no cardiac deaths and no myocardial

Table 1
OPCAB Conduits Studied

Conduit	*No.*
LIMA	269
Saphenous vein graft	423
Radial	36
RIMA	8
Free RIMA	1

Table 2
OPCAB Fitsgibbon Scores by Conduit

Conduit	*A*	*B*	*A + B*	*O*	*Total*
LIMA	247	21	99.6%	1	263
Saphenous vein graft	408	7	98.1%	8	423
Radial	33	3	100.0%	0	36
RIMA	8	0	100.0%	0	8
Free RIMA	1	0	100.0%	0	1

Table 3
OPCAB Target Vessels Studies (n = 785)

Target	*No.*	*%*
LAD	278	35.4
Diagonal	13	16.6
D1	114	14.5
D2	16	2
Ramus	13	1.7
OM1	36	4.6
OM2	95	12.1
OM3	18	2.3
PLOM	21	2.7
RCA	44	5.6
PDA	127	16.2

Table 4
OPCAB Fitzgibbon Scores by Target Vessel

Target	*A*	*B*	*A + B*	*O*	*Total*
LAD	256	21	99.6%	1	278
Diagonal	126	2	98.5%	2	130
Ramus	13	0	100.0%	0	13
Marginal	159	7	97.6%	4	170
RCA	82	2	97.7%	2	86
PDA	85	0	100.0%	0	85
Other	22	0	97.7%	1	23
Total	723	32	98.7	10	785

infarctions. Seven patients (1.8%) required cardiac catheterization, showing a total of five occluded grafts. Four patients (1.1%) had PTCA, two of which were for new lesions in unbypassed coronary arteries. Six patients (1.6%) had late non-cardiac-related deaths, 1–18 mo after discharge. All other patients were alive and well without angina.

Results of Intermediate-Term (1–12 mo) Angiography After OPCAB

In one of the earliest accounts of angiographic evaluation of patients undergoing OPCAB, Calafiore and his colleagues *(30)* described angiographic patency in 271 of 434 patients of (62%) undergoing left internal thoracic artery (LITA) to left anterior descending (LAD) artery grafting via MIDCAB. Postoperative angiography was performed during the first year after surgery with an overall angiographic patency rate of 94%. Furthermore, they note that anastomotic quality improved over the course of this series of patients, such that in the last 190 patients, 134 (71%) underwent postoperative coronary angiography and had a 99% patency rate.

Possati et al. *(50)* studied 76 of 77 patients (99%) with postoperative angiograms at a mean of 1.7 ± 2.8 months. In 66 cases (87%) the LIMA graft, the LIMA–LAD anastomosis, and the LAD adjacent to the anastomotic site were normal. In one case (1%), the LIMA was occluded. In the remaining nine cases (12%) the LIMA was patent, but anomalies of the LIMA course, the anastomosis, or the adjacent LAD were present. Of these nine patients, three required reoperation and subsequent repair of the anastomosis using conventional coronary surgery and one patient underwent successful PTCA of an anastomotic stenosis. When they analyzed their results with respect to the type of instrumentation used at surgery (either specifically designed for beating-heart surgery or not), the authors noted a 100% patency rate for those patients with dedicated chest retractors and coronary stabilizers compared to 82% for those without dedicated OPCAB instrumentation.

In 1998, Mohr and his colleagues *(51)* reviewed their experience in 195 patients undergoing single LIMA-to-LAD coronary artery bypass via a left anterolateral thoracotomy incision (MIDCAB). Postoperative angiography prior to discharge was completed in 191 patients (91%) and revealed an overall patency rate of 97%. The results of a midterm (6 mo) follow-up coronary angiogram in the first 58 patients revealed a patency rate of 98%.

While most preceding series evaluated single-vessel coronary artery bypass (LIMA-to-LAD) via the thoracotomy incision, Calafiore *(52)* described his initial experience using a median sternotomy with two or more arterial conduits in 122 primary coronary patients. Sixty-seven patients (55%) underwent 185 distal anastomoses and postoperative angiography was performed at a mean of 33 ± 35 d after the operation. The overall patency rate was 98.9% (183 of 185 grafts); the (FitzGibbon grade A patency rate was 98% (182 of 185 grafts). These data demonstrated that precise arterial grafting of all the regions of the heart is possible without cardiopulmonary bypass.

In an innovative series of robotic-assisted IMA harvesting and direct CABG through a 5-cm thoracotomy incision without the use of cardiopulmonary bypass, Vassiliades et al. *(53)* assessed angiographic graft patency in 45 of 66 consecutive patients 6 mo (range 2–15 mo) postoperatively. The overall patency rate for the study group was 98%, demonstrating that beating-heart coronary artery bypass surgery using thoracoscopic IMA harvesting can achieve effective intermediate-term revascularization.

In a study evaluating early and mid-term angiographic patency of 55 coronary anastomosis constructed on 51 patients undergoing beating-heart surgery without the benefit of mechanical stabilization, Gill et al. *(54)* noted that overall patency was 96% (53 of 55 sites) at 4–6 h following surgery. Follow-up angiography at a mean of 9.6±4.5 mo (range 3–19 mo) in 32 of 51 patients (64%) revealed a 94% (30 of 32 patients) anastomotic patency rate. Although these data recount anastomotic patency prior to the widespread utilization of mechanical stabilization, they do describe acceptable longer-term angiographic follow-up for beating-heart coronary grafting.

Results of Late (> 1 yr) Angiography After OPCAB

In a controversial paper, Ömero{gg}lu and his colleagues *(55)* reported the long-term angiographic patency of 70 randomly chosen patients (10%) from a total population of 696 patients who had beating-heart surgery at their institution. The interval from operation to angiography varied from 24 to 61 mo (mean, 36 ± 11 mo). They noted a 96% patency (65 of 68 patients) of the LIMA-to-LAD anastomoses, but only a 47% patency (16 of 34 patients) in saphenous vein grafts (SVG). The angiography study population consisted of only 10% of the overall beating-heart surgery population and 3% of the total hospital CABG experience over 7 yr. Nevertheless, the low saphenous vein graft 3-yr angiographic patency rate is of concern. In conventional coronary bypass, FitzGibbon et al. *(56)* have previously described a patency rate in 1170 saphenous vein grafts of 81% at 1 yr, 75% at 5 yr, and 50% at greater than 15 yr.

More recently, Kim and associates *(57)* have analyzed the results of 122 consecutive, nonrandomized OPCAB cases compared with those of 65 consecutive conventional CABG cases. The average number of distal anastomoses between groups was comparable (OPCAB: 3.1 ± 1.1 vs conventional CABG: 3.7 ± 0.9). In the OPCAB group, coronary angiograms prior to discharge were performed in 92% (121 of 122) of patients revealing a 96% (162 of 168 grafts) patency rate for arterial grafts and 86% (160 of 187 grafts) for SVG. One-year follow-up coronary angiograms in the OPCAB group were performed in 74% of patients (90 of 122) and the patency rate was 98% (132 of 135 grafts) for arterial grafts and 68% (106 of 156 grafts) for SVG. One-year follow-up in conventional bypass patients was performed in 65% of patients (42 of 65). The patency rate was 94%, in the authors' hands (43 of 46 grafts) for arterial grafts and 88% (98 of 111 grafts) for SVG. This small series suggests that early patency of vein grafts after OPCAB is less than that for arterial grafts, and also suggests a lower patency rate in 1-yr postoperative angiograms for OPCAB vein grafts compared to vein grafts constructed utilizing conventional CABG on CPB. In contrast, our series of postoperative coronary angiograms prior to hospital discharge (Table 3) does not reveal a significant difference between arterial and vein graft patency rates.

Currently, there is little information and no standardization of the angiographic findings of OPCAB bypass grafts in the postoperative period *(3)*. The most commonly used classification to assess the quality of grafts following cardiac surgery is the aforementioned FitzGibbon classification (Fitz O grafts are occluded; Fitz B are grafts with stenosis resulting in a diameter less than 50% of the target vessel diameter; and Fitz A are grafts without stenoses) *(58)*. Although this classification alone does not adequately describe all the findings and its lack of robustness hinders its use as a prognostic tool, it is the most commonly used angiographic classification.

FUTURE TECHNOLOGIES TO EVALUATE POSTOPERATIVE GRAFT PATENCY

Despite its "gold standard" status for patency analysis, limitations of angiography have spawned great interest in new technologies to assess patency of postoperative coronary artery bypass grafts. Refinements and advancements in electron-beam computed tomogaphy (EBT) have effectively detected coronary calcifications and stenoses and evaluated coronary artery bypass graft patency *(59–63)*. More recently, a novel, multislice, helical computed tomography (CT) scanner with four detector rows for 3-D reconstruction has been introduced for visualization of postoperative coronary grafts *(64)*. Magnetic resonance angiography *(65,66)* and high-frequency transthoracic echocardiography *(67)* have also been evaluated as alternatives to standard contrast angiography and cardiac catheterization. None of these techniques is presently able to provide the resolution and detail of angiography, but technological advances may allow of these to supplant angiography as the technique of choice for graft assessment in the future.

SUMMARY

Surgical techniques for multivessel OPCAB continue to evolve and improve. The techniques utilized in performing multivessel OPCAB remain diverse *(68–70)*. Careful maintenance of myocardial protection during off-pump coronary revascularization is of central importance and will lead to reduced morbidity and mortality. Intraoperative or postoperative coronary angiography remains the "gold standard" in the evaluation of graft patency. Notwithstanding, controversies remain regarding performance, cost, and clinical decision making with this technique. The advantage of obtaining an intraoperative angiogram is the ability to document graft patency before leaving the operating room. However, the presence of an angiographic abnormality may lead to an unnecessary revision, since some early angiographic lesions may be due to transient intramural hematomas or spasm. Postoperative angiography offers the benefit of being able to document graft patency before discharge, but involves an additional procedure with the associated additional morbidity and expense. Advances in standardization and ease with which noninvasive techniques can be utilized by cardiac surgeons intraoperatively and postoperatively may improve the assessment of coronary distal anastomoses following beating-heart coronary surgery.

REFERENCES

1. Puskas JD, Wright CE, Ronson RS, Brown WM, Gott JP, Guyton RA. Clinical outcomes and angiographic patency in 125 consecutive off-pump coronary bypass patients. Heart Surg Forum 1999;2:216–221.
2. Puskas JD, Thourani VH, Marshall JJ, et al. Clinical outcomes, angiographic patency, and resource utilization in 200 consecutive off-pump coronary bypass patients. Ann Thorac Surg 2001;71:1477–1483.
3. Mack MJ, Osborne JA, Shennib H. Arterial graft patency in coronary artery bypass grafting: what do we really know? Ann Thorac Surg 1998;66:1055–1059.
4. Louagie YAG, Haxhe JP, Jamart J, Buche M, Schoevaerdts JC. Doppler flow measurement in coronary-artery bypass grafts and early postoperative clinical outcome. Thorac Cardiovasc Surg 1994;42:175–181.
5. Walpoth BH, Bosshard A, Genyk I, et al. Transit-time flow measurement for detection of early graft failure during myocardial revascularization. Ann Thorac Surg 1998;66:1097–1100.
6. D'Ancona G, Karamanoukian HL, Ricci M, Bergsland J, Salerno TA. Graft patency verification in coronary artery bypass grafting: principles and clinical applications of transit time flow measurement. Angiology 2000;51:725–731.
7. VanHimbergen DJ, Koenig SC, Jaber SF, Cerrito PB, Spence PA. A review of transit-time flow measurement for assessing graft patency. Heart Surg Forum 1999;2:226–229.
8. Franklin DL, Ellis RS, Rushmir RF. Ultrasonic transit time flowmeter. IRE Trans Biomed Engl 1962;9:44–49.
9. D'Ancona G, Karamanoukian HL, Ricci M, et al. Graft revision after transit time flow measurements in off-pump coronary artery bypass grafting. Eur J Cardiothorac Surg 2000;17:287–293.

10. Ricci M, Karamanoukian HL, Salerno TA, D'Ancona G, Bergsland J. Role of coronary graft flow measurement during reoperations for early graft failure after off-pump coronary revascularization. J Card Surg 1999;14:342–347.
11. Jaber SF, Koenig SC, BhaskerRao B, VanHimbergen DJ, Spence PA. Can visual assessment of flow waveform morphology detect anastomotic error in off-pump coronary artery bypass grafting? Eur J Cardiothorac Surg 1998;14:476–479.
12. Koenig S, VanHimbergen DJ, Jaber SF, Ewert D, Cerrito P, Spence PA. Spectral analysis of graft flow for anastomotic error detection in off-pump CABG. Eur J Cardiothoracic Surg 1999;16:S83–S87.
13. Cerrito P, Koenig SC, VanHimbergen DJ, Jaber SF, Ewert DL, Spence PA. Neural network pattern recognition analysis of graft flow characteristics improves intra-operative anastomotic error detection in minimally invasive CABG. Eur J Cardiothoracic Surg 1999;16:88–89.
14. Bergsland J, D'Ancona G, Karamanoukian HL, Ricci M, Schmid S, Salerno TA. Technical tips and pitfalls in OPCAB surgery: the Buffalo experience. Heart Surg Forum 2000;3:189–193.
15. D'Ancona G, Karamanoukian HL, Salerno TA, Schmid S, Bergsland J. Flow measurement in coronary surgery. Heart Surg Forum 1999;2:121–124.
16. D'Ancona G, Karamanoukian HL, Soltoski P, Salerno TA, Bergsland J. Changing referral pattern in off-pump coronary artery bypass surgery: a strategy for improving surgical results. Heart Surg Forum 1999;2:246–249.
17. D'Ancona G, Karamanoukian H, Ricci M, Bergsland J, Salerno TA. Preoperative angiography and intraoperative transit time flow measurement to detect coronary graft patency in reoperations: an integrated approach. Angiology 2000;51:777–780.
18. Takami Y, Ina H. Relation of intraoperative flow measurement with postoperative quantitative angiographic assessment of coronary artery bypass grafting. Ann Thorac Surg 2001;72:1270–1274.
19. Takami Y, Ina H. A simple method to determine anastomotic quality of coronary artery bypass grafting in the operating room. Cardiovasc Surg 2001;9:499–503.
20. Hol PK, Fosse E, Mørk BE, et al. Graft control by transit time flow measurement and intraoperative angiography in coronary artery bypass surgery. Heart Surg Forum 2001;4:254–258.
21. Louagie YAG, Haxhe JP, Jamart J, Buche M, Schoevaerdts JC. Intraoperative assessment of coronary artery bypass grafts using a pulsed Doppler flowmeter. Ann Thorac Surg 1994;58:742–749.
22. Louagie YAG, Brockmann CE, Jamart J, et al. Pulsed Doppler intraoperative flow assessment and midterm coronary graft patency. Ann Thorac Surg 1998;66:1282–1288.
23. Louagie YAG, Haxhe JP, Buche M, Schoevaerdts JC. Intraoperative electromagnetic flowmeter measurements in coronary artery bypass grafts. Ann Thorac Surg 1994;57:357–364.
24. Bandyk DF, Galbraith TA, Haasler GB, Almassi GH. Blood flow velocity of internal mammary artery and saphenous vein grafts to the coronary arteries. J Surg Res 1988;44:342–351.
25. Oda K, Hirose K, Nishimori H, Sato K, Yamashiro T, Ogoshi S. Assessment of internal thoracic artery graft with intraoperative color Doppler ultrasonography. Ann Thorac Surg 1998;66:79–81.
26. Takayama T, Suma H, Wanibuchi Y, Tohda E, Matsunaka T, Yamashita S. Physiological and pharmacological responses of arterial graft flow after coronary-artery bypass-grafting measured with an implantable ultrasonic Doppler miniprobe. Circulation 1992;86:217–223.
27. Elbeery JR, Brown PM, Chitwood WR. Intraoperative MIDCABG arteriography via the left radial artery: a comparison with Doppler ultrasound for assessment of graft patency. Ann Thorac Surg 1998;66:51–55.
28. Lin JC, Fisher DL, Szwerc MF, Magovern JA. Evaluation of graft patency during minimally invasive coronary artery bypass grafting with Doppler flow analysis. Ann Thorac Surg 2000;70:1350–1354.
29. Calafiore AM, Gallina S, Iaco A, et al. Minimally invasive mammary artery Doppler flow velocity evaluation in minimally invasive coronary operations. Ann Thorac Surg 1998;66:1236–1241.
30. Calafiore AM, Di Giammarco G, Teodori G, et al. Midterm results after minimally invasive coronary surgery (LAST operation). J Thorac Cardiovasc Surg 1998;115:763–771.
31. Elbeery JR, Chitwood WR. Intraoperative catheterization of the left internal mammary artery via the left radial artery. Ann Thorac Surg 1997;64:1840–1842.
32. Barstad RM, Fosse E, Vatne K, et al. Intraoperative angiography in minimally invasive direct coronary artery bypass grafting. Ann Thorac Surg 1997;64:1835–1839.
33. Izzat MB, Khaw KS, Atassi W, Yim APC, Wan Wan S, El-Zufari MH. Routine intraoperative angiography improves the early patency of coronary grafts performed on the beating heart. Chest 1999;115:987–990.
34. Izzat MB, Yim APC. MIDCABG: lessons learned from routing "on-table" angiography. Ann Thorac Surg 1997;64:1872–1874.

35. Lazzara RR, Kidwell FE, Griffith R. A new technique for intraoperative greaft angiography utilizing the radial artery stump. Heart Surg Forum 2000;3:123–126.
36. Lazzara RR, McLellan BA, Kidwel FE, et al. Intraoperative angiography during minimally invasive direct coronary artery bypass operations. Ann Thorac Surg 1997;64:1725–1727.
37. Suma H, Isomura T, Horii T, Sato T. Intraoperative coronary artery imaging with infrared camera in off-pump CABG. Ann Thorac Surg 2000;70:1741–1742.
38. Takayama T, Wanibuchi Y, Suma H, et al. Intraoperative coronary angiography using fluorescein. Ann Thorac Surg 1991;51:140–143.
39. Shabbo FP, Rees GM. Thermography in assessing coronary artery saphenous graft patency and blood flow. Cardiovasc Res 1982;16:158–162.
40. Mohr FW, Matloff J, Grundfest W, et al. Thermal coronary angiography: a method for assessing graft aptency and coronary anatomy in coronary bypass surgery. Ann Thorac Surg 1989;47:441–449.
41. Lawson W, BenEliyahu D, Meinken L, et al. Infrared thermography in the detection and management of coronary artery disease. Am J Cardiol 1993;72:894–896.
42. Falk V, Walther T, Philippi A, et al. Thermal coronary angiography for intraoperative patency control of arterial and saphenous vein coronary artery bypass grafts: results in 370 patients. J Card Surg 1995;10:147–160.
43. Schaff HV, Cable DG, Rihal CS, Daly RC, Orszulak TA. Minimial thoracotomy for coronary artery bypass: value of immediate postprocedure graft angiography. Circulation 1996;94(suppl 1):51.
44. Subramanian VA, McCabe JC, Geller CM. Minimally invasive direct coronary artery bypass grafting: two-year clinical experience. Ann Thorac Surg 1997;64:1648–1655.
45. Poirier NC, Carrier M, Lespérance J, et al. Quantitative angiographic assessment of coronary anastomoses performed without cardiopulmonary bypass. J Thorac Cardiovasc Surg 1999;117:292–297.
46. Mack MJ, Magovern JA, Acuff TA, et al. Results of graft patency by immediate angiography in minimally invasive coronary artery surgery. Ann Thorac Surg 1999;68:383–390.
47. Gill IS, FitzGibbon GM, Higginson LAJ, Valji A, Keon WJ. Minimally invasive coronary artery bypass: a series with early qualitative angiographic follow-up. Ann Thorac Surg 1997;64:710–714.
48. Puskas JD, Wright CE, Ronson RS, Brown WM, Gott JP, Guyton RA. Off-pump multivessel coronary bypass via sternotomy is safe and effective. Ann Thorac Surg 1998;66:1068–1072.
49. Thourani VH, Puskas JD, Marshall JJ, et al. Postoperative graft patency and clinical outcomes in 378 consecutive off-pump coronary bypass patients. Ann Thorac Surg, to be published.
50. Possati G, Gaudino M, Alessandrini F, Zimarino M, Glieca F, Luciani N. Systemic clinical and angiographic follow-up of patients undergoing minimally invasive coronary artery bypass. J Thorac Cardiovasc Surg 1998;115:785–790.
51. Diegeler A, Falk V, Matin M, et al. Minimally invasive coronary artery bypass grafting without cardiopulmonary bypass: early experience and follow-up. Ann Thorac Surg 1998;66:1022–1025.
52. Calafiore AM, Teodori G, Di Giammarco G, et al. Multiple arterial conduits without cardiopulmonary bypass: early angiographic results. Ann Thorac Surg 1999;67:450-6.
53. Vassiliades TA Jr, Rogers EW, Nielson JL, Lonquist JL. Minimally invasive direct coronary artery bypass grafting: intermediate-term results. Ann Thorac Surg 2000;70:1063–1065.
54. Gill IS, Higginson LA, Maharajh GS, Keon WJ. Early and follow-up angiography in minimally invasive coronary bypass without mechanical stabilization. Ann Thorac Surg 2000;69:56–60.
55. Ömero{gg}lu SN, Kirali K, Güler M, et al. Midterm angiographic assessment of coronary artery bypass grafting without cardiopulmonary bypass. Ann Thorac Surg 2000;70:884–850.
56. FitzGibbon GM, Leach AJ, Keon WJ, Burton JR, Kafka HP. Coronary bypass fate. J Thorac Cardiovasc Surg 1986;91:773–778.
57. Kim K-B, Lim C, Lee C, et al. Off-pump coronary artery bypass may decrease the patency of saphenous ven grafts. Ann Thorac Surg 2001;72:S1033–S1037.
58. FitzGibbon GM, Kafka HP, Leach AJ. Coronary bypass graft fate and patient outcome: angiographic follow-up of 5,065 grafts related to survival and reoperation in 1,388 patients during 25 years. J Am Coll Cardiol 1996;28:616–626.
59. Gulbins H, Reichenspurner H, Becker C, et al. Preoperative 3D-reconstructions of ultrafast-CT images for the planning of minimally invasive direct coronary artery bypass operation (MIDCAB). Heart Surg Forum 1998;1:111–115.
60. Hernigou A, Challande P, Boudeville JC, Sene V, Grataloup C, Planfosse MC. Reproducibility of coronary calcification detection with electron-beam computed tomography. Eur Radiol 1996;6: 210–216.

61. Moshage W, Achenbach S, Seese B, Bachman K. Non-invasive coronary diagnosis with EBT (electon beam tomography). Population screening for coronary heart disease (reliability imaging of coronary stenoses). Fortschr Med 1997;115:45–49.
62. Ruping D, Shaoxiong Z, Bin L, et al. Three-dimensional reconstruction of electron beam computed tomograhy angiography for evaluating coronary artery bypass grafts. Chinese Med J 1998;111:588–592.
63. Lu B, Dai R-P, Jing B-L, et al. Evaluation of coronary artery bypass graft patency using three-dimensional reconstruction and flow study on electron beam tomography. J Comput Assisted Tomogr 2000;24:663–670.
64. Sawamura Y, Takase K, Saito H, Kikuchi S, Ito T. Noninvasive postoperative angiography for internal mammary artery grafts. Circulation 2001;104:373–374.
65. Boehm DH, Wintersperger BJ, Reichenspurner H, et al. Contrast-enhanced magnetic resonance angiography for control of minimally invasive coronary artery bypass conduits (MIDCAB/OPCAB). Heart Surg Forum 1999;2:222–225.
66. Vetter HO, Driever R, Mertens H, Kempkes U, Cramer BM. Contrast-enhanced magnetic resonance angiography of mammary artery grafts after minimally invasive coronary bypass surgery. Ann Thorac Surg 2001;71:1229–1232.
67. De Simone L, Caso P, Severino S, et al. Noninvasive assessment of left and right internal mammary artery graft patency with high-frequency transthoracic echocardiography. J Am Soc Echocardiogr 1999;12:841–849.
68. Flameng W. Role of myocardial protection for coronary artery bypass grafting on the beating heart. Ann Thorac Surg 1997;63:S18–S22.
69. Puskas JP, Vinten-Johansen J, Muraki S, Guyton RA. Myocardial protection for off-pump coronary artery bypass surgery. Sem Thorac Cardiovasc Surg 2001;13(1):82–88.
70. Chitwood WR Jr, Wixon CL, Elbeery JR, et al. Minimally invasive cardiac operation: adapting cardioprotective strategies. Ann Thorac Surg 1999;68:1974–1977.

14 Minimally Invasive Conduit Harvesting

Kevin D. Accola, MD, *Mike Butkus,* PA-C,
and Brenda Dickey, RN

Contents

Introduction
Direct Limited-Access Saphenous Vein Harvest
Endoscopic Saphenous Vein Harvest
Techniques of Minimally Invasive Radial Artery Harvest
Summary
References

INTRODUCTION

More than 500,000 coronary artery bypass grafting (CABG) procedures were performed last year in the United States. The greater saphenous vein (GSV) was used as a bypass conduit in approx 95% of these cases *(1)*. The traditional method of harvesting the GSV for either CABG or for peripheral arterial bypass involves making a long incision along the length of the patient's lower extremity. Much literature has been written about the pain associated with the vein harvest site incision as compared to the lesser discomfort of the primary sternotomy incision. The associated pain and morbidity that results from harvesting of the vein via the conventional approach may begin shortly after surgery and may last for years. Numerous reports have also documented potential major and minor complications that may result from GSV harvesting *(2–6)*. Major complications include infection, dehiscence, or necrosis requiring debridement, skin grafting, arterial revascularization, or even amputation *(6)* (**Figs. 1** and **2**). Minor complications, reported to occur in 0.5–31% of patients, include cellulitis, hematoma, seroma, and edema.

Minimally invasive saphenous vein harvesting has been shown to be associated with decreased postoperative pain, earlier ambulation, and decreased hospital stay as compared to conventional vein harvesting *(1,7–14)*. It also provides patients with an improved cosmetic result secondary to the smaller incision. With the availability of the internet and increased access to information, patients have become better informed

From: *Contemporary Cardiology: Minimally Invasive Cardiac Surgery, Second Edition*
Edited by: D. J. Goldstein and M. C. Oz © Humana Press Inc., Totowa, NJ

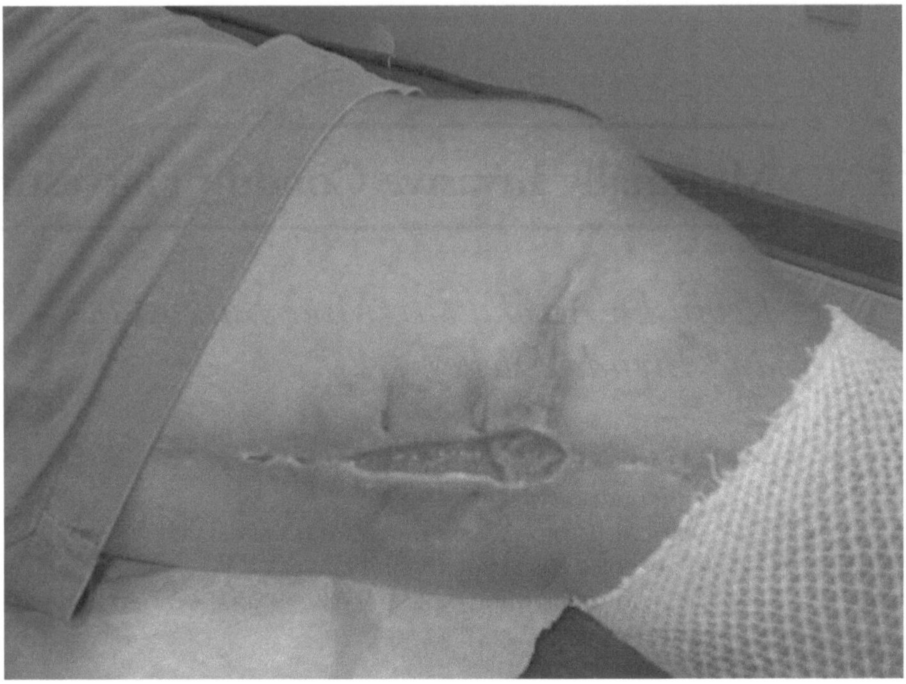

Fig. 1. Saphenous wound site dehiscence.

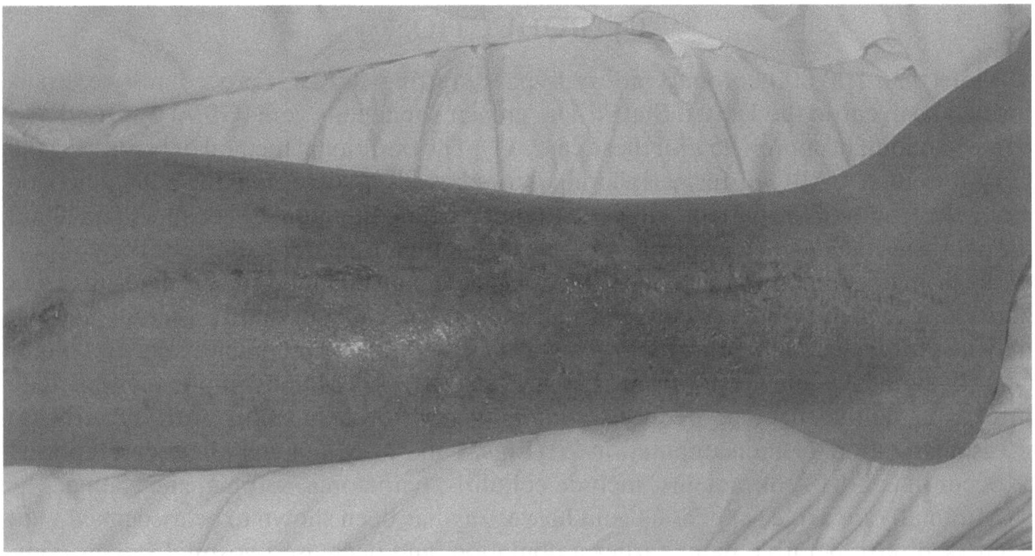

Fig. 2. Severe infection of saphenous wound site with erythema, lymphedema, and cellulitis.

regarding minimally invasive harvesting techniques and often present to their surgeon requesting a minimally invasive approach.

This chapter discusses direct limited-access and video-assisted endoscopic vein harvesting, two minimally invasive techniques used for harvesting the GSV. Each of these techniques will be outlined separately, with comments on their advantages and limitations.

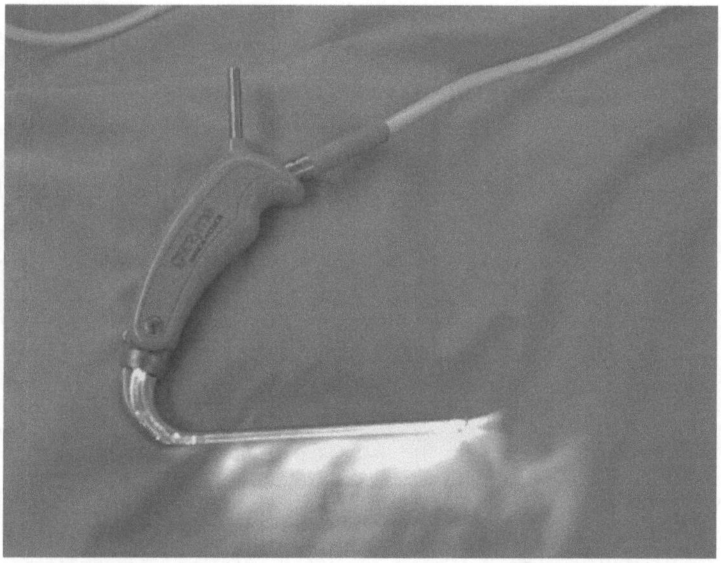

Fig. 3. The Genzyme BioSurgical SaphLite hand-held lighted retractor.

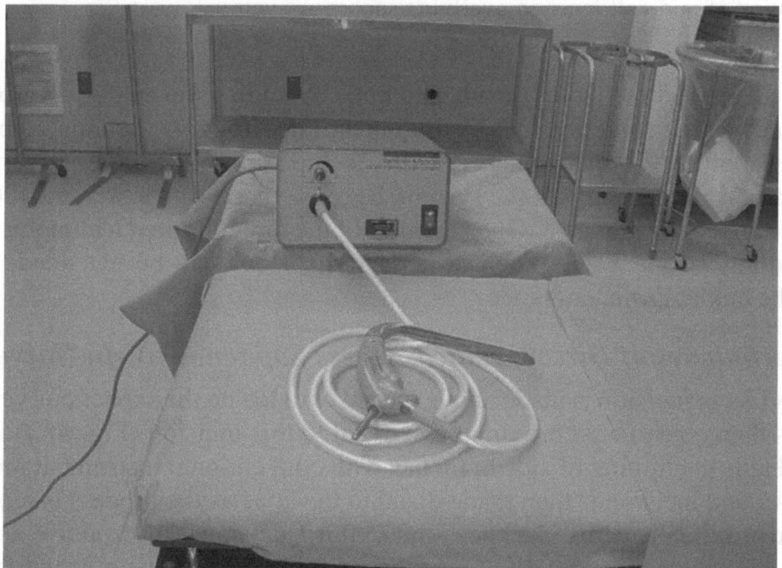

Fig. 4. The Genzyme BioSurgical SaphLite console.

DIRECT LIMITED-ACCESS SAPHENOUS VEIN HARVEST

The technique of skin bridging for saphenous vein harvesting represents an attempt to minimize overall incision length, in which a series of multiple incisions is interspersed with "bridges" of skin. Direct limited-access harvesting of saphenous veins is a modification of this technique. A retractor with a light source provides a "lighted" tunnel and an opportunity to decrease the number of skin incisions necessary (Genzyme BioSurgical SaphLite) (**Figs. 3** and **4**). With this approach, the primary objectives are to avoid inci-

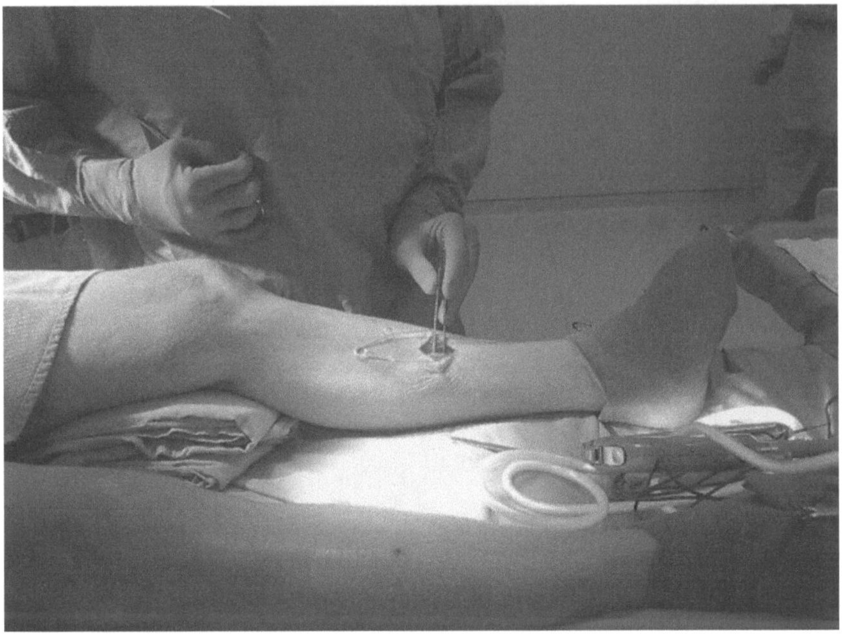

Fig. 5. Creation of mid-calf incision overlying saphenous vein.

sions over the medial malleolus, groin, and knee. Avoiding the ankle and groin reduces infection and healing complications. Avoiding the knee improves healing, joint mobility, and patient comfort. The advantages of this technique are the ease and simplicity of instrumentation and mobility of the system. Because there is no tower, the retractor and light source are easily movable. One can modify the direct limited technique depending on the anatomy of the vein. When necessary, incisions can be extended, while still avoiding the ankle, groin, and knee.

Techniques of Direct Limited-Access Saphenous Vein Harvest

A 10- to 12-cm incision is made above the ankle to locate the saphenous vein (**Fig. 5**). A tunnel is then constructed proximal and distal to this incision (**Fig. 6**). A retractor is placed and aids in clipping of side branches with conventional instrumentation (**Figs. 7** and **8**). A second incision is then made distal to the knee as the process is repeated both distally and proximally across the knee joint. A third incision is made above the knee, and the tunnel is extended proximally. Once the desired length of vein is achieved, a stab incision is made near the ankle and the groin. The saphenous vein is then clipped and tied (**Fig. 9**). Hemostasis is achieved during this dissection using electrocautery.

The wound is closed with running subcuticular suture and a topical dressing is placed over it (**Fig. 10**). Circumferential wrapping of the harvest site is recommended during the bypass procedure to ensure hemostasis (**Fig. 11**). Hemostasis should be rechecked once the patient is separated from cardiopulmonary bypass and heparin has been reversed. Some centers recommend a leg wrap for 24 h, although the reported incidence of post-operative hematomas and seromas in the perioperative period has not been shown to be increased if a compressive wrap is not used.

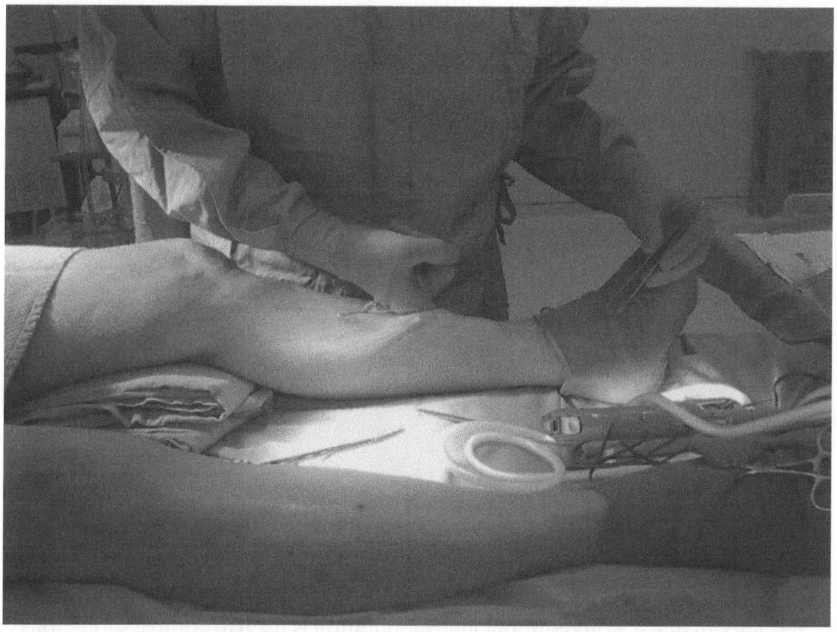

Fig. 6. Digital creation of saphenous tunnel.

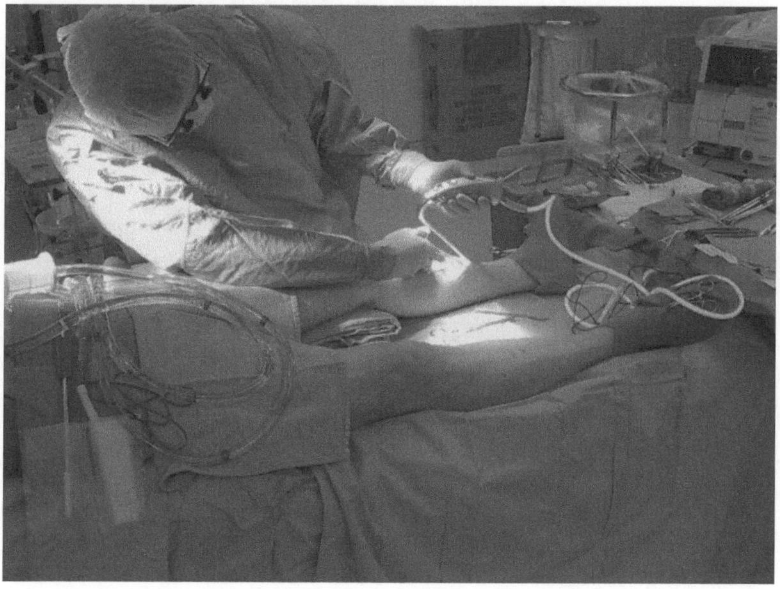

Fig. 7. Lighted retractor is placed to localize branches.

ENDOSCOPIC SAPHENOUS VEIN HARVEST

The technology for endoscopic saphenous vein harvesting continues to evolve *(15)*. There is a significant learning curve in becoming proficient in this technique. Once

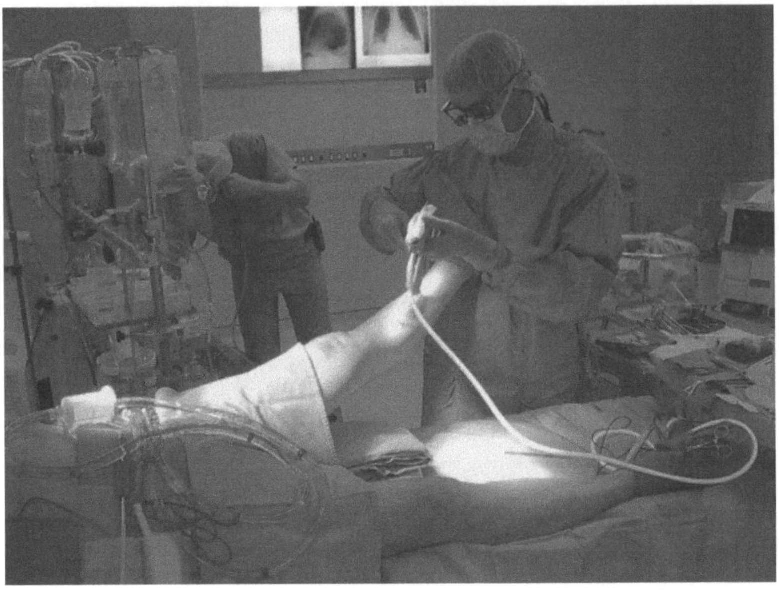

Fig. 8. With retractor in place, conventional instrumentation is used to control saphenous tributaries.

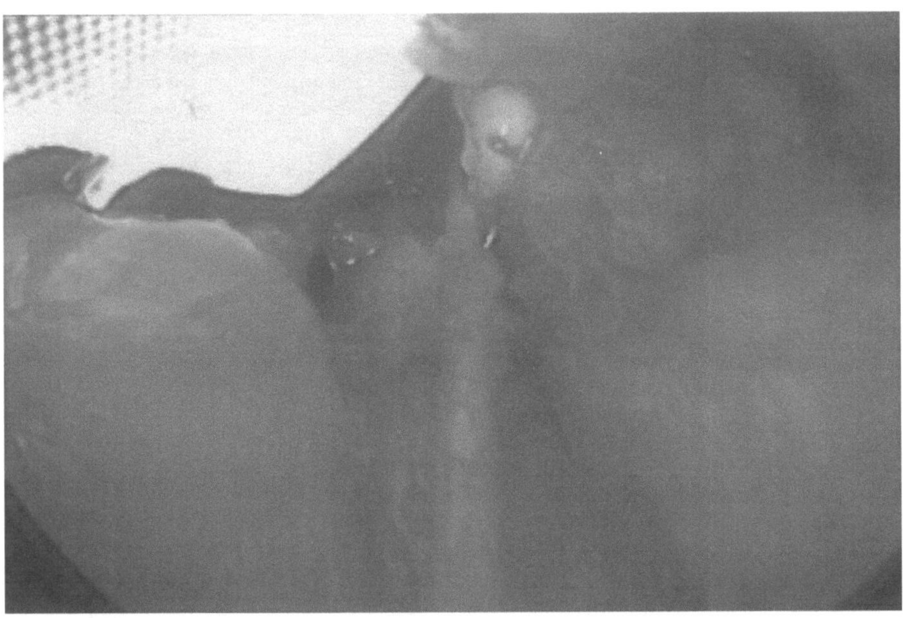

Fig. 9. The vein harvest has been completed through three small incisions.

proficiency is established, however, this technique allows the entire length of saphenous vein to be harvested from a single incision site above the knee.

Techniques of Endoscopic Saphenous Vein Harvest

The instrumentation that we employ is the Guidant Vasoview Uniport Plus System (**Fig. 12**), which involves videoscopic viewing and CO_2 insufflation. The incision is

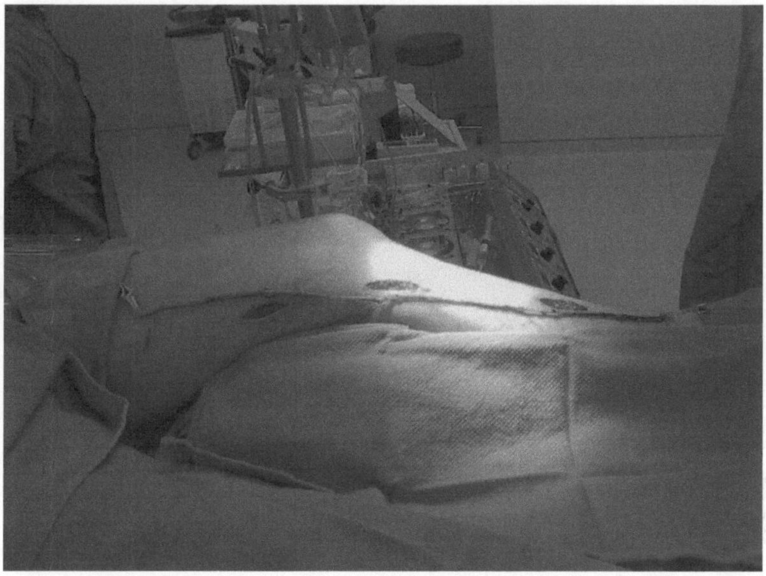

Fig. 10. Subcuticular suture and topical dressing on wound site.

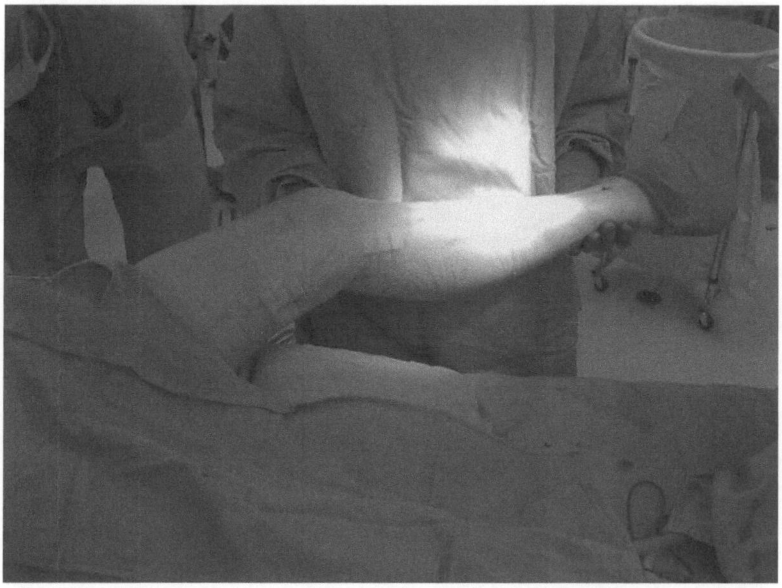

Fig. 11. Circumferential wrapping to reduce chance of postoperative hematomas.

typically made above the knee, through which the dissection takes place. A seal is made with the skin around the insufflator port. The insufflator is placed in the incision, followed by an injection, enabling visualization of the vein. Continuous insufflation of CO_2 maintains a "window" to circumferentially dissect the vein and has not been found to negatively affect the quality of the vein *(16)*. The insertion site of the dissection cannula must remain airtight to maintain CO_2 insufflation pressure. Dissection is performed under direct endoscopic guidance using endoscopic instruments (**Figs. 13–16**). An endoscopic

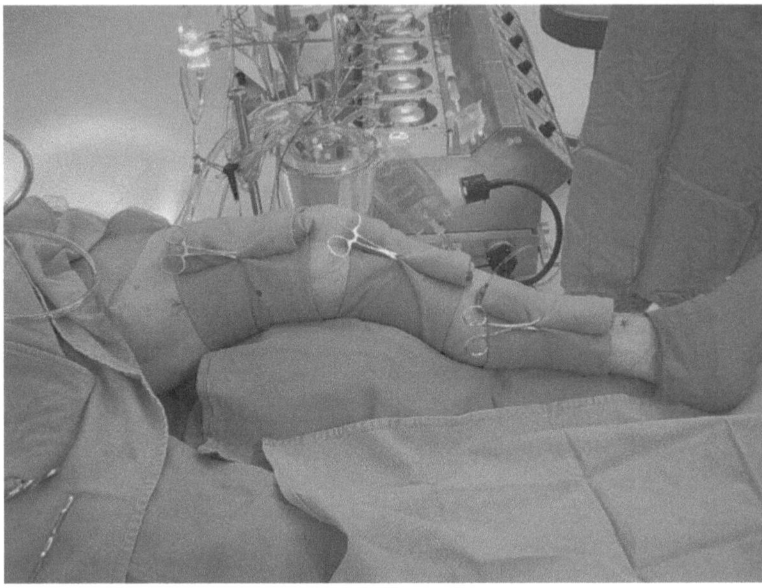

Fig. 12. The Guidant Vasoview Uniport Plus system. (Reproduced with permission of Guidant Corporation.)

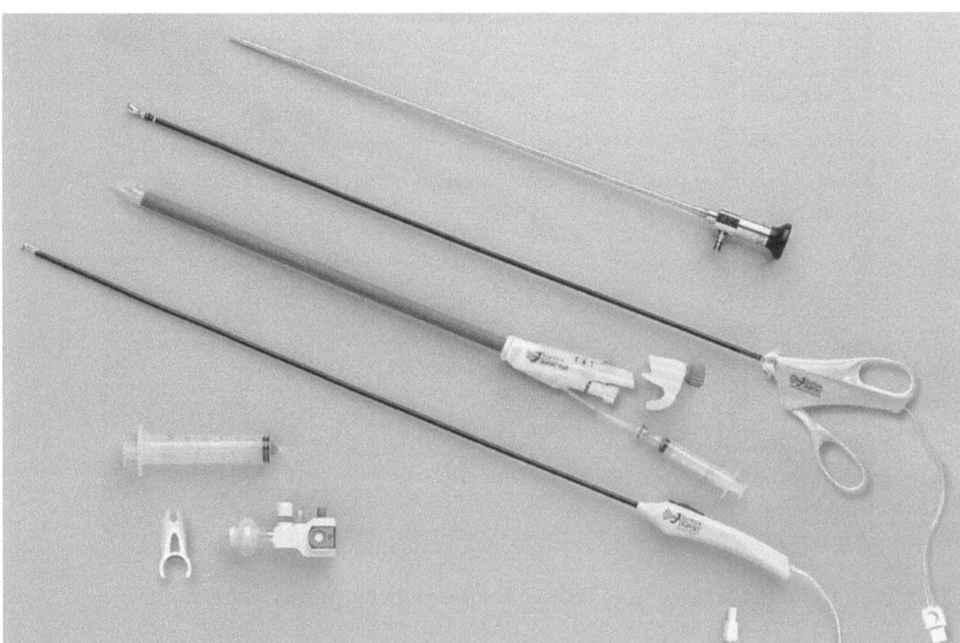

Fig. 13. The videoscope is introduced into the wound.

view seen through the videoscope is demonstrated in **Fig. 17**. The vein is typically dissected proximally and then distally, depending on the length of conduit that is required. Cautery scissors can be placed into the insufflator port to maintain adequate

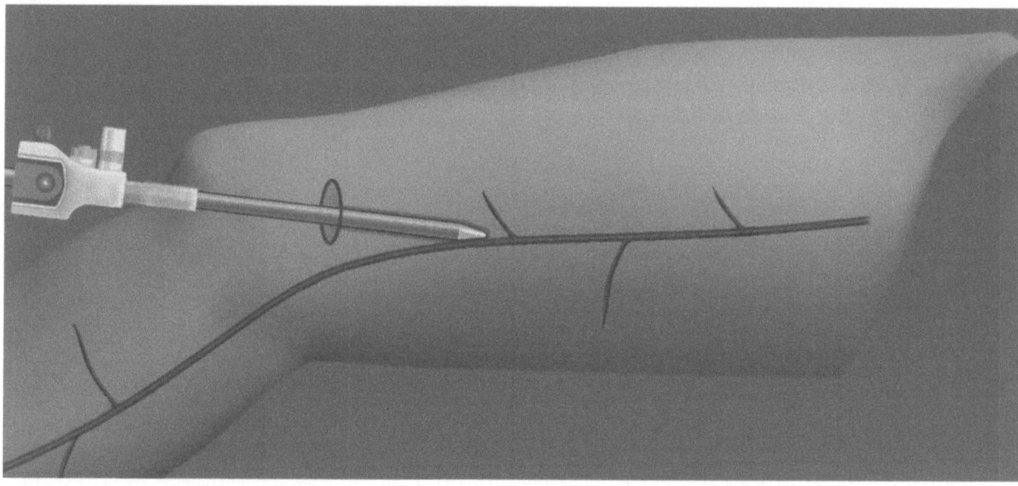

Fig. 14. Insufflator is enabled to create tunnel and allow visualization.

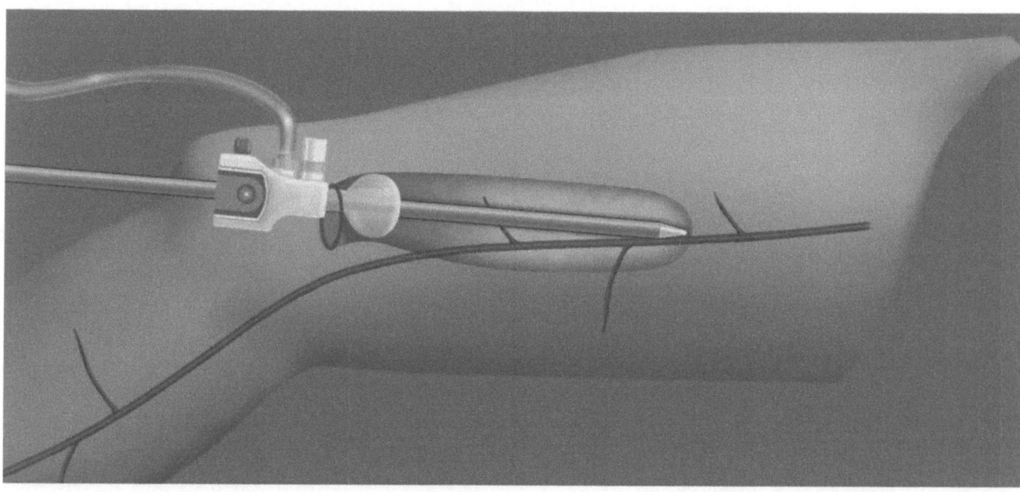

Fig. 15. Dissection progresses distally.

hemostasis as well as to aid in the dissection process. Small clip applicators can be used to control side branches during dissection.

Proximal and distal division of the vein is performed with an endoscopic scissors and vein-clipping apparatus. Division of the vein can also be performed through a small incision over the most proximal and distal sites with ligation of the vein. Once the vein is removed from the leg, conventional operative techniques are utilized.

Results of Minimally Invasive Saphenous Vein Harvest

Many studies in the literature have demonstrated a variety of benefits associated with a minimally invasive harvesting approach as compared to open *(7–14)*. A prospective, randomized trial by Allen revealed a decreased wound complication rate of 4% for endoscopic harvest as compared to 19% for open, as well as decreased hospital stay for

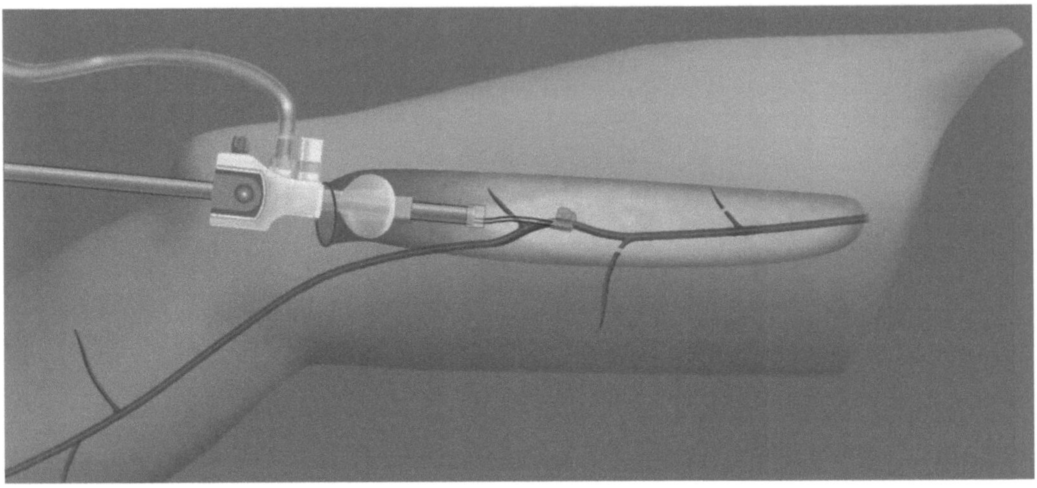

Fig. 16. Endoscopic clip applicator is inserted to control side branches.

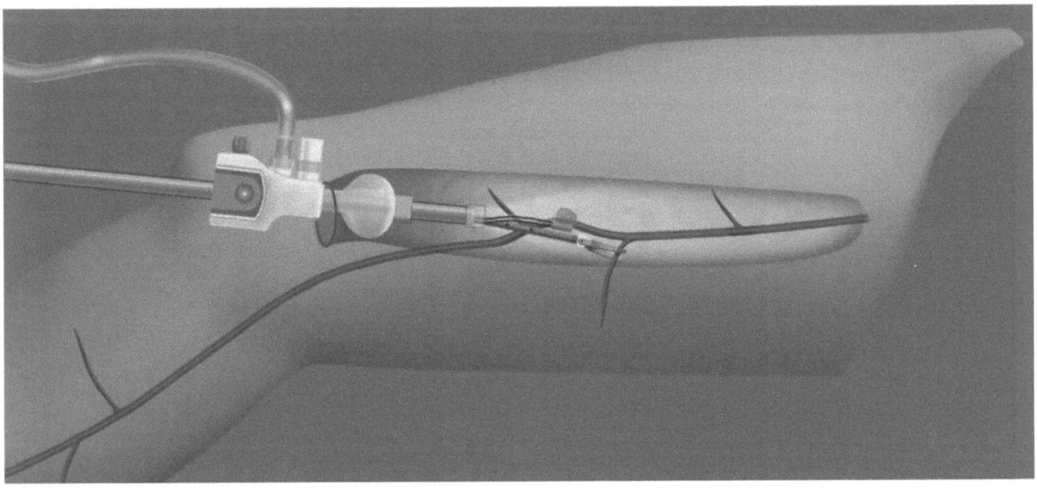

Fig. 17. Endoscopic view of saphenous vein.

endoscopic patients ($p < 0.05$) *(7)*. Puskas also prospectively randomized open and endoscopic patients and demonstrated improvement in postoperative discomfort with an endoscopic approach *(8)*.

In our series, the incidence of leg wound infections was less than 2%, with no deep wound infections or any cases requiring operative intervention or debridement. Other studies have also shown a decreased wound infection rate in endoscopic as compared to open harvesting (Table 1).

Several studies have compared endoscopic and bridged approaches *(1,10)*. Patel et al. reported on 200 CABG patients who were prospectively studied after undergoing either bridged or endoscopic GSV harvest. There was a significantly lower incidence of wound complications in the endoscopic group—2% vs 12% ($p<0.05$). Endoscopic patients also ambulated earlier and had a significantly decreased hospital stay ($p < 0.05$) *(1)*. Some

Table 1
Comparison of Infection Rates between Endoscopically and Coinventionally Harvested SVG

		Wound Infection Rate (%)		
Author	*Year*	*Endoscopic*	*Conventional*	*p-value*
Bitondo et al.	2002	6.8	28.3	<0.001
Allen et al.	1998	4	19	<0.02

Table 2
Comparison of Infection Rates between Endoscopically and Bridge Approaches

		Wound Infection Rate (%)		
Author	*Year*	*Endoscopic*	*Bridge*	*p-value*
Horvath et al.	1998	32	3	<0.005
Patel et al.	2001	2	12	<0.05

studies have confirmed these conclusions, while others have shown a bridged approach to be associated with an improved outcome (Table 2).

Although minimally invasive harvesting techniques have associated benefits, until recently, many questioned the quality and integrity of the vein with such an approach. Several studies have addressed this concern *(17,18)*. Griffith et al. studied 178 patients who underwent either open or endoscopic vein harvest *(17)*. Veins were analyzed for histological abnormalities using hematoxylin–eosin, trichrome, and elastin staining. No differences were found between veins harvested via an open or endoscopic approach with regard to intimal endothelial continuity ($p = 0.45$), elastic lamina continuity ($p = 0.27$), medial connective tissue uniformity ($p = 0.91$), medial smooth muscle continuity ($p = 0.16$), or adventitial connective tissue uniformity ($p = 0.92$).

This observation was also noted by Meyer et al., who compared veins harvested via an endoscopic approach with those harvested via an open approach *(18)*. No significant abnormalities were found in the intimal, medial, or adventitial layers of the veins in either of the groups. Additional immunohistochemical studies for factors VIII:vWF and CD 34 also showed no difference between the groups.

Studies have also investigated whether there is a difference in smooth muscle reactivity and vasomotor function between veins harvested via an open vs an endoscopic approach *(19–21)*. Black et al. prospectively randomized 40 patients into open or endoscopic vein harvest and studied smooth muscle function of the harvested veins *(19)*. Smooth muscle baseline contractile function was assessed by responses to potassium chloride and phenylephrine, and relaxation was assessed by receptor-dependent agonists (acetylcholine and bradykinin) as well as receptor-independent agonists (calcium ionophore and sodium nitroprusside) ($p = 0.3$). No difference was found between the two groups, implying that there is preservation of endothelial and smooth muscle cell function. Cable et al. also evaluated the functional state of the endothelium in veins harvested via an endoscopic approach and found similar results *(20)*.

In a randomized study performed in our institution comparing direct-lighted retractor vs conventional harvest techniques, subjective benefits were noted using minimally invasive techniques. Patients ambulated earlier and with considerably less pain. The study was terminated prematurely due to an overwhelming patient satisfaction both in comfort and cosmesis with minimally invasive harvesting.

Disadvantages of Minimally Invasive Saphenous Vein Harvest

Another possible disadvantage associated with a minimally invasive approach may be inadequate exposure and lighting. The lighted retractor or video-assisted equipment does not always yield optimal visualization of the vein. This occurs most often in obese patients, when the anatomy of the vein is abnormal, and when there is extensive branching of the vein. When there is inadequate visualization or lighting, it is often necessary to extend the initial incision to obtain adequate visualization and to ensure that the vein quality is not compromised. It may be necessary to make a mid-thigh incision to better delineate anomalous anatomy. A direct-lighted retractor technique may have a benefit in these patients, as it does not rely on insufflated venous tunnels. If the harvest requires opening the leg partially, the remainder of the vein can be removed utilizing the lighted retractor in a more "limited access" fashion.

Several other factors can limit the use of minimally invasive vein harvest procedures. Varicosities cause a significant amount of bleeding and obscure visualization through the tunnel. Superficial veins, close to the dermal edge, will not accommodate an adequate-sized tunnel to work within. This not only obscures visualization but also limits the space for optimal vein dissection. Additionally, delicate or friable saphenous veins must be approached with caution and may, in some cases, be a contraindication to a minimally invasive approach. When these situations are encountered, the decision must be made whether the limiting factors will compromise the quality of the vein.

In emergency cases, when it is necessary to harvest the vein rapidly, we typically pursue a conventional leg incision. We utilize the direct-lighted retractor across the knee joint and then extend the incision up into the groin to limit postoperative infection and knee pain.

Possible Postoperative Complications of Minimally Invasive Saphenous Vein Harvest

Although wound infections are uncommon with a minimally invasive approach, when they occur, they may be associated with an infected tunnel hematoma. This may require opening of the tunnel with irrigation, although there are reports of effective closed-space irrigation *(22)*.

Postoperative hematomas need to be evacuated from the tunnel site. This can typically be accomplished with a small stab incision over the hematoma site and application of pressure. A pressure dressing is then applied and maintained as a wrap for 24–36 h.

Seromas occur in 1–2% of patients and typically occur 2–3 wk postoperatively in patients with previous hematomas. They are generally treated with needle aspiration and a pressure dressing, although there are occasions when a small incision with packing of the seroma site may be required.

Direct injury to the saphenous vein can also occur, although not more frequently as compared to a conventional approach. In a prospective randomized study at our institution, the necessity of conduit repair was less in minimally invasive harvested conduits as compared to those harvested by conventional techniques.

Table 3
Scoring System for Saphenous Vein Graft Intraluminal Lesions

Score	*Grading*
0	No endoluminal surface lesions
1	A. Isolated simple fibrous strands < 5
	B. Hemorrhagic staining < 3
	C. Grade 0 with spasm
2	A. Multiple simple fibrous strands 5–10
	B. Complex fibrous strands < 5
	C. Hemorrhagic staining >3
	D. Grade 1 with spasm
3	A. Diffuse strands > 10
	B. Complex fibrous strands > 5
	C. Thrombus
	D. Grade 2 with spasm

Angioscopy for Monitoring of Intraluminal Lesions

We recently began performing intraoperative angioscopy on harvested veins to evaluate for intraluminal pathology. Using a 2.2-mm Olympus angioscope, a variety of lesions have been identified that include simple fibrous strands, complex fibrous strands, hemorrhagic staining, and thrombus. We devised a scoring system ranging from 0 to 3, with 3 being associated with the greatest number of intraluminal lesions (Table 3). Intraoperative angioscopy is recorded and viewed by three surgeons after the operation, and veins are scored based on the number and severity of intraluminal lesions. Each vein is scored before and after saline irrigation. A ratio of the number of lesions postirrigation divided by the number of lesions preirrigation is calculated. A ratio of the number of lesions before and after irrigation divided by the length of vein is also calculated. We recently began comparing scores of open and endoscopic veins. Preliminary data indicate that the majority of lesions tend to flush out with saline irrigation, with an improvement in the postirrigation score. There seems to be no significant difference in the number of lesions postirrigation or the postirrigation scores of open vs endoscopic.

TECHNIQUES OF MINIMALLY INVASIVE RADIAL ARTERY HARVEST

Minimally invasive techniques have been applied to harvesting of the radial artery (RA) as well. Several studies evaluating endoscopic RA harvest have demonstrated favorable results with regard to arterial patency. However, this approach is not widely used because there is a relatively high incidence of complications. Possible complications include direct injury to the artery, dissection, and hematoma with subsequent compartment syndrome. Other complications include cellulitis and dorsal thenar sensory numbness. In a series of 300 patients who underwent endoscopic RA harvest, the incidence of cellulitis and dorsal thenar sensory numbness was 1.6% and 8.7%, respectively *(23,24)*.

SUMMARY

Saphenous vein harvesting can be performed safely using minimally invasive techniques. These minimally invasive approaches are associated with improvement in cosmetic results, decreased wound complications, shorter hospital stay, and patient satisfaction. We believe that these techniques will continue to evolve as technology continues to improve.

REFERENCES

1. Patel AN, Hebeler RF, Hamman BL, et al. Prospective analysis of endoscopic vein harvesting. Am J Surg 2001;182:716–719.
2. DeLaria GA, Hunter JA, Goldin MD, Serry C, Javid H, Najafi H. Leg wound complications associated with coronary revascularization. J Thorac Cardiovasc Surg 1981;81:403–407.
3. Baddour, LM, Bisno AL. Recurrent cellulitis after saphenous venectomy for coronary bypass surgery. Ann Intern Med 1982;97:493–496.
4. Reifsnyder T, Bandyk D, Seabrook G, et al. Wound complications of the in-situ saphenous vein bypass technique. J Vasc Surg 1992;15:843–850.
5. Wipke-Tevis DD, Stotts NA, Skov P, Carrieri-Kohlman V. Frequency, manifestations, and correlates of impaired healing of saphenous vein harvest incisions. Heart Lung 1996;25:108–116.
6. Lee KS, Reinstein L. Lower limb amputation of the donor site extremity after coronary artery bypass graft surgery. Arch Phys Med Rehabil 1986;67:564–565.
7. Allen KB, Griffith GL, Heimansohn DA, et al. Endoscopic versus traditional saphenous vein harvesting: a prospective randomized trial. Ann Thorac Surg 1998;66:26–32.
8. Puskas J, Wright C, Miller P, et al. A randomized trial of endoscopic versus open saphenous vein harvest in coronary bypass surgery. Ann Thorac Surg 1999;68:1509–1512.
9. Crouch JD, O'Hair DP, Keuler JP, Barragry TP, Wermer PN, Kleinman LN. Open versus endoscopic saphenous vein harvesting: wound complications and vein quality. Ann Thorac Surg 1999;68:1513–1516.
10. Horvath KD, Gray D, Benton L, Hill J, Swanstrom LL. Operative outcomes of minimally invasive saphenous vein harvest. Am J Surg 1998;175:391–395.
11. Davis Z, Jacobs HK, Zhang M, Thomas C, Castellanos Y. Endoscopic vein harvest for coronary artery bypass grafting: technique and outcomes. J Thorac Cardiovasc Surg 1998:116:228–235.
12. Morris RJ, Butler MT, Samuels LE. Minimally invasive saphenous vein harvesting. Ann Thorac Surg 1998;66:1026–1028.
13. Hayward TZ, Hey LA, Newman LL, et al. Endoscopic versus open saphenous vein harvest: the effect on postoperative outcomes. Ann Thorac Surg 1999;68:2107–2111.
14. Kan C, Luo C. Endoscopic saphenous vein harvest decreases leg wound complication in coronary artery bypass grafting patients. J Card Surg 1999;14:157–162.
15. Allen KB, Shaar CJ. Endoscopic saphenous vein harvesting. Ann Thor Surg 1997;64:265–266.
16. Vitali RM, Reddy RC, Molinaro PJ, Sabado MF, Jacobowitz IJ. Hemodynamic effects of carbon dioxide insufflation during endoscopic vein harvesting. Ann Thorac Surg 2000;70:1098–1099.
17. Griffith GL, Allen KB, Waller BF, et al. Endoscopic and traditional saphenous vein harvest: a histologic comparison. Ann Thorac Surg 2000;69:520–523.
18. Meyer DM, Rogers TE, Jessen ME, Estrera AS, Chin AK. Histologic evidence of the safety of endoscopic saphenous vein graft preparation. Ann Thorac Surg 200;70:487–491.
19. Black EA, Guzik TJ, West NRJ, et al. Minimally invasive saphenous vein harvesting: effects on endothelial and smooth muscle function . Ann Thorac Surg 2001;71:1503–1507.
20. Cable DG, Dearani JA, Pfeifer EA, Daly RC, Schaff HV. Minimally invasive saphenous vein harvesting: endothelial integrity and early clinical results. Ann Thorac Surg 1998;66:139–143.
21. Fabricius AM, Oser A, Diegeler A, Rauch T, Mohr FW. Endothelial function of human vena saphena magna prepared with different minimally invasive harvesting techniques. Eur J Cardiothorac Surg 2000;18:400–403.
22. Allen KB, Fitzgerald EB, Heimansohn DA, Shaar CJ. Management of closed space infections associated with endoscopic vein harvest. Ann Thorac Surg 2000;69:960–961.
23. Connolly MW, Torrillo MD, Stauder MJ, et al. Endoscopic radial artery harvesting: results of the first 300 patients. Ann Thorac Surg 2002;74(2):502–505.
24. Terada Y, Uchida A, Fukuda I, Hochberg J, Mitsui T, Sato F. Endoscopic harvesting of the radial artery as a coronary artery bypass graft. Ann Thorac Surg 1998;66:2123–2124.

15 Hybrid Revascularization

Uwe Klima, MD *and Axel Haverich*, MD

Contents

Introduction
Patients and Methods
Operative Procedure: MIDCAB
Percutaneous Intervention
Case Scenarios
Results
Discussion
Summary
References

INTRODUCTION

Revascularization with the left internal mammary artery (LIMA) and additional radial artery and/or vein grafts via a median sternotomy is the generally accepted surgical approach to multivessel coronary artery disease. Cardiopulmonary bypass (CPB) with cardioplegic arrest still represents the standard technique for coronary artery surgery in most centers worldwide. However, as this book underscores, there is a strong trend toward beating-heart surgery in an effort to avoid potential complications caused by CPB *(1,2)*. Minimally invasive direct coronary artery bypass (MIDCAB) grafting without cardiopulmonary bypass through an anterolateral minithoracotomy has become a therapeutic option, especially in multimorbid, elderly, and redo patients with single-vessel disease *(3)*. However, owing to limited access through the minithoracotomy, this approach cannot be applied to multivessel revascularization without additional incisions or use of CPB. To expand the benefits of the MIDCAB approach to patients with multivessel disease, a "hybrid" procedure combining MIDCAB surgical revascularization of the left anterior descending artery (LAD) with catheter-based interventional procedures (PTCA; percutanous transluminal coronary angioplasty ± stent) for additional coronary lesions is increasingly being considered as an attractive therapeutic option *(4)*.

From: *Contemporary Cardiology: Minimally Invasive Cardiac Surgery, Second Edition*
Edited by: D. J. Goldstein and M. C. Oz © Humana Press Inc., Totowa, NJ

Table 1
Demographics and Extent of Coronary Artery Disease Among 33 Patients Undergoing Hybrid Revascularization

Demographic	
Age (yr)	62.1 ± 8.5
Sex (M/F)	27/6
Unstable angina	6 (18.2%)
Previous MI[a]	15 (45.5%)
One–vessel disease[b]	6 (18.2%)
Two–vessel disease	18 (54.5%)
Three–vessel disease	9 (27.3%)
Previous PTCA[c]/stent	3 (9.1%)
Proximal LAD[d] disease	33 (100%)

[a]Myocardial infarction.
[b]Diseased vessel is the LAD and PTCA is to the diagonal branch of the LAD.
[c]Percutaneous coronary transluminal angioplasty.
[d]Left anterior descending.

Our preliminary results using a "hybrid" approach to myocardial revascularization suggest that this concept is a safe and effective method of complete revascularization for selected patients with multivessel involvement. Very old patients and redo patients with significant comorbidity are likely to benefit most from this approach. However, even younger patients with aggressive disease, for whom repeat coronary revascularization procedures seem likely in the future, should also benefit. Such patients will avoid the risk of CPB, and the discomfort and possible complications of median sternotomy.

In this chapter, we present our preliminary results in 33 consecutive cases undergoing a "hybrid" procedure consisting of an initial MIDCAB surgical revascularization of the LAD with subsequent angioplasty of additional coronary lesions.

PATIENTS AND METHODS

Between June 1996 and September 2001 a total of 530 MIDCAB procedures were performed at Hannover Medical School. Thirty-three (6.2%) of these patients had an elective hybrid procedure. Following MIDCAB revascularization of the LAD, 33 patients had PTCA of an additional 48 coronary lesions after a median of 7 d. Patient characteristics, cardiac performance, and comorbidities of those 33 patients are summarized in Tables 1 and 2.

OPERATIVE PROCEDURE: MIDCAB

After induction of general anesthesia with standard intravenous agents, the left chest is exposed by placing the patient on the right side in the 30° decubitus position. The left lung is collapsed by use of a bronchial blocker. An indicator dilution catheter is placed for hemodynamic measurements. A short (8–10 cm), left fourth- or fifth-intercostal space incision is made using the chest radiograph, for estimating the better level for exposing the anterolateral surface of the heart. The LIMA pedicle is then dissected from the chest wall. It is important to dissect a sufficient length to obviate tension on the anastomosis.

Table 2
Comorbidities Among 33 Patients Undergoing Hybrid Revascularization

Comorbidity	*No. (%) of patients*
Peripheral vascular disease	2 (6.1%)
Deep venous thrombosis	1 (3%)
Left ventricular aneurysm	1 (3%)
Chronic renal failure	2 (6.1%)
Cerebrovascular accident	2 (6.1%)
Diabetes	9 (27.3%)
COPD[a]	3 (9.2%)
Tuberculosis	2 (6.1%)
Hyperthyroidism	1 (3%)
Melanoma	1 (3%)
Morbid obesity	2 (6.1%)

[a]Chronic obstructive pulmonary disease.

At least 8 cm and, with a large heart or a very distal anastomosis, as much as 15 cm may be required. Proximal dissection may reach the subclavian origin of the LIMA. Dilute papaverine is sprayed onto the pedicle frequently to avert conduit spasm.

After dissection of the LIMA is completed, the patient is systemically heparinized (100 IU/kg body weight) and the distal end of the LIMA pedicle is divided between clips. The pericardium is opened with a "T"-incision and a pericardial sling is formed with strategically placed stay sutures to elevate and position the heart for optimum exposure of the LAD. The appropriate site for an arteriotomy is selected and that region of the heart is fixed and rendered relatively motionless by use of a semielliptical, atraumatic, stabilizing retractor. To provide a bloodless field, we have used a commercially available mist machine and 4-0 polypropylene snares looped around the LIMA. For the first 200 MIDCAB patients we used snares both proximal and distal to the arteriotomy.

It was later shown that snare trauma may presage arterial stenosis in the native vessel at the snare site; thereafter we modified our technique to omit the distal snare. In the present study group of 33 patients, the first 15 patients had both proximal and distal snares. Hemodynamics were evaluated for 2 min after tightening the snare. If the heart tolerated this, the anastomosis was undertaken using 8-0 polypropylene sutures. During the snaring period, two patients in the study had hemodynamic instability unresponsive to inotropes and a temporary intraluminal shunt was inserted to bridge the arteriotomy and afford distal myocardial perfusion during the performance of the anastomosis. At the completion of the anastomosis the snare is released and removed. Protamine is then given at a dose calculated to yield a 50% reversal of the administered heparin. Fibrin glue is applied to the anastomosis for further hemostatic assurance, and is used to fix the pedicle to the epicardium in a gentle curve without tension, torsion, or angulations. The pericardium is loosely closed. A single chest tube is placed in the costophrenic sulcus. The interspace incision is closed in layers in standard fashion.

PERCUTANEOUS INTERVENTION

Each patient was recatheterized between postoperative d 3 and 9. Patients were instructed to take 500 mg of aspirin at 24 h and again 1 h before recatheterization. The

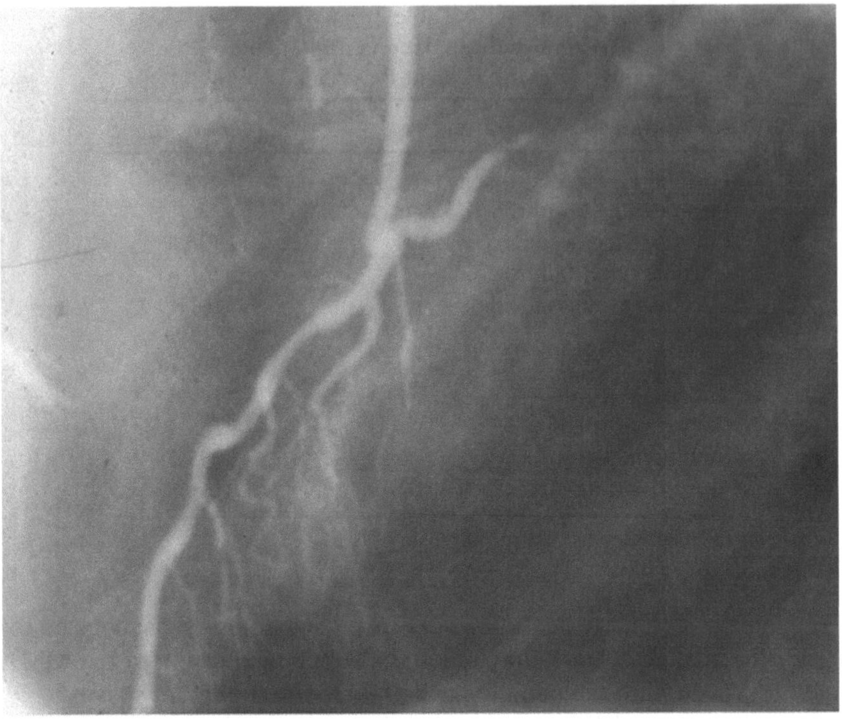

Fig. 1. Completed LIMA to LAD anastomosis.

transfemoral approach was used. All LIMA grafts were demonstrated to show good to excellent flow (**Fig. 1**). Assured of good flow in the LIMA–LAD distribution, attention was then directed to the additional known coronary lesions, which were confirmed by reinjection. Each patient was then given 15,000 IU of heparin through the intra-arterial catheter. If a stent was used, 250 mg of ticlopidine was also administered. A guide catheter (7 or 8 F), suitable for angioplasty, was positioned appropriately for each additional lesion of concern. Balloon dilatations were then performed over a 0.0014 guide wire. If any lesion had a residual stenosis of over 35%, the lesion was stented. A final coronary arteriogram documented the success of the PTCA/stenting procedure (**Fig. 2**).

CASE SCENARIOS

Several clinical scenarios led to our decision to perform hybrid procedures in our patients. In the following paragraphs, three "typical" patients are described in whom we utilized the two-pronged surgical and interventional approach.

Case 1

A 58-yr-old male patient had suffered recurrent angina after previous surgical myocardial revascularization. At cardiac evaluation the vein graft to the right coronary artery was patent and well functioning. However, vein grafts to both the circumflex and left anterior descending artery were closed, and both native coronaries showed significant proximal stenosis. Because the LIMA was still available, the patient was reoperated upon by MIDCAB technique. On the fifth postoperative day, a repeat angiogram showed a

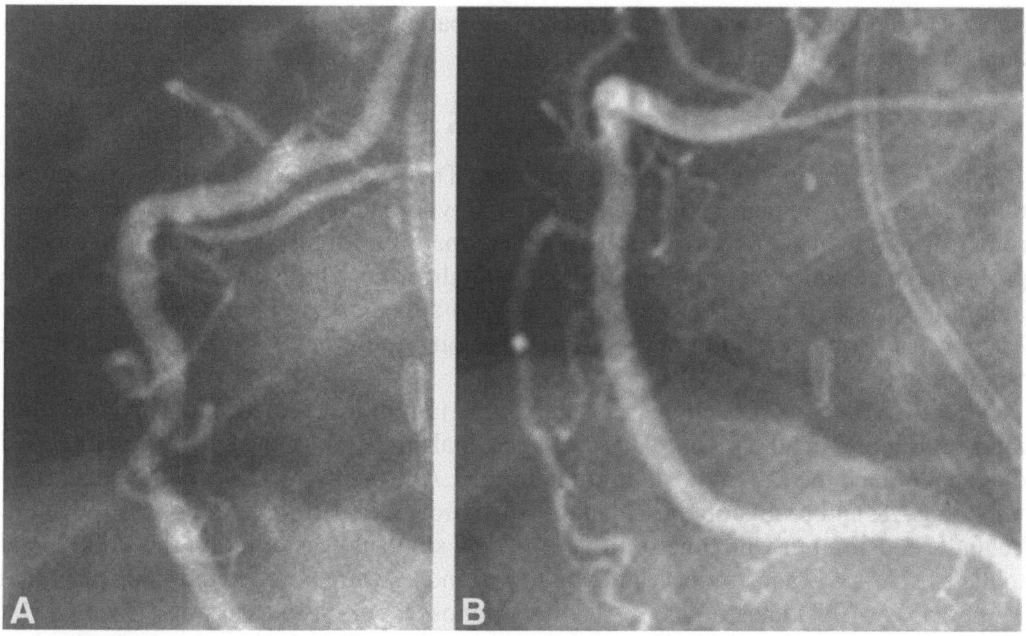

Fig. 2. Successful PTCA of right coronary artery: (**A**) Stenosis before and (**B**) after intervention.

patent LIMA-to-LAD anastomosis. The proximal circumflex stenosis was dilated and stented successfully. Three years after the hybrid procedure the patient remains free of angina.

Case 2

A 49-year-old female patient underwent cardiac transplantation 2 yr before for dilated cardiomyopathy. Although she remained free of cardiac failure, on her second annual follow-up catheterization severe triple-vessel transplant vasculopathy was diagnosed. The right coronary artery supplied no significant area of myocardium and was not treated. A dominant obtuse marginal branch was significantly stenosed, as was the mid-LAD. After performing a LIMA-to-LAD MIDCAB procedure, the stenosis in the obtuse marginal branch of the circumflex artery was successfully stented 5 d after the MIDCAB.

Case 3

A 79-year-old female patient with unstable angina had significant comorbidity. In addition to angina, her cardiac evaluation showed that her left ventricular ejection fraction was less than 25%. She had advanced pulmonary obstructive disease with a forced expiratory volume at 1 s (FEV1) of 600 mL. Her CT scan showed a porcelain aorta. She had insulin-dependent diabetes. These findings excluded her from consideration for conventional revascularization. The preoperative cardiac angiogram revealed severe triple-vessel disease with a severe obstruction in the proximal portion of the right coronary artery, a subtotal proximal LAD occlusion, and multiple stenoses in the circumflex. Medical management was unsuccessful, as the patient could not be weaned from continuous intravenous nitroglycerin and heparin. Hence, we performed a MIDCAB procedure, followed by stenting of the proximal right coronary artery on the seventh day postoperatively. Both procedures were successful and the patient was discharged to rehabilitation on the ninth postoperative day.

RESULTS

There were no intra- or perioperative deaths. There were no conversions to a sternotomy. There were no major complications (i.e., myocardial infarction, stroke, other neurological deficit, bleeding sufficient to require reoperation, or respiratory failure requiring prolonged mechanical ventilation) during hospitalization. These patients did not require inotropic support. Blood loss was minimal, with a mean of 450 ± 120 mL per patient. There was no major (> 1 unit of blood) transfusion requirement. Average postoperative ventilation time was 8.5 ± 4.1 h.

After the MIDCAB procedures, coronary reangiography revealed patent and functioning LIMA grafts in all patients. There was one mal-insertion of the LIMA into a second diagonal branch instead of the main trunk of the LAD, but there was excellent backflow into the LAD and perfusion of its distal distribution. One LIMA pedicle was judged to be under tension but was functioning. One new stenosis was noted in the LAD distal to the LIMA–LAD anastomosis and two new stenoses were noted in the LAD proximal to the LIMA–LAD anastomosis. All these stenoses were less than 50%. Two LIMA pedicles were found to be fixed to the chest wall but were functioning. Angiography data are summarized in Table 3.

No further deterioration of organ function occurred in patients with preexisting comorbidity of lungs, kidneys, or central nervous system. Subsequent PTCA, and stenting were required ($n = 14$). A total of 45 additional lesions were treated successfully. There were no major complications related to these procedures. Two patients had groin hematomas that did not require surgical management. Mean follow-up time was 54 ± 9.2 mo. Thirty-one patients (94 %) are alive and free of angina. One patient died of a myocardial infarction 16 mo after the hybrid procedure. The cause of death in the one additional patient is unknown; one patient suffered a myocardial infarction (posterior wall) during follow-up 12 mo after the operation. There have been seven nonelective percutaneous interventions during the long-term follow-up. One of these was a repeat PTCA (12 mo postoperatively) of a lesion previously dilated as part of an initial hybrid procedure. Six were dilatations of new lesions in lateral or posterior wall coronary branches.

DISCUSSION

MIDCAB has become an accepted therapeutic option worldwide for the management of single-vessel disease, especially in patients with high proximal stenosis of the left anterior descending coronary artery *(5)*. Major advantages have been realized because of the avoidance of extracorporeal circulation and sternotomy incision. This has been particularly true for elderly patients and patients with extensive comorbidities. Because the results have been so favorable for MIDCAB alone, additional applications have been sought. As a result, the combined surgical (MIDCAB) and catheter-type intervention emerged *(6,7)*, called the "hybrid" approach. This strategy is gaining increasing acceptance as a method to perform a protected left main coronary stenosis angioplasty *(8)*.

In our series, the patients had numerous comorbid factors. All these comorbidities are by themselves, or in combination, risk factors for increased perioperative morbidity and mortality. However, in our patients undergoing a hybrid procedure, no intra- or

Table 3
Angiographic Results After MIDCAB LIMA-to-LAD Anastomosis

LIMA–LAD Anastomosis	*n*	*Native LAD*	*n*
Tension	1	New proximal stenosis (< 50%)	2
Dissection	0	New distal stenosis (< 50%)	1
Competitive flow	0		
Occlusion	0		
Fixation to chest wall	2		
Narrowing	2		
Stenosis	0		
Malinsertion to D1	1		

perioperative death occurred and none of our patients suffered a major complication during hospitalization. Neuropsychiatric complications, including perioperative stroke, are frequently seen complications following coronary artery bypass grafting. Trehan and coworkers *(9)* evaluated the use of an individualized surgical approach including the hybrid procedure for reducing neurological injury in patients undergoing CABG who were at high risk of stroke because of aortic atherosclerosis or carotid artery disease. They concluded that selective surgical techniques, including hybrid procedures, can prevent adverse neurological sequelae while achieving complete myocardial revascularization, even in a group of high-risk patients. Our patients had no postoperative strokes, other neurological complications, or psychoses.

At the present time, MIDCAB is used predominantly for grafting of vessels on the anterior surface of the heart. Vessels on the lateral or posterior left ventricular walls are operated on through a mid-sternotomy using a beating-heart technique or conventional CPB-supported surgery. Can we select certain patients with multiple lesions who might benefit more from a hybrid procedure than from conventional surgery or PTCA-stenting alone? A patient with a specific contraindication to CPB, who in the past might have had only a MIDCAB to the LAD, would be left with incomplete revascularization. Because it has been well demonstrated that incomplete revascularization carries an increased risk of myocardial infarction, repeated angioplasties or stenting procedures, and redo surgery, we believe that additional efforts should be made to do as complete a revascularization as possible. Patients with an LAD not amenable to PTCA-stenting who in addition have an unacceptable risk for CPB are clearly candidates for the hybrid procedure.

Two factors determine the long-term efficacy of the hybrid procedure: the long-term patency of the MIDCAB LIMA–LAD graft and the duration of benefit from the PTCA-stenting procedure. Previous experience has shown LIMA–LAD surgery to be superior in long-term patency, freedom from significant cardiac events, survival, and relief of symptoms, to catheter intervention techniques. Also PTCA-stenting has a better record regarding restenosis when applied to the right coronary artery or to lesions in the circumflex system than the 20% first-year failure rate, even with stenting, when similar interventions are applied to the LAD. The hybrid procedure combines the best features of both the surgical and the interventional techniques. It permits the benefits of MIDCAB surgery to be extended to a wider spectrum of patients. Certain patients with two-vessel disease in which the LAD stenosis is considered to be a type C lesion are known to be unfavorable candidates for PTCA-stenting and are also recognized to have a progressive form of coronary disease in which repeated interventions and redo surgery are all too often the rule. An initial MIDCAB LIMA–LAD would avoid redo surgery through a midsternotomy whenever the likely recurrence of symptoms develops. A particularly elegant application of the hybrid principle is in the patient with a left main coronary artery stenosis who is also an unacceptable risk for conventional surgery. A preliminary MIDCAB LIMA–LAD affords protection from myocardial ischemia during the subsequent catheter intervention.

There is current debate regarding the proper sequence of the two segments of the hybrid procedure. If the percutaneous intervention is done first, conventional surgery could possibly treat the actual coronary artery disease and manage the complication at the same time. Supporters of that sequence also mention that the extensive anticoagulation required after catheterization complications and after stenting might lead to bleeding difficulties in the previous MIDCAB operative site. However, complications of interventional techniques such as intimal tears, plaque disruption, acute thrombosis, and distal embolization are rare. If the catheter procedure requires the use of high-dose, multiagent anticoagulant and antiplatelet therapy, there may be a significant and detrimental delay in performing the MIDCAB. We believe that the LAD lesion is likely to be the most significant ischemic lesion and should be treated first by MIDCAB LIMA–LAD. The catheter intervention for additional lesions should follow at a convenient early date thereafter. We also believe that the ultimate goal should be the performance of the two phases of the hybrid procedure on the same day, in the same operative theater, with the MIDCAB preceding the catheter intervention. For a variety of reasons this is impractical in most hospitals today.

Mid- and long-term patency and an uneventful clinical course are important factors in evaluating the efficacy of this relatively new procedure. After a mean follow-up time of 54 ± 9.2 mo, all patients had a clinical reevaluation or, if that was not possible, answered a standardized questionnaire. Analysis of the data was encouraging: 31 patients (94%) were alive and free of angina. Considering that this subset of patients has severe comorbidity, the results are very promising. Similar results have been reported by other groups *(7,10,11)* with 11.4–24 mo follow-up. Table 4 delineates the outcomes of five most recent series investigating hybrid approaches to revascularization *(12–16)*.

SUMMARY

The combination of an initial MIDCAB LIMA–LAD followed, in 3–9 d, by PTCA-stenting for additional coronary obstructive lesions, is called the hybrid approach to myocardial revasularization. We have found the hybrid approach to be safe, with low morbidity, and effective in establishing complete revascularization in patients with double- and triple-vessel coronary disease. It has been particularly helpful in the very old patient, the patient with extensive associated disease, and in those patients who are at high risk for CPB or mid-sternotomy. Younger patients whose coronary anatomy or type of atherosclerotic coronary artery disease makes them unsuitable for standard interventional or standard surgical procedures may also be considered for the hybrid approach.

REFERENCES

1. Puskas JD, Wright CE, Ronson RS, Brown WM 3rd, Gott JP, Guyton RA. Clinical outcomes and angiographic patency in 125 consecutive off-pump coronary bypass patients. Heart Surg Forum 1999;2(3):216–221.

Table 4
Most Recent Series Investigating the Results of Hybrid Revascularization

Author (Ref.)	*No. of Patients*	*Order of Intervention*	*Mean Age (yr)*	*Mortality*	*Early Graft Patency (%)*	*Reintervention PTCA or CABG*
Matsumoto *(12)*	11	PTCA first	70 ± 9	0	100.0	27% of PTCA lesions
Presbitero *(13)*	42	na	na	4.70%	92.3	4.7% of LIMA–LAD grafts
Riess *(14)*	57	MIDCAB first	65 ± 8	0	98.0	23.5% of PTCA lesions
Cisowski *(15)*	50	MIDCAB first	55 ± 20	0	100.0	10% of PTCA lesions 2% of LIMA–LAD grafts

2. Isomura T, Suma H, Horii T, Sato T, Kobashi T, Kanemitsu H. Minimally invasive coronary artery revascularization: off-pump bypass grafting and the hybrid procedure. Ann Thorac Surg 2000;70(6):2017–2022.
3. Cremer JT, Wittwer T, Boning A, et al. Minimally invasive coronary artery revascularization on the beating heart. Ann Thorac Surg 2000;69(6):1787–1791.
4. Wittwer T, Cremer J, Boonstra P, et al. Myocardial "hybrid" revascularisation with minimally invasive direct coronary artery bypass grafting combined with coronary angioplasty: preliminary results of a multicentre study. Heart 2000;83(1):58–63.
5. Diegeler A. Left internal mammary artery grafting to left anterior descending coronary artery by minimally invasive direct coronary artery bypass approach. Curr Cardiol Rep 1999;1(4):323–330.
6. Riess FC, Schofer J, Kremer P, et al. Beating heart operations including hybrid revascularization: initial experiences. Ann Thorac Surg 1998;66(3):1076–1081.
7. De Canniere D, Jansens JL, Goldschmidt-Clermont P, Barvais L, Decrol P, Stoupel E. Combination of minimally invasive coronary bypass and percutaneous transluminal coronary angioplasty in the treatment of double-vessel coronary disease: two-year follow-up of a new hybrid procedure compared with "on-pump" double bypass grafting Am Heart J 2001;142(4):563–570.
8. Mack MJ, Brown DL, Sankaran A. Minimallly invasive coronary bypass for protected left main coronary stenosis angioplasty. Ann Thorac Surg 1998;64(5):1313–1315.
9. Trehan N, Mishra M, Kasliwal RR, Mishra A. Surgical strategies in patients at high risk for stroke undergoing coronary artery bypass grafting. Ann Thorac Surg 2000;70(3):1037–1045.
10. Wittwer T, Haverich A, Cremer J, Boonstra P, Franke U, Wahlers T. Follow-up experience with coronary hybrid-revascularisation. Thorac Cardiovasc Surg 2000;48(6):356–359.
11. Wittwer T, Haverich A, Cremer JT, Boonstra PW. The hybrid procedure for myocardial revascularisation: intermediate results. Ann Thorac Surg 1999;69(3):975.
12. Matsumoto Y, Endo M, Kasashima F, et al. Hybrid revascularization feasibility in minimally invasive direct coronary artery bypass grafting combined with percutaneous transluminal coronary angioplasty in patients with acute coronary syndrome and multivessel disease. Jpn J Cardiovasc Surg 2001;49:700–705.
13. Presbitero P, Nicolini F, Maiello L, et al. "Hybrid" percutaneous and surgical coronary revascularization: selection criteria from a single-center experience. Ital Heart J 2001;2:369–371.
14. Riess FC, Bader R, Kremer P, et al. Coronary hybrid revascularization from January 1997 to January 2001: a clinical follow up. Ann Thorac Surg 2002;73:1849–1855.
15. Cisowski M, Morawski W, Drzewiecki J, et al. Integrated minimally invasive direct coronary artery bypass grafting and angioplasty for coronary artery revascularization. Eur J Cardiothorac Surg 2002;22:261–265.

16 Neurocognitive Issues in Off-Pump CABG

Ronald M. Lazar, PHD
and Daniel F. Heitjan, PHD

CONTENTS

INTRODUCTION
NEUROLOGICAL ASPECTS
NEUROCOGNITIVE ASPECTS
NEUROBEHAVIORAL OUTCOMES AFTER OFF-PUMP CORONARY ARTERY SURGERY
CLINICAL MANAGEMENT
REFERENCES

INTRODUCTION

Since its introduction in 1968, coronary artery bypass grafting (CABG) has resulted in superior survival and a better quality of life for specific subgroups of patients with coronary artery disease when compared to medical therapy *(1)*. For most patients, CABG and the combined use of cardiopulmonary bypass (CPB) have resulted in clinically undetectable deficits, but in a significant minority the results have been more serious *(2)*. Of all the adverse consequences associated with bypass grafting, neurological outcomes represent an important proportion *(3)*. Given that more than 650,000 people in the United States and 800,000 worldwide undergo CABG *(4)*, improvements in surgical techniques and patient management stand to have an impact on significant numbers of patients with respect to both medical costs and quality of life.

The purpose of this chapter is to demonstrate that one impetus for the trend toward the use of off-pump CABG is the neurogenic morbidity that can be associated with on-pump surgery. The following material thus represents a discussion of the broad neurological

From: *Contemporary Cardiology: Minimally Invasive Cardiac Surgery, Second Edition*
Edited by: D. J. Goldstein and M. C. Oz © Humana Press Inc., Totowa, NJ

and neurocognitive issues. Suggestions regarding pre- and postoperative evaluations will be made.

NEUROLOGICAL ASPECTS

Cerebrovascular morbidity is a well-documented complication of (on-pump) CABG, with the rate of perioperative cerebral infarction ranging from 2% to 6% in studies conducted over the past 20 years *(5–10)*. In a large, multicenter prospective study, Roach and colleagues studied 2108 patients in which the overall stroke rate following CABG was 3.0%, with an additional 3.1% suffering prolonged unconsciousness, seizures, or encephalopathy *(4)*. The mortality rate of patients with stroke, stupor, or coma was 21% compared to 2% for those without. Age and duration of cardiopulmonary bypass were the factors most significantly correlated with adverse neurological events. Tuman's group found an overall stroke rate of 2.8% among 2000 prospective patients undergoing CABG; patients under the age of 65 had a rate of 0.9% while those over 75 had an incidence of 9.0% *(11)*. Like other studies, duration of CPB and prior stroke were also significant risk factors.

In one of the largest studies to date, Stamou and his group at the Washington Hospital Center found that among 16,528 consecutive patients undergoing on-pump CABG over a 10-yr period, 333 (2%) had postoperative stroke *(12)*. Patients who suffered these events were older, but several important operative characteristics were predictive. Indeed, the crossclamp and cardiopulmonary bypass times were significantly longer in those who developed postoperative stroke than in those who did not.

Two pathophysiological mechanisms have been proposed to underlie major neurological events arising from CABG associated with CPB: multiple emboli and cerebral hypoperfusion arising from intraoperative hypotension. With respect to macroembolization, possible mechanisms include air, valve, and aortic atheroma *(13)*. Wijdicks and Jack evaluated the clinical and brain-imaging (CT) features of 25 patients with ischemic stroke following CABG, with events occurring from 1 to 22 d after surgery *(14)*. No patient had watershed infarcts. Rather, the imaging and clinical course of these patients suggested that post-CABG stroke was consistent with embolic phenomena, related to retained cardiac thrombi, new-onset atrial fibrillation, or intimal damage of the aorta during clamping. Indeed, there are new data supporting the importance of premorbid aortic disease in CABG that makes off-pump surgery an attractive alternative. Trehan et al. prospectively screened 3660 patients undergoing CABG with transesophageal echocardiography (TEE) and found 104 patients with plaque with a mobile element (grade III) *(15)*. Using intraoperative TEE, they found no embolic events in the subgroup of 88 patients who underwent off-pump CABG. The other possible mechanism, hypotension, is thought to occur in some cases, but is considered much less common *(16)*. It is not yet clear whether embolism in the brain circulation in the context of a transient, hypoperfused state and/or during a postsurgical inflammatory period accelerates the ischemic cascade.

The coexistence of coronary and carotid atherosclerosis continues to be documented, yet controversy still surrounds the prophylactic application of carotid endarterectomy prior to CABG *(17,18)*. Nevertheless, Yoon et al. found among 201 prospectively studied (on-pump) CABG patients that 52.4% had extracranial carotid disease (≥70% stenosis) and/or intracranial carotid disease (≥50% stenosis) *(19)*. More important, on multivariate analysis, intracranial carotid disease had an independent association with the development of CNS complications. Such studies have yet to be performed with off-pump patients.

NEUROCOGNITIVE ASPECTS

Neuropsychological function refers to the complex set of cognitive tasks subserved by the brain involving such spheres as language, memory, attention, visual perception, and executive skills *(20)*. The terms "neuropsychological" and "neurocognitive" are generally used interchangeably. It has been suggested that the assessment of neurocognition is probably a more sensitive index of brain integrity with cerebrovascular disease than sensorimotor function or coordination *(21–23)*, and is dissociable from depression *(24)*. It is therefore not surprising that, in contrast to major neurological complications, the reported incidence of cognitive changes following CABG, especially with CPB, is much higher. Except in cases of frank ischemic stroke, cortical deficits such as aphasia, apraxia, agnosia, and amnesia are rarely found. Rather, alteration of cognitive function following CABG resembles that found in chronic, small-vessel cerebrovascular disease in the periventricular and subcortical white matter *(25)*.

Both short- and long-term deficits have been identified, but there is considerable variation across studies *(26)*. Early studies demosntrated that the incidence of decline in the first 2 wk postoperatively ranged from 30% to 79%, and when extended to 6-mo follow-up, decline ranged from 24% to 57% *(27)*. Mahanna et al. summarized the literature from 1980 to 1994, encompassing 21 studies with 1864 CABG patients, and found that the variability occurred from factors such as surgical technique, type of anesthesia, cognitive instruments used, severity of illness, and patient demographics *(28)*. In addition, the operational definition of cognitive impairment also affected the reported incidence of postsurgical dysfunction. These studies, however, led to two important consensus conferences outlining such needs as having a baseline, presurgical testing; an evaluation of a comprehensive range of function; an assessment at least 3 mo postoperatively; the importance of identifying change scores in individual patients; and consideration of "practice effects" in the analysis of findings *(29,30)*.

McKann et al. studied eight cognitive domains in 127 CABG patients at 1 mo and 1 yr after surgery *(27)* . All but 12% of patients demonstrated decline in cognitive function. While functions such as language declined and then improved, approx 10% had persistent declines in verbal memory, visual memory, attention, and visuoconstruction, and 24% had late, further decline in visuoconstruction. More recently, another prospective study of 127 patients from the same investigator group showed that surgery-related factors correlated with cognitive impairment at 3 mo, but at 1 yr, only medical history variables were related to such dysfunction, all of which suggested that there may be different determinants of cognitive change at different postoperative time points *(31)*. It was pointed out, however, that only 127 of the original 172 patients were successfully evaluated at all study points.

The longest-term study to date assessing the neurocognitive consequences of on-pump CABG comes from Newman and his group at Duke *(32)*. They followed 261 patients who underwent CABG by administering a neurocognitive battery preoperatively, before discharge, 6 wk, 6 mo, and 5 yr after surgery. The authors performed a statistical analysis of the baseline (presurgical) scores to eliminate concern about the redundancy of tests and derived four "noncorrelated" domains of function: (1) verbal memory and language comprehension; (2) abstraction and visual–spatial orientation; (3) attention, psychomotor processing speed, and concentration; and (4) visual memory. Cognitive decline was defined as a loss of one standard deviation in performance in any one of the four domains. It was found among the 172 patients who completed the study that 52% had cognitive decline at discharge, 36% at 6 wk, 24% at 6 mo, and 42% at 5 yr. Predictors of decline at 5 yr included older age, higher baseline neurocognitive function, lower educational level, and cognitive decline at discharge. Interestingly, duration of cardiopulmonary bypass and duration of aortic crossclamping were not significant predictors in this study.

Analogous to major neurological events following conventional CABG, microembolism is said to account for most of the cognitive changes seen after surgery *(33)*. Moody and colleagues found fatty material containing aluminum in the brain microvasculature from autopsy specimens of patients who had died shortly after CABG with CPB and who had cognitive impairment *(34)*. Using intraoperative transcranial Doppler (TCD), Jacobs et al. found that high-intensity transient signals (HITS) in 18 CABG patients occurred primarily during cardiopulmonary bypass and to a lesser extent during aortic manipulation and were correlated with cognitive changes 8–12 d postoperatively *(35)*. It was also seen that such neuropsychological deficits were not correlated with the total number of HITS, suggesting that the location of brain injury was more important for the development of such deficits, a notion that is also supported by brain SPECT *(36)*.

One method for detecting brain ischemic disease is magnetic resonance imaging (MRI) *(37)*. Sylivris and colleagues studied 41 patients undergoing CABG both with intraoperative TCD and pre- and postsurgery MRI *(38)*. TCD confirmed that most microemboli occurred during cardiopulmonary bypass, but MRI failed to show a relationship between new-onset small-vessel disease and subsequent neuropsychological deficits. They proposed that neuropsychological testing may be more sensitive than radiological detection of vascular events as a result of the limit in the resolution of conventional MRI to detect very small strokes.

A new method for the early detection of brain ischemia is diffusion-weighted MRI (DWI), which has been shown capable of detecting neurovascular changes as quickly as 105 min after the onset of a clinical event, with the ability to discriminate old vs new lesions *(39)*. Moreover, it has been found that DWI is not only more sensitive than conventional MRI in detecting acute lesions, but that lesion volume on early DWI correlates significantly with clinical outcome ratings on the NIH Stroke Scale, the Barthel Index, and the Rankin Scale *(40)*. Recently, DWI was reported in 14 post-CABG (on-pump) cases of acute stroke *(41)*. Whereas CT detected 5/12 ischemic events, infarcts were seen in 10/14 patients with DWI, with radiographic findings suggestive of multiple embolic infarcts involving multiple vascular territories.

To illustrate the sensitivity of this new radiographic technique, we present in **Fig. 1** two cases of patients who underwent CABG, one off-pump (above) and one on-pump (below), as part of an ongoing clinical trial. The T_2-weighted image obtained shortly after surgery in both cases shows the presence of old strokes. In the off-pump case, the DWI shows no new event, but there is a new lesion in the left thalamus of the patient who underwent on-pump surgery. To our knowledge, this new imaging technology has the potential to identify highly subtle changes in brain integrity that could elucidate further the underlying mechanisms.

One of the important as yet unsettled issues in the detection of neurocognitive change after CABG is the operational definition of abnormality: What standard should be used as an index of an alteration of function? There seem to be two major approaches in this regard. Both have in common the notion that there must be a presurgical baseline, and that

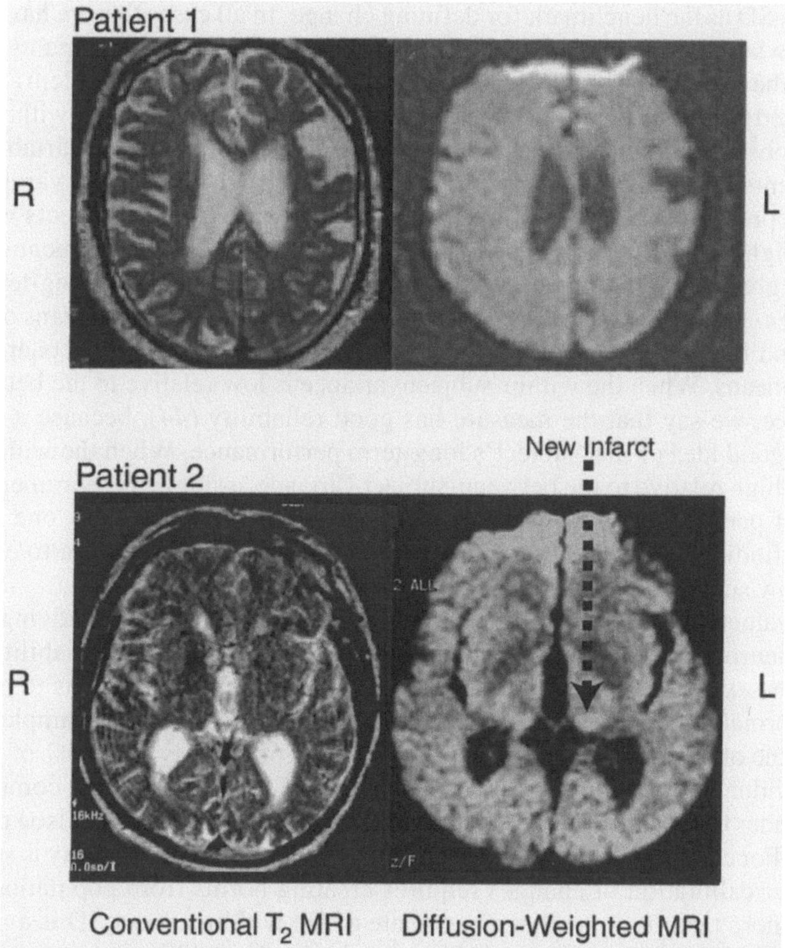

Fig. 1. Magnetic resonance imaging of the brain on two patients within 72 h after CABG surgery, with T_2-weighted images on the left and diffusion-weighted images (DWI) on the right. Patient 1 had off-pump CABG and Patient 2 had on-pump CABG. The black arrow points to a new infarct in the left thalamus.

with repeated testing over time there is at least some degree of practice effect. One line of investigation has used a one-standard-deviation (SD) decline on either a particular test or a group of tests clustered into a domain of function. As pointed out in the review by Symes et al., problems with this form of measurement include the likelihood of "floor effects" in patients whose scores are so low at baseline that further decline is difficult to detect and that declines in high baseline scores require a greater degree change *(42)*. Within this framework, there has never been a consensus as to the number of tests or domains that need to change. The other definition has been a 20% change on 20% of the tests employed, which some consider more sensitive in the identification of cognitive loss *(28)*. The problem with this method, however, is that it does not take into account the greater degree of normal variation as patients get older, especially on tests that are timed and/or require manual dexterity *(43)*.

A major implication of the way in which decline is defined bears on the statistical analysis needed in a clinical trial. As indicated above, some investigators have used a decline of 1 SD as the benchmark for defining change. In all cases that we have seen, the standard deviation was estimated from a pool of subjects (study participants or normal subjects in the population), each evaluated on a single occasion. The problem arises when this estimated standard deviation is used to evaluate longitudinal changes within subjects. When one observes repeated measurements on a population, the total variability in the measurements has two components: one representing within-subject variability and the other representing between-subject variability. That is, some subjects will generally give high values, with some variability around their long-term means, whereas others will give low values, again with some variability around their long-term means. The between-subject SD measures variability between the long-term means of different subjects, and the within-subject SD measures variability within subjects around their long-term means. When the within-subject variance is low relative to the between-subject variance, we say that the measure has good reliability *(44)*, because a single test provides a good idea of that subject's long-term performance. When the within-subject variance is high relative to the between-subject variance, a single measurement is a poor indicator of performance, and we say that the reliability is low. Thus, one reason for discrepant findings across neurocognitive studies may lie in the failure to establish in advance how such patients perform on the same test over time.

When evaluating change over time within subjects, as we intend in studying treatment effects on neurocognition, it is preferable to use only within-subject variability, because it gauges the expected level of variation within a subject and allows us to distinguish between normal temporal variability and real treatment effects. For example, a change from baseline of 3 within-subject SDs or more would occur only about 5% of the time in stable individuals. We cannot calibrate changes based on the SD that we commonly use, which includes both within- and between-subject components, without also knowing the reliability: For example, even a 1 SD change may be large if the reliability is sufficiently high. Proper calibration of changes requires creating norms from populations that are measured more than once, so that an estimate of the within-subject SD is available.

A second issue that arises in establishing standards of variability for measuring change within subjects is the source of the estimated SD. Some studies (e.g., Newman, et al. *[32]*) have estimated the SD from the study's own baseline observations. Aside from the issues discussed above, this can create a practical problem for data analysis. In clinical trials, it is common to perform one or more interim analyses with the objective of stopping early should the data lean strongly one way or the other. If the primary outcome is, say, the percentage of patients who experience a decline of 1 SD or more, and the SD is based on baseline data from the study itself, then this SD will change as more subjects are accrued. So unless accrual is complete by the time of the first interim analysis, the SD is bound to change from one interim analysis to the next. This creates an ambiguity in the data analysis that is not desirable in a clinical trial. From this perspective, it is clearly preferable to use a prespecified set of norms, rather than the accruing study data itself, to determine the measure of variability for a neurocognitive endpoint in a clinical trial.

While previous neurocognitive studies have suggested possible mechanisms for alterations of functioning, the clinical importance of detecting these cognitive changes, sometimes referred to as "ecological validity," is unresolved *(45,46)*. A major contribution to our understanding of the short- and long-term effects of CABG with cardiopulmonary bypass, or to compare it with other surgical techniques, would be the relationship between specific neuropsychological deficits and the outcomes of validated quality-of-life instruments. The paucity of such correlational data to date may also account for the lack of agreement in the definition of cognitive abnormality found in the literature.

Another group of relatively new markers of neuronal injury associated with on-pump CABG is the specific brain-originated proteins that include protein S-100B and neuron-specific enolase (NSE), easily assessed from blood samples *(47,48)*. Kilminster et al. found a statistical association between increased S-100 release during and 5 h after the onset of cardiopulmonary bypass and poorer neuropsychological performance 6–8 wk following surgery *(49)*. More recently, Herrmann et al., studying patients undergoing either on-pump CABG or valve-replacement surgery, found similar early correlations between increased NSE and S-100B and neuropsychological impairment. Unfortunately, only two patients were seen at the planned 6-mo follow-up. In contrast, Wimmer-Greinecker et al. found that increases in NSE and S-100B protein during and immediately after surgery did not predict impairment in neuropsychological scores 5 d or 2 mo postsurgery. Thus, the brain protein data to date are suggestive but not yet convincing as predictors of cognitive problems, but the effects may only be related to short-term, transient impairment.

NEUROBEHAVIORAL OUTCOMES AFTER OFF-PUMP CORONARY ARTERY SURGERY

The presence of central nervous system complications, whether gross or subtle, has led to a few recent preliminary efforts to compare coronary artery surgery with and without CPB. Hernandez and his colleagues compared outcomes between 445 patients undergoing conventional CABG with 322 off-pump patients. There were no differences in perioperative stroke or in-hospital mortality, but cognitive status was not reported *(50)*. In a Brazilian study, 81 patients (48 with CPB and 33 without) were evaluated neurologically and cognitively before and 5–7 d after surgery *(51)*. Of the 81 patients, 5 died. There were otherwise no statistical differences in outcomes between the two groups. It should be noted, however, that only patients with diagonal, left anterior descending, and right coronary artery lesions were eligible for the non-CPB group, thus precluding a randomized design. In addition, 49 patients were either illiterate or had less than a fifth-grade education, so it was unlikely that significant deficits in cognition function could be detected.

Andrew and colleagues compared pre- and postoperative neuropsychological dysfunction among three groups of patients: minimally invasive direct coronary bypass grafting (MIDCAB) patients ($n = 7$), single-graft CABG/CPB recipients ($n = 9$) patients, and multiple-graft CABG/CPB ($n = 27$) *(52)*. Postsurgery follow-up occurred before discharge. It was found that the multiple-graft CPB group had a significantly higher incidence of cognitive decline than the MIDCAB or single-graft groups. There was, however, no longer-term follow-up.

Murkin's group in Western Ontario published results of an ongoing study comparing 33 on-pump CABG patients with 35 off-pump CABG patients *(53)*. The preliminary data showed no clinically apparent strokes in either group. At the fifth postoperative day, there was a significantly lower incidence of cognitive dysfunction in the off-pump cases. At 3 mo postoperatively, 50% of the on-pump patients had cognitive deficits, compared to 5% in the off-pump group.

Finally, Diegeler et al. randomized 40 patients to either on- or off-pump CABG *(54)*. During surgery, there were a significantly greater number of high-intensity transient

Table 1
Domains of Neurocognitive Function and Representative Tests That Can Comprise a Neuropsychological Test Battery

Domain	*Test (Ref.)*
Global mental status	Mini-Mental State Examination *(55)*
Verbal memory	Rey Auditory Verbal Learning Test *(57)*
	California Verbal Learning Test *(58)*
Visual memory	Wechsler Memory Scale—Third Edition *(56)*
	Rey Complex Figure Test (Recall) *(59)*
Language	Boston Diagnostic Aphasia Examination *(60)*
	Boston Naming Test *(61)*
Attention	Digit Span *(62)*
Visuoconstruction	Rey Complex Figure (Copy) *(54)*
	Block Design *(57)*
Executive function	Trail Making Test *(63)*
	Stroop Test *(64)*
Motor speed	Purdue Pegboard *(65)*
	Grooved Pegboard *(66)*

signals (HITS) in the conventional group compared to the off-pump patients. Using a cognitive function scale validated for Alzheimer's disease, they found that on d 7 after surgery, 90% of the on-pump patients had abnormal cognitive scores, with no abnormality in the off-pump group. There was, however, no long-term follow-up of these patients, and it was acknowledged that perioperative mental and physical stress can have an early effect.

CLINICAL MANAGEMENT

The data are highly suggestive that conventional coronary artery bypass surgery poses neurological and neurocognitive risk for patients, mainly due to embolism. Although the incidence of frank stroke has diminished with advances in surgical equipment and technology, patients can be left with injury that is less physically apparent but equally disabling.

The patients at risk for neurological/neuropsychological insult appear, in particular, to be older individuals with a prior history of stroke or TIA, carotid artery disease, and atherosclerosis of the ascending aorta. Of course, the presence of other risk factors for stroke and cardiac disease, in general, must be taken into consideration, such as hypertension, diabetes, hypercholesterolemia, smoking, atrial fibrillation, and so forth. It would therefore seem prudent that all patients with elevated cerebrovascular risk undergo neurological examination, carotid duplex Doppler, and transcranial Doppler (TCD) prior to surgery. Conventional MRI can detect the presence of old strokes. The onset of strokelike symptoms should be evaluated by diffusion-weighted MRI (DWI), which is capable of differentiating between acute and chronic lesions. CT can show larger strokes but is less sensitive to small-vessel disease.

With respect to neurocognitive function, patients who have any degree of premorbid decline of higher cognitive function or have significant risk for stroke should undergo baseline neuropsychological examination, not simply the administration of a single screening test. Table 1 shows the broad spectrum of domains that should be evaluated, and representative tests for each sphere of function that should be administered by a qualified neuropsychologist. Lezak's review of neuropsychological tests *(20)* is among the most comprehensive compendia of well-validated, standardized measures in the field. Depending on the index of suspicion of premorbid deficits and the time available for testing, such batteries can last from 1 to 8 h. It is not advisable to have patients perform such tests late in the evening prior to the day of surgery. There can be nonspecific cognitive changes just after surgery, so follow-up should not be done until the time of discharge, only if specifically indicated, with a more valid evaluation occurring no earlier than 4 wk postsurgery, and preferrably at 8–12 wk. If depression appears to be a part of the clinical picture, then a psychiatric consultation is indicated.

REFERENCES

1. The Veterans Administration Coronary Artery Bypass Surgery Cooperative Study Group. Eleven-year survival in the Veterans Administration randomized trial of coronary bypass surgery for stable angina. N Engl J Med 1984;311:1333–1339.
2. Murkin JM, Boyd WD, Ganapathy S, et al. Beating heart surgery: why expect less central system morbidity? Ann Thorac Surg 1999;68:1498–1501.
3. Brillman J. Central nervous system complications in coronary artery bypass graft surgery. Neurol Clin 1993;11:475–495.
4. Roach GW, Kanchuger M, Mangano CM, et al. Adverse cerebral outcomes after coronary bypass surgery. N Engl J Med 1996;335;1857–1863.
5. Gardner TJ, Horneffer PJ, Manolio TA, et al. Major stroke after coronary artery bypass graft surgery: changing magnitude of the problem. J Vasc Surg 1986;3:684–694.
6. Loop FD, Cosgrove CM, Lytle BW, et al. An 11-year evolution of coronary arterial surgery (1968–1978). Ann Surg 1979;190:444–455.
7. Reed GL, Singer DE, Picard EH, et al. Stroke following coronary artery bypass surgery. N Eng J Med 1988;319:1246–1250.
8. Bull DA, Neumayer LA, Hunter GC, et al. Risk factors for stroke in patients undergoing coronary artery bypass grafting. Cardiovasc Surg 1993;1:182–185.
9. Breuer AC, Furlan AJ, Hanson MR, et al. Central nervous system complications of coronary artery bypass graft surgery: prospective analysis of 421 patients. Stroke 1983;14(5):682.
10. Murkin JM, Martzke JS, Buchan AM, et al. A randomized study of the influence of perfusion technique and pH management strategy in 316 patients undergoing coronary artery bypass surgery. II. Neurologic and cognitive outcomes. J Thorac Cardiovasc Surg 1995;110:349–362.
11. Tuman KJ, McCarthy RJ, Najafi H, et al. Differential effects of advanced age on neurologic and cardiac risks of coronary operations. J Thorac Cardiovasc Surg 1992;104:1510–1517.
12. Stamou SC, Hill PC, Dangas G. Stroke after coronary artery bypass: incidence, predictors, and clinical outcome. Stroke 2001;32:1508–1513.
13. Shaw PJ, Bates D, Cartlidge NEF, et al. Neurologic and neuropsychological morbidity following major surgery-comparison of coronary artery bypass and peripheral vascular surgery. Stroke 1987;18:700–707.
14. Wijdicks EFM, Jack CR. Coronary artery bypass grafting-associated ischemic stroke. J Neuroimag 1996;6:20–22.
15. Trehan N, Mishra M, Kasliwal RR, et al. Reduced neurological injury during CABG in patients with mobile aortic atheromas: a five-year follow-up study. Ann Thorac Surg 2000;70:1558–1564.
16. Sotaniemi KA. Long-term neurologic outcome after cardiac operation. Ann Thorac Surg 1995;59:1336–1339.
17. Mackey WC, Khabbaz K, Bojar R, et al. Simultaneous carotid endarterectomy and coronary bypass: perioperative risk and long term survival. J Vasc Surg 1996;24:58–64.
18. Jahangiri M, Rees M, Edmondson SJ, et al. A surgical approach to coexistent coronary and carotid artery disease. Heart 1997:77;164–167.
19. Yoon B-Y, Bae H-J, Kang D-W, et al. Intracranial cerebral artery disease as a risk factor for central nervous system complications of coronary artery bypass graft surgery. Stroke 2001;32:94–99.
20. Lezak M. Neuropsychological Assessment. 3rd ed. New York: Oxford, 1995.
21. Lazar RM, Marshall RS, Pile-Spellman J, Young WL, Sloan RP, Mohr JP. Continuous time estimation as a behavioral index of human cerebral ischemia during temporary occlusion of the internal carotid artery. J Neurol Neurosurg Psychiatr 1996; 60:559–563.
22. Lazar RM, Connaire C, Marshall RS, Pile-Spelman J, Hacein-Bey L, Solomon RA, Sisti MB, Young WL, Mohr JP. Developmental learning disorders in adult patients with cerebral arteriovenous malformations. Arch Neurology 1999;56:103–106.

23. Mohr JP. Acute clinical trials: an expression of concern Cerebrovasc Dis 1999(suppl);3:45–50.
24. McKhann GM, Borowicz LM, Goldborough MA, et al. Depression and cognitive decline after coronary artery bypass grafting. Lancet 1997;349:1282–1284.
25. de Groot JC, de Leeuw FE, Oudkerk M, et al. Cerebral white matter lesions and cognitive function: the Rotterdam Scan Study. Ann Neurol 2000(Feb);47:145–151.
26. Selnes OA, Goldsborough MA, Borowicz LM, McKann GM. Neurobehavioural sequelae of cardiopulmonary bypass. Lancet 1999;353:1601–1606.
27. McKann GM, Goldsborough MA, Borowicz LM, et al. Cognitive outcome after coronary artery bypass: A one-year prospective study. Ann Thorac Surg 1997;63:510–515.
28. Mahanna EP, Blumenthal JA, White WD, et al. Defining neuropsychological dysfunction after coronary artery bypass grafting. Ann Thorac Surg 1996;61:1342–1347
29. Murkin JM, Newman SP, Stump DA, et al. Statement of consensus on assessment of neurobehavioral outcomes after cardiac surgery. Ann Thorac Surg 1995;59:1289–1295.
30. Murkin JM, Stump DA, Blumenthal JA, et al. Defining dysfunction: group means versus incidence analysis—a statement of consensus. Ann Thorac Surg 1997;64:904–905.
31. Selnes OA, Goldborough MA, Borowicz LM, et al. Determinants of cognitive change after coronary artery bypass surgery: a multifactorial problem. Ann Thor Surg 1999;67:1669–1676.
32. Newman MF, Kirchner JL, Jerry L, et al. Longitudinal assessment of neurocognitive function after coronary-artery bypass surgery. N Engl J Med 2001;344:395–402.
33. Stump DA, Rogers AT, Hammon JW, et al. Cerebral emboli and cognitive outcome after cardiac surgery. J Cardio Vasc Anesth 1996;10:113–119.
34. Moody DM, Brown WR, Challa VR, et al. Brain microemboli associated with cardiopulmonary bypass: a histologic and magnetic resonance imaging study. Ann Thorac Surg 1995;59;1304–1307.
35. Jacobs A, Neveling M, Horst M, et al. Alterations of neuropsychological function and cerebral glucose metabolism after cardiac surgery are not related only to intraoperative microembolic events. Stroke 1998;29:660–667.
36. Degirmenci B, Durak H, Hazan E, et al. The effect of coronary artery bypass surgery on brain perfusion. J Nucl Med 1998;39:587–591.
37. DeLaPaz RL, Mohr JP. Magnetic resonance imaging. In Barnett HJM, Mohr JP, Stein BM, Yatsu FM, eds. Stroke: Pathophysiology, Diagnosis, and Management. 3rd ed. New York: Churchill-Livingstone, 1998;227–256.
38. Sylivris S, Levi C, Matalanis G, et al. Pattern and significance of cerebral microemboli during coronary artery bypass grafting. Ann Thorac Surg 1998;66:1674–1678.
39. Warach S, Chen D, Li W, Ronthal M, Edelman RR. Fast magnetic resonance imaging of acute human stroke. Neurology 1992;42:1717–1723.
40. van Everdingen KJ, van der Grond J, Kappelle LJ, et al. Diffusion-weighted magnetic resonance imaging in acute stroke. Stroke 1998;29:1783–1790.
41. Wityk RJ, Goldsborough MA, Hillis A. Diffusion and perfusion-weighted magnetic resonance imaging in patients with neurological complications after cardiac surgery. Arch Neurol 2001;58:571–576.
42. Symes ES, Maruff P, Ajani A, et al. Issues associated with the identification of cognitive change following coronary artery bypass grafting. Austral N Z J Psychiatr 2000;34:770–784.
43. Lazar RM, Heitjan DH, Kurlansky P, et al. Randomized trial of on- vs off-pump CABG reveals baseline memory dysfunction. Circulation 2001;104:II-815.
44. Fleiss J. The Design and Analysis of Clinical Experiments. New York: Wiley, 1986.
45. Makatura TJ, Lam CS, Leahy BJ, Castillo MT, Kalpakjian CZ. Standardized memory tests and the appraisal of everyday memory. Brain Injury 1999;13:355–367.
46. Burgess PW. Alderman N. Evans J. Emslie H. Wilson BA. The ecological validity of tests of executive function. J Int Neuropsychol Soc 1998;4:547–558.
47. Johnsson P, Lundqvist C, Lindgren A, et al. Cerebral complications after cardiac surgery assessed by S100 and NSE levels in blood. J Cardiothorac Vasc Anesth 1995;9:694–699.
48. Kumar P, Dhital K. Hossein-Nia M, et al. S-100 protein release in a range of cardiothoracic surgical procedures. J Thorac Cardiovasc Surg 1997;113:953–954.
49. Kilminster S, Treasure T, McMillan T, et al. Neuropsychological change and S-100 protein release in 130 unselected patients undergoing cardiac surgery. Stroke 1999;30:1869–1874.
50. Hernandez F, Clough RA, Klemperer JD, et al. Off-pump coronary artery bypass grafting: initial experience at one community hospital. Ann Thorac Surg 2000;70:1070–1072.

51. Malheiros SMF, Brucki SMD, Gabbai AA, et al. Neurological outcome in coronary artery surgery with and without cardiopulmonary bypass. Acta Neurol Scand 1995;92:256–260.
52. Andrew MJ, Baker RA, Kneebone AC, et al. Neuropsychological dysfunction after minimally invasive direct coronary artery bypass grafting. Ann Thorac Surg 1998;66:1611–1617.
53. Murkin JM, Boyd WD, Ganapathy S, et al. Beating heart surgery: why expect less central nervous system morbidity? Ann Thorac Surg 1999;68:1498–1501.
54. Diegeler A, Hirsh R., Schneider F, et al. Neuromonitoring and neurocognitive outcome in off-pump versus conventional coronary bypass operation. Ann Thorac Surg 2000;69:1162–1166.
55. Folstein MF, Folstein SE, McHugh PR. "Mini-mental state." J Psychiat Res 1975;12:189–198.
56. Wechsler D. WMS-III Manual. San Antonio, TX: The Psychological Corporation, 1997.
57. Schmidt M. Rey auditory verbal learning test. Los Angeles: Western Psychological Services, 1996.
58. Delis DC, Kramer JH, Kaplan E, et al. California Verbal Learning Test—second edition. San Antonio, TX: The Psychological Corporation, 2000.
59. Meyers JE, Meyers KR. Rey Complex Figure Test and Recognition Trial. Odessa, FL, 1995.
60. Goodglass H, Kaplan E, Barresi B. The Assessment of Aphasia and Related Disorders. 3rd ed. Hagerstown, MD: Lippincott Williams & Wilkins, 2000.
61. Kaplan E, Goodglass H, Weintraub S. The Boston Naming Test. 2nd ed. Hagerstown, MD: Lippincott Williams & Wilkins, 2000.
62. Wechsler D. WAIS-III Manual. San Antonio, TX: The Psychological Corporation, 1997.
63. Reitan RM, Wolfson D. The Halstead-Reitan Neuropsychological Test Battery: theory and clinical interpretation. Tucson, AZ: Neuropsychology Press, 1985.
64. Sachs TL, Clark CR, Pols RG, et al. Comparability and stability of performance on six alternate forms of the Dodrill-Stroop color-word test. Clin Neuropsychol 1991;5:220–225.
65. Lafayette Instrument Company. Lafayette, IN.
66. Lafayette Instrument Company. Lafayett, IN.

17 Multivessel Off-Pump Revascularization in High-Risk Patients

Severe Left Ventricular Dysfunction

Daniel J. Goldstein, MD,
Robert B. Beauford, MD, *Patricia Garland*, MD,
and Craig R. Saunders, MD

Contents

Introduction
Methods
Patients
Operative Technique
Results
Quality of Life
Discussion
References

INTRODUCTION

Off-pump coronary artery bypass grafting (OPCAB) is increasingly being applied as an alternative to conventional cardiopulmonary bypass-supported myocardial revascularization. Indeed, the last harvest of the Society of Thoracic Surgeons database demonstrates that in the year 2001, nearly 19% of patients who had isolated coronary revascularization underwent a beating-heart procedure (Table 1). Despite the rising enthusiasm for the clinical use of OPCAB, there has been a reluctance to apply this approach to patients with severe left ventricular dysfunction, for fear of hemodynamic instability and increased morbidity and mortality.

From: *Contemporary Cardiology: Minimally Invasive Cardiac Surgery, Second Edition*
Edited by: D. J. Goldstein and M. C. Oz © Humana Press Inc., Totowa, NJ

Table 1
Proportion of Isolated Coronary Bypass Surgery Procedures Performed Off-Pump According to Society of Thoracic Surgeons Database, 1998–2001

	1998	*1999*	*2000*	*2001*
No. of isolated coronary bypass procedures	181,774	155,581	138,826	128,530
Percent off-pump	2.5	6.9	13.7	18.6

It is well known that patients with impaired left ventricular function undergoing revascularization on cardiopulmonary bypass have increased mortality and morbidity when compared to patients with normal left ventricular function *(1)*. It has been speculated that extracorporeal circulation may exacerbate myocardial damage in compromised left ventricles as a result of: (1) activation of inflammatory mediators *(2)*; (2) nonphysiological ventricular geometry of the empty heart impeding collateral flow to ischemic areas *(3)*; and (3) worsened preservation of interventricular septal movement *(4)*. In view of these factors and because patients with depressed left ventricular function often have several accompanying comorbidities, we hypothesized that beating-heart revascularization may impact favorably on the suboptimal early and intermediate outcomes associated with cardiopulmonary bypass-supported revascularization in this ill group of patients. To this effect, we review our institutional experience and that in the literature to shed light on the safety and feasibility of this approach in this high-risk cohort of patients.

METHODS

We interrogated our prospectively (daily) updated database (CAOS, Intelligent Business Solutions, Clemmons, NC) to identify all patients who underwent OPCAB at our institution between January 1, 1999, and July 31, 2001, and who had a preoperative left ventricular ejection fraction (LVEF) of 30% or less as measured by echocardiography, nuclear imaging, and/or ventriculography. The chosen dates ensured that all surgeons' learning curves had been overcome and that the technique was standardized among all surgeons.

The incidence of adverse events among this high-risk group were compared to the Society of Thoracic Surgeons (STS) benchmarks for *all CABG* patients, as those for patients with severe left ventricular dysfunction in the database were not available to us. National STS guidelines and definitions were used to define adverse events and outcomes. Patients and referring cardiologists were contacted for follow-up data.

While no formal quality-of-life instruments (MLHF, SF-36) were used, we contacted each patient to assess for surrogates of quality-of-life factors. In particular, we investigated the incidence of recurrent angina, hospital readmission, hospital readmission for cardiac causes, need for recatheterization, and need for repeat CABG. We also inquired of the patients whether they would undergo surgery again knowing what it entailed.

PATIENTS

During the study period, 1624 patients underwent coronary artery bypass grafting as an isolated procedure or accompanied by transmyocardial laser revascularization or carotid endarterectomy. Of these, 911 (56%) were performed as off-pump procedures.

Among these, 811 (89%) patients had an LVEF of greater than 30% and 100 (11%) had an LVEF less or equal to 30%. The latter constitutes the study group.

Patients' demographic profile is depicted in Table 2. The mean age was 67 yr and the typical patient was a Caucasian male. Hypertension, previous myocardial infarction, and a history of smoking were prevalent comorbidities. Approximately half of the patients were receiving β-blockers, angiotensin-converting-enzyme inhibitors, and diuretics, but the duration of treatment with these agents was not available. Mean LVEF was 26 ± 4.6%. The majority of patients presented with symptoms of congestive heart failure. For those patients without angina, efforts were made to determine viability on nuclear imaging studies or dobutamine stress echocardiography. Left main disease, defined as >50% stenosis, and triple-vessel disease, were rather prevalent in this population.

OPERATIVE TECHNIQUE

All patients underwent general endotracheal anesthesia with placement of continuous output Swan–Ganz catheter monitoring, transesophageal echocardiography (TEE), and arterial pressure monitoring. A thorough TEE evaluation was undertaken in each patient to assess wall-motion abnormalities, presence and degree of mitral regurgitation, severity of atherosclerotic disease of the aorta, and right and left ventricular function. Significant atherosclerotic disease of the aortic arch and/or descending aorta prompted evaluation of the ascending aorta with epicardial echo probe. Presence of more than 2+ mitral insufficiency was a contraindication to off-pump revascularization. Those patients were placed on cardiopulmonary bypass and underwent conventional revascularization and mitral valve repair.

After harvest of conduits, the pericardium was opened. Extent of disease, epicardial anatomy (i.e., intramuscular?), and size of target vessels as well as size of the heart were assessed. Presence of extensive calcification, deep intramyocardial vessel, small target (<1.5 mm) and/or significant cardiomegaly were relative contraindications to proceed with off pump grafting.

After the decision had been made to undertake off-pump grafting, four deep pericardial sutures with snare protectors were placed in a straight line between the left inferior pulmonary vein and the inferior vena cava. The snare protectors served to avoid erosion of the taut sutures through the epicardium. The right pleura was routinely opened, and pericardial sutures were not used on the right side of the heart.

In general, distal anastomoses were performed first and the aorta was partially occluded only once. On rare occasions, a proximal anastomosis was performed first if a severely disease aorta required use of a facilitating anastomotic device. In most instances, the left internal mammary artery-to-LAD anastomosis was performed first, unless a totally occluded right coronary artery was present, in which case the latter was revascularized first. Full systemic heparinization and complete protamine reversal were used in most instances. No antifibrinolytic therapy (i.e., aminocaproic acid, aprotinin) was used. Intracoronary shunts were rarely used. No partial bypass circuits or adjunctive retracting devices were used.

Intraoperative Doppler graft flow assessment (Medi-Stim Butterly Flowmeter, Medtronic, MN) was performed on a selective basis at the discretion of the surgeon. EKG tracing, transesophageal wall motion assessment, visual and manual inspection of the graft as well as Doppler flow interrogation were all used to determine need to revise an anastomosis.

Table 2
Demographic Profile of Patients (n = 100) with Severe Left Ventricular Dysfunction Undergoing OPCAB

Age	67 ± 10
% Female	21
Race (%)	
Caucasian	69
Black	21
Hispanic	7
Asian	3
CAD[a] risk factors (%)	
Hypertension	77
Diabetes	37
Family history	14
Smoking	
Current	27
Former	50
Never	22
Unknown	1
Previous MI[b]	49
Obesity	14
Medication use (%)	
β-blockers	57
Diuretics	55
ACE inhibitors	48
Intravenous nitrates	32
Digoxin	19
Inotropes	11
Renal insufficiency[c] (%)	16
LVEF[d] (%)	26 ± 4.6
NYHA[e] class	2.4 ± 0.6
Congestive heart failure (%)	65
Left main disease > 50%	37
Surgical priority (%)	
Elective	24
Urgent	67
Emergent	8
Salvage	1

[a]Coronary artery disease.
[b]Myocardial infarction.
[c]Defined as preoperative creatinine greater than 1.5 mg/dL.
[d]Left ventricular ejection fraction.
[e]New York Heart Association.

RESULTS

One hundred consecutive patients with LVEF ≤ 30% underwent OPCAB. One additional patient was converted to conventional CABG because of severe cardiomegaly. Intraoperative details are summarized in Table 3. Most patients underwent isolated OPCAB, but a few patients had concomitant transmyocardial laser revascularization or

Table 3
Intraoperative Variables

Prior CABG (%)	4
Hemodynamic instability (%)	10
Intraaortic balloon pump (%)	
Preoperative	16
Intraoperative	6
Operation (%)	
OPCAB[a]	89
Redo OPCAB	4
OPCAB + TMR[b]	5
OPCAB + CEA[c]	2
Number of grafts	
Mean	3.5 ± 1.3
Range	1–7
% Internal mammary artery use	83
Mean skin-to-skin OR time	3 h, 57 min

[a]Off-pump coronary artery bypass.
[b]Transmyocardial revascularization.
[c]Carotid endarterectomy.

Table 4
Incidence of Major Complications and Comparison to STS Database Benchmark Figures for all CABG Patients

Complication	*Study*	*STS National Database Benchmark for all CABG*
Reoperation for bleeding	4%	2.32%
Atrial fibrillation	20%	19.37%
Q-wave MI	0%	1.08%
Stroke	1%	1.65%
Transient ischemic attack	1%	0.74%
Prolonged ventilation[a]	26%	5.46%
Mediastinis	1%	0.70%
Renal failure[b]	3%	3.14%
Reoperation for graft occlusion	0%	0.15%
Readmission within 30 d	6%	5.22%

[a]Defined as greater than 24 h.
[b]Defined as 50% rise in baseline creatinine or new need for dialysis.

carotid endarterectomy. Intra-aortic balloon support was prevalent. Sixteen percent of patients had a balloon placed preoperatively, and 6% intraoperatively. Emphasis was placed on the use of arterial grafts (internal mammary and radial arteries) and on complete revascularization.

The incidence of adverse events is displayed in Table 4. These are compared to the STS database benchmarks for all CABG patients regardless of left ventricular function. Median postoperative length of stay was 7 d (range 4–88 days). Six patients were readmitted

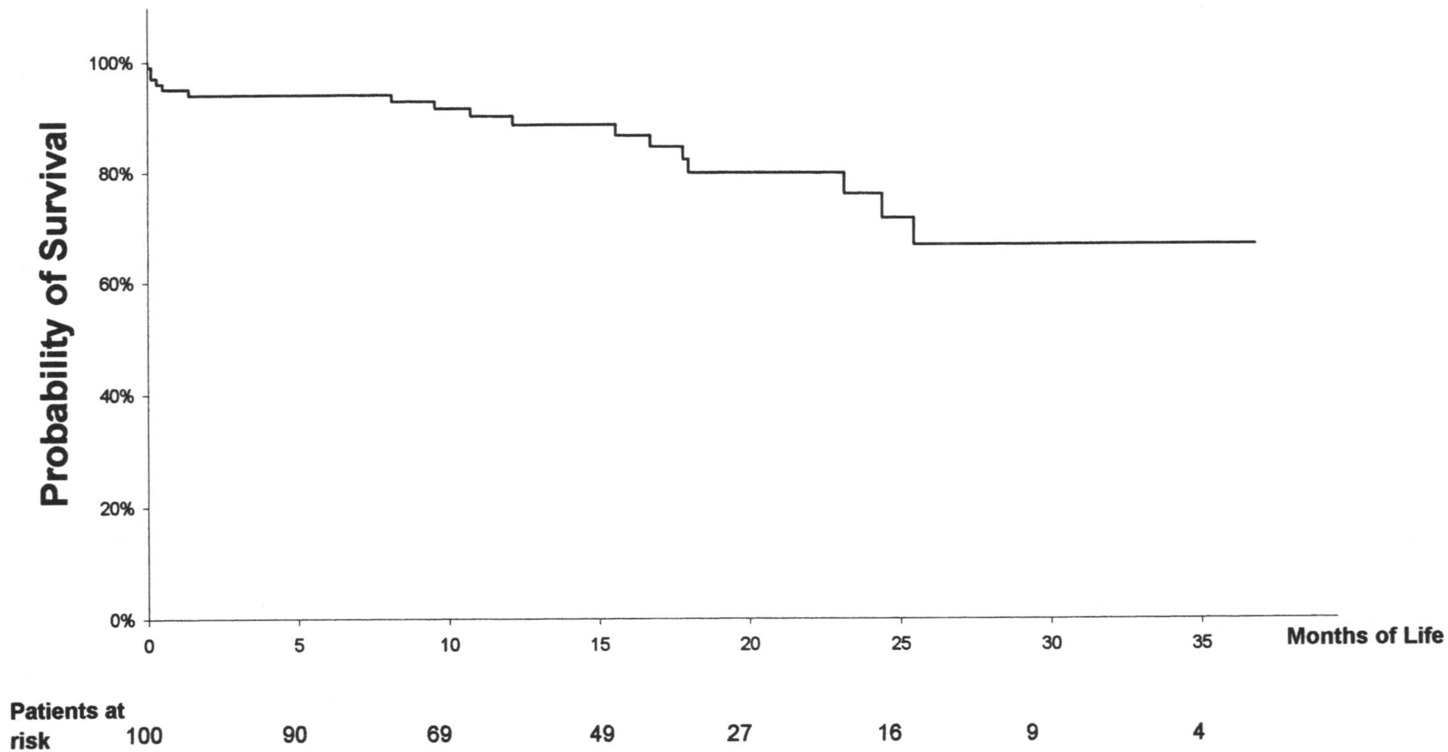

Fig. 1. Kaplan–Meier estimates of survival for patients with severe left ventricular dysfunction undergoing multivessel OPCAB.

Table 5
Quality-of-Life Events Following OPCAB

Quality-of-Life Event	
Rehospitalization *(%)*	
None	*63*
Cardiac-related	7
Non-cardiac-related	6
Unknown	10
Angina (%)	
Yes	16
No	75
Unknown	10
Recatheterization for recurrent angina (%)	
Yes	1
No	89
Unknown	10
Would have surgery again?	
Yes	77
No	8
Not Sure	5
Unknown	10

Figures are rounded to nearest number and may not add up to 100%.

within 30 d of surgery. Reasons included sternal dehiscence (2), wound infection (2), near-syncope (1), and recurrent angina (1). Observed mortality was 3%, while the predicted (STS) mortality was 5.3%, with an observed-to-expected (O/E) ratio of 0.56. Individual predicted STS mortalities ranged from 0.41% to 50.9%.

The three deaths were due to low-output syndromes, one on the day of surgery and two on postoperative d 4. There were 13 late deaths over a mean follow-up time of 13.5 mo. Causes of late death were cardiac-related in 11, a stroke in 1 patient, and unknown in 1 patient. Kaplan–Meier estimates of survival are depicted in **Fig. 1**. Six- and 12-mo survivals were 94% and 88%, respectively.

QUALITY OF LIFE

Follow-up was 90% complete. Mean follow-up was 13.5 ± 9 mo. Freedom from recurrent angina was 83%, freedom from hospital readmission was 69%, and freedom from readmission for cardiac causes was 92%. One patient underwent recatheterization. No patients required repeat surgical revascularization. When asked if they would have surgery again knowing what the process entailed, 77% answered yes, 8% answered no, and 5% were unsure. Ten patients could not be reached (see Table 5).

DISCUSSION

The introduction of enabling technologies in the mid-1990s paved the way for the dissemination of beating-heart revascularization. Prior to this, OPCAB procedures had been largely in the realm of a few pioneering groups in South America *(5,6)* and limited to patients with one- or two-vessel (noncircumflex) disease.

Most of the literature addressing beating-heart revascularization is focused on the application of this technology to low-risk patients. In fact, the six published randomized trials comparing coronary bypass grafting with and without cardiopulmonary bypass *(7–12)* did not include any patients with severe left ventricular dysfunction. This, we believe, reflects a skepticism regarding the safety of off-pump surgery in patients with compromised left ventricular function. Many investigators, including our group, feel that the greatest benefits derived from avoidance of extracorporeal circulation will become manifest not in low-risk individuals, but in patients with significant comorbidities.

Extensive literature exists evaluating the outcomes of conventional bypass grafting in patients with severe left ventricular dysfunction *(13–15)*, but a limited number of such patients has been submitted to off-pump revascularization. Sternik et al. *(16)* retrospectively compared 64 patients operated on without cardiopulmonary bypass to 53 who underwent conventional operation. Mean number of grafts was much lower in the off-pump group (1.9 grafts/patient) vs the conventional group (3.5 grafts/patient), with almost no patients receiving circumflex revascularization in the former group. The early and midterm survival were better for the off-pump cohort, but this probably reflects the lesser severity of disease present in the off-pump population. Another report from the same group *(17)*, again investigating the safety of beating-heart approaches in patients with compromised left ventricular function, described 75 patients with ejection fraction less than 35%. There was a 2.7% mortality rate and 1.3% stroke rate. Again, a mean of 1.9 grafts were performed, suggesting less extensive disease or incomplete revascularization.

Arom and colleagues *(18)* compared in retrospective fashion 45 OPCAB vs 132 conventional CABG recipients with ejection fraction less than 30%. The authors highlighted, as we do, that cardiac displacement is well tolerated in these patients. Fewer grafts were performed in the OPCAB group, which benefited from reduced postoperative blood loss. The incidence of adverse events in both groups was comparable for all variables studied. Meharwal and colleagues *(19)* published the largest study to date. The authors reported on 355 patients with ejection fractions of 30% or less, with an average age of 58 yr, who underwent OPCAB. Mean number of grafts was 2.8 (vs 3.3 in the on-pump cohort) and mortality was 3.9%. The incidence of atrial fibrillation, prolonged ventilation, and hospital stay was reduced in off-pump recipients. This group of patients from India appear to be younger and with less triple-vessel disease than that reported in most CABG series in the recent literature.

In an effort to enhance the limited experience available describing patients with compromised left ventricular function undergoing beating-heart coronary bypass, we report on the use of off-pump coronary bypass in 100 consecutive patients with severe (LVEF < 30%) ventricular dysfunction. Unlike the aforementioned studies, our population of patients had a very high incidence of triple-vessel disease. Moreover, the mean number of grafts performed in our patients (3.5 per patient) is much higher than that achieved in the literature and is highly indicative of complete revascularization. In contrast to these earlier studies, revascularization of the circumflex territory was routine. We were very pleased with the low incidence of adverse events, which parallel the benchmark incidence of these events for *all CABG* patients, regardless of ejection fraction, in the STS database. We presume that the incidence of adverse events for patients with LVEF ≤ 30 in the database would be much higher, but these data were not available to us. We did not fare so well with early extubation, probably a result of the high use of balloon pumps and inotropes in the early postoperative setting in combination with a high prevalence of active or recent smoking (77%) in our population of patients.

Only three perioperative deaths (3% mortality) were observed despite an expected 5.3% mortality. The incidence of early hospital readmission was remarkably low and was mostly related to wound complications. No instances of acute graft occlusion occurred and no patients have required a reoperation.

The low perioperative mortality and incidence of adverse events in this series can be attributed to several factors. First is the achievement of complete revascularization. Completeness of revascularization has been found to improve early survival in young *(20)* and elderly *(21)* patients, and we believe it to be a critical factor in patients with left ventricular dysfunction. Second, the liberal use of balloon pump support stabilizes hemodynamics and allows the cardiac mobilization necessary for exposure of lateral and inferior wall targets. It is of interest that Dietl et al. documented improved survival for the cohort patients with ejection fractions less than 25% who underwent conventional CABG with preoperative balloon insertion as compared to those who did not receive counterpulsation support *(22)*. Finally, and perhaps most important, is the presence of a dedicated cardiac anesthesiologist constantly vigilant of hemodynamics and progress of the operation, who can alert the surgeon to the need to return the verticalized heart to a more physiological position and to rapidly create a proximal anastomosis or to insert a shunt for hemodynamically compromising ischemia. Moreover, the experienced off-pump anesthesiologist is adept at using inotropes and pressors as necessary based on hemodynamics and continuous TEE evaluation of the degree of mitral regurgitation and can anticipate the next step in the operation and adjust vasoactive drips and bed positioning as necessary to ensure a smooth operation.

On follow-up, most of the patients were free from angina, rehospitalization, and recatheterization at a mean of 13.5 mo postoperatively. When asked if they would go through the procedure again, the majority of patients responded affirmatively. The 88% 1-yr survival and good quality of life achieved in this ill group of patients lends validity to the safety and efficacy of beating-heart revascularization for patients with severely compromised left ventricular function.

While the present study represents one of the largest series of consecutive patients with severe left ventricular dysfunction undergoing OPCAB with multivessel revascularization, several limitations of the study deserve mention. First, because of its retrospective design, no concurrent conventional CABG cohort exists for comparison. A concurrent retrospective cohort comparison was not available. A second and probably most significant limitation is the introduction of selection bias. The decision to proceed with OPCAB or conventional CABG was the sole decision of the operating surgeon, made at the time of operation, based usually on anatomy or clinical findings. Recently, however, we approach all patients for revascularization as potential off-pump candidates and tend to select patients for OPCAB preferentially when we think they would benefit most from elimination of CPB. These tend to be the sicker, more morbid patients. As with many other surgical undertakings, we doubt that a randomized trial evaluating the safety and efficacy of OPCAB in severe left ventricular dysfunction will ever be realized, and the best alternative is the accumulation of large series of consecutive patients with prospectively collected data. Second, no long-term follow-up is available to confirm the encouraging early results. The addition of formal instruments to measure quality of life would be of great interest to enhance our understanding of the benefits of off-pump revascularization in this ill group of patients.

In our hands, OPCAB is a safe and effective approach for revascularization of the patient with severe left ventricular dysfunction. Liberal use of intra-aortic balloon pump is recommended, and complete revascularization is achievable and desirable. To confirm the benefit of this approach, long-term follow-up is mandatory, but we believe that every coronary surgeon should have equal expertise in on- and off-pump revascularization so that the bypass operation can be optimally tailored to any individual patient, regardless of anatomy or comorbidities.

REFERENCES

1. O'Connor GT, Pume SK, Olmstead EM, et al. Multivariate prediction of in-hospital mortality associated with coronary artery bypass graft surgery. Circulation 1992;85:2110–2118.
2. Moshkovitz Y, Sternik L, Paz Y, et al. Primary coronary artery bypass grafting without cardiopulmonary bypass in impaired left ventricular function. Ann Thorac Surg 1997;63:S44–S47.
3. Kirklin JW, Barrat-Boyes BG, eds. Cardiac Surgery, 2nd ed. New York: Churchill-Livingstone, 1993:83–97.
4. Akins CW, Boucher CA, Pohost GM. Preservation of interventricular septal function in patients having coronary artery bypass with cardiopulmonary bypass. Am Heart J 1984;107:304–309.
5. Benetti FJ, Naselli G, Wood M, Gefner L. Direct myocardial revascularization without extracorporeal circulation. Chest 1991;100:312–316.
6. Gomes LF. Coronary artery bypass grafting without cardiopulmonary bypass. Ann Thorac Surg 1996;61:63–66.
7. van Dijk D, Jansen EW, Hijman R, et al. Cognitive outcome after off-pump and on-pump coronary artery bypass graft surgery. JAMA 2002;287:1405–1412.
8. Diegeler A, Hirsch R, Schneider F, et al. Neuromonitoring and neurocognitive outcome in off-pump versus conventional coronary bypass operation. Ann Thorac Surg 2000;69:1162–1166.
9. Ascione R, Lloyd CT, Underwood MJ, Lotto AA, Pitsis AA, Angelini GD. Inflammatory response after coronary revascularization with of without cardiopulmonary bypass. Ann Thorac Surg 2000;69:1198–1204.
10. Ascione R, Caputo M, Calori G, Lloyd CT, Underwood MJ, Angelini GD. Predictors of atrial fibrillation after conventional and beating heart coronary surgery. Circulation 2000;102;1530–1535.
11. Wandschneider W, Thalmann M, Trampitsch E, Ziervogel G, Kobinia G. Off pump coronary bypass operations significantly reduce S100 release: an indicatory for less cerebral damage? Ann Thorac Surg 2000;70:1577–1579.
12. van Dijk D, Nierich AP, Jansen EW, et al. Early outcome after off-pump versus on-pump coronary bypass surgery. Circulation 2001;104:1761–1766.
13. Mickleborough LL, Carson S, Tamariz M, Ivanov J. Results of revascularization in patients with severe left ventricular dysfunction. J Thorac Cardiovasc Surg 2000;119(3):550–557.
14. Trachiotis GD, Weintraub WS, Johnston TS, Jones EL, Guyton RA, Craver JM. Coronary artery bypass grafting in patients with advanced left ventricular dysfunction. Ann Thorac Surg 1998;66:1632–1639.
15. Elefteriades JA, Morales DM, Gradel C, Tollis G Jr., Levi E, Zaret BL. Results of coronary artery bypass grafting by a single surgeon in patients with left ventricular ejection fractions < or = 30%. Am J Cardiol 1997;79:1573–1578.
16. Sternik L, Moshkovitz Y, Hod H, Mohr R. Comparison of myocardial revascularization without cardiopulmonary bypass to standard open heart technique in patients with left ventricular dysfunction. Eur J Cardiothorac Surg 1997;11:123–128.
17. Moshkovitz Y, Sternik L, Paz Y, et al. Primary coronary artery bypass grafting without cardiopulmonary bypass in impaired left ventricular function. Ann Thorac Surg 1997;63:S44–S47.
18. Arom KV, Flavin TF, Emery RW, Kshettry VR, Petersen RJ, Janey PA. Is low ejection fraction safe for off-pump coronary bypass operation ? Ann Thorac Surg 2000;70:1021–1025.
19. Meharwal ZS, Trehan N. Off-pump coronary artery bypass grafting in patients with left ventricular dysfunction. Heart Surg Forum 2002;5(1):41–45.
20. Osswald BR, Tochtermann U, Schweiger P, Thomas G, Vahl CF, Hagl S. Does the completeness of revascularization contribute to an improved early survival in patients up to 70 years of age? Thorac Cardiovasc Surg 2001;49:373–377.

21. Osswald BR, Blackstone EH, Tochtermann U, et al. Does the completeness of revascularization affect early survival after coronary artery bypass grafting in elderly patients? Eur J Cardiothorac Surg 2001;20:120–125.
22. Dietl CA, Berkheimer MD, Woods EL, Gilbert CL, Pharr WF, Benoit CH. Efficacy and cost-effectiveness of preoperative IABP in patients with ejection fraction of 0.25 or less. Ann Thorac Surg 1996;62:401–408.

18 Multivessel Off-Pump Revascularization in High-Risk Populations

Octogenarians

Frederic Sardari, MD,
Robert B. Beauford, MD,
and Daniel J. Goldstein, MD

CONTENTS

INTRODUCTION
PATIENTS AND METHODS
RESULTS
SUMMARY
REFERENCES

INTRODUCTION

The elderly population in the United States is growing exponentially. It is estimated that by the year 2050 there will be 38 million octogenarians (up from 9 million in 2002) *(1)*. Increasingly, government initiatives are being created in an attempt to qualify their health status, ascertain their functional limitations, and identify their morbidity and mortality. It is well known that 25% of octogenarians have severe functional limitations secondary to cardiovascular disease *(2)*. Furthermore, cardiovascular disease has been, and continues to be, the number one cause of death in people over 65 yr of age *(3)*. Many of these patients have disease refractory to medical therapy, which has led to a marked increase in the number of elderly patients being referred for coronary revascularization. Over the last decade, numerous investigators have reported on the feasibility and efficacy of cardiac surgery in this population. Most remarkably, the preponderance of studies underscore the high-risk profile of elderly patients with their higher prevalence of

From: *Contemporary Cardiology: Minimally Invasive Cardiac Surgery, Second Edition*
Edited by: D. J. Goldstein and M. C. Oz © Humana Press Inc., Totowa, NJ

comorbidities and left ventricular dysfunction as well as the greater severity of coronary artery disease *(4–10)*. Several reports indicate that coronary revascularization can be performed with an acceptable mortality in octogenarians *(4,6,7,11)* and efforts are now aimed at further decreasing morbidity and mortality after coronary bypass in this older population.

The growing popularity of off-pump coronary artery bypass (OPCAB) has been fueled by developments in enabling technologies and by early data suggesting improved coronary surgery outcomes by avoidance of extracorporeal circulation. Several comparative studies have documented reduced transfusion requirements, shortened length of stay, and reduced hospital costs for OPCAB recipients when compared to those undergoing conventional coronary artery bypass *(12–18)*.

Octogenarian patients represent a particularly attractive target for application of OPCAB. The prevalence of comorbidities and the propensity for neurological dysfunction place octogenarians at higher risk for cardiopulmonary bypass (CPB)-induced morbidity and mortality. Despite this, scarce data exist documenting the safety and efficacy of OPCAB in these elderly patients. To this effect we report our recent experience with a large series of octogenarian patients undergoing beating-heart revascularization.

PATIENTS AND METHODS

Our prospectively (daily) updated database (CAOS, Intelligent Business Solutions, Clemmons, NC) was queried to identify all patients who underwent bypass grafting at Newark Beth Israel Medical Center and Saint Barnabas Hospital. Between January 1, 1999, and July 31, 2001, a total of 1624 were identified. Of these, 911 (56%) had OPCAB procedures, including 113 octogenarians. The latter represents our study group.

Demographics, clinical profiles, and adverse outcomes were collected. Complications were compared to STS benchmarks for *all CABG* patients. Follow-up was obtained by telephone interviews with patients and referring cardiologists. Information was gathered regarding quality-of-life surrogates including anginal symptoms, subsequent hospitalizations and/or procedures, and date and cause of death where applicable. Additionally, the patients were also asked whether, in retrospect, they would undergo the procedure again.

Operative Technique

All patients underwent OPCAB under general endotracheal anesthesia. Continuous output Swan–Ganz catheter, transesophageal echocardiography (TEE) probe, and arterial pressure monitoring lines were placed. A thorough TEE exam was performed to assess wall-motion abnormalities, presence and degree of mitral regurgitation, severity of atherosclerotic disease of the aorta, and right and left ventricular function. Significant atherosclerotic disease (i.e., mobile atheromata, wall thickening, etc.) of the aortic arch and/or descending aorta prompted evaluation of the ascending aorta with epicardial echo probe. Presence of more than 2+ mitral insufficiency precluded an off-pump procedure, and conventional cardiopulmonary bypass was undertaken with mitral valve repair. Other relative contraindications to OPCAB included extensively calcified, deep intramyocardial, or small target (<1.5 mm) vessels, as well as significant cardiomegaly.

All operations were performed through a median sternotomy incision. Briefly, the conduits (left internal mammary artery, radial artery, or saphenous vein) were harvested and the pericardium was opened widely. Elevation and stabilization of the heart was accomplished using four deep pericardial sutures with snare protectors. The right pleura was opened widely. Pericardial sutures were not routinely used on the right side of the heart. In general, distal anastomoses were performed first and the aorta was partially occluded only once. The anastomoses were performed with the aid of the Octopus 2 (Medtronic, Inc., Minneapolis, MN) stabilizing system, and their order was flexible. Full systemic heparinization and complete protamine reversal were used in most instances. No antifibrinolytic therapy (i.e., aminocaproic acid, aprotinin) was used. Intracoronary shunts were rarely used. No partial bypass circuits or adjunctive apical retracting devices were used.

Intraoperative Doppler graft flow assessment (Medi-Stim Butterly Flowmeter, Medtronic, Minneapolis, MN) was performed at the discretion of the operating surgeon. Transesophageal wall motion, EKG tracing, and visual and manual inspection of the grafts were all considered in evaluation of the conduits. Failure to obtain pulsatility indices between 1 and 5 or flows greater than 15 cc/min usually led to immediate graft revision.

RESULTS

One hundred thirteen consecutive octogenarians underwent OPCAB. The demographic profile and clinical characteristics are depicted in Table 1. Mean age was 83 ± 2.5 yr. The majority (81%) of patients had a history of hypertension. Previous myocardial infarct, tobacco use, diabetes, and congestive heart failure were also prevalent comorbidities. The mean left ventricular ejection fraction (LVEF) was 51 ± 11%, and 11% had a history of previous neurological event.

The operative profile is summarized in Table 2. Three patients underwent concomitant transmyocardial laser revascularization or carotid endarterectomy; all other patients underwent isolated OPCAB. Intra-aortic balloon support was rarely used. Emphasis was placed on internal mammary artery use and on complete revascularization as illustrated by the mean number of grafts performed.

Adverse events are depicted in Table 3 and are compared to the STS database benchmarks for all CABG patients, *regardless* of age. The most prevalent complication was development of atrial fibrillation postoperatively, which occurred in 43% of the patients. Postoperative cerebrovascular accident occurred in four patients (3.6%).

The postoperative length of stay ranged from 4 to 33 d with a mean of 9 d. There were nine readmissions within 30 d. Of these, three were cardiac-related, two were pulmonary-related, and two were wound-related. Altered mental status and a toe amputation comprised the other two.

In this series, there was only one postoperative death. Our observed mortality was 0.9, which compares favorably to the STS predicted mortality of 6.0%, resulting in an observed-to-expected (O/E) ratio of 0.15. This death occurred on postoperative d 33 and was due to a cerebrovascular accident. There were three late deaths over a mean follow-up time of 13.2 mo. One death was cardiac-related, the other two were secondary to malignancy. Kaplan–Meier estimates of survival are depicted in **Fig. 1**. Six-, 12-, and 24-mo survivals were 99%, 96%, and 90%, respectively.

Quality of Life

Mean follow-up was 13.2 ± 7 mo and was complete in 90% of the study group (Table 4). Eighty-five of 98 patients (87%) available for follow-up were free from

Table 1
Demographic Profile and Clinical Characteristics of Octogenarians Undergoing OPCAB[a] (n = 113)

Variable	*N*	*(%)*
Age (yr)		
Mean	83 ± 2	
Gender		
Male	67	(59)
Female	46	(41)
Race		
Caucasian	97	(86)
African-American	8	(7)
Hispanic	3	(3)
Asian	5	(4)
Comorbidities		
Hypertension	92	(81)
Previous MI[b]	45	(40)
Smoker	43	(38)
Diabetes	39	(35)
CHF[c]	35	(31)
Obesity	17	(15)
Previous CVA[d]	12	(11)
Renal insufficiency[e]	16	(14)
Family history	6	(5)
Medication use		
β-Blockers	74	(65)
ACE inhibitors	42	(37)
Diuretics	37	(33)
Intravenous nitrates	31	(27)
Digoxin	16	(14)
Inotropes	5	(4)
Mean LVEF[f]	51 ± 11%	
Left main disease > 50%	53	(47)
Priority		
Elective	21	(19)
Urgent	85	(75)
Emergency	7	(6)

[a]Off-pump coronary artery bypass.
[b]Myocardial Infarct.
[c]Congestive heart failure.
[d]Cerebrovascular accident.
[e]Defined and creatinine >1.5.
[f]Left ventricular ejection fraction.

recurrent angina at the time of telephone survey. Sixty-six percent of contacted patients were free from hospital readmission for any reason, and 90% were free from readmission for cardiac causes. Recatheterization was required in seven patients, but none required surgical revascularization. When asked if, in retrospect, they would undergo the surgery again knowing what it entailed, most of the patients answered in the affirmative.

Table 2
Operative Profile for Study Population

Variable	*N*	*(%)*
Operation		
OPCAB[a]	110	(97)
OPCAB/TMR[b]	1	(1)
Redo OPCAB/TMR	1	(1)
OPCAB/CEA[c]	1	(1)
Intra-aortic balloon pump		
Pre-op/intra-op	5 / 2	(6)
Internal mammary artery use	94	(83)
Number of grafts		
Mean	3.3 ± 1	
Range	2 to 6	
Mean skin-to-skin OR time	3 h, 34 min	

[a]Off pump coronary artery bypass.
[b]Transmyocardial revascularization.
[c]Carotid endarterectomy.

Table 3
Incidence of Major Complications in the Study Population and Comparison to STS National Database Figures for All CABG Patients

Complication	*Study N*	*(%)*	*STS National Database Benchmark for All CABG[b] (%)*
Atrial fibrillation	49	43%	19.4%
Readmission within 30 d	9	8%	5.2%
New renal failure[a]	6	5%	3.1%
Reexploration for bleeding	5	4%	2.3%
Neurological complication (CVA)	4	4%	1.7%
Q-wave myocardial infarction	1	1%	1.1%
Mediastinitis	1	1%	0.7%
Reexploration for graft occlusion	0	0%	0.2%

[a]Defined as 50% rise in baseline creatinine or new need for dialysis.
[b]Regardless of age.

SUMMARY

The explosive growth of off-pump bypass grafting parallels the growth of elderly patients being referred for revascularization. Most of the literature, however, addresses the use of OPCAB in younger patients with lower risk profiles, highlighting the trend to exclude this population of patients when considering newer technologies. As the learning curve with OPCAB has been overcome and technical skill with the procedure has been enhanced, many investigators, including our group, feel that the greatest benefit derived from avoidance of cardiopulmonary bypass will be realized not in low-risk individuals but in those patients who fall into a higher-risk profile, including those with multiple comorbidities and the elderly.

Table 4
Quality of Life

Mean follow-up 13.2 ± 7 mo (n = 98)[a]	
Rehospitalization	
None	66%
Cardiac-related	10%
Non-cardiac-related	23%
Angina	
Yes	13%
No	87%
Recatheterization	
Yes	7%
No	93%
Would have surgery again[b]	
Yes	66%
No	26%
Undecided	9%

[a]15 patients lost to follow-up, including 4 deaths.
[b](*n* = 93) 5 patients were followed up exclusively through the cardiologist's office; this subjective information was therefore not available.

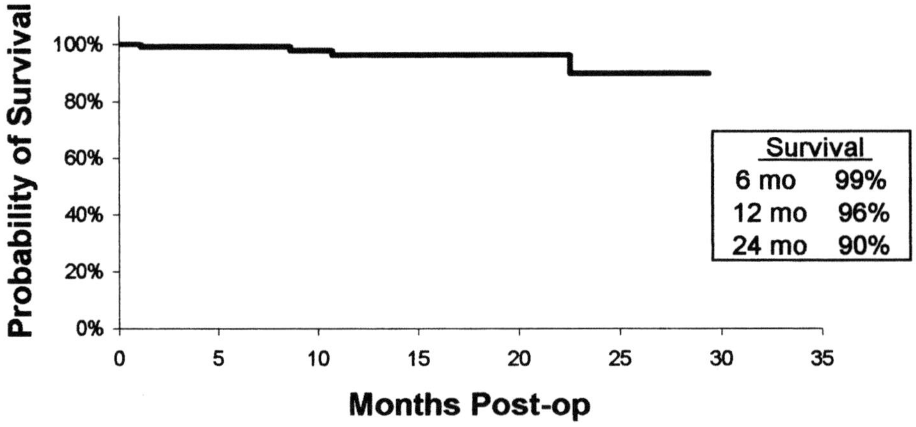

Figure 1

An extensive body of literature exists documenting the experience with conventional CABG in octogenarians. The largest study to date was conducted by Peterson et al. *(19)*. The authors surveyed the Medicare Provider Analysis and Review file from 1987 to 1990 and returned 24,461 octogenarians undergoing cardiac revascularization. This study documented a 67% increase in the national use of bypass surgery for octogenarians. Noted was a significant escalation in the lengths of stay and hospital costs as well as in-hospital and short-term (3-yr) mortality when compared with younger patients (ages

65–70). Their 30-d, 1-yr, and 3-yr mortality rates were 11.5%, 19.3%, and 28.8%, respectively. Interestingly, the long-term mortality for patients in this population was similar to that of the general octogenarian population. Predictors of mortality prior to this study were depressed left ventricular function, diabetes mellitus in combination with ventricular dysfunction, and presence of congestive heart failure or need for urgent surgery. Peterson and colleagues noted that these predictions were based on single-institution experiences with relatively small numbers of patients (maximum of 159). Using national Medicare data, this group had access to more than 24,000 patients, from which predictors of mortality could be extrapolated. They found that increasing age, female sex, preoperative myocardial infarction, and congestive heart failure identified patients with higher 30-d and 3-yr mortality. Chronic renal disease, peripheral vascular disease, and cerebral vascular disease also independently predicted patients with higher short- and long-term mortality. Diabetes mellitus and pulmonary disease, though not predictive of increased 30-d mortality, were predictive of octogenarians with worse long-term outcomes.

Morris and colleagues *(20)* investigated coronary artery bypass grafting in octogenarians at Hahnemann University between 1987 and 1994 ($n = 474$). Though their focus was the efficacy of conduits, this still represents one of the largest octogenarian study populations since the benchmark study by Peterson and colleagues. They reported a mortality rate of 7.8%. Comparatively, a cohort of younger patients (<80 yr old) had a mortality rate of 3.5%. This further documents the age-associated increase in mortality. In their patients, as for most octogenarians referred for coronary revascularization, they saw a trend of increased comorbidities and greater severity of disease. Their most prevalent morbidity was respiratory failure (9.8% patients). Postoperative cerebrovascular accident was seen in 6.9% of patients and myocardial infarct was noted in the postoperative period in 4.4%. Follow-up in this study averaged 46 mo and was complete in 92% of patients. The long-term survival was approx 68% at 5 yr.

Pliam et al. *(4)* scrutinized their recent improvements in the results of coronary bypass surgery in octogenarians. Their search for all octogenarians undergoing CABG at the San Francisco Heart Institute between 1985 and 1996 yielded 404 patients. They divided this study group into two groups of 202 to compare their old and more recent experience. They report statistically significant decreases in postoperative days to extubation, days in the intensive care unit, and lengths of stay in hospital. Also significantly decreased were rates of complications [34.2% vs 22.8% ($p = 0.03$)] and mortality [12.9% vs 5.4% ($p = 0.01$)].

Williams and colleagues *(6)* specifically investigated determinants of mortality in octogenarians undergoing coronary bypass. Their investigation at Miami's Mount Sinai Medical Center yielded 300 octogenarians undergoing isolated CABG. Their major morbidities included pulmonary complications (20%), renal dysfunction (13%), and cerebrovascular accident (CVA) (2.3%). Their principal determinants of mortality were preoperative renal dysfunction and postoperative pulmonary insufficiency, renal dysfunction, intraoperative aortic balloon pump use, and sternal wound infection. Surgical priority was also a major determinant of mortality, as their elective surgery mortality rate was 9.6% and that of their emergent operations was 33%. Their overall mortality rate was 11%. Their actuarial survival for patients discharged from the hospital was 74.6% ± 5.6% at 54 mo.

In short, there is no debate that the number of octogenarians being referred for revascularization has increased significantly in recent years. Additionally, these patients tend to have more comorbidities, more significant left ventricular dysfunction, and more

Table 5
Published Series of Mortality Rates and CVA Rates in Octogenarians Who Had OPCAB

Author	*n*	*Mean No. of Grafts*	*Mortality*	*CVA %*
Ricci et al. 2000 *(23)*	97	1.8	10.3%	0.0%
Stamou et al. 2000 *(24)*	71	1.6	6.0%	3.0%
Yokoyama et al. 2000 *(26)*	28	3.2	0.0%	7.1%
Present study, 2002	113	3.3	0.9%	3.5%

severe symptomatology. The literature also collectively suggests that CABG in octogenarians is a safe operation with acceptable mortality and long-term survival.

Scarce data exist, however, on the use of OPCAB in octogenarians (Table 5). Ricci et al. *(21)* retrospectively reviewed myocardial revascularization in octogenarians with and without bypass. Of 269 octogenarians who had coronary revascularization at SUNY Buffalo between 1995 and 1999, 197 were done conventionally and 97 without cardiopulmonary bypass. This study noted a significant incidence of postoperative complications in elderly patients compared to younger patients, but noted that elderly patients displayed a significantly higher rate of freedom from complications after OPCAB. Eighty-five percent of off-pump octogenarians were free from postoperative complications, compared with 75% of the CPB group. Most notable, however, was a 0% stroke rate in the OPCAB group (vs 9.3%). They did, however, note that there was a trend toward a higher mortality rate (10.3%).

Stamou and colleagues *(22)* reported on their experience with all patients undergoing OPCAB who were 60 years of age and older. Among their 71 octogenarians, they report a CVA rate of 3% as compared to 1% in patients 70–79 yr old and 0.3% in patients and 60–69. More significant findings were higher incidence of pneumonia, postoperative atrial fibrillation, and the need for inotropic support in the older age group. Similar to that published in the conventional CABG literature for this age group, the postoperative length of stay is prolonged compared to younger patients. They reported predictors of prolonged length of stay including preoperative congestive heart failure (CHF), previous CVA, ejection fraction less than 34%, and postoperative atrial fibrillation and inotropic support. Octogenarians in this study had a mortality rate of 6%, which was statistically significant compared to 3% and 0.3% seen in the 70–79-yr-olds and the 60–69-yr-olds, respectively.

It is notable that both Ricci and colleagues and Stamou et al. included MIDCAB patients in their patient population. Additionally, their mean number of grafts was less than 2, which in our opinion is a different study group from the octogenarians we studied, who had a mean number of grafts over 3.

Finally, Yokoyama et al. *(23)* investigated coronary bypass in high-risk subgroups. Though this series was not designed specifically for octogenarians, they did report 28 octogenarians who underwent OPCAB who had a mean of 3.2 grafts per patient. The authors reported reductions in renal complications, postoperative bleeding, and days in the ICU or on the ventilator. This study documented a 7.1% stroke rate and a 0% mortality rate. They concluded that eliminating cardiopulmonary bypass reduced the overall incidence of postoperative complications.

To our knowledge, our series of 113 patients represents the largest series of consecutive octogenarians undergoing multivessel OPCAB reported in the literature. In analyzing our results it is worth pointing out that surgical intervention was undertaken in an urgent or emergency manner in 92 patients (81%). This factor alone is considered an independent risk factor for morbidity in cardiac surgery patients *(24–26)*. Moreover, the mean number of grafts was 3.3 per patient, which is commensurate with data for conventional coronary artery bypass and significantly higher than that reported in the literature with OPCAB.

Our most prevalent complication was the development of postoperative atrial fibrillation. It is well known that the overall incidence of atrial fibrillation increases incrementally with age, and this factor is multiplied in patients with coronary artery disease *(27,28)*. With the exception of atrial fibrillation, the rate of complications was very low. These results (Table 3) parallel the STS benchmark data for all CABG patients, regardless of age. Although not available, we presume that the morbidity in *octogenarians* in the STS database would likely be magnified given their higher risk profile.

Stroke is reported to occur in 1–9% of patients undergoing myocardial revascularization, and increasing age is reported to be the leading risk factor *(29–32)*. In a 24-institution randomized trial, Roach et al. *(29)* report the incidence of stroke after revascularization was approximately 6% in all patients. In this study they note an incidence of neurological events in octogenarians to be approx 8%. In the small retrospective studies referenced in the present study, the general consensus is that there is a significant reduction in stroke rate after OPCAB compared with conventional revascularization with cardiopulmonary bypass *(9,21–23,31–34)*. Our results further support these findings. A previous history of neurological event, seen in 11% (12) of our patients preoperatively, and the incidence of atrial fibrillation postoperatively, seen in 43% of our patients (49), have both been reported as independent risk factors for CVA *(29)*, yet our postoperative stroke rate was 3.5% (4 patients).

Despite an expected high mortality, only one patient died in the perioperative period (0.9% mortality rate). During sternal closure, this patient was noted to have ischemic changes on EKG and was hemodynamically unstable, ultimately requiring cardiopulmonary bypass support and redo of one of the grafts. Though the patient recovered from the acute episode, she suffered a CVA later in the hospital course and ultimately died on postoperative d 33. There were only 3 late deaths (1 cardiac), which brings the 1-yr mortality rate to 3.6%.

There are limited data regarding follow up in octogenarians after OPCAB. Our early-outcome analysis correlates strongly with the literature for conventional CABG in that octogenarians can lead event-free lifestyles after this major operation, evidenced by 80% of our patients living chest-pain-free and only 9% necessitating readmission for reasons related to the surgery or for chest pain. The best indicator of our octogenarians' satisfaction with the surgery is the fact that the majority would have the surgery again knowing what was involved.

In spite of our satisfying results, several limitations exist that warrant mention. This study was a retrospective review, and while a randomized study comparing conventional CABG to OPCAB would be ideal, it is unlikely to occur. Additionally, serial neurological exams, head imaging, or formal neurocognitive evaluations were not conducted on our series of patients, and hence, minor events, e.g., clinically silent strokes, could have gone unrecognized.

The results of the present study strongly suggest that off-pump multivessel revascularization in octogenarians is associated with excellent early and intermediate outcomes and provides a highly satisfactory quality of life. While extended follow-up is mandatory to confirm these encouraging early findings, we preferentially approach all octogenarians as potential off-pump candidates.

REFERENCES

1. Health United States: 2001; Current Population Reports, "Americans with Disabilities, 1997" P70-73, February 2001, and related Internet data; Internet releases of the Census Bureau and the National Center on Health Statistics; and unpublished tables from the Bureau of Labor Statistics.
2. Van Nostrand JF, Furrier SE, Suzman R, eds. Health data on older Americans in the United States, 1992. National Center for Health Statistics. Vital Health Stat 1993;3(27).
3. Sahyoun NR, Lentzner H, Hoyert D, Robinson KN. Trends in causes of death among the elderly. Aging Trends; No.1. Hyattsville, MD: National Center for Health Statistics, 2001.
4. Pliam MB, Zapolanski A, Ryan CJ, Shaw RE, Mengarelli L. Recent improvement in results of coronary bypass surgery in octogenarians. J Invas Cardiol 1999;11:281–289.
5. Sollano JA, Rose EA, Williams DL, et al. Cost-effectiveness of coronary artery bypass surgery in octogenarians. Ann Surg 1998;228(3):297–306.
6. Williams DB, Carrillo RG, Traad EA, et al. Determinants of operative mortality in octogenarians undergoing coronary bypass. Ann Thorac Surg 1995;60(4):1038–1043.
7. Deiwick M, Tandler R, Mollhoff T, et al. Heart surgery in patients aged eighty years and above: determinants of morbidity and mortality. Thorac Cardiovasc Surgeon 1997;45(3):119–126.
8. Naunheim KS, Dean PA, Fiore AC, et al. Cardiac surgery in the octogenarian. Eur J Cardiothorac Surg 1990;4(3):130–135.
9. D'Ancona G, Karamanoukian H, Kawaguchi AT, Ricci M, Salerno TA, Bergsland J. Myocardial revascularization of the beating heart in high-risk patients. J Card Surg 2001;16(2):132–139.
10. Batchelor WB, Anstrom KJ, Muhlbaier LH, et al. Contemporary outcome trends in the elderly undergoing percutaneous coronary interventions: results in 7,472 octogenarians. National Cardiovascular Network Collaboration. J Am College Cardiol 2000;36(3):723–730.
11. Mullany CJ, Darling GE, Pluth JR, et al. Early and late results after isolated coronary artery bypass surgery in 159 patients aged 80 years and older. Circulation 1990;82(5 Suppl):IV229–236.
12. Hart JC. A review of 140 Octopus off-pump bypass patients over the age of seventy: procedure of choice? Heart Surg Forum 2001;4 Suppl 1:S24–29.
13. Prifti E, Bonacchi M, Giunti G, et al. Does on-pump/beating-heart coronary artery bypass grafting offer better outcome in end-stage coronary artery disease patients? J Card Surg 2000;15(6):403–410.
14. Cleveland JC Jr, Shroyer AL, Chen AY, Peterson E, Grover FL. Off-pump coronary artery bypass grafting decreases risk-adjusted mortality and morbidity. J Ann Thorac Surg 2001;72(4):1282–1288.
15. Weintraub WS, Craver JM, Cohen CL, Jones EL, Guyton RA. Influence of age on results of coronary artery surgery. Circulation 1991;84(Suppl 3):226–235.
16. Kilger E, Weis FC, Goetz AE, et al. Intensive care after minimally invasive and conventional coronary surgery: a prospective comparison. Intensive Care Med 2001;27(3):534–539.
17. Bittner HB, Savitt MA, McKeown PP, Lucke JC. Off-pump coronary artery bypass grafting. Excellent results in a group of selected high-risk patients. J Cardiovasc Surg 2001;42(4):451–456.
18. Demers P, Cartier R. Multivessel off-pump coronary artery bypass surgery in the elderly. Eur J Cardio-Thorac Surg 2001;20(5):908–912.
19. Peterson ED, Cowper PA, Jollis JG, et al. Outcomes of coronary artery bypass graft surgery in 24,461 patients aged 80 years or older. Circulation 1995;92(9 Suppl):II85–91.
20. Morris RJ, Strong MD, Grunewald KE, et al. Internal thoracic artery for coronary artery grafting in octogenarians. Ann Thorac Surg 1996;62(1):16–22.
21. Ricci M, Karamanoukian HL, Abraham R, et al. Stroke in octogenarians undergoing coronary artery surgery with and without cardiopulmonary bypass. Ann Thorac Surg 2000;69(5):1471–1475.
22. Stamou SC, Dangas G, Dullum MK, et al. Beating heart surgery in octogenarians: perioperative outcome and comparison with younger age groups. Ann Thorac Surg 2000;69(4):1140–1145.
23. Yokoyama T, Baumgartner FJ, Gheissari A, Capouya ER, Panagiotides GP, Declusin RJ. Off-pump versus on-pump coronary bypass in high-risk subgroups. Ann Thorac Surg 2000;70(5):1546–1550.

24. Gersh BJ, Kronmal RA, Frye RL, et al. Coronary arteriography and coronary artery bypass surgery: morbidity and mortality in patients ages 65 years or older. A report from the Coronary Artery Surgery Study. Circulation 1983;67(3):483–491.
25. Tasdemir O, Vural K, Karagoz H, Bayazit K. Coronary artery bypass grafting on the beating heart without the use of extracorporeal circulation: review of 2052 cases. J Thorac Cardiovasc Surg 1998;116:68–73.
26. Hirose H, Amano A, Takahashi A. Coronary artery bypass grafting for octogenarians: Experience in a private hospital and review of literature. Ann Thorac Cardiovasc Surg 2001;7:282–291.
27. Aranki SF, Shaw DP, Adams DH, et al. Predictors of atrial fibrillation after coronary artery surgery. Current trends and impact on hospital resources. Circulation. 1997;96(6):2084–2085.
28. Furberg CD, Psaty BM, Manolio TA, Gardin JM, Smith VE, Rautaharju PM. Prevalence of atrial fibrillation in elderly subjects (the Cardiovascular Health Study). Am J Cardiol 1994;74(3):236–241.
29. Roach GW, Kanchuger M, Mangano CM, et al. Adverse cerebral outcomes after coronary bypass surgery. Multicenter study of perioperative ischemia research group and the Ischemia Research and Education Foundation Investigators. N Engl J Med 1996;335(25):1857–1863.
30. Tuman KJ, McCarthy RJ, Najafi H, Ivankovich AD. Differential effects of advanced age on neurologic and cardiac risks of coronary artery operations. J Thorac Cardiovasc Surg 1992;104(6):1510–1517.
31. Gardner TJ, Horneffer PJ, Manolio TA, Hoff SJ, Pearson TA. Major stroke after coronary bypass surgery: changing magnitude of the problem. J Vasc Surg 1986;3684–3687.
32. Iglesias I, Murkin JM. Beating heart surgery or conventional CABG: are neurologic outcomes different? Semin Thorac Cardiovasc Surg 2001;13(2):158–169.
33. Hirose H, Amano A, Takahashi A. Off-pump coronary artery bypass grafting for elderly patients. Ann Thorac Surg 2001;72(6):2013–2019.
34. Koutlas TC, Elbeery JR, Williams JM, Moran JF, Francalancia NA, Chitwood WR Jr. Myocardial revascularization in the elderly using beating heart coronary artery bypass surgery. Ann Thorac Surg 2000;69(4):1042–1047.

III Minimally Invasive Valvular Surgery

19 Minimally Invasive Mitral Valve Surgery

Victor F. Chu, MD, *L. Wiley Nifong*, MD,
and W. Randolph Chitwood, Jr., MD

Contents

Introduction
Minimally Invasive Mitral Surgery: Evolution
The "Micro-Mitral Operation"
Clinical Experience
Discussion
References

INTRODUCTION

Interest in minimally invasive cardiac surgery in general, and mitral valve surgery in particular, has grown exponentially among cardiac surgeons and their patients. This enthusiasm can be attributed to improved enabling technologies, excellent clinical results, and enhanced communication. The authors believe that a truly "minimally invasive approach" is a philosophy and it consists of: (1) limited or no cardiopulmonary perfusion; (2) very small incisions; (3) minimal musculoskeletal retraction; (4) careful hemostasis; and (5) meticulous blood conservation. At present, mitral valve operations require cardiopulmonary bypass (CPB) support and thus, we have directed our focus toward "minimalism" by the use of small incisions, videoscopic vision, robotic assistance, modified perfusion techniques, simplified aortic occlusion, and optimal myocardial preservation during mitral valve surgery. This chapter provides a synopsis of our mid-term minimally invasive mitral valve surgery experience along with a description of new methodologies.

MINIMALLY INVASIVE MITRAL SURGERY: EVOLUTION

Developments in minimally invasive mitral surgery began in the mid-1990s with the pioneering work of Cohn *(1)*, Cosgrove *(2)*, Navia *(3)*, and others. Technological

From: *Contemporary Cardiology: Minimally Invasive Cardiac Surgery, Second Edition*
Edited by: D. J. Goldstein and M. C. Oz © Humana Press Inc., Totowa, NJ

Table 1
Carpentier-Loulmet Classificaion of Degrees of Surgical Invasiveness

Level I	
	Mini-incision (10–12 cm)
	Direct vision
Level II	
	Micro-incision (4–6 cm)
	Video-assisted
Level III	
	Micro or port incision (1–2 cm)
	Video-directed
Level IV	
	Port incision with robotic instruments
	Video-directed

advancements in instrumentation, assisted vision, and CPB support have followed closely and have expedited this evolutionary process. Within a few short years we have gone from simple modifications of conventional techniques to near totally endoscopic operations, using computer-based telemanipulation, and assisted vision. Although a myriad of approaches have arisen, these procedures can be best classified using the Carpentier/Loulmet nomenclature, which is based on incision size and visualization methods (Table 1). In this scheme, higher classification levels denote smaller incision sizes and increased reliance on visual assistance technology. Of course, the uncompromised objective is to preserve the same quality of valve repair or replacement as is achieved with traditional sternotomy, full-access operations.

Level I: Mini-Incision and Direct Vision

Level I operations differ from traditional "open" approaches in that mini-incisions (10–12 cm) are used instead of either a full median sternotomy or thoracotomy (20–30 cm). A variety of reduced incisions, including mini-sternotomies, para-sternotomies, and mini-thoracotomies, have been shown to provide adequate mitral valve exposure. Using "mini-incisions" and direct vision, simple modifications of standard techniques and instruments alone are required, thus facilitating a surgeon's transition from the traditional sternotomy. Numerous groups *(1,2,4,5)* independently have reported encouraging results with low mortalities (1–3%) and little morbidity using these methods. In 1994, surgeons at Stanford University first deployed a peripheral perfusion system with intra-aortic occlusion balloon for mitral valve surgery *(6)*. Thereafter, this Port-Access™ system was used successfully by a number of surgeons to perform Level I mitral repairs and replacements. Early reports suggested more surgical complications (retrograde aortic dissection) than expected with this device; however, operator experience and improved guidewires have reduced this risk for later models. Many centers, ours included, believe that intra-aortic balloon occlusion is associated with unnecessary increases in cost and complexity. Instead, our group has favored transthoracic aortic clamp occlusion as a safe, economical, and simple method for performing routine limited-access procedures *(7,8)*.

Level I operations, with or without the Port-Access method, have produced results comparable to that of the "open" or conventional sternotomy operations *(9–11)*. Importantly, the success of Level I procedures has served as a new "comfort zone" and helped launch more advanced techniques in minimization.

Level II: Micro-Incisions and Video-Assisted Vision

Level II operations rely on video-assisted vision to facilitate exposure through even smaller incisions (4–6 cm). Interestingly, this idea is not new and, in fact, Cutler *(12)* and Sakakibara *(13)* used cardioscopy clinically earlier in the twentieth century, but technical limitations at the time precluded widespread adoption. In 1996, Kaneko first used video assistance during a sternotomy-based mitral valve replacement *(14)*. Carpentier performed the first true video-assisted mitral valve repair in early 1996, through a mini-thoracotomy using cold fibrillatory arrest *(15)*. A few months later, our group in East Carolina University (ECU) performed a mitral valve replacement using a transthoracic aortic clamp and retrograde cardioplegia *(8)*. In these early videoscopic operations an assistant manipulated the telescopic camera.

Level III and IV: Micro- or Port-Incision and Video-Directed, Robotic Operation

The addition of a voice-activated robot (AESOP 3000™) for camera control now enables smoother, more precise video control, which further facilitates these operations. The clinical series from ECU *(7)* and other groups *(16,17)* have demonstrated safety and efficacy in using video assistance with micro-incisions for valve repairs. Moreover, complex repairs with good results have become routine. Repair techniques have included quadrangular resections, sliding valvuloplasties, chordal replacements, and transfers, as well as edge-to-edge (Alfieri) leaflet approximations. After operators gain experience, both anterior and posterior, as well as annular, pathology become repairable with this technique. Currently, the AESOP 3000 video-assisted mini-thoracotomy approach is our standard operation for primary and reoperative mitral valve operations.

Computer-assisted robotic systems potentially enable surgeons to overcome the limitations of operating through small ports with long instruments. Telemanipulation is the last step toward a totally endoscopic mitral valve operation. Mitral repairs using the da Vinci™ Surgical System (Intuitive Surgical, Inc., Sunnyvale, CA) were first performed in May 1997 by Carpentier in Paris and by Mohr in Leipzig *(15,17)*. The first complete robotic mitral repair with an annuloplasty ring in North America was performed at our center using the da Vinci system *(18)*. A somewhat similar *Zeus*™ system (Computer Motion, Inc., Santa Barbara, CA) has been used by the New York University group to perform partial mitral repairs *(19)*. This system is reviewed in detail in Chapter 30. We recently completed a 20-patient Phase I FDA mitral valve repair trial using the da Vinci system. Moreover, a 10-center, FDA-approved robotic mitral surgery trial is well underway using this system. Over 75 completely robotic mitral operations have been performed successfully in this trial to date. This study should elucidate both the benefits and difficulties associated with robotic mitral surgery done by multiple surgeons in their home institutions. With the aid of surgical robotic systems, it is now possible to perform complex mitral operations using near-port incisions. With continuous development of adjunctive innovations, it is possible to foresee totally endoscopic mitral operations in the near future.

THE "MICRO-MITRAL OPERATION"

Since 1996, ECU surgeons have used a standardized minimally invasive video-assisted approach, or micro-mitral operation (MMO), for mitral valve procedures. With the exception of the da Vinci FDA trial patients, all isolated mitral valve surgery is performed by this method. Key elements of MMO include: (1) mini-thoracotomy access;

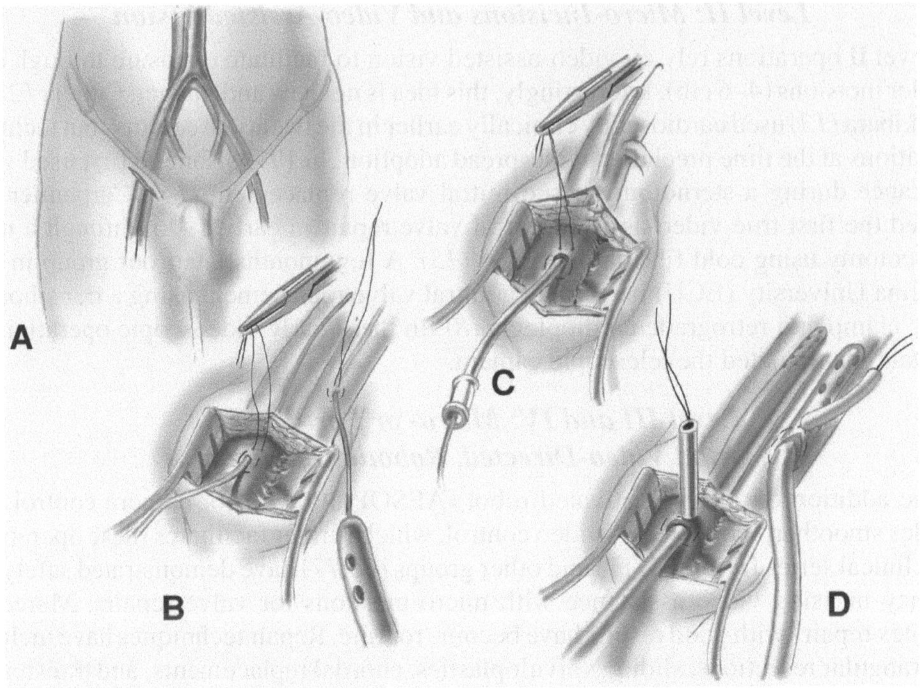

Fig. 1. Minimally invasive technique for cannulating right femoral artery and vein.

(2) direct transthoracic aortic clamping; (3) telescopic video assistance; and (4) peripheral arterial perfusion and assisted venous return. Specialized surgical instruments have been either developed or modified from other ones to perform these operations.

Preoperative Preparation

Independent left lung ventilation is obtained using either a double-lumen endotracheal tube or a right-sided bronchial blocker. Subsequently, the patient is positioned on the operating table with the right chest elevated by 40° and the shoulders tilted back. The right arm is suspended carefully over the head on a padded holder. Alternatively, the right arm can be positioned along the side, residing behind the posterior axillary line. External defibrillator pads are positioned posterior to the right scapula and at the left anterior axillary line near the fifth interspace, thereby subtending the greatest cardiac mass. A transesophageal echocardiographic (TEE) probe is inserted and a baseline study obtained. Patients are prepared in a similar manner for either the MMO or the robotic operations.

Technical Considerations

A 3-cm incision is made just below the right inguinal fold and the anterior femoral artery and vein are exposed with minimal dissection. Circumferential dissection and clamping of both vessels are avoided and oval purse-string sutures (4-0 monofilament) are placed longitudinally. Following heparinization, a 17–19 fr. Biomedicus™ (Medtronic, Minneapolis, MN) arterial cannula is advanced into the proximal iliac artery using the Seldinger technique (**Fig. 1**). When femoral cannulation is contraindicated or impossible, central aortic cannulation is performed. In this instance, a purse-string suture

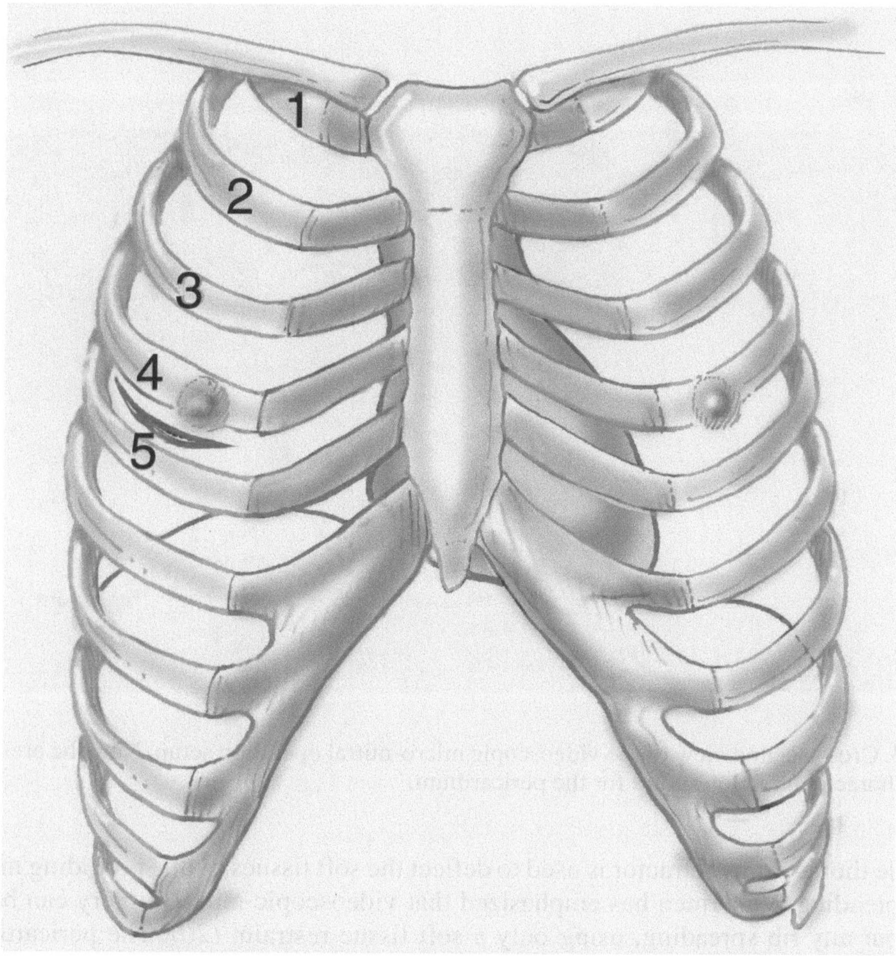

Fig. 2. Sub mammary right mini-thoracotomy in the fourth intercostal space.

is placed just proximal to the innominate artery and the arterial cannula introduced under videoscopic assistance using the Seldinger technique, either via the incision or through a thoracoport. Specialized transthoracic cannulas (Straightshot™ and EndoDirect™, Cardiovations, Inc., Sommerville, NJ) have been developed for this purpose. Both are deployed without a guidewire, and this maneuver is facilitated by a retractable intraluminal blade tip. Alternatively, the right axillary artery can be exposed, and a short segment of 8-mm synthetic graft attached end-to-side. A conventional straight arterial cannula is then inserted into the graft.

The anesthesia team inserts a 17 fr percutaneous cannula into the right internal jugular vein to augment superior vena caval drainage. For the majority of cases, a 19–23 fr Biomedicus femoral venous cannula is passed over a guide wire to the right atrium under TEE visualization. Echo guidance is essential to confirm correct luminal passage and destination of the venous cannula. A Biomedicus centrifugal pump is used for kinetic bicaval drainage. When femoral vein insertion is contraindicated or catheter passage is difficult, the right atrium can be cannulated directly.

A right 5-cm anterior axillary line submammary skin incision is made and the pectoralis muscles are mobilized for fourth intercostal space thoracic entry (**Fig. 2**). A low-

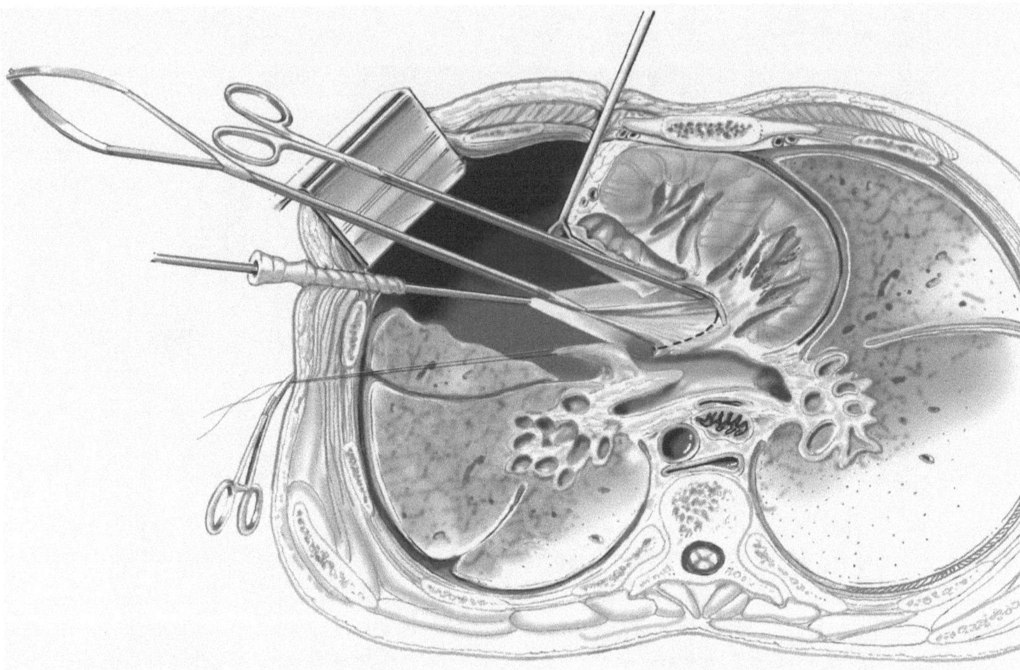

Fig. 3. Cross-section view of the videoscopic micro-mitral operation setup. Note the presence of transthoracic retraction suture for the pericardium.

profile thoracotomy retractor is used to deflect the soft tissues, while providing minimal rib spreading. Vanermen has emphasized that videoscopic mitral surgery can be done without any rib spreading, using only a soft tissue restraint *(20)*. The pericardium is opened 2-cm ventral to the phrenic nerve under direct vision and carried cephalad to the aortic reflection. The anterior edge of the pericardium is tacked to incision edges using silk sutures, while the posterior edge is distracted posterolaterally using transthoracic sutures (**Fig. 3**). This maneuver rotates the heart counterclockwise, effectively displacing the left atrium laterally and ventrad. This arrangement provides direct-vision exposure and access to the aortic origin, atriocaval junction, and right superior pulmonary vein.

For camera placement, a 5-mm thoracoport (Genzyme-DSP, Boston, MA) is inserted through the fourth intercostal space just dorsal to the incision. The port should be positioned with the tip ventral to the pericardial edge and parallel to the superior pulmonary vein. A 5-mm 0° telescopic camera is then passed through the port and attached to the Aesop 3000 robotic arm (**Figs. 4** and **5**). For da Vinci cases the camera is inserted through the incision and the arm ports are placed in the second and fourth interspaces.

With videoscopic assistance, a purse-string suture is placed along the anterior ascending aorta, just distal to the right coronary origin. This is easier to accomplish with the patient on full CPB and the right atrium decompressed. A suction-vent cardioplegia catheter is inserted either through the thoracotomy or via a separate port incision. The transthoracic clamp is inserted directly through the third intercostal space along the mid-axillary line. Under videoscopic guidance, and with care not to injure either the right pulmonary artery or the left atrial appendage, the clamp is positioned with the posterior fixed-tine, directed through the transverse sinus (**Fig. 6**). Proper positioning of the clamp

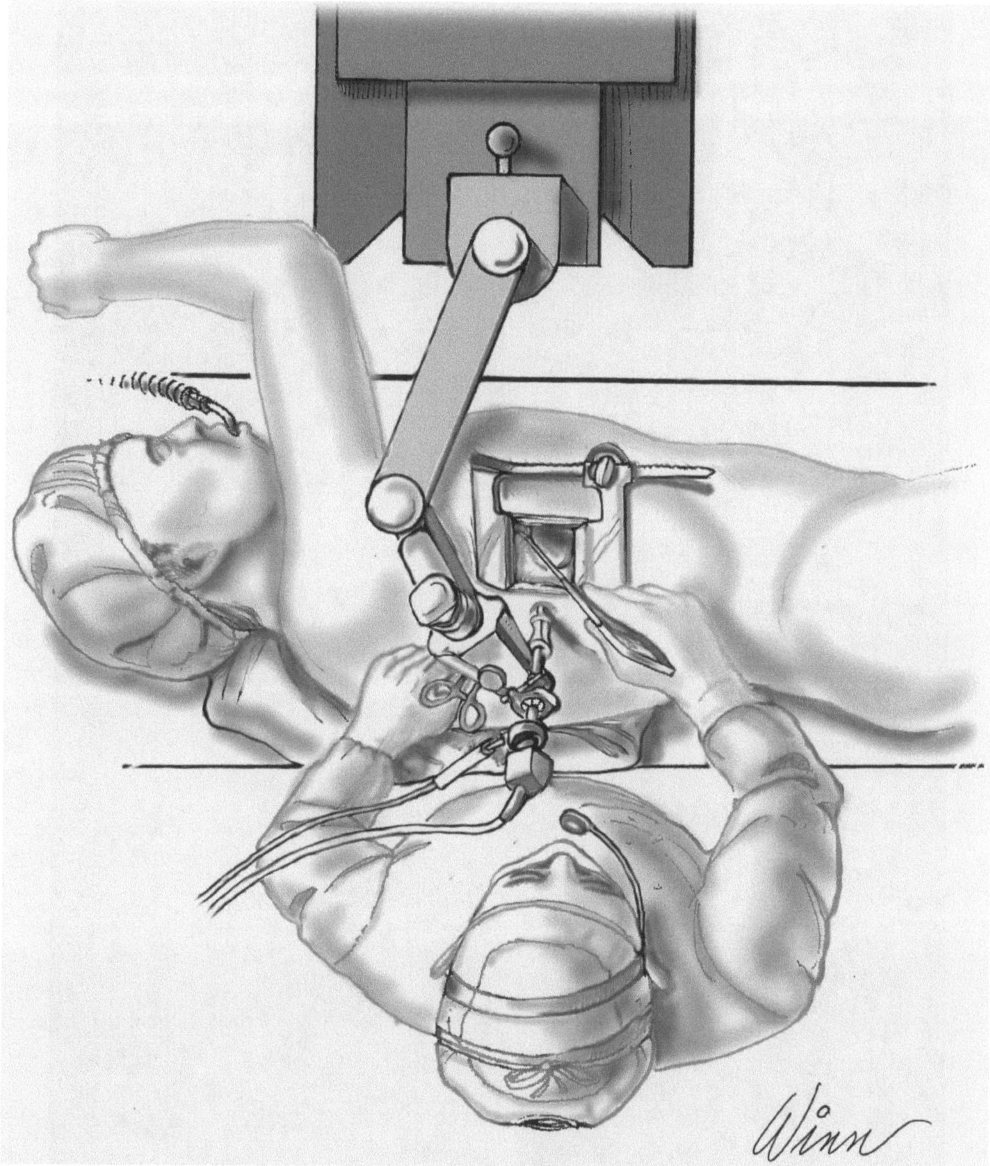

Fig. 4. Patient setup for Aesop 3000-assisted videoscopic micro-mitral operation.

should be confirmed with the video camera. Compared to the traditional approach, transthoracic aortic clamping minimizes aortic and cardiac distortion and maintains aortic valve competency. Consequently, intermittent antegrade cardioplegia can be used and provides superb myocardial protection. If desired, a retrograde cardioplegia catheter can be positioned into the coronary sinus under TEE guidance, either directly through the atrial wall or percutaneously via the jugular vein.

Intrathoracic CO_2 insufflation is begun before the atriotomy is performed, and is maintained until the atriotomy is closed. Sondergaard's interatrial groove is dissected over only 1–2 cm, and the small left atriotomy should be made just medial to the right superior pulmonary vein entrance. A fourth interspace transthoracic retractor (Heartport™

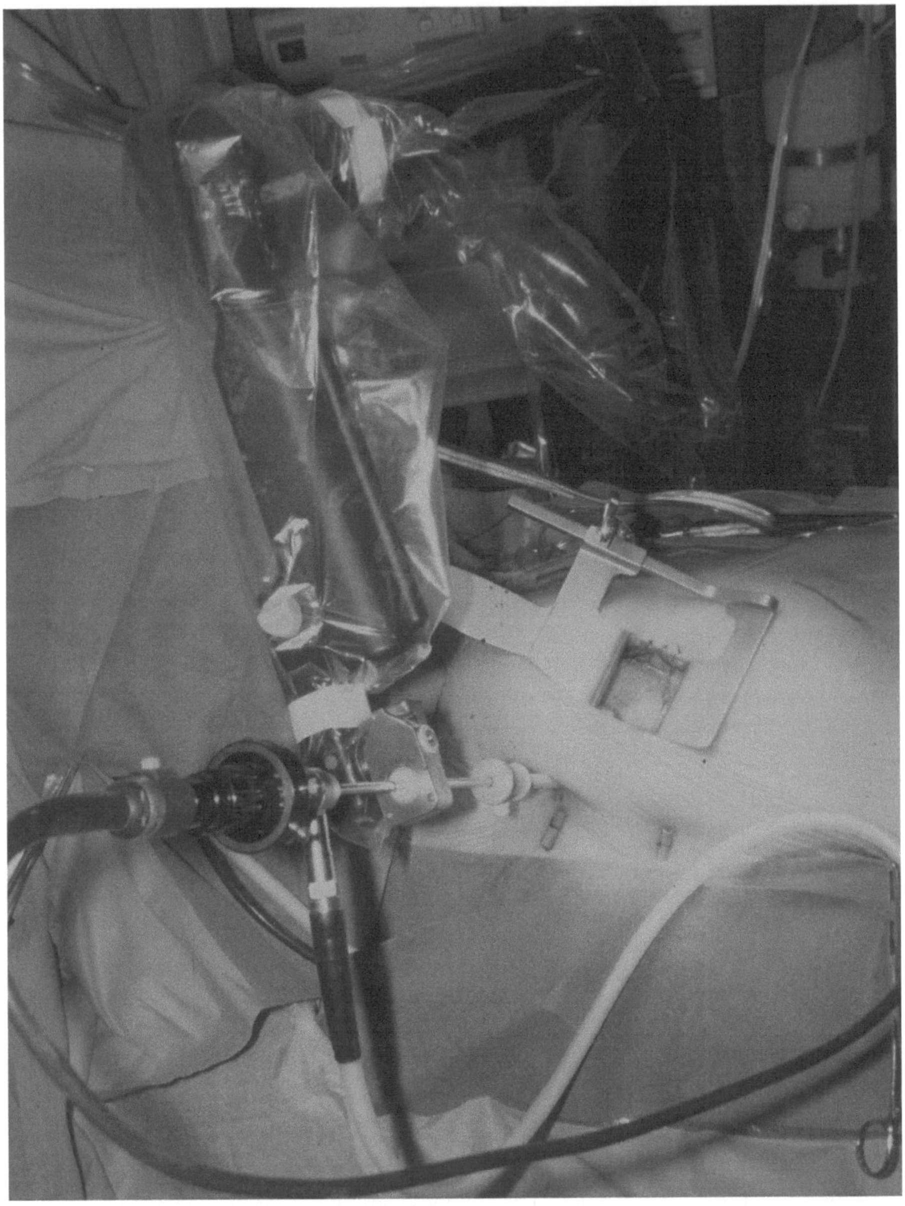

Fig. 5. Aesop 3000-controlled videoscopic assistance.

Inc.) is used to provide valve exposure by "toeing in," which elevates the interatrial septum toward the sternum, encouraging the anterior mitral leaflet to hang freely. In the presence of large left atria, the lateral walls tend to collapse. Hence, early placement of commissural sutures reestablishes anatomical orientation and exposure of the valve.

For mitral valve repairs, we prefer using both Carpentier–Edwards Physio™ annuloplasty rings and Cosgrove–Edwards™ bands. As the latter prosthesis extends only posteriorly between the fibrous trigones, fewer sutures are required. Often all annular sutures are placed before beginning leaflet or chordal repairs as visualization becomes progressively improved. Sutures are placed in a counterclockwise fashion, beginning at the right (posterior) fibrous trigone. The sutures are arranged serially and maintained in

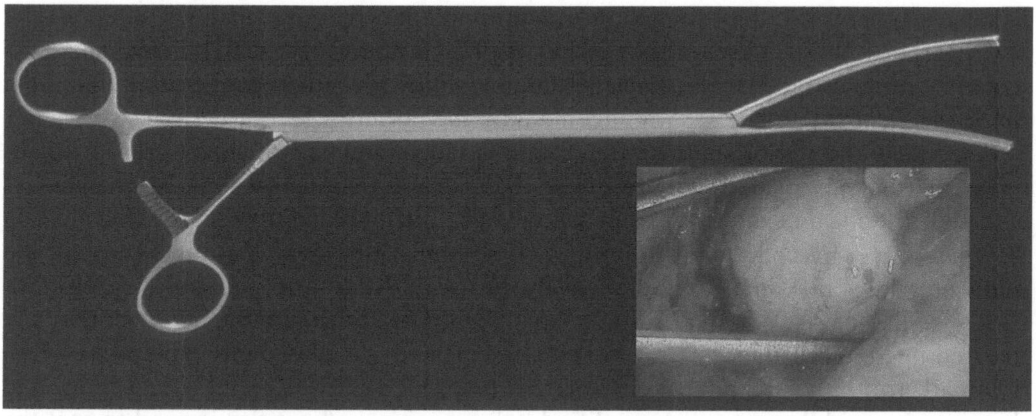

Fig. 6. Transthoracic (Chitwood) aortic clamp. (*Inset*) Videoscopic confirmation of clamp placement through transverse sinus.

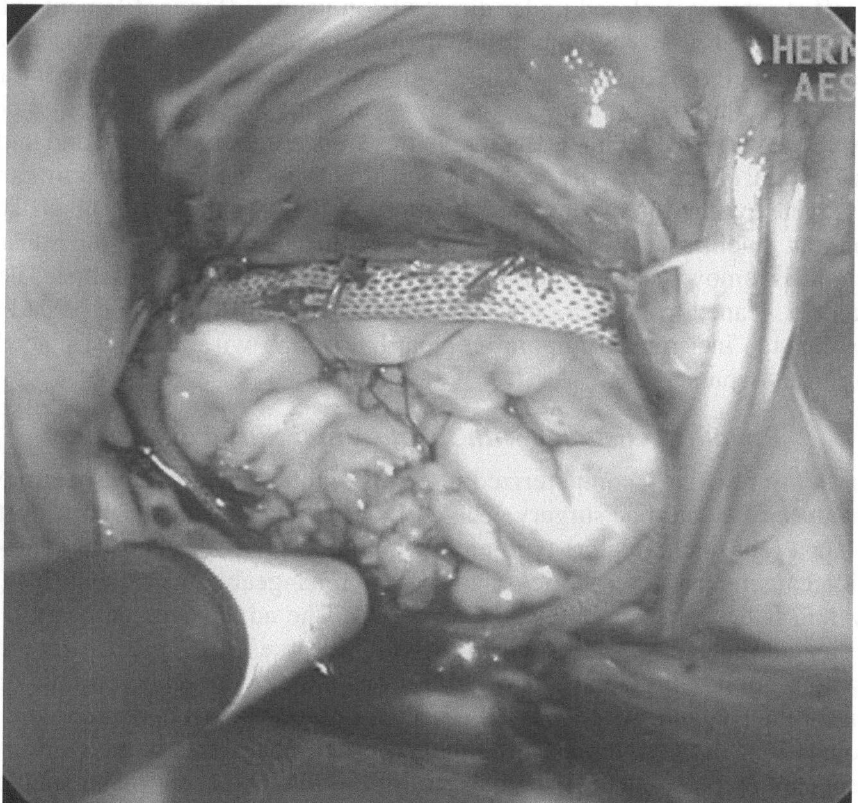

Fig. 7. Endoscopic view of completed quadrangular resection with a posterior sliding plasty ring annuloplasty.

external suture guides. **Figure 7** depicts a completed P_1 and P_3 sliding plasty after a posterior leaflet quadrangular resection with chordal transfers to A2. For mitral valve replacements, subannular pledgeted 2-0 sutures are placed serially, while the anterior leaflet is progressively "snipped" in a counterclockwise fashion. The posterior leaflet and subvalvar apparatus are always left intact to optimize ventricular function. Along some annular segments we may transition to supra-annular everting mattress sutures. The combination of these suture techniques has resulted in no early perivalvular leakage. This method facilitates videoscopic anterior annular suture placement while minimizing the risk of mechanical prostheses impingement by the posterior leaflet.

Placement of anterior sutures often requires video assistance, whereas posterior sutures can usually be placed either by direct vision or endoscopically. Suturing maneuvers at the left trigone and anterior commissure can be difficult and may require the aid of a 30° telescope. Optimal needle stability is essential while placing sutures through the mitral annulus. This can be best achieved by the use of a short grip, shafted "Heartport™-type" needle holder. When all sutures have been passed through the annulus, they are inserted into the prosthesis extrathoracically before it is lowered into position through the small atriotomy. The left trigone suture is tied first, followed by the right trigone and the posterior middle sutures. A modified valve positioner/knot tier is used to seat the valve and secure the knots. It is critical that the first two knots slip in order to achieve ideal prosthesis to annular tissue apposition. Using a guillotine-type suture cutter, the remaining sutures are cut to a uniform length.

The left atriotomy is closed under direct vision using 3-0 monofilament sutures. A transvalvular vent is used routinely following valve replacements. Prior to aortic clamp release, venous return is decreased, while both lungs are ventilated, and the intracardiac air is evacuated through both the atriotomy suture line and aortic vent. All de-airing maneuvers are performed with the patient in the Trendelenburg position and under TEE guidance. Partial release of aortic occlusion and direct ventricular massage are carried out until complete evacuation of air is documented. With continuous CO_2 insufflation, we have found it much easier to achieve complete cardiac deairing. After the transthoracic aortic clamp is removed, the posterior aorta is examined with the videoscope. Thereafter, the patient is weaned from CPB, and two small thoracostomy tubes are placed through the existing stab incisions. Temporary epicardial pacing wires are best placed before weaning from bypass.

Robotic Assistance with the da Vinci Surgical System

Over the last few years, computerized surgical "robotic" systems have been developed and introduced into cardiac surgery. The current da Vinci surgical robotic system is a master–slave (console–effector)-type telemanipulation device that consists of a 3-D high-resolution camera and two robotic arms with interchangeable instrument tips (**Fig. 8**). This system is described in detail in Chapter 31. The advantages of surgical robotic systems include enhanced 3-D visualization with "tele-presence," precise micromanipulation with motion scaling and tremor "filtration," along with an ergonomic operating position for the surgeon. As of May, 2003, a total of 81 patients had undergone robotic mitral operations in ECU, representing the largest clinical series in the world.

Patients are prepared as described above for the MMO, except that a smaller, 4-cm chest incision is used. After the valve is inspected, ergonomic trajectories from the chest wall to valve annulus are determined prior to insertion of left and right robotic arms. Most frequently, the right trocar is placed in the fourth or fifth intercostal space, posterior-lateral to the incision and parallel to the right superior pulmonary vein. The left trocar generally is placed 6 cm cephalad and medial to the right trocar, ensuring sufficient clearance between arms to avoid both external and internal arm conflicts. Optimal geometric positioning avoids obtuse converging angles between arms, which decreases left atrial wall tearing with instrument manipulation. The 3-D endoscope is placed through

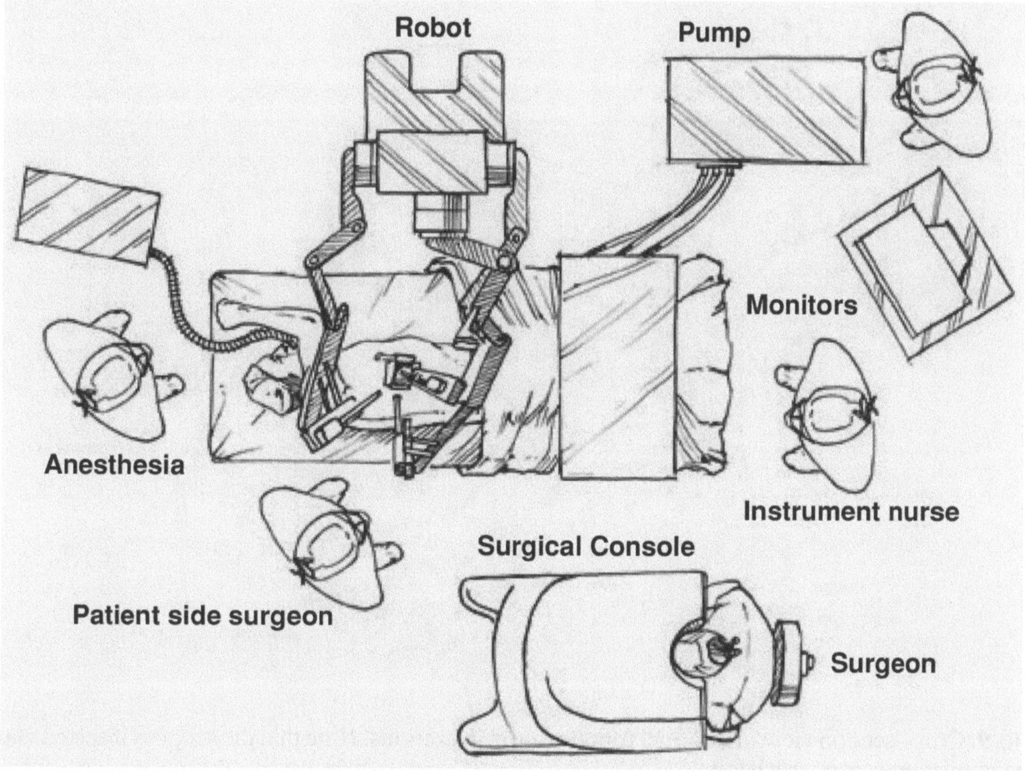

Fig. 8. Operating room floor plan for da Vinci robotic mitral operations.

the medial portion of the mini-thoracotomy, and the patient-side assistant uses the remainder of the incision as a working port (**Fig. 9**). A magnetic suture retriever and large-bore suture vacuum enable the assistant in delivering supplies and removing refuse rapidly. Surgeons operate from the console, placed 10 ft from the patient, which houses the 3-D video screen and the master-control hand pieces (**Fig. 10** and inset). In addition, foot controls enable ergonomic hand repositioning and dynamic camera manipulations. A variety of mitral repairs have been performed, including complex anterior leaflet reconstructive procedures. In all da Vinci cases, a Cosgrove annuloplasty band was used. Upon completion of the repair, robotic devices are removed from the operating table and the atrium is closed under direct vision. Standard deairing and weaning procedures are identical to that of the micro-mitral operations. **Figure 11** depicts a da Vinci mitral valve repair employing a posterior leaflet quadrangular resection.

CLINICAL EXPERIENCE

Our most recently published videoscopic mitral surgery experience includes 127 micro-mitral operations, of which 72 employed the Aesop 3000 voice-activated robotic camera and 38 used the complete robotic (da Vinci) system *(7,21)*. Table 2 shows the demographic data for both groups. For comparison, retrospective analyses of 100 consecutive patients who underwent traditional mitral operations at our institution are included. Preoperative gender, New York Heart Association functional class (NYHA), left ventricular ejection function (EF), and cardiac risk factors were similar among all groups (p = ns). Operative techniques and perioperative data for all cohorts are shown in

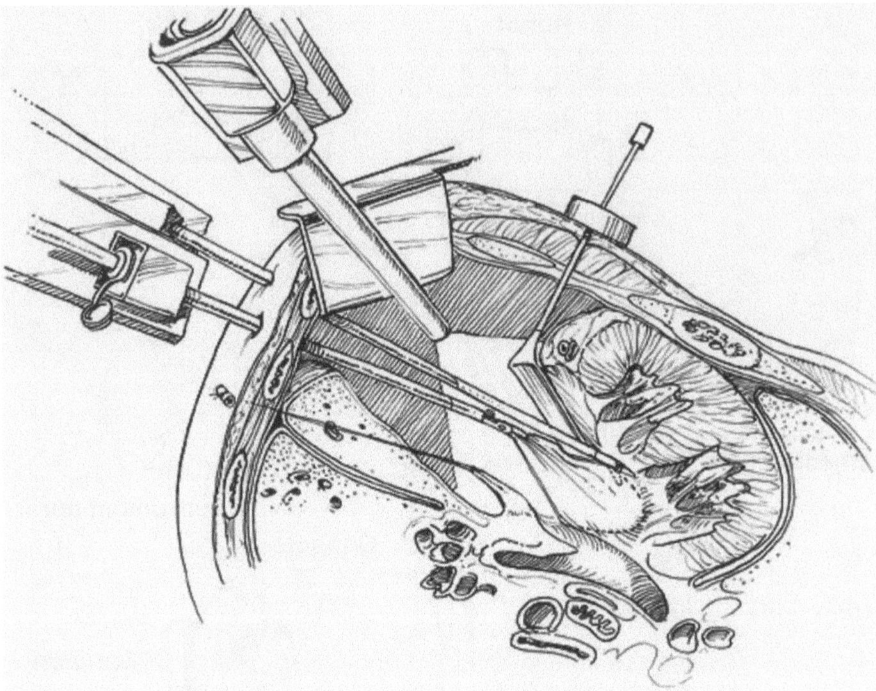

Fig. 9. Cross-section view of da Vinci robotic mitral operations. Note that the scope is inserted via the mini-thoracotomy incision.

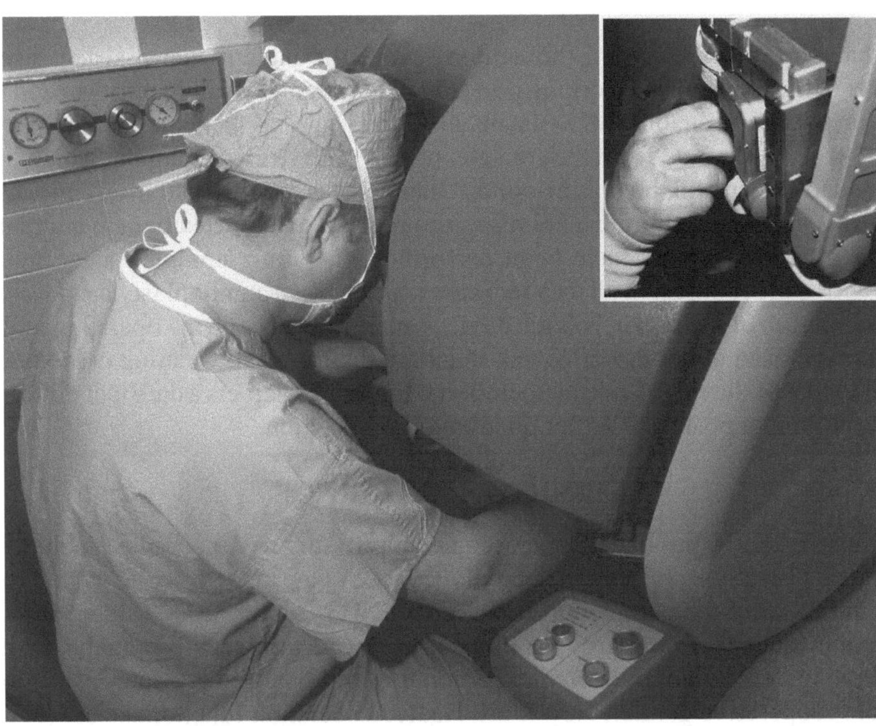

Fig. 10. Surgeon operating at the console during da Vinci robotic mitral operation. (*Inset*) Close-up view of the hand control unit.

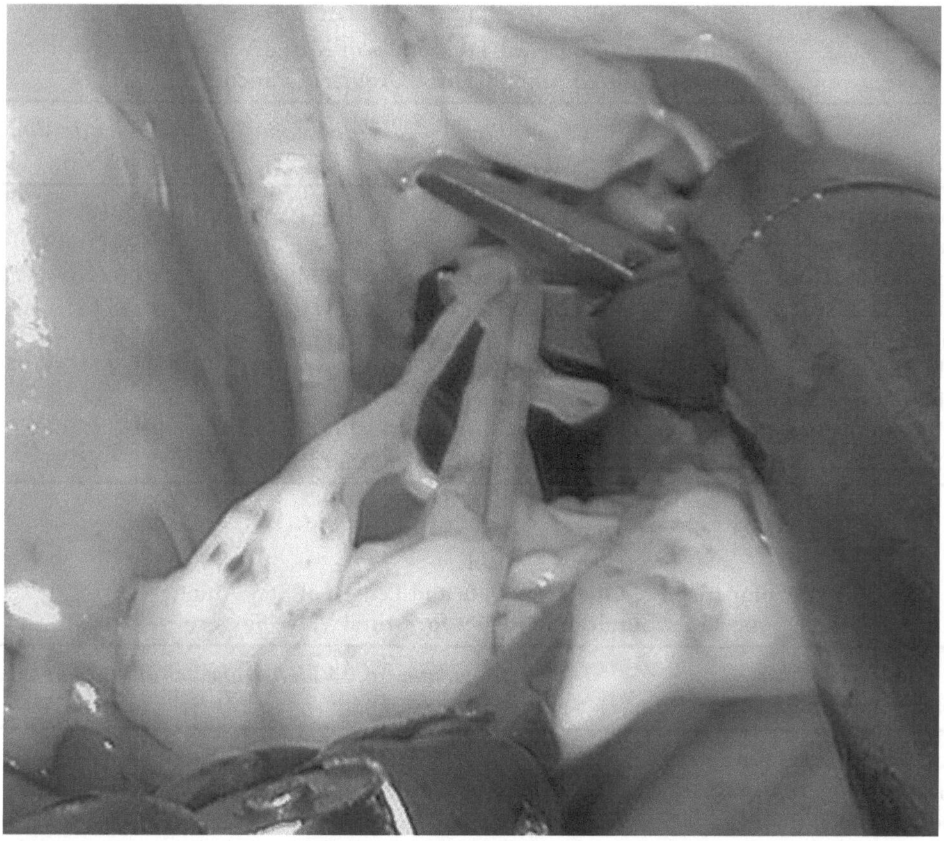

Fig. 11. Close-up view of the mitral valve leaflet and subvalvar apparatus during da Vinci robotic operation.

Table 2
Comparison of Patient Demographics Among the Three Groups of Patients Undergoing Mitral Valve

Demographics	*Conventional (n = 100)*	*Videoscopic (n = 127)*	*Robotic (da Vinci) (n = 38)*
Age (yr)	62	57	56
% Female	48	50	31
NYHA I (%)	3	7	N/A[a]
NYHA II (%)	41	46	N/A
NYHA III (%)	49	42	N/A
NYHA IV (%)	7	5	N/A
LVEF (%)	54 ± 1.2	55 ± 1.2	53 ± 1.3
Reop (%)	0	8.6	0

[a]Not available.

Tables 3 and 4, respectively. The only difference between the MMO and the da Vinci groups was defined by the 39 prosthetic valve replacements in the former series. For both videoscopic and da Vinci groups there was a progressive decline in both operative and

Table 3
Comparison of Surgical Techniques of Mitral Valve Surgery Utilized Among Three Groups of Patients

Surgical Technique	*Conventional (n = 100)*	*Videoscopic (n = 127)*	*Robotic (da Vinci) (n = 38)*
Replacement	46 (46%)	39 (31%)	0
Repair	54 (54%)	88 (69%)	38 (100%)
Annuloplasty only	10 (10%)	43 (34%)	6 (16%)
Quadrangular resection	29 (29%)	33 (26%)	18 (47%)
Sliding plasty	0	3 (2%)	5 (13%)
Chordal transfer	6 (6%)	0	2 (5%)
Chordal replacement	0	2 (1.6%)	3 (8%)
Alfieri (edge-to-edge) repair	0	2 (1.6%)	3 (8%)
Other	9 (9%)	3 (2%)	1 (3%)

Table 4
Comparison of Operative Data and Length of Stay Among the Three Surgical Strategies for Mitral Valve Surgery

Operative Data	*Conventional (n = 100)*	*Videoscopic (n = 127)*	*Robotic (da Vinci) (n = 38)*
Crossclamp time (min)	84.4 ± 2.7	106.5 ± 4.5	143 ± 5
Cardiopulmonary bypass time (min)	108.4 ± 3.6	155.9 ± 5.7	178 ± 6.5
Operation time (h)	3.1 ± 0.9	4.5 ± 0.1	4.8 ± 0.1
Ventilator time (h)	23 ± 4.7	15 ± 3.5	10.4 ± 1.1
ICU length of stay (d)	1.6 ± 0.2	1.1 ± 0.1	0.9 ± 0.1
Hospital length of stay (d)	7.9 ± 0.6	4.7 ± 0.4	3.8 ± 0.6
Patients transfused (%)	32	34	16
Units PRBC[a] transfused/patient	1.1	1	3.5
Units FFP[b] transfused/patient	0.7	0.2	N/A[c]
Units platelets transfused/patient	1.2	0.1	N/A
Units cryoprecipitate transfused/patient	0.1	0	N/A

[a]Packed red blood cells.
[b]Fresh frozen plasma.
[c]Not applicable.

crossclamp times. Our latest operative times for the videoscopic group are approaching that of the conventional group *(7)*. We now have performed over 200 video-assisted mitral operations using long instruments.

Postoperative chest tube drainage was significantly less in patients who underwent videoscopic operations. However, no group differences existed, either in percentage of patients receiving transfusions or total amount of packed red blood cells, fresh frozen plasma, or platelets transfused. Rank-order analysis of variance of ventilator dependency revealed a significant difference between conventional and videoscopic cases, but not between the later cohort and the robotic group. Both minimally invasive groups had similar intensive care periods and shorter hospital lengths of stay compared to the cohort of patients who underwent conventional mitral surgery. Comparative crossclamp and perfusion times are shown in **Figs. 12** and **13**.

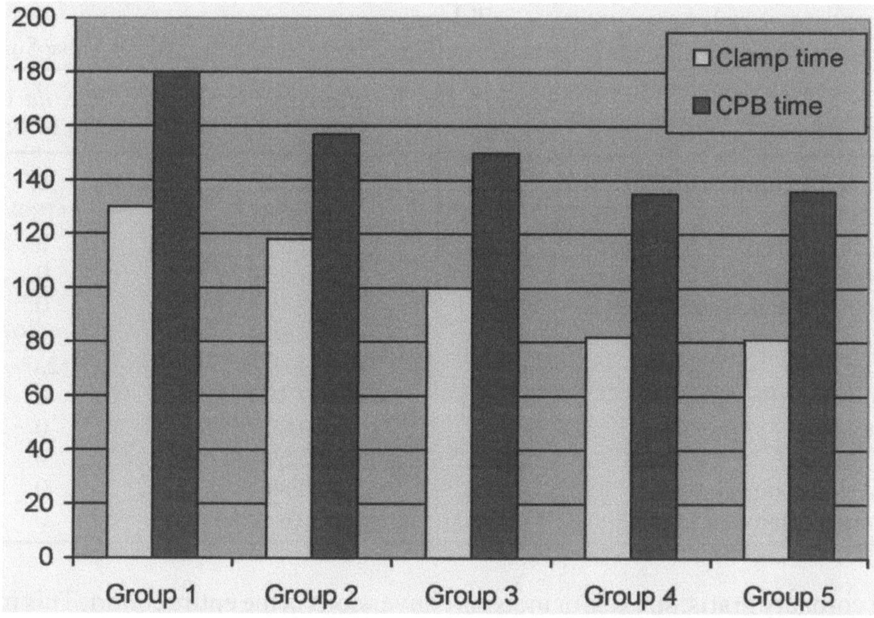

Fig. 12. The 127 videoscopic micro-mitral patients were separated into 5 consecutive cohorts of 25 patients. There was a consistent decline of CPB time and crossclamp time from the earliest cohort (Group 1) to the latest cohort (Group 2).

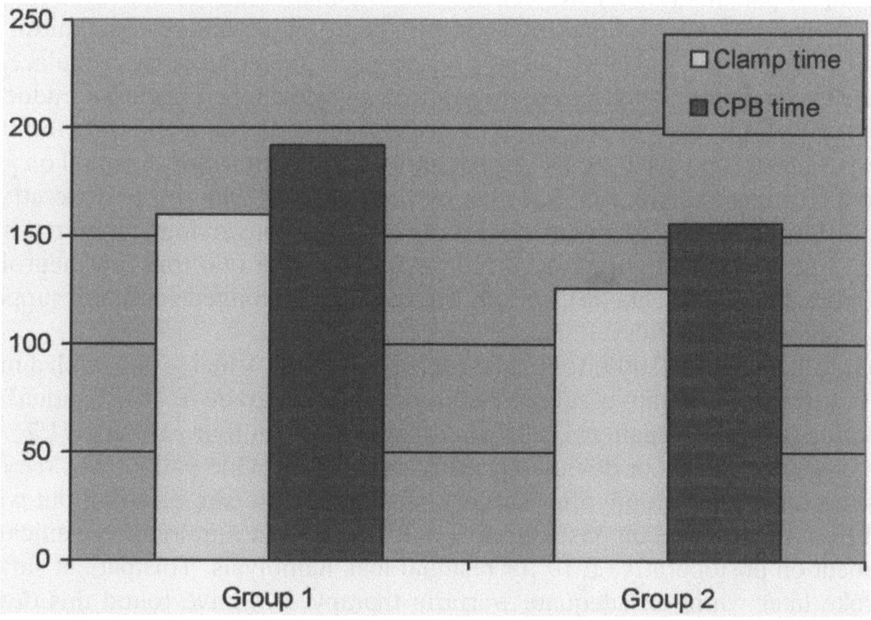

Fig. 13. Comparison of CPB time and crossclamp time between the first 19 da Vinci robotic patients (Group 1) and the last 19 patients (Group 2).

Seventeen patients in this cohort were *reoperations*, and there was one perioperative death (5.8%) from postoperative pneumonia. Thirteen of these operations were performed under hypothermic fibrillatory arrest without aortic crossclamping. The average operative time and CPB times were 4.6 and 2.7 h, respectively. There were no injuries to

Table 5
Comparison of Adverse Events Among Three Operative Strategies for Mitral Valve Surgery

Adverse Event	*Conventional (n = 100)*	*Videoscopic (n = 127)*	*Robotic (da Vinci) (n = 38)*
Conversion to sternotomy	0	2 (1.5%)	0
Atrial fibrillation	27 (27%)	27 (21%)	7 (18%)
Sternal infection	1 (1%)	1 (0.8%)	0
Groin infection	0	1 (0.8%)	0
Transient ischemic attack	2 (2%)	1 (0.8%)	0
Stroke	1 (1%)	1 (0.8%)	1 (2.6%)
Bleeding	7 (7%)	1 (0.8%)	1 (2.6%)
Prolonged ventilation	13 (13%)	1 (0.8%)	0
Pneumonia	2 (2%)	1 (0.8%)	0
Renal failure	2 (2%)	1 (0.8%)	0
Deep vein thrombosis	0	1 (0.8%)	0
Myocardial infarction	1 (1%)	0	0

existing coronary grafts, strokes, or incision conversions in the entire cohort. This method is quite effective when mitral valve operations are required in patients having prior coronary surgery.

Table 5 shows comparative adverse everts. Total videoscopic MMO patient follow-up was 90% complete at 25.1 ± 3.6 mo. Most recently, 97 patients (85.1%) were NYHA class 0-I and 9 patients (7.9%) were class II. Five patients (5.1%) had initial improvements of their symptoms but later returned with heart failure and residual mitral regurgitation. Of these, three had late (>38 mo) recurrences and required valve replacements. The other two patients were dialysis-dependent and developed bacterial endocarditis requiring valve replacements at 1 and 2 mo following repair. Overall 30-d mortality for the videoscopic group was 2.3% (3/127 patients). One death was in-hospital on postoperative d 28 from pneumonia and the other two were home deaths on postoperative d 15 and d 29 from presumed arrhythmias. There were two conversions to sternotomy for bleeding. One permanent stroke occurred, and there were two transient neurological sequelae (brachial plexus, ataxia). One patient required prolonged ventilator support (32 d) from a phrenic nerve palsy.

Patient follow-up was 100% for the 38 patients in the da Vinci group, with a mean of 10.7 ± 0.9 mo. Postoperative echocardiograms showed grade 1 or 0 residual mitral regurgitation (MR) in 34 patients (89%) and grade 2 MR in four patients (11%). There were no operative deaths or device related complications. One patient was reexplored through the same incision 6 h after surgery for pacing wire site bleeding but was discharged from the hospital on postoperative d 3. One patient required mechanical valve replacement on postoperative d 19 for residual leak hemolysis. This patient suffered a fatal stroke later while on adequate warfarin therapy. We have found this device to facilitate complex mitral reconstructions and operative times are beginning to fall progressively. In the last 20 da Vinci mitral valve repairs, crossclamp time has averaged 126 min.

DISCUSSION

The authors believe that smaller incisions are beneficial to patients, and can provide an uncompromised, quality operation. This has been demonstrated by our experiences both with the video-assisted micro-mitral operations as well as with the da Vinci-performed procedures. Using video assistance, we have been able to achieve superior mitral valve exposure with a 4–5-cm skin incision without resecting ribs or cartilage. A small skin incision also limits soft tissue dissection and rib retraction, which in turn minimizes overall surgical trauma. Compared to patients with traditional sternotomy approaches, our patients generally require less blood product transfusions, have less postoperative pain, recover faster, and are discharged earlier.

We have identified several technical elements that are crucial for the success of these videoscopic operations. Peripheral cannulation and assisted venous drainage in combination with transthoracic direct aortic clamping have provided excellent exposure and cardiac protection. With the addition of the SVC drainage catheter via the internal jugular vein, we have had no problems with cardiac decompression, even with smaller percutaneous femoral catheters. Transthoracic aortic clamping is simple, safe, and reliable. Using a mini-thoracotomy and videoscope, the mitral valve can be exposed through a small atriotomy without tense retraction on the heart. Not only is the visualization of the valve and the subvalvar apparatus superior, the aortic valve remains relatively competent, permitting effective antegrade cardioplegia delivery in most cases.

Specially designed minimally invasive surgical instruments, such as the custom atrial retractors, long-shafted forceps and needle drivers, as well as the valve pusher/knot tier, are required to facilitate the MMO. As stated previously, the micro-mitral videoscopic approach is our standard choice for isolated mitral operations. The da Vinci device obviates the need for these long instruments, as the operative action is at the valvular site. We believe that there are very few absolute contraindications to using these innovative approaches. However, relative contraindications include: (1) a previous right thoracotomy, (2) previous radiation to right thorax, (3) severe pulmonary dysfunction, and (4) severe pulmonary hypertension. A full sternotomy still affords the most options for dealing with potential complications of severe pulmonary hypertension. Generally we do not use either minimally invasive approach in patients with pulmonary systolic pressures either over half-systemic or greater than 70 mmHg.

Based on our experience, as well as inference from past general surgical endoscopic history, there is clearly a learning curve in the transition from conventional to videoscopic mitral operations. Our operative and perfusion times in the latest videoscopic cases are comparable to that of our conventional approach *(7)*. Above all, obtaining the best operation should take primacy over the approach, and quality should never be compromised for any reason. It is our belief that postoperative quality of life, including satisfaction with the procedure, return to work, level of discomfort, and performance of daily activities, are improved by these minimally invasive approaches. However, large-scale prospective studies are needed to confirm our impressions. Only time and cumulative clinical volume will be able to prove irrefutably the benefits of an operative strategy aimed at reducing surgical trauma. However, it is clear that progress is being made daily. The concept of a totally endoscopic mitral repair for complex mitral pathology seemingly is becoming a reality.

REFERENCES

1. Cohn LH, et al. Minimally invasive cardiac valve surgery improves patient satisfaction while reducing costs of cardiac valve replacement and repair. Ann Surg 1997;226(4):421–426; discussion 427–428.
2. Cosgrove DM, Sabik JF, Navia JL. Minimally invasive valve operations. Ann Thorac Surg 1998;65(6):1535–1538; discussion 1538–1539.

3. Navia JL, Cosgrove DM. Minimally invasive mitral valve operations. Ann Thorac Surg 1996.;62(5):1542–1544.
4. Arom KV, Emery RW. Minimally invasive mitral operations. Ann Thorac Surg 1997;63(4):1219–1220.
5. Gundry SR, et al. Facile minimally invasive cardiac surgery via ministernotomy. Ann Thorac Surg 1998;65(4):1100–1104.
6. Pompili MF, et al. Port-access mitral valve replacement in dogs. J Thorac Cardiovasc Surg 1996;112(5):1268–1274.
7. Felger JE, et al. Evolution of mitral valve surgery: toward a totally endoscopic approach. Ann Thorac Surg 2001;72(4):1203–1208; discussion 1208–1209.
8. Chitwood WR Jr, et al. Video-assisted minimally invasive mitral valve surgery. J Thorac Cardiovasc Surg 1997;114(5):773–780; discussion 780–782.
9. Gillinov AM, Banbury MK, Cosgrove DM, et al. Hemisternotomy approach for aortic and mitral valve surgery. J Card Surg 2000;15(1):15–20.
10. Glower DD, et al. Predictors of outcome in a multicenter port-access valve registry. Ann Thorac Surg 2000;70(3):1054–1059.
11. Byrne JG, et al. Minimally invasive direct access heart valve surgery. J Card Surg 2000;15(1):21–34.
12. Cutler E, Beck C. Surgery of the heart and pericardium. In (Nelson, ed.) Loose Leaf Surgery, New York: Thos. Nelson & Sons, 1927.
13. Sakakibara S, et al. Direct visual operation of aortic stenosis with a cardioscope: studies on cardioscope no. 2. Bull Heart Inst Jap 1958;2:1–21.
14. Kaneko Y, et al. Video-assisted observation in mitral valve surgery. J Thorac Cardiovasc Surg 1996;111(1):279–280.
15. Carpentier A, et al. [Computer assisted open heart surgery. First case operated on with success]. C R Acad Sci III 1998;321(5):437–442.
16. Reichenspurner H, et al. Three-dimensional video and robot-assisted port-access mitral valve operation. Ann Thorac Surg 2000;69(4):1176–1181; discussion 1181–1182.
17. Falk V, et al. Robot-assisted minimally invasive solo mitral valve operation. J Thorac Cardiovasc Surg 1998;115(2):470–471.
18. Chitwood WR Jr, et al. Robotic mitral valve repair: trapezoidal resection and prosthetic annuloplasty with the da vinci surgical system. J Thorac Cardiovasc Surg 2000;120(6):1171–1172.
19. Grossi EA, et al. Case report of robotic instrument-enhanced mitral valve surgery. J Thorac Cardiovasc Surg 2000;120(6):1169–1171.
20. Vanermen H, et al. Video-assisted Port-Access mitral valve surgery: from debut to routine surgery, Will Trocar-Port-Access cardiac surgery lead to robotic surgery? Semin Thorac Cardiovasc Surg 1999;11:223–234.
21. Nifong LW, Chu VF, Bailey BM, et al. Robotic mitral valve repair: experience with the da Vinci system. Ann Thorac Surg 2003;75(2):438–442.

20 Port-Access Mitral Valve Surgery

Ashish S. Shah, MD *and Donald D. Glower,* MD

CONTENTS

INTRODUCTION
PATIENT SELECTION
OPERATIVE TECHNIQUE
INCISIONS
FEMORAL ARTERY CANNULATION
CENTRAL AORTIC CANNULATION
AORTIC OCCLUSION/CARDIOPLEGIA
COMPLETION OF PROCEDURE
POSTOPERATIVE CARE
POTENTIAL PITFALLS
RESULTS
CONCLUSIONS
FUTURE
REFERENCES

INTRODUCTION

Port access, a term originally coined by the founders of Heartport, Inc. (Redwood City, CA), was intended to describe a totally endoscopic approach to cardiac surgery using cardiopulmonary bypass *(1,2)*. While the founders of Heartport ultimately concluded in the mid-1990s that totally endoscopic cardiac surgery was not technically feasible at the time, the term port access was retained and applied to minimally invasive cardiac surgical procedures using a small thoracotomy and any combination of catheters developed by Heartport. The system consists of endoclamps, catheters for percutaneous retrograde cardioplegia and pulmonary artery venting, femoral venous cannulation, direct aortic cannulation, and femoral arterial cannulation.

Once animal studies at Stanford University and New York University demonstrated the feasibility of applying port access to mitral valve operations *(1,3,4)*, port-access

From: *Contemporary Cardiology: Minimally Invasive Cardiac Surgery, Second Edition*
Edited by: D. J. Goldstein and M. C. Oz © Humana Press Inc., Totowa, NJ

mitral valve procedures were performed at Stanford University and New York University in 1996 as part of a U.S. Food and Drug Administration (FDA)-approved clinical trial *(5,6)*. Simultaneously, port-access mitral valve procedures were performed in Germany, Singapore, and several other sites worldwide *(7)*. In October 1996, the FDA approved port-access devices for clinical use in the United States, and over 100 sites in the United States and Europe began to apply port-access techniques to mitral valve surgery. Initial users of port access underwent training on animals and proctoring *(8)*. Subsequent users adopted port access after visiting established sites and by proctoring. As of the end of the year 2000, over 18,000 port-access valve and coronary procedures had been performed worldwide.

Other approaches to the mitral valve using a small thoracotomy were developed in parallel with port access *(9–13)*. The best-known approach is the Chitwood mini-mitral procedure *(14–16)*, described by the author in Chapter 19. These approaches all include a small right thoracotomy and an external aortic clamp, generally with femoral arterial and venous cannulation. Other investigators favor a slightly larger right thoracotomy using standard equipment *(17–20)*.

Now that port access has been established clinically, port access continues to be applied with a growing number of modifications to the original technique. Appropriately, the port-access approach (which was originally intended for totally endoscopic robotic procedures) is once again being applied to robotic mitral valve surgery *(21–23)*. To date, a small number of totally endoscopic robotic mitral valve procedures have been performed in the United States and Europe using port-access techniques. The viability of the port-access approach today (despite diverse economic and technological pressures) attests to the flexibility and validity of the original concept behind port access.

PATIENT SELECTION

When given the choice, most patients will choose port access or a small thoracotomy over standard median sternotomy. In the experience of one surgeon at Duke University, 252 of 268 (94%) of all isolated mitral valve patients were considered candidates for the port-access approach and underwent mitral operation using port access.

Relative indications for port access include desire for improved cosmesis (especially in young women), previous median sternotomy (especially with patent bypass grafts), and any factors that increase risk of sternotomy complications such as obesity, chronic steroid use, lung disease, and diabetes. Data supporting these relative indications for port access are presented later in this chapter and are based primarily on the lack of sternal wound complications and the limited mediastinal dissection associated with port access.

Relative contraindications include previous right thoracotomy, severe pectus excavatum, and need for concurrent coronary or aortic valve operation. Of those patients excluded from port access at Duke University, 13 of 16 (81%) were excluded because of possibly needing concurrent aortic or coronary operation.

OPERATIVE TECHNIQUE

Patients are positioned supine with the right shoulder elevated and with the right arm at the patient's side *(6,24)*. Alternatively, the right arm may be supported over the head *(25)*. External defibrillator pads should be placed prior to skin preparation to allow defibrillation in the presence of severe pericardial adhesions. One defibrillator lead is placed over the left anterolateral chest, and the other lead is placed under the right shoulder.

If central aortic cannulation is anticipated, the ability to deflate the right lung is generally necessary. These patients should be intubated with a dual-lumen endotracheal tube or with an endobronchial blocker placed in the right mainstem bronchus. In those patients in whom the right lung cannot be deflated for technical reasons or because of significant lung disease, cannulation of the femoral artery and femoral vein will be necessary to initiate cardiopulmonary bypass prior to dissecting the mediastinum. The combination of lung disease precluding one-lung ventilation and the inability to cannulate the femoral artery would be a contraindication to the port-access or thoracotomy approach.

Anesthetic management of port-access mitral patients differs from that of sternotomy patients in several regards *(26)*. First is the need to obtain single-lung ventilation if aortic cannulation is planned. Second, if the endoclamp is placed from the femoral artery with the possibility of endoclamp balloon migration, bilateral radial artery arterial lines should be placed to detect occlusion of the innominate artery should the endoclamp migrate distally. If central aortic cannulation is planned, only a single radial arterial line is needed. Third, several other pressure transducers are needed for use of the endoclamp, and these include lines for aortic root pressure, endoclamp balloon pressure, and coronary sinus pressure. Finally, if desired, the anesthesiologist may place a percutaneous catheter (EP, CardioVations, Sommerville, NJ) into the coronary sinus during line placement *(27)*. This technique has the advantage of providing retrograde cardioplegia without having an additional catheter in the surgical field. The disadvantages to percutaneous coronary sinus catheter placement include the learning curve in catheter placement, the variability of coronary sinus anatomy, and the additional cost of the coronary sinus catheter. In experienced hands, the coronary sinus catheter can be placed percutaneously 80% of the time. Also available is a pulmonary artery vent catheter (CardioVations, Sommerville, NJ), which can be inserted by the anesthesiologist into the pulmonary artery through a venous sheath. In the future, anesthetic management of port-access patients may include regional analgesia such as paravertebral blocks to assist in the postoperative course.

INCISIONS

Several different incisions have been used for mitral and tricuspid valve operations using port access. The first incision is placed just lateral to the nipple over the fourth intercostal space (above the nipple in men and in the inframammary crease in most women) (**Fig. 1**). This anterolateral incision has the advantage of providing excellent access for central aortic cannulation and also provides the most direct and most lateral view of the mitral valve. The disadvantages of this incision are that it places the surgeon at a greater distance from the mitral valve and that more lateral cutaneous nerves may be injured, providing a somewhat wider area of medial numbness and paresthesia in some patients. The second commonly used incision is placed in the inframammary crease directly inferior to the nipple and just lateral to the mammary artery. This incision has the advantages of placing the surgeon closer to the mitral valve and of causing less medial paresthesia. Disadvantages include less access to the ascending aorta and a less favorable angle to view the mitral valve and subvalvular apparatus. The more medial incision is often used with femoral arterial cannulation and with greater use of the video camera to visualize the mitral valve (video-directed surgery) *(28)* rather than direct vision through the incision. Incisions can be made as small as 4 cm if the femoral artery is cannulated, and cannulation of the ascending aorta generally requires a 6-cm incision. An additional adjunct to provide exposure of the ascending aorta is to divide the fourth rib medially at the costochondral junction and then to enter the bed of the fourth rib. The rib is repaired

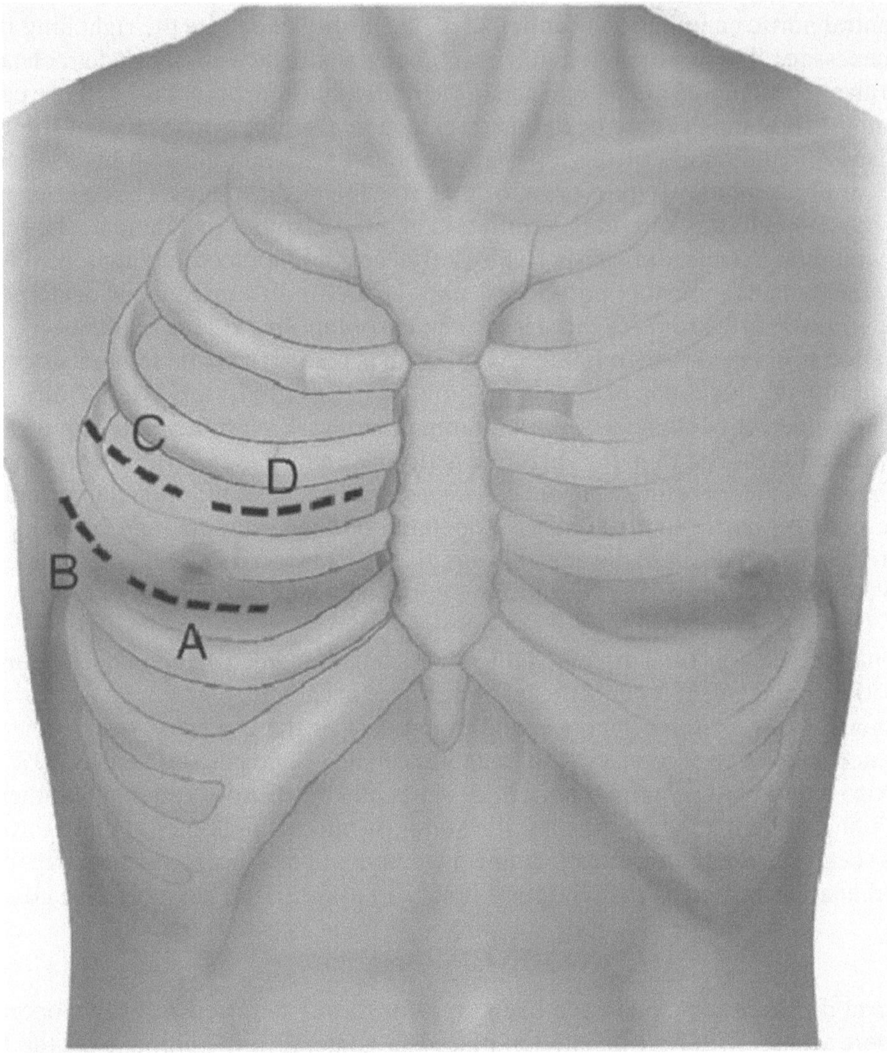

Fig. 1. Four different incisions applicable to port access mitral procedures: (**A**) inframammary, (**B**) infralateral, (**C**) supralateral, and (**D**) supramedial. The supramedial incision (**D**) is in the third intercostal space, and all others are in the fourth intercostal space.

at the end of the procedure. A third approach to the mitral valve is to enter the right third intercostal space just lateral to the sternum if combined mitral and aortic valve procedures are planned *(29)*.

The pericardium is opened vertically from the diaphragm to the ascending aorta, keeping the incision at least 1–2 cm anterior to the phrenic nerve. If the ascending aorta is to be cannulated, the incision should be carried up to the innominate vein. Three lateral retraction sutures are placed on the posterior pericardial edge. The first is placed over the right superior pulmonary vein and is secured to the lateral corner of the skin incision. The second is placed halfway to the diaphragm and is passed through the chest wall using a 12-gage needle, a small hook, and a small clamp to secure the suture. The third suture is

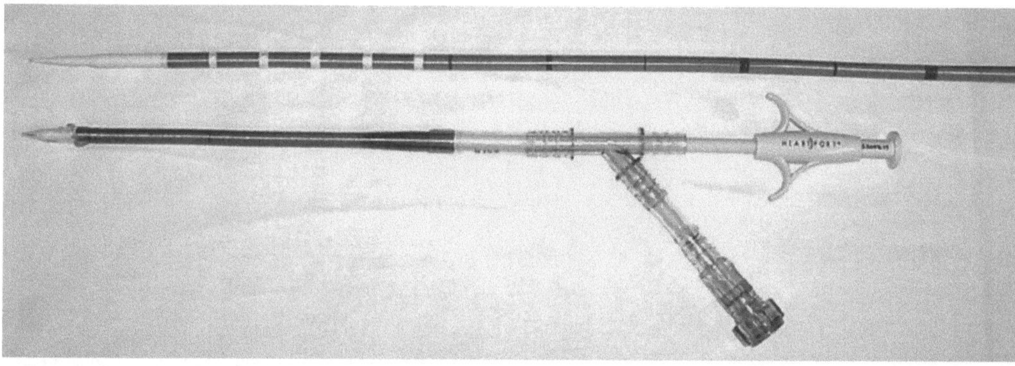

Fig. 2. Venous cannula with serial dilators suitable for percutaneous access (above), and aortic cannula with knife-tipped introducer (below). Note the side arm on the aortic cannula for insertion of the endoclamp into the arterial line.

placed at the level of the superior vena cava and is passed through the third intercostal space as laterally as possible. If the ascending aorta is to be cannulated, the medial pericardium at the mid-ascending aorta is secured to the posterior sternum to provide aortic exposure.

FEMORAL ARTERY CANNULATION

Femoral arterial cannulation is performed through a small 3- to 4-cm transverse incision in the groin between the inguinal crease and the inguinal ligament. The femoral artery and femoral vein are exposed and encircled with tapes, although tape placement is not necessary in a scarred and previously operated groin. Two concentric purse strings are placed in the femoral vein and artery using 5-0 polypropylene suture secured using tourniquets *(30)*.The femoral venous cannula is generally placed first. After heparinization, a guidewire is passed up the femoral vein into the superior vena cava using either echocardiography, direct palpation, or direct vision. The 22 or 25 fr femoral venous cannula (QD-22 or QD-25, CardioVations, Sommerville, NJ) (**Fig. 2**) is then passed over the wire and through the purse strings to place the tip of the cannula 2 cm into the superior vena cava. The two 5-0 polypropylene suture tourniquets are then secured, and tapes on the proximal and distal vein are released, allowing continuous venous drainage of the leg and excellent hemostasis. Two concentric 5-0 polypropylene sutures are similarly placed in the common femoral artery, being careful that the diameter of the purse strings is less than one-half the diameter of the vessel to avoid vessel stenosis. After controlling the artery proximally and distally, an arteriotomy is made within the purse strings and is dilated to a diameter large enough to pass the arterial cannula. A 21 or 23 fr arterial cannula (ER-23 or ER-21, CardioVations Sommerville, NJ) is then passed over a wire into the femoral artery, placing the cannula tip at least 2 cm into the femoral artery and away from any plaques or bends in the femoral artery. The 5-0 polypropylene tourniquets are then secured, and all tapes on the femoral artery are released so that the leg will be continuously perfused around the cannula. Both the arterial and venous cannulas can be placed as above if no difficulties are apparent, otherwise fluoroscopy may be necessary. Fluoroscopy is rarely needed for port access in experienced centers today.

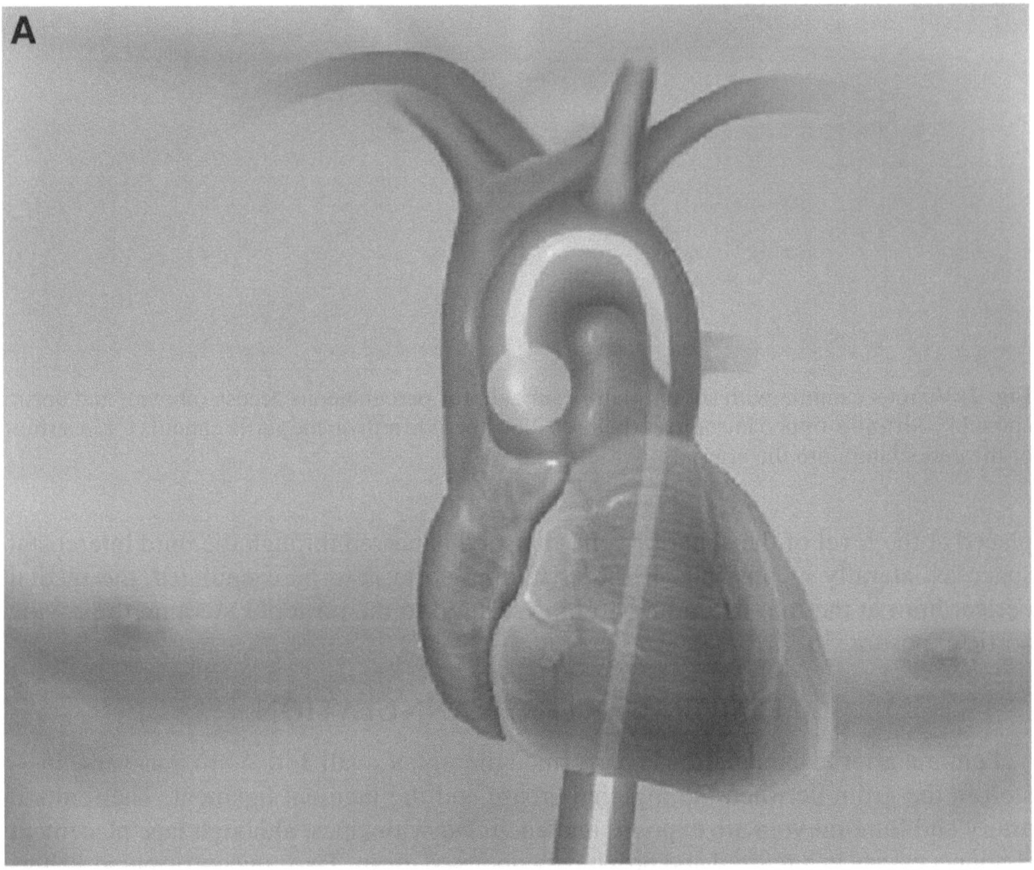
A

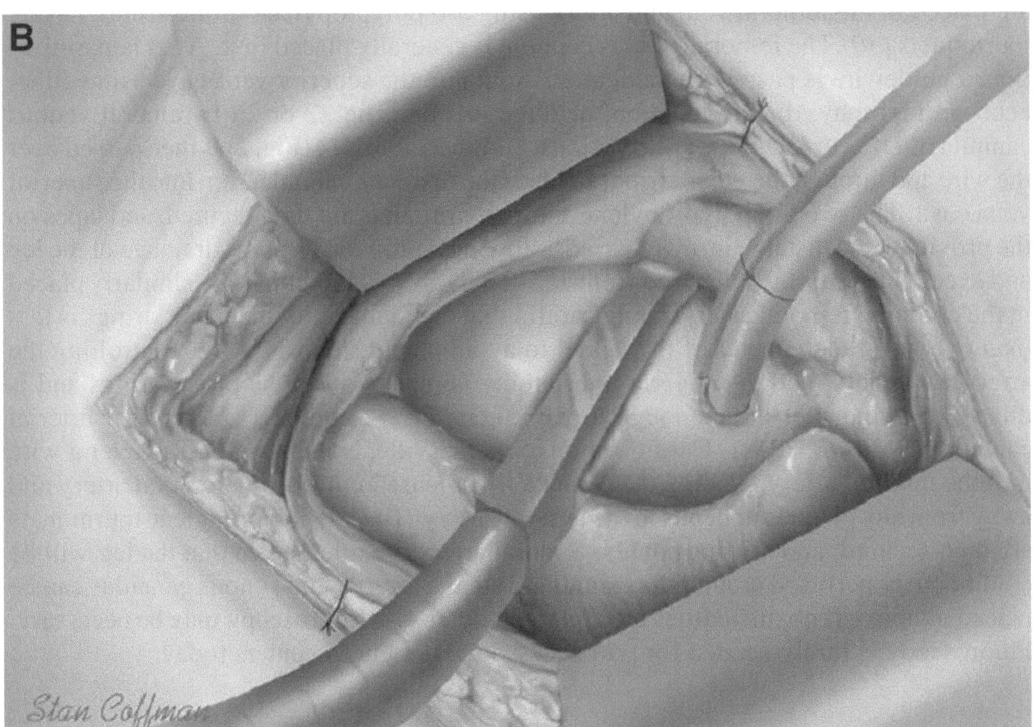
B
Stan Coffman

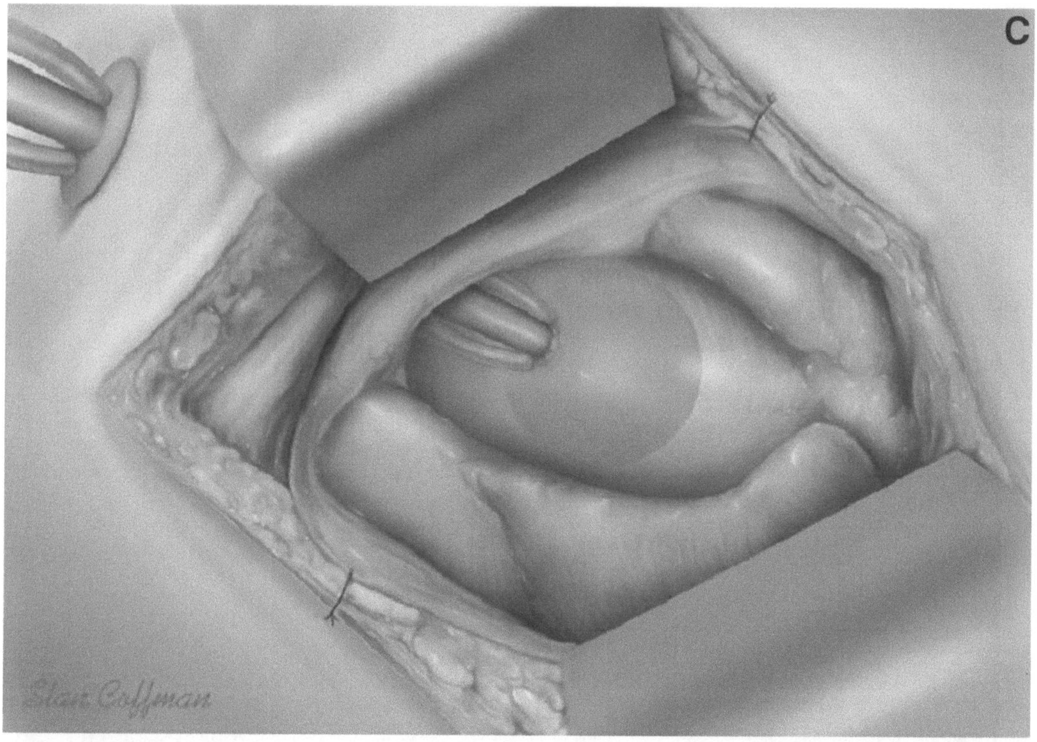

Fig. 3. Three different options to obain aortic occlusion: (**A**) transfemoral endoclamp, (**B**) external aortic clamp, and (**C**) transaortic endoclamp.

CENTRAL AORTIC CANNULATION

Central aortic cannulation has the advantages of eliminating endoclamp balloon migration, avoiding embolization and/or dissection due to aortic or peripheral vascular disease, avoiding femoral arterial injury, limb ischemia, and groin incision complications (seroma, infection, hematoma) *(31)*. Central aortic cannulation has the disadvantage of requiring a somewhat larger incision and requiring the additional hardware of a specifically designed aortic cannula. Once the thoracotomy incision is made, the chest wall retractor is placed. A reusable-type retractor may be desirable here, as opposed to the earlier soft tissue retractor, to provide greater exposure of the ascending aorta by lifting upward on the superior chest wall. A 16-gage 6-in. needle is then passed through the first intercostal space at the midclavicular level, angling toward the desired cannulation site on ascending aorta to identify the optimal placement of the arterial line port. Care is needed to avoid the right internal mammary artery and vein. The arterial cannula should enter the aorta 1–2 cm proximal to the innominate artery with the aortic cannula directed toward the aortic valve. Angulation toward the aortic valve ensures that the endoclamp will pass toward the aortic valve and not down the aortic arch. Once this approach line is demonstrated with the 16-gage needle, a 2.5-cm transverse skin incision is made at the 16-gage needle puncture site, and an 11.5-mm trocar is passed through the former 16-gage needle track to provide a direct port for the aortic cannula. This port should point directly at the desired aortic cannulation site. The aortic cannula (DF-K-24, CardioVations, Sommerville, NJ) (**Fig. 3A–C**) is then passed through the 11.5-mm port to ascertain that direct access to the desired cannulation site is possible without torque on the cannula (**Fig. 4**).

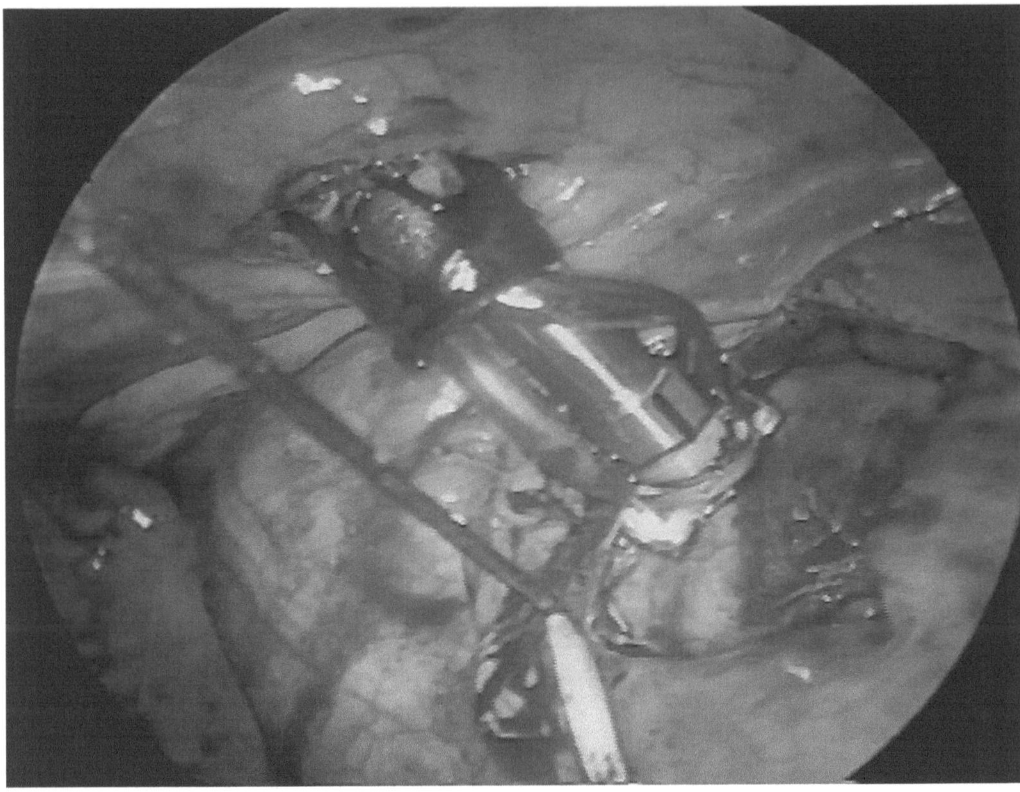

Fig. 4. Surgeon's view of the aortic cannula placed through a port in the first intercostal space. Tourniquets on the aortic purse-string sutures pass through the trocar for stability.

Attention is then turned to the femoral vein, which can be accessed percutaneously to avoid a groin incision. After heparinization, the common femoral vein is cannulated as described previously. Once the femoral vein is cannulated, a standard aortic purse string is placed at the desired cannulation site on the ascending aorta using two concentric 2-0 polyester sutures. The aortic cannula (DF-K-24, CardioVations, Sommerville, NJ) (**Fig. 3**) is passed through the 11.5-mm trocar in the first intercostal space so that the cannula introducer is centered in the aortic purse-string suture. The knife tip on the aortic cannula introducer is deployed only long enough to allow the introducer to reach the aortic wall. The introducer knife tip is then immediately withdrawn (to avoid injury to the back wall of the aorta), and the introducer and cannula are easily passed with a twisting motion into the ascending aorta. The 2-0 purse-string sutures are then passed through the 11.5-mm trocar and secured using plastic tourniquets placed through the trocar and secured with a heavy suture. Excellent aortic cannula stability is obtained (**Fig. 4**). The placement of the venous cannula prior to aortic cannulation provides an additional source of vascular access should any bleeding be encountered. If an endoclamp is not to be used, then alternative aortic cannulas (SS-23-A-K or SS-23-S-K, CardioVations, Sommerville, NJ) can be used that do not have a side arm for an endoclamp but that still have the knife-tipped introducer.

Additional alternatives in venous cannulation include placement of a second venous catheter into the superior vena cava via the right internal jugular vein *(25,28)*. This is generally a 17 fr arterial-type cannula placed over a wire. Otherwise, a 28 fr angled plastic

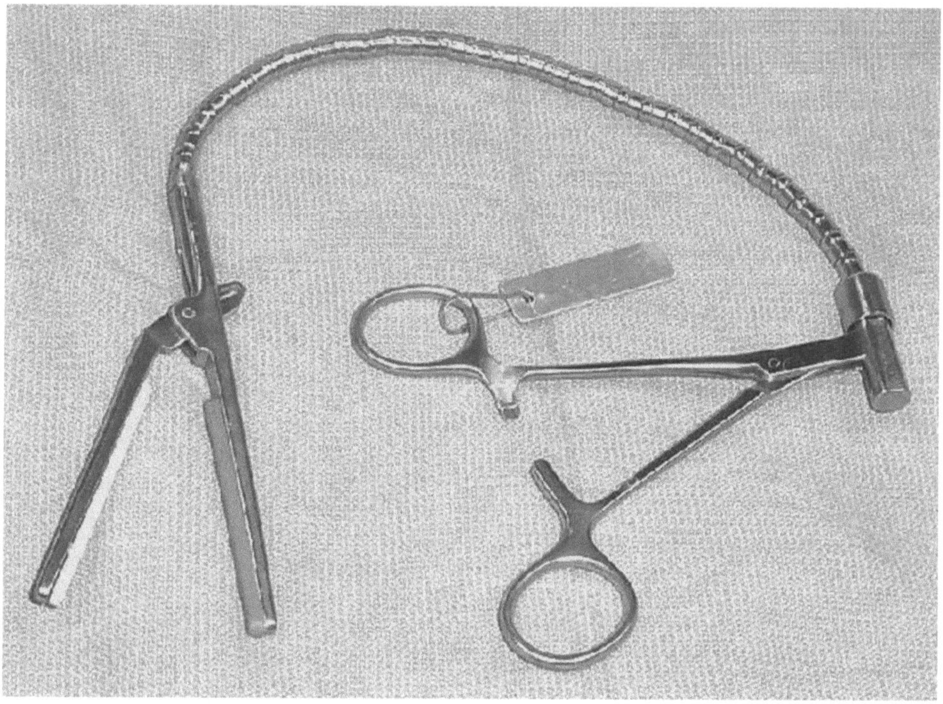

Fig. 5. A flexible Cosgrove external aortic clamp that may be used as an alternative to an external Chitwood clamp or an endoclamp.

venous cannula can be placed through the chest wall or through the thoracotomy incision to provide standard cannulation of the superior vena cava. In this instance, a standard purse-string suture would be placed in the right atrium or in the superior vena cava after withdrawing the femoral venous cannula into the body of the right atrium. In those patients in whom femoral venous cannulation is not possible or desirable, the inferior vena cava can be cannulated through a right atrial purse-string suture with the cannula passed through the chest wall or through the thoracotomy incision. It is important that venous cannulation provide adequate drainage of the superior vena cava when the left atrium is retracted anteriorly, so that obstruction of the superior vena cava does not result. Assisted venous return should generally be used either via vacuum assist or by use of a Biomedicus centrifugal pump in the venous line.

AORTIC OCCLUSION/CARDIOPLEGIA

Several alternatives exist for aortic occlusion. First, ventricular fibrillation may be used when the ascending aorta is not easily occluded. This may be desirable when open bypass grafts (especially left internal mammary grafts) are present and are not easily or safely accessible. Second, the ascending aorta can be occluded with an external clamp of either the Cosgrove (**Fig. 5**) or Chitwood *(14–16)* variety (**Figs. 3** and **6**). These aortic clamps can be passed through the incision or through a separate stab wound lateral to the incision. If an external clamp is used, anterograde cardioplegia may be delivered through a standard cardioplegia cannula secured with purse-string sutures in the ascending aorta. Alternatively, a single dose of anterograde cardioplegia can be given using a spinal needle passed through the chest wall into the ascending aorta.

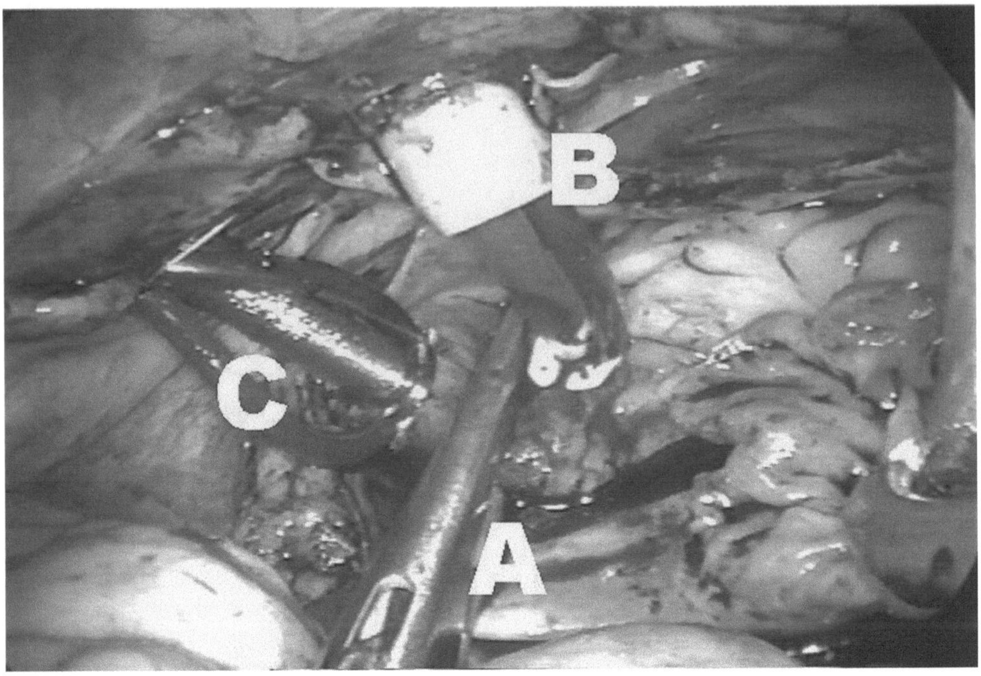

Fig. 6. External clamping (A) of the ascending aorta. Note the cannula (B) in the aortic root for cardioplegia/venting. The ascending aorta may be cannulated (C) for arterial access as seen here, or the femoral artery may be used.

Finally, the aorta can be occluded using an endoclamp passed through the aortic or femoral arterial cannula (**Fig. 3**). Once the arterial cannula is placed, an endoclamp (EC-65 or EC-100, CardioVations, Sommerville, NJ) (**Fig. 7**) is passed through the "Y"-limb in the arterial cannula to position the end of clamp in the ascending aorta just above the aortic valve. Transesophageal echo or fluoroscopy can be used. If a femoral arterial cannula is employed, the endoclamp is passed over a wire. For direct cannulation of the ascending aorta, a wire is unnecessary. Once in the endoclamp is positioned, cardiopulmonary bypass is initiated using assisted venous drainage. With the transaortic endoclamp, the balloon is partially inflated, pulled back snugly against the tip of the aortic cannula, and then inflated to a volume sufficient to occlude the ascending aorta as demonstrated by transesophageal echo and/or direct palpation and inspection. With femoral cannulation, the endoclamp is inflated using transesophageal echo or fluoroscopy to ascertain positioning at least 1 cm above the aortic valve but proximal to the innominate artery. Once in place, slack on the femoral endoclamp catheter is tightened enough to prevent proximal balloon migration, without being so tight as to cause distal endoclamp balloon migration.

Similarly, cardioplegia delivery can be handled in several ways. Ventricular fibrillation is an option when aortic occlusion cannot be obtained or when anterograde and retrograde cardioplegia are not feasible. Anterograde cardioplegia can be delivered through the endoclamp catheter or through a needle in the aortic root if an external clamp is used. Finally, retrograde cardioplegia can be delivered through a percutaneous coronary sinus catheter or through a retrograde coronary sinus catheter placed directly through a purse string in the right atrium.

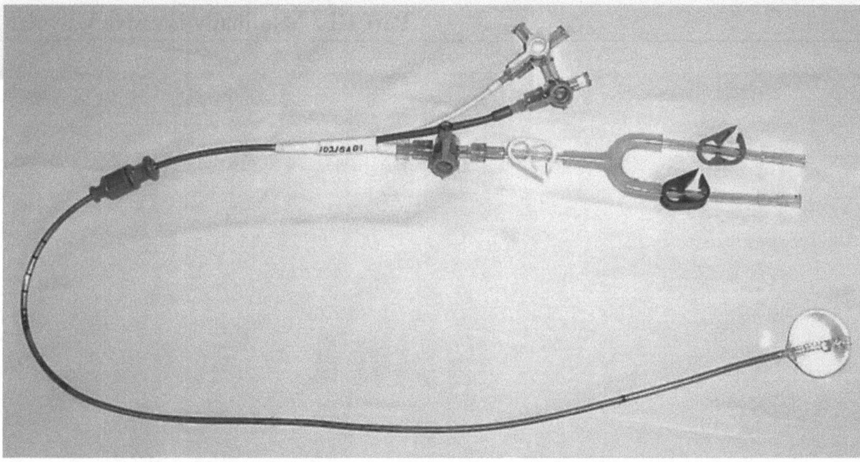

Fig. 7. Transaortic balloon endoclamp (65 cm). The transfemoral endoclamp is similar but longer (100 cm). Note the three catheter lumens for cardioplegia/venting (proximal Y connector), balloon inflation (dark stopcock), and monitoring of aortic root pressure (white stopcock).

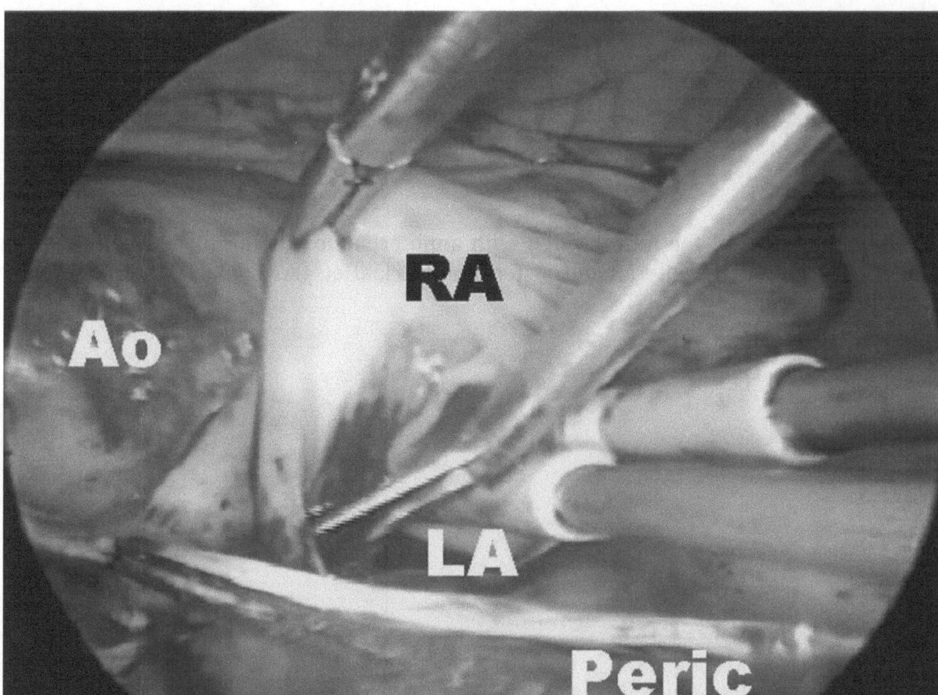

Fig. 8. Opening the left atrium (LA) through the interatrial groove. Suckers are in the left atrium. The right atrium (RA) is retracted toward the aorta (Ao) with forceps. The pericardium (Peric) and phrenic nerve are below.

COMPLETION OF PROCEDURE

With the heart arrested on cardiopulmonary bypass, the left atrium is opened adjacent to the interatrial groove (**Fig. 8**). If needed, the left atriotomy can be extended superiorly behind the superior vena cava and inferiorly behind the inferior vena cava. The view of

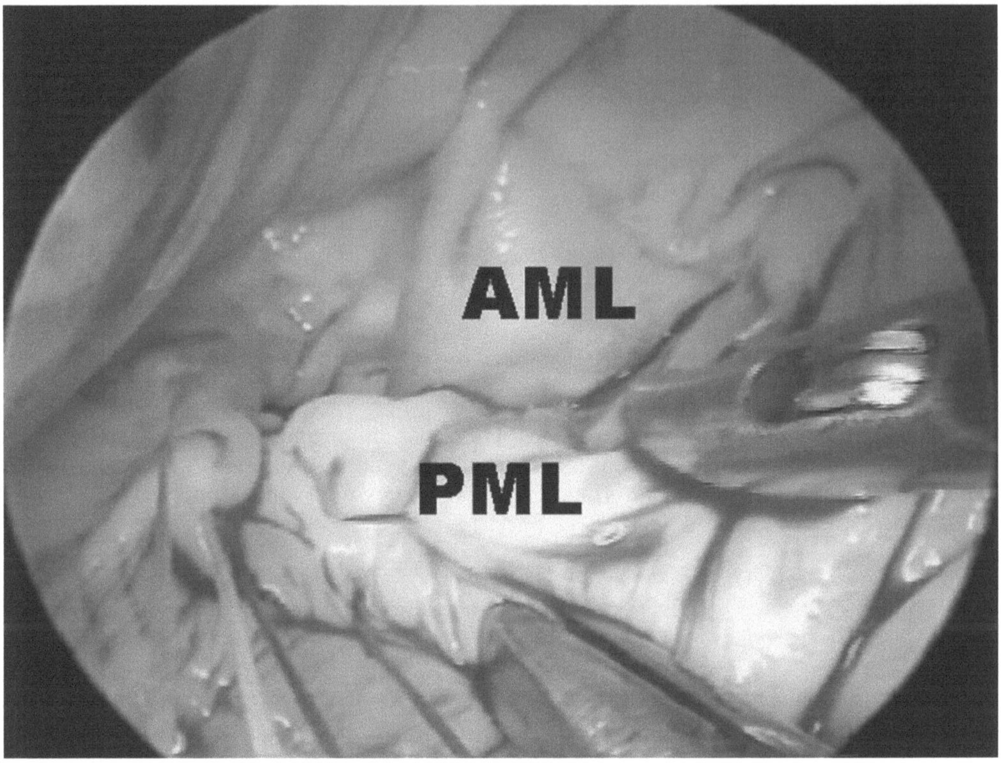

Fig. 9. Operative view of the mitral valve with annular sutures being placed with endoscopic instruments. The view of the anterior and posterior mitral leaflets (AML and PML) and subvalvular apparatus is excellent.

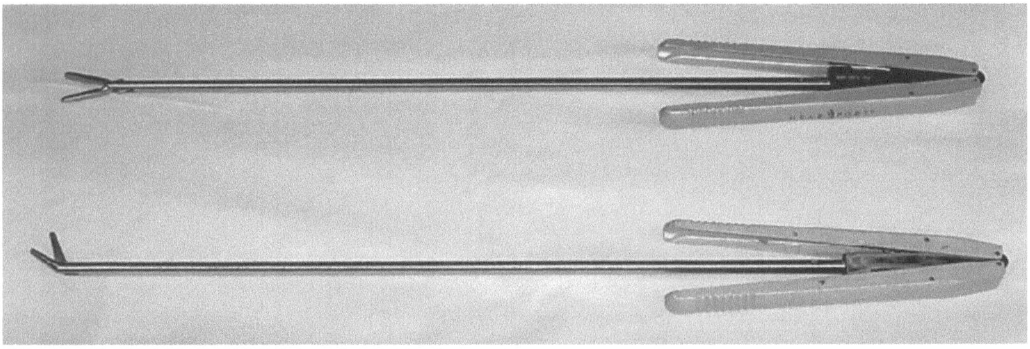

Fig. 10. Typical endoscopic instruments (forceps above and scissors below) used to reach the mitral valve.

the left atrium and mitral valve is generally excellent and sufficient to perform complex repairs of the mitral valve and subvalvular apparatus. The mitral procedure itself is performed in a manner identical to that with sternotomy, with the exception that endoscopic instruments are required due to the distance to the mitral valve and due to the limited incision (**Fig. 9**). These endoscopic instruments include endoscopic forceps, endoscopic needle drivers, endoscopic scissors, and endoscopic knot pushers (**Fig. 10**).

Upon completion of the mitral procedure, the left atrium is closed in a standard fashion with a left ventricular vent passed through the left atrial incision, through the mitral valve, and into the left ventricle. Several important adjuncts are used to air the heart. First, the entire thoracotomy field may be flooded with carbon dioxide throughout the case *(32)*. Second, with the left atrium closed around the left ventricular vent by a tourniquet, suction is applied to the left ventricular vent with the aorta is still clamped. Ideally, some of the vent cannula holes should be in the left ventricle, and some holes should also be in the left atrium. Third, the patient is turned side to side while the perfusionist fills the heart with blood. Once the heart appears to be adequately de-aired on transesophageal echo, the patient is placed in Trendelenberg position, suction is applied to the aortic root vent, and the aorta is unclamped. The patient is maintained in Trendelenberg position for 2 min after a weaning from cardiopulmonary bypass. Any residual air on echo can be aspirated through the aortic root vent or cleared down the right coronary artery. Once the heart is well de-aired on echo, the ventricular vent is removed, closure of the left atriotomy is completed, and the patient is weaned from cardiopulmonary bypass.

Aortic decannulation is performed by tying the dual aortic purse-string sutures directly through the thoracotomy incision. The percutaneous venous cannula is simply withdrawn and the subcutaneous tissue closed with absorbable suture. If a groin incision is used, the arterial and venous purse strings are tied, and the groin incision is closed in a standard fashion. The surgeon should have a low threshold to repair or patch any small, diseased, or narrowed femoral artery. A single 19 fr rubber drain may be placed in the pericardium and brought through the chest wall. The drain is placed so that both the pericardial space and the pleural space are drained postoperatively. A single 36 fr chest tube is left in the pleural space for the first 12–24 h. The fourth rib is repaired with a #4 sternal wire if the rib was divided. The skin incision and any other port sites are closed with absorbable sutures.

POSTOPERATIVE CARE

Postoperative management differs little from that of standard sternotomy patients. Because bleeding is generally minimal, the pleural drain is usually removed within 12 h and the 19 fr drain is removed after 3–5 d. Postoperative pain appears to be similar to sternotomy for the first 1–3 d, and thereafter appears to be less than with sternotomy *(33)*. Patients appear to have greater arm use and earlier mobility than with sternotomy *(24)*. Thoracotomy pain in the first 48 h responds well to anti-inflammatory agents, but at the risk of renal complications. All patients are given an intravenous bolus of 750 mg of procainamide while on cardiopulmonary bypass and are maintained on a procainamide (or quinidine) drip until oral antiarrhythmic agents can be started on the second postoperative day. If patients are discharged in sinus rhythm, the antiarrhythmic therapy is continued for 2–3 wk or longer, depending on the likelihood of postoperative atrial fibrillation. Anticoagulation is used only for those patients at risk for atrial fibrillation after discharge or with mechanical prostheses. All patients are discharged on aspirin. Median hospital stay in our experience is 5 d. Patients are advised to return to driving in 2 wk and may return to working in 3–6 wk depending on their overall condition.

POTENTIAL PITFALLS

As mentioned previously, body habitus can preclude the port-access approach or can require a modified approach. Body habitus can preclude either aortic or femoral cannulation, requiring the alternative technique. In patients with lung disease who cannot tolerate single-lung ventilation, or in patients in whom one-lung ventilation cannot be obtained, femoral arterial cannulation would be the next alternative. Patients with disease of the femoral artery, iliac artery, or abdominal or thoracic aorta may be better candidates for central aortic cannulation.

The endoclamp may have difficulty occluding an ascending aorta of 3.5 cm or larger diameter. In these patients, ventricular fibrillation or an external aortic clamp should be used. If the femoral venous cannula cannot be placed into the superior vena cava on cardiopulmonary bypass, a separate cannula should be placed in the superior vena cava to guarantee drainage of the superior vena cava and right atrium while retracting on the left atrium. In patients with preexisting pericardial adhesions, placement of temporary ventricular pacing wires may be difficult or impossible. On rare occasions, a small left thoracotomy can be performed in the left fourth intercostal space to place permanent epicardial pacing leads on the left ventricle.

A number of techniques are available to handle intraoperative difficulties. Coronary sinus perforation can generally be repaired while on cardiopulmonary bypass by exposing the coronary sinus posterior to the inferior vena cava through the right thoracotomy incision. In the event of more serious cardiac injury or problems inaccessible from a small right thoracotomy, the thoracotomy incision can be extended medially and laterally into a full right anterolateral thoracotomy. The incision can also be extended across the midline into a transverse sternotomy, or the thoracotomy can be abandoned and a standard median sternotomy performed. Bleeding most commonly comes from the right chest wall, so all accessible wounds and puncture sites should be examined closely for hemostasis prior to closing the chest. Ascending aortas 4 cm or more in diameter ideally should not be cannulated through the thoracotomy due to the difficulty repairing any injury to a dilated and abnormal aorta.

RESULTS

Early feasibility studies generated initial enthusiasm for port-access techniques. By the year 2001, over 18,000 port-access procedures had been performed worldwide. There has since been a progression to evaluate this technology critically, comparing port access to conventional surgery with respect to patient outcomes. As of 2001, a small number of totally endoscopic mitral valve operations have been performed using robotics to perform the mitral valve procedure, while the port-access platform provides femoral vein-to-femoral artery cardiopulmonary bypass and cardioplegic arrest with an endoclamp.

Intraoperative Factors

Recent reviews of port-access mitral valve surgery at single institutions and the Port Access International Registry (PAIR) have looked at intraoperative and patients outcomes following port-access mitral surgery, with excellent results (Table 1). Both mitral valve repair and replacement have been performed with cardiopulmonary bypass times that range from 135 to 212 min and crossclamp times from 95 to 133 min. Despite the age of this technology, conversion to a median sternotomy has had reported rates of 0–9.5%.

Hospital Outcomes

Similarly, in-hospital results following port-access mitral surgery have been outstanding in light of the age of this technology. Thirty-day mortality ranged from 1.1 to 5.0% with ICU stays of 1–1.8 d and mean hospital length of stay between 5 and 11 d (Table 1).

Table 1
Outcomes of Mitral Operations in Largest Clinical Series Using Port-Access Approach

Author, Year (Ref.)	*No. of Patients*	*Mean Age*	*Mitral Valve Repair*	*Mitral Valve Replacement*	*CPB[a] Time (min)*	*Crossclamp Time (min)*	*Conversion Rate[b] (%)*	*Mortality*	*ICU LOS[c]*	*Hospital LOS*	*Atrial Fibril. (%)*	*Stroke (%)*
Glower, 1998 (24)	21	60	13	8	212	133	5	0	NA[d]	6	28	0
Mohr, 1998 *(7)*	51	58	28	23	133	72	12	9.8	2	13	NA	NA
Gulielmos, 2000 *(34,35)*	33	64	9	24	NA	108	10	3	1	10	NA	NA
Glower, 2000 *(36)*	1059	58	491	568	127	92	4	1.6–5.5	0.9	5	10	2.6
Chaney, 2000 *(37)*	19	57	NA	NA	145	105	NA	NA	1.3	6.1	11	NA
Reichenspurner, 2000 *(39,40)*	50	61	26	24	125	83	NA	0	1.5	9	NA	NA
Vanerman, 2000 *(28)*	121	60	75	46	140	101	4	2	2.1	8.7	NA	1
Grossi, 2001 *(38)*	100	56	100	NA	135	NA	0	0	NA	NA	NA	2

[a]Cardiopulmonary bypass time.
[b]Conversion to full sternotomy.
[c]Intensive care unit length of stay.
[d]Not available/reported.

Table 2
Institutional Experience with Port-Access Mitral Valve Surgery

	Mitral Valve		
	Repair	*Replacement*	*Total*
No. of patients	191	111	302
Age (yr)	58 ± 14	58 ± 14	58 ± 15
Intraoperative date			
Crossclamp time (min)	104 ± 57	90 ± 65	99 ± 60
Cardiopulmonary bypass time (min)	181 ± 49	194 ± 54	186 ± 51
Surgery time (min)	332 ± 62	353 ± 75	339 ± 67
Postoperative data			
Transfusion (units)	2 ± 4	2 ± 2	2 ± 3
Chest tube output (mL)	422 ± 470	330 ± 274	389 ± 413
Intubation time (h)	8 ± 5	11 ± 12	9 ± 8
Length of stay (d)	7 ± 10	7 ± 4	7 ± 8
Adverse events			
Aortic dissection	0 (%)	0 (0%)	0 (0%)
Wound infection	0 (0%)	1 (1%)	1 (0.3%)
New pacemaker	2 (1%)	3 (3%)	5 (2%)
Stroke	1 (1%)	3 (3%)	4 (1%)
Reop for bleeding	10 (5%)	1 (1%)	11 (4%)
Conversion to sternotomy	3 (2%)	2 (2%0	5 (2%)
Reop on mitral valve	4 (2%)	1 (1%)	5 (2%)
Mortality	1 (1%)	0 (0%)	1 (0.3%)

In the PAIR study, the incidence of stroke was 2.6% and 2.8% for mitral valve repair and replacement, respectively. The incidence of renal failure and new atrial fibrillation was 2.1% and 10.4% for mitral repair and 3.3% and 10.0% for mitral replacement *(36)*. Early reports of aortic dissection have dramatically decreased with the use of direct aortic cannulation *(7,36,41)*. A multivariable analysis of the PAIR data showed that the major predictors of death were reoperation, older age, and mitral valve replacement *(36)*. Importantly, low case volume did not appear to be significantly associated with adverse outcomes. Using port access, complex repairs of the anterior mitral chordeae yields initial and early (2 yr) success rates equivalent to those after simple annuloplasty using port access *(42,43)*. Although difficult to quantify, cosmesis is generally superior with a small thoracotomy than with standard sternotomy, and cosmesis may be more relevant to the patient than to the physician.

Blood Transfusion

Transfusion practices vary among institutions, but several reports have documented median blood transfusion of 1–3 units (Table 2) *(24,38)*. When compared to conventional mitral valve repair or replacement, two case-controlled series demonstrated significantly less blood use in port access patients *(24,38)*. Trends have been for less chest tube output with port access relative to sternotomy *(24)*.

Comparison to Other Approaches

Port-access mitral valve surgery has been compared to conventional approaches in several case series. Postoperative pain scores were found to be significantly less between postoperative d 3 and 7 with port access relative to sternotomy *(33)*. Hospital stay has been similar or slightly decreased with port access *(24,38)*, with fewer wound or septic complications in all patients *(38)* and in elderly patients *(44)*. Port-access patients have returned to normal activity four weeks earlier than did sternotomy patients *(24)*. Alternatively, cardiopulmonary bypass, cross-clamp, and operative times are universally longer with port access as compared to conventional mitral surgery *(24,38,45)* (Table 1). The frequency of cerebral microemboli has not been different between techniques *(46)*.

Arom et al. *(47,48)* compared port access to partial sternotomy in 65 patients having aortic or mitral valve operation. Port-access patients had longer clamp time and longer surgery time. However, port-access patients had less atrial fibrillation and returned to work 4 wk earlier. In a comparison of port access to the Chitwood mini-mitral procedure, Aybek et al. *(49)* found that port access had longer clamp time, longer pump time, longer procedure time, and more blood loss.

Learning Curves

As described above, operative times are consistently longer for port-access procedures, and as with any new technology there is significant interest in learning curves and the effect of institutional volumes on outcomes. A recent study from PAIR data examined the determinants of operative times looking at institutional experience, case volumes, and procedure type *(36)*. Interestingly, institutional case volume was not a determinant of operative time. Instead, procedure type (mitral valve repairs particularly) was an important factor. A multivariable analysis of registry data also showed that institutional volume was not significantly associated with death, stroke, or reoperation for bleeding *(36,50)*. Interestingly, time spent off-pump accounted for significant variation among institutions. Furthermore, operative times continued to decrease beyond 100 cases, suggesting that learning in port-access surgery is a continuing process *(50)*.

CONCLUSIONS

Port-access approaches to the mitral valve have been shown to be safe and effective. Relative to sternotomy, port access may have the advantages of better cosmesis, earlier postoperative patient mobilization, less sepsis and wound complications, and possibly less blood loss and use. Port access may be especially advantageous in patients (1) with prior sternotomy, (2) at risk for sternal complications, (3) with impaired mobility, and (4) placing a high value on cosmesis. These advantages are at the expense of longer operating time, longer learning curve, and greater equipment costs.

Port access is applicable in over 90% of isolated mitral procedures, and even complex mitral repairs can be performed with excellent short-term outcome. The driving forces at institutions applying port access to the mitral valve include patient biases toward minimally invasive approaches, a desire to improve patient outcome and further technology, and perhaps a desire to obtain a marketing advantage. Ultimately, broader application of port-access technology may be limited. There are certainly specific applications for port-access techniques, particularly in reoperative situations where a right chest approach is easier. Furthermore, port-access techniques have been considered a transition to total endoscopic or robotic repairs of the mitral valve. Nonetheless, port-access approaches to mitral reconstruction offer important alternatives to conventional techniques and are associated with excellent outcomes.

FUTURE

In a few short years, port-access technology has proven to be a safe and effective method to operate on the mitral valve. Benchmark comparisons to conventional surgery have shown similar efficacy and modest improvements in patient recovery and satisfaction. Importantly, as experience grows, specific indications for port access (such as reoperative surgery) will be better refined. Nonetheless, the future of port-access mitral surgery is unclear. Many continue to advocate that port access is simply a stepping stone to a totally endoscopic repair of the mitral valve. The goal of totally endoscopic mitral surgery is becoming possible using port access, but only with robotic assistance *(22,28,51–54)*. At several institutions, port access has been used to perform mitral operations through a small thoracotomy using robotic assistance to manipulate the camera or surgical instruments *(39–41,51–53)*. Robotics in turn could greatly facilitate training of younger surgeons in minimally invasive techniques. Robotics can for the first time allow remote surgery with the operating surgeon and the patient in two different locations *(55)*. However, current robotic procedures have disadvantages of expensive and bulky instrumentation, longer operating times, need for a groin incision, and remaining technical issues such as limited facility with knot tying.

The ultimate market share enjoyed by port access for isolated mitral valve surgery will be a balance between patient demand for the procedure vs limited time, limited resources, and limited experience of providing physicians and hospitals. Efforts to simplify the port-access platform will continue over the next few years as robotic technology evolves. As instrumentation and imaging improve, port-access approaches to the mitral valve may have broader appeal. It is clear that subsets of patients can benefit from the port-access approach to mitral operations, and continued development of techniques, equipment, and education will help define these cohorts.

REFERENCES

1. Pompili MF, Stevens JH, Burdon TA, et al. Port-access mitral valve replacement in dogs. J Thorac Cardiovasc Surg 1996;112:1268–1274.
2. Pompili MF, Yakub A, Siegel LC, Stevens JH, Awang Y, Burdon TA. Port-access mitral valve replacement: initial clinical experience [abstr]. Circulation 1996;94:I-533.
3. Schwartz DS, Ribakove GH, Grossi EA, et al. Minimally invasive mitral valve replacement: port-access technique, feasibility, and myocardial functional preservation. J Thorac Cardiovasc Surg 1997;113:1022–1031.
4. Schwartz DS, Ribakove GH, Grossi EA, et al. Minimally invasive cardiopulmonary bypass with cardioplegic arrest: a closed chest technique with equivalent myocardial protection. J Thorac Cardiovasc Surg 1996;111:556–566.
5. Galloway AC, Ribakove GH, Miller JS, et al. Minimally invasive port-access valvular surgery: initial clinical experience [abstr]. Circulation 1997; I-508.
6. Fann JI, Pompili MF, Burdon TA, Stevens JH, St. Ghoar FG, Reitz BA. Minimally invasive mitral valve surgery. Semin Thorac Cardiovasc Surg 1997;9:320–330.
7. Mohr FW, Falk V, Diegeler A, Walther T, van Son JAM, Autschbach R. Minimally invasive port-access mitral valve surgery. J Thorac Cardiovasc Surg 1998;115:567–576.
8. Galloway AC, Shemin RJ, Glower DD, et al. First report of the Port Access International Registry. Ann Thorac Surg 1999;67:51–58.
9. Carpentier A, Loulmet D, Carpentier A, LeBret E, Haugades B, Petal D. Chirurgie a coeur ouvert par video-chirurgie et minithoracotomie—premier cas (valvuloplastie mitrale) opere avec success. L'Academie des Sciences: Sciences de la vie 1996;319:219–223.
10. Loulmet DF, Carpentier A, Cho PW, et al. Less invasive techniques for mitral valve surgery. J Thorac Cardiovasc Surg 1998;115:772–779.

11. Zapolanski A, Korver K, Pliam MB, Mengarelli L. Mitral valve surgery via a right anterior minithoracotomy with central aortic cannulation and no endoscopic assistance [abstr]. Heart Surg Forum 2001;4:S80.
12. Mishra YK, Malhotra R, Mehta Y, Sharma KK, Kasliwal RR, Trehan N. Minimally invasive mitral valve surgery through right anterolateral minithoracotomy. Ann Thorac Surg 1999;68:1520–1524.
13. El-Fiky MM, El-Sayegh T, El-Beishry AS, et al. Limited right anterolateral thoracotomy for mitral valve surgery. Eur J Cardiothorac Surg 2000;17:710–713.
14. Chitwood WR Jr, Elbeery JR, Chapman WHH, et al. Video-assisted minimally invasive mitral valve surgery: the "micro-mitral" operation. J Thorac Cardiovasc Surg 1997;113:413–414.
15. Chitwood WR Jr, Elbeery JR, Moran JF. Minimally invasive mitral valve repair using transthoracic aortic occlusion. Ann Thorac Surg 1997;63:1477–1479.
16. Chitwood WR Jr, Wixon CL, Elbeery JR, Moran JF, Chapman WHH, Lust RM. Video-assisted minimally invasive mitral valve surgery. J Thorac Cardiovasc Surg 1997;114:773–782.
17. Holman WL, Goldberg SP, Early LJ, et al. Right thoracotomy for mitral reoperation: analysis of technique and outcome. Ann Thorac Surg 2000;70:1970–1973.
18. Braxton JH, Higgins RS, Schwann TA, et al. Reoperative mitral valve surgery via right thoracotomy: decreased blood loss and improved hemodynamics. J Heart Valve Dis 1996;5:169–173.
19. Cohn LH. Right thoracotomy, femorofemoral bypass, and deep hypothermia for re-replacement of the mitral valve. Ann Thorac Surg 1997;64:578–579.
20. Srivastava AK, Garg SK, Ganjoo AK. Approach for primary mitral valve surgery: right anterolateral thoracotomy or median sternotomy. J Heart Valve Dis 1998;7:370–375.
21. Reichenspurner H, Boehm D, Reichart B. Minimally invasive mitral valve surgery using three-dimensional video and robotic assistance. Semin Thorac Cardiovasc Surg 1999;11:235–243.
22. Chitwood WR Jr. Video-assisted and robotic mitral valve surgery: toward an endoscopic surgery. Semin Thor Cardiovasc Surg 1999;11:191–205.
23. Vanerman H, Wellens F, DeGeest R, Degrieck I, VanPraet F. Video-assisted port-access mitral valve surgery: from debut to routine surgery. Will trocar-port- access cardiac surgery ultimately lead to robotic cardiac surgery? Semin Thorac Cardiovasc Surg 1999;11:223–234.
24. Glower DD, Landolfo KP, Clements F, et al. Mitral valve operation via Port Access versus median sternotomy. Eur J Cardiothorac Surg 1998;14:S143–S147.
25. Chitwood WR Jr. Video-assisted mitral valve surgery: using the Chitwood Clamp. Op Tech Thorac Cardiovasc Surg 2000;5:190–202.
26. Peters WS, Burdon TA, Pompili MF. Port-access cardiac surgery: a system analysis. Perfusion 1998;13:253–258.
27. Grossi EA, Ribakove G, Galloway AC, Colvin SB. Minimally invasive mitral valve surgery with endovascular balloon technique. Op Tech Cardiovasc Surg 2000;5:176–189.
28. Vanerman H, Farhat F, Wellens F, et al. Minimally invasive video-assisted mitral valve surgery: from port-access towards a totally endoscopic procedure. J Card Surg 2000;15:51–60.
29. Colvin SB, Grossi EA, Ribakove G, Galloway AC. Minimally invasive aortic and mitral valve operation. Op Tech Cardiovasc Surg 2000;5:212–220.
30. Chitwood WR Jr, Nifong LW. Minimally invasive videoscopic mitral valve surgery: the current role of surgical robotics. J Card Surg 2000;15:61–75.
31. Glower DD, Komtebedde J, Clements FM, Debruijn NP, Stafford-Smith M, Newman MF. Direct aortic cannulation for Port-Access mitral or coronary bypass operations. Ann Thorac Surg 1999;68:1878–1880.
32. Gillinov AM, Cosgrove DM. Minimally invasive mitral valve surgery: mini- sternotomy with extended transseptal approach. Semin Thorac Cardiovasc Surg 1999;11:206–211.
33. Walther T, Falk V, Metz S, et al. Pain and quality of life after minimally invasive versus conventional cardiac surgery. Ann Thorac Surg 1999;67:1643–1647.
34. Gulielmos V, Tugtekin SM, Kappert U, et al. Three-year follow-up after port access mitral valve surgery. J Card Surg 2000;15:43–50.
35. Gulielmos V, Wunderlich J, Dangel M, et al. Minimally invasive mitral valve surgery—clinical experiences with a Port Access system. Eur J Cardiothorac Surg 1998;14:S148–S153.
36. Glower DD, Siegel LC, Frischmeyer KJ, et al. Predictors of outcome in a multicenter Port-Access valve registry. Ann Thorac Surg 2000;70:1054–1059.
37. Chaney MA, Durazo-Arvizu RA, Fluder EM, et al. Port-access minimally invasive cardiac surgery increases surgical complexity, increases operating room time, and facilitates early postoperative hospital discharge. Anesthesiology 2000;92:1637–1645.

38. Grossi EA, Galloway AC, Ribakove GH, et al. Impact of minimally invasive valvular heart surgery: a case-control study. Ann Thorac Surg 2001;71:807–810.
39. Reichenspurner H, Boehm DH, Gulbins H, et al. Three-dimensional video and robot-assisted port-access mitral valve operation. Ann Thorac Surg 2000;69:1181–1182.
40. Reichenspurner H, Weltz A, GulielmosV, Boehm DH, Reichart B. Port-Access cardiac surgery using endovascular cardiolpumonary bypass: theory, practice, and results. J Card Surg 1999;14:275–280.
41. Mohr FW, Onnasch JF, Falk V, et al. The evolution of minimally invasive mitral valve surgery - 2 year experience. Eur J Cardiovasc Surg 1999;17:233–239.
42. Glower DD, Siegel LC, Galloway AC, et al. Predictors of operative time in multicenter Port-Access valve registry: institutional differences in learning. Heart Surg Forum 2001;4:40–46.
43. Grossi EA, LaPietra A, Ribakove GH, et al. Minimally invasive versus sternotomy approaches for mitral reconstruction: comparison of intermediate-term results. J Thorac Cardiovasc Surg 2001;1221:708–713.
44. Grossi EA, Galloway AC, Ribakove GH, et al. Minimally invasive port access surgery reduces operative morbidity for valve replacement in the elderly. Heart Surg Forum 1999;2:212–215.
45. Ferdinand FD, Trace C, Priest BP, Sutter FP, Kowey PR. Minimally invasive mitral valve surgery: less may be more [abstr]. Heart Surg Forum 2001;4:S81.
46. Schneider F, Onnasch JF, Falk V, Walther T, Autschbach R, Mohr FW. Cerebral microemboli during minimally invasive and conventional mitral valve operations. Ann Thorac Surg 2000;70:1094–1097.
47. Arom KV, Emery RW, Kshettry VR, Dubois KA. Evaluation of two new heart valve surgery techniques: partial sternotomy and port-access approaches. Eur J Cardiothorac Surg 1999;16:S99–S102.
48. Arom KV, Emery RW, Kshettry VR, Janey PA. Comparison between port-access and less invasive valve surgery. Ann Thorac Surg 2000;68:1525–1528.
49. Aybek T, Dogan S, Wimmer-Greinecker G, Westphal K, Moritz A. The micro- mitral operation comparing the Port-Access technique and the transthoracic clamp technique. J Card Surg 2000;15:76–81.
50. Glower D, Landolfo K, Kypson A, Bashore T, Harrison K, Wang A. Is port- access applicable to complex mitral valve repair? [abstr]. Heart Surg Forum 2001;4:S73.
51. Onnasch JF, Falk V, Schneider F, Diegler A, Autschbach R, Mohr FW. Minimally invasive mitral valve surgery—experience in 361 patients [abstr]. Heart Surg Forum 2001;4:S81.
52. Chitwood WR Jr, Nifong LW, Elbeery JE, et al. Robotic mitral valve repair: trapezoidal resection and prosthetic annuloplasty with the da Vinci surgical system. J Thorac Cardiovasc Surg 2000;120:1171–1172.
53. Falk V, Autschbach R, Krakor R, et al. Computer-enhanced mitral valve surgery: toward a total endoscopic procedure. Semin Thorac Cardiovasc Surg 1999;11:244–249.
54. Carpentier A, Loulmet D, Aupecle B, Berrebi A, Relland J. Computer-assisted cardiac surgery. Lancet 1999;353:379–380.
55. Autschbach R, Onnasch JF, Falk V, et al. The Liepzig experience with robotic valve surgery. J Card Surg 2000;15:82–87.

21 Minimally Invasive Aortic Valve Surgery

Jerome Sepic, MD *and Lawrence H. Cohn,* MD

CONTENTS

INTRODUCTION
OPERATIVE TECHNIQUES
INSTITUTIONAL EXPERIENCE
CONCLUSION
REFERENCES

INTRODUCTION

Corrective aortic valve surgery, both replacement and repair, has been a significant advancement in modern medical science. These operations have given countless patients with aortic stenosis and aortic regurgitation longer and more productive lives. Starting with the aortic prosthetic valves developed by Harken and Starr and extending to the current era of mechanical, bioprosthetic, and biological valves (including homografts and autografts), aortic valve replacement surgery has evolved considerably and has proven to be efficacious *(1,2)*. In addition, numerous reparative techniques such as commissurotomy, debridement, and prolapse reduction have been developed to, when possible, preserve the native aortic valve.

In the last 30 years, aortic valve surgery typically has been performed using a full median sternotomy with cardiopulmonary bypass (CPB), with direct aortic and right atrial or bicaval cannulation. Outcomes have improved dramatically with the use of varying degrees of systemic hypothermia and myocardial protection with antegrade cardioplegia and, more recently, retrograde cardioplegia via coronary sinus catheters.

Since the first report by Cosgrove in 1996, minimally invasive aortic valve surgery has continued to be an evolving concept *(3)*. Its goals include reducing incision size, decreasing surgical trauma and pain, and improving cosmesis, patient satisfaction, and recovery times. However, the most important goal of minimally invasive aortic valve surgery must be to maintain or improve the efficacy and safety of conventional aortic valve surgery. Unlike minimally invasive coronary artery bypass grafting, which includes off-pump

From: *Contemporary Cardiology: Minimally Invasive Cardiac Surgery, Second Edition*
Edited by: D. J. Goldstein and M. C. Oz © Humana Press Inc., Totowa, NJ

coronary artery bypass (OPCAB), all aortic valve surgery to date requires the use of CPB. Therefore, minimally invasive aortic valve replacement and repair (MIAVR) technique developments have centered on different operative exposures and cannulation strategies.

Although numerous different MIAVR techniques have been proposed, characteristics of some techniques make them more feasible and more easily adopted then others. Ideally, low-morbidity techniques that have a relatively quick learning curve, use conventional instrumentation or economical variations, and provide versatile exposure and cannulation combinations are preferable. Additionally, these techniques should be applicable to a wide variety of first-time and reoperative patient candidates and should allow for all types of aortic valve replacements and repairs, as well as possible aortic root procedures when needed. If the necessity arises, conversion to full sternotomy exposure should be practical.

In this chapter, we will review the different operative techniques for MIAVR. Emphasis will be placed on detailed descriptions of varying surgical approaches and instrumentation. In addition, we will report our 365-patient experience with MIAVR at the Brigham and Women's Hospital from July 1996 to July 2001.

OPERATIVE TECHNIQUES

Preoperative Preparation

Each patient must be assessed on an individual basis when considering a minimally invasive approach. The patient's body habitus, operative history, and posteroanterior and lateral chest X-ray films should be carefully reviewed. Although not routinely necessary, spiral computed tomography (CT) can be an accurate preoperative study to assess aortic annulus position *(4)*. Obtaining adequate exposure can be complicated by marked obesity, significant chest wall abnormalities (pectus excavatum, deep anteroposterior diameter), and unusual cardiac orientation (extremely vertical or horizontal, left shift) *(5)*. The need for aortic valve surgery and concomitant procedures, such as coronary grafting or additional valve procedures, may not be amenable to some or all minimally invasive approaches. Transesophageal echocardiography is recommended for guiding cannulation, clearing intracardiac air, and assessing the technical results. Pulmonary artery catheter use is varied but, in general, recommended in elderly patients, those with decreased left ventricular function, and those with severe pulmonary hypertension. Transcutaneous defibrillator pads placed on patients may be useful.

Incisions

In general, there have been four operative approaches presented for minimally invasive aortic valve surgery. All four approaches utilize a less-than-10-cm incision and include the right parasternal incision, the right anterolateral thoracotomy, the transverse sternotomy, and variations of the mini-sternotomy. Numerous cannulation combinations are possible, including the aorta, atrium, axillary artery/vein, innominate vein, and femoral artery/vein.

Right Parasternal Incision

The right parasternal incision, as presented by Cosgrove in 1996, was the first reported MIAVR technique (**Fig. 1**) *(3)*. A 5–10-cm incision is made, extending from the lower border of the second costal cartilage to the upper border of the fifth costal cartilage. Once the pectoralis major muscle is divided, the second and third costal cartilages are exposed

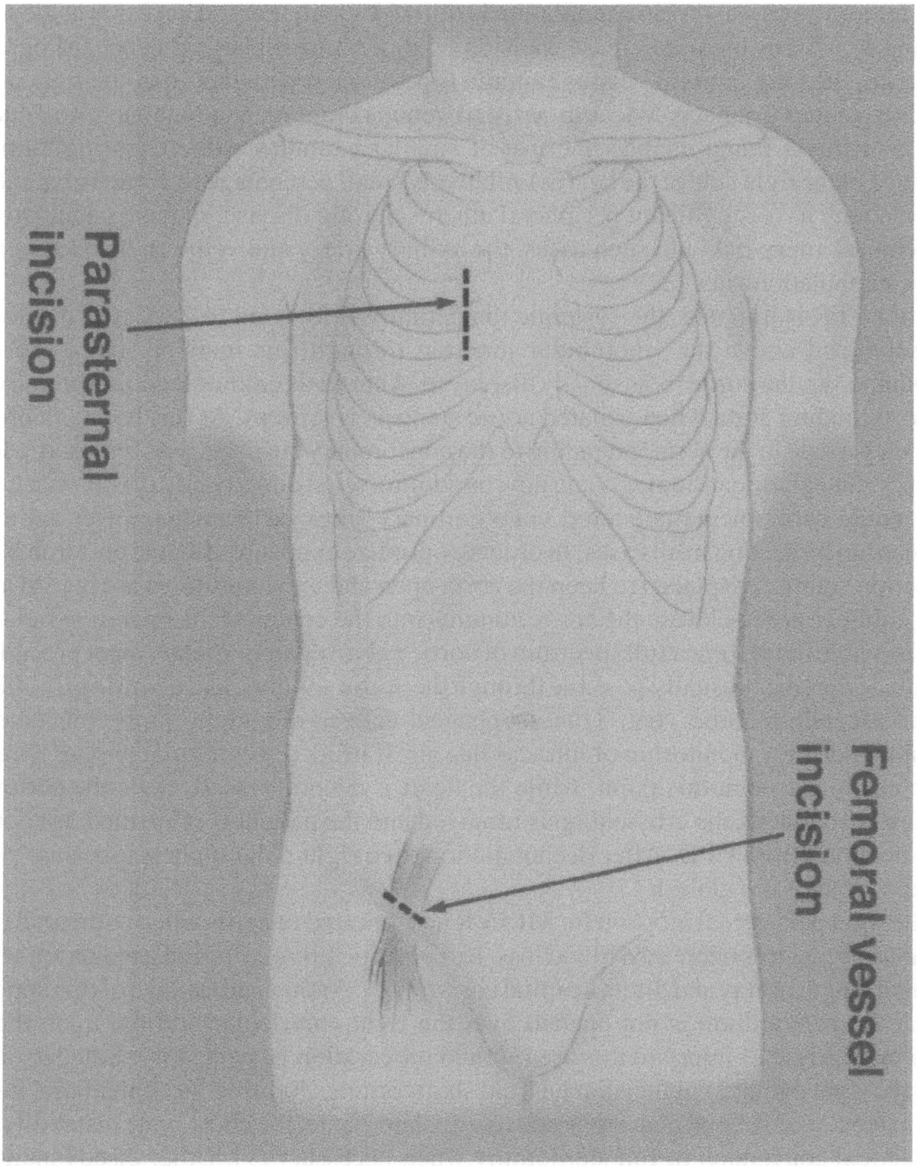

Fig. 1. A right parasternal skin incision over the second and third costal cartilages for aortic valve exposure is illustrated. The femoral vessels are exposed through an incision made 1 cm above the groin crease.

and totally excised. Of note, a costal cartilage sparing variation of this procedure, reported by Minale, involves cutting and retracting the third and fourth costal cartilages for exposure without excision *(6)*. Next, the right pleura is opened to prevent postoperative pericardial effusions. The intact right internal thoracic artery is retracted laterally and the pericardium is incised and marsupialized to the wound edges with multiple retraction sutures *(7)*. At this point the aorta is exposed along with the right atrium, which can be used for direct cannulation if needed, and the superior pulmonary vein, which can be used for venting if needed. In most cases, after heparinization, either percutaneous or open right femoral artery and vein cannulation is utilized. Open femoral access is achieved by making a 3–5-cm inguinal crease incision. Using transesophageal echocardiographic guidance, the long femoral venous cannula is positioned with the tip in the right atrium for CPB venous drainage. Vacuum-assisted venous drainage via regulated wall suction or a centrifugal pump enables the use of smaller cannulas while ensuring complete drainage of the right side of the heart. A relatively small percentage of aortic valve surgery patients may have significant peripheral atherosclerotic disease, making cannulation of the femoral artery risky. In such cases, the axillary artery and vein can be used as alternative cannulation sites *(8)*.

After CPB is initiated, the systemic temperature is lowered to 28°C and the aorta is crossclamped above the sinotubular junction through this incision. Once the heart decompresses, the aortic root is easily displayed. Antegrade cardioplegia can be delivered in the ascending aorta when isolated aortic stenosis is present. At this point, an oblique incision is made in the aorta, extending to the noncoronary cusp. In cases with aortic insufficiency, antegrade cardioplegia can now be administered directly into the coronary ostia. Retrograde cardioplegia delivered via a coronary sinus catheter may offer additional myocardial protection in all cases. In order to optimize exposure after the aortotomy, four retraction sutures are placed to keep the aorta open and tension sutures are placed above each commissure to elevate the aortic annulus into the center of the operative field. It is now possible to perform a full spectrum of aortic valve repair or replacement procedures. Adequate venting is usually possible through the aortic annulus, and de-airing is achieved via an ascending aortic vent. Transesophageal echocardiography probe placement is recommended for monitoring of intracardiac air. If needed, ventricular pacing wires are more easily placed at this point, while the heart is decompressed. Once the aortotomy closure is complete, the crossclamp is removed and the patient is rewarmed, transfused, and separated from CPB. After decannulation, two right pleural chest tubes are placed and the wounds are closed.

The right parasternal incision for MIAVR has reported benefits when compared to full sternotomy, such as decreased blood loss, less postoperative pain, and a reduction of both hospital length of stay and direct hospital costs *(9,10)*. Another advantage of this approach is that the pericardium is not opened over the right ventricular outflow tract, thereby reducing the risk of injury to this area should reoperation be necessary. Since its inception, the right parasternal incision has had shortcomings limiting its clinical use, including instances of suboptimal aortic valve exposure, anterior chest wall instability, and impractical conversion to full sternotomy when necessary *(9)*. Other disadvantages of this approach include complications associated with femorofemoral cannulation, frequently necessary due to incision constraints limiting direct cannulation. Owing to the above-mentioned disadvantages and the subsequent development of more versatile approaches, the right parasternal incision is no longer extensively used for MIAVR.

Right Anterolateral Thoracotomy

A right anterolateral thoracotomy for MIAVR was first described by Benetti in 1997 *(11)*. For this approach, the patient is either positioned on the operating table in a 30° left lateral decubitus position with the right arm elevated above the head or in the standard supine position. A 5–7-cm incision is made through the third intercostal space and an adapted rib spreader (Access Platform, CTS, Inc., Menlo Park, CA) is used to expose the aortic root, the right atrium, and the right superior pulmonary vein. CPB cannulation is established via the right femoral artery and the right atrium. Alternatively, a long femoral venous cannula positioned in the right atrium can be used, as previously described. Venting is performed through the right superior pulmonary vein. Upon completion of a transverse aortotomy and placement of commissural sutures, aortic valve replacement or repair is completed.

Avoidance of rib fractures when establishing exposure with this technique limits postoperative pain. Benetti contends that the right anterolateral thoracotomy is a less traumatic and painful approach because removal of rib or cartilage fragments is not required *(11)*. This approach is useful when combined aortic and mitral valve procedures are necessary *(12)*. However, the right anterolateral thoracotomy for isolated aortic valve procedures provides some exposure limitations and is not practical for conversion to full sternotomy, if necessary. Overall, this approach has not been widely adopted for MIAVR.

Transverse Sternotomy

The transverse sternotomy for MIAVR consists of a small vertical or horizontal skin incision with the sternum being transected at the level of the third intercostal space. Both internal thoracic arteries are ligated and divided. A small retractor allows access to aortic root, the superior vena cava, and the right atrium. CPB is established by directly cannulating the aorta and the right atrium (a superior vena caval cannula can be added). Alternatively, venous drainage can be performed using a long femoral vein cannula, as previously described. Once the diseased aortic valve is repaired or replaced, the sternotomy is closed with two interrupted steel wires.

The benefits of the transverse sternotomy for MIAVR include good exposure of the aortic valve and the possibility of direct cannulation for CPB through the incision. Although only a small percentage of isolated aortic valve surgery patients will eventually require coronary revascularization, the sacrifice of both internal thoracic arteries is potentially detrimental should coronary artery bypass grafting ever be necessary *(13)*. This approach can result in sternal instability in some cases. Should full sternotomy be necessary, the combination of these two approaches would result in four-piece fragmentation of the sternum and a more complex sternal closure. In at least one small series, comparing the transverse sternotomy to median sternotomy for aortic valve replacement, the authors found unacceptably high mortality and morbidity rates with the transverse sternotomy *(14)*. In general, the transverse sternotomy approach has not been adopted on a wide scale for MIAVR.

Mini-sternotomy

Since the T mini-sternotomy was first popularized by Gundry, numerous variations of the mini-sternotomy approach for MIAVR have been proposed *(15)*. The T mini-sternotomy consists of a 6–10-cm midline skin incision and a reverse T sternal midline incision made into the second, third, or fourth intercostal space (**Fig. 2**). Other commonly used variations of the mini-sternotomy include the "j," the "J" or reverse "C," and the hemi-sternotomy without horizontal transection. Svensson described the "j" sternotomy as consisting of an upper midline sternotomy that extends to a right intercostal space, preserving the left sternum. This approach is especially useful when good exposure of the ascending aorta or aortic arch is required. The "J" or reverse "C" sternotomy, also described by Svensson, preserves the upper sternum by using an incision of the right sternum at the first intercostal space *(16)*. Tam has described a hemi-sternotomy approach that consists of a partial upper sternotomy without transection of the sternum *(17)*. With these exposures, it is relatively easy to cannulate the right atrium or innominate

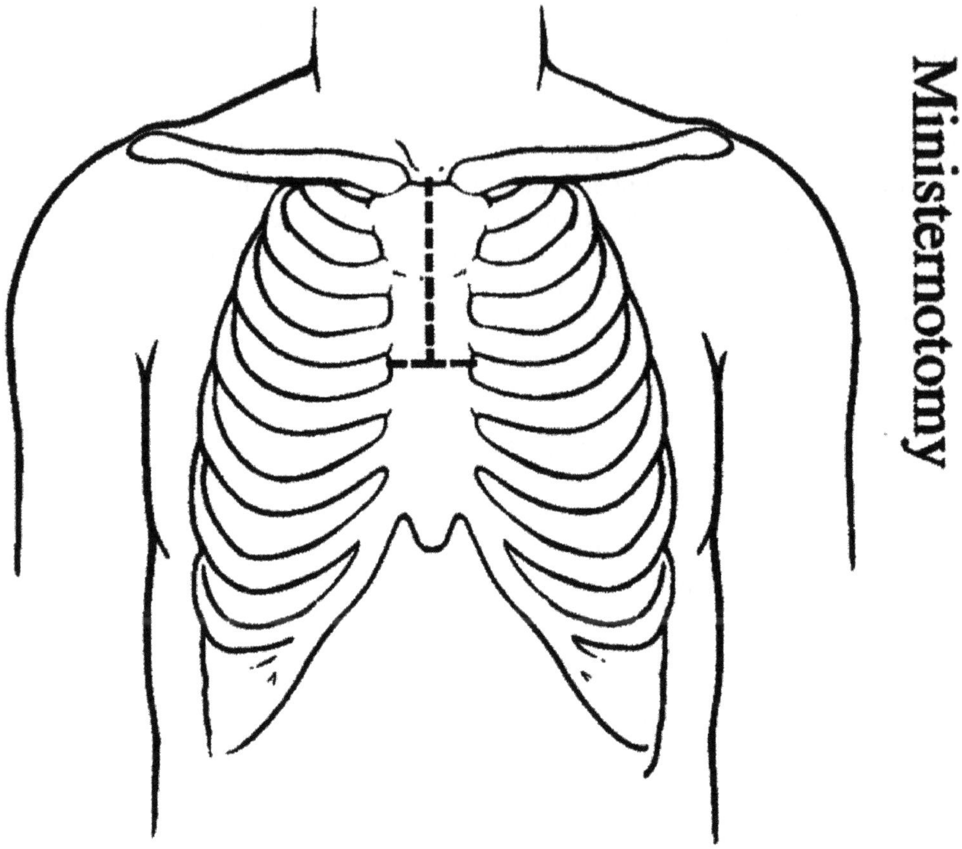

Fig. 2. An upper T mini-sternotomy for aortic valve exposure.

vein and the distal ascending aorta directly. Vents can be placed either transannular or in the right superior pulmonary vein.

The mini-sternotomy approach allows for good exposure during MIAVR and a variety of aortic root procedures, including full root, hemi-root, and subcoronary techniques for implantation of homografts or stentless bioprostheses, as well as valved conduits *(18)*. This approach, compared to full sternotomy for aortic valve operations, has been reported to reduce incisional trauma and duration of ventilation, decrease blood loss and postoperative pain, and result in a cosmetically superior wound (**Fig. 3**) *(19,20)*. The mini-sternotomy is particularly useful in reoperative aortic valve operations. In this group, peripheral cannulation should be done before the mini-sternotomy is performed, in case of injury to vital structures adherent to the underside of the sternum. In a comparison between reoperative aortic valve replacement with partial upper mini-sternotomy vs full sternotomy, the minimal incision avoided unnecessary lower mediastinal dissection, thereby reducing blood loss, transfusion requirements, and total operative times *(21)*. Additional benefits of mini-sternotomy include direct cannulation (avoiding possible complications associated with femoral cannulation) and easy conversion to full sternotomy, if necessary. The mini-sternotomy is currently the most popular approach for minimally invasive aortic valve and aortic root procedures.

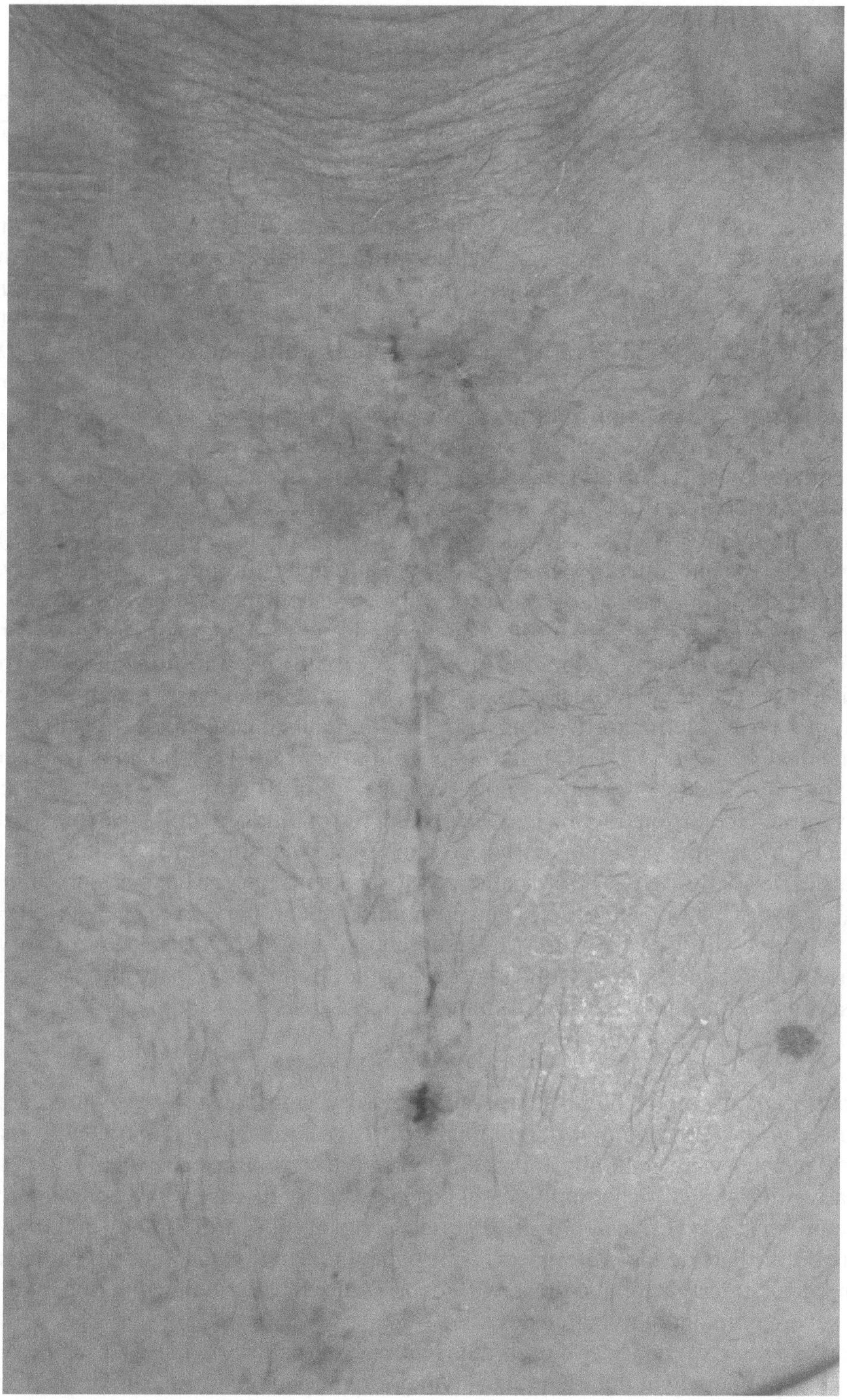

Fig. 3. A mini-sternotomy incision scar after aortic valve replacement.

MINIMALLY INVASIVE AORTIC VALVE SURGERY: A 5-YR EXPERIENCE

In this section, we will summarize our 5-yr experience with minimally invasive aortic valve replacement and repair at the Brigham and Women's Hospital through July 2001.

Methods

Between July 1996 and July 2001, 365 patients (mean age 63.4 ± 14.5 yr) underwent minimally invasive aortic valve surgery through either an upper mini-sternotomy ($n = 326$, 89%), a right parasternal incision ($n = 37$, 10.1%), or a right thoracotomy ($n = 2$, 0.5%). Two hundred twenty-six (63.7%) were males and 47 (12.9%) were reoperations. Of the 365 patients, 363 (99.5%) underwent aortic valve replacement and 2 (0.5%) underwent aortic valve repair. The most common concomitant procedures performed included 17 (4.7%) ascending aorta repairs and 4 (1.1%) single-vessel coronary artery bypass graftings. In the 363 patient aortic valve replacement group, 174 (47.7%) received Carpentier–Edwards (Baxter Healthcare Corp., Santa Ana, CA) pericardial valves, 109 (29.9%) received St. Jude (St. Paul, MN) mechanical valves, 55 (15%) received homografts, and 23 (6.3%) received Hancock (Medtronic, Inc., Minneapolis, MN) porcine valves. The only operation that we have not attempted through a minimally invasive incision is the pulmonary autograft aortic valve replacement (Ross procedure).

The indication for surgery in this patient group was isolated aortic stenosis in 183 (50.3%), isolated aortic regurgitation in 99 (27.1%), and mixed aortic stenosis and regurgitation in 83 (22.7%). In order of frequency, the most common causes of aortic valve pathology were calcific aortic stenosis ($n = 244$, 66.8%), congenital ($n = 66$, 18.1%), rheumatic disease ($n = 17$, 4.7%), and endocarditis ($n = 15$, 4.1%). A majority of patients had New York Heart Association Functional Class II or III symptoms (mean 2.4 ± 0.6). Left ventricular ejection fraction (EF) was preserved or mildly depressed in most patients (mean EF 57.1 ± 11.1%). Preoperative rhythm was normal sinus in 324 (88.8%) patients and atrial fibrillation in 32 (8.8%) patients. Most patients underwent coronary angiography ($n = 296$, 81.1%), 238 (65.2%) had no significant coronary disease, 51 (14.0%) had one- to two-vessel disease requiring no intervention, and 7 (1.9%) had one- to two-vessel disease with preoperative angioplasty or stenting. Preoperative patient characteristics and surgical procedure details are summarized in Tables 1, 2, and 3.

Operative Techniques

Each patient's body habitus, operative history, and chest X-ray were carefully reviewed prior to proceeding with minimally invasive aortic valve surgery. High-risk and elderly patients were generally approached via a full sternotomy to expedite bypass and operative times. Significant multivessel coronary artery disease was a contraindication to the minimally invasive approach. Transesophageal echocardiography and transcutaneous defibrillator pads were used in all patients. A pulmonary artery catheter was reserved for elderly patients, those with depressed left ventricular function, and those with severe pulmonary hypertension.

Early in our experience, we used the right parasternal ($n = 37$, 10.1%) approach, as described previously in this chapter. The majority of patients were cannulated for CPB through a small (2–4-cm) incision above and parallel to the right groin crease. The most common cannulae we used included a 20F cannula (Sarns, Inc., Ann Arbor, MI) in the right femoral artery, and a long 23 to 27 fr Bio-Medicus cannula (Medtronic Bio-Medicus,

Table 1
Demographics Among Patients Undergoing Minimally Invasive Aortic Valve Surgery at One Institution

Demographics	*n*	*(%)*
Number of patients	365	
Age (yr)		
Mean	63.4 ± 14.5	
Range	25–93	
Men	226	63.7
NYHA[a] functional class	2.4 ± 0.6	
Aortic valve pathophysiology		
Aortic regurgitation	99	27.1
Aortic stenosis	183	50.3
Mixed	83	22.7
Aortic valve pathology		
Calcific	244	66.8
Congenital	66	18.1
Rheumatic	17	4.7
Endocarditis	15	4.1
Structural valve degeneration (reop)	11	3.0
Nonstructural valve degeneration (reop)	4	1.1
Periprosthetic Leak (reop)	2	0.5
Annulo-aortic ectasia	3	0.8
Dissection	1	0.3
Myxomatous	2	0.5
Left ventricular function		
Mean ejection fraction (EF, %)	57.1 ± 11.1	
Preserved function (EF > 50%)	294	80.5
Mild dysfunction (EF = 40–50%)	41	11.2
Moderate dysfunction (EF = 30–39%)	18	4.9
Severe dysfunction (EF < 30%)	12	3.3
Preoperatrive rhythm		
Normal sinus rhythm	324	88.8
Atrial fibrillation	32	8.8
Paced	9	2.5
Coronary artery disease		
None	238	65.2
One- to two-vessel, no intervention	51	14.0
One- to two-vessel, preoperative PTCA[b]	7	1.9
Coronary angiogram not performed	69	18.9

[a]New York Heart Association.
[b]Percutaneous transluminal coronary angioplasty.

Eden Prairie, MN) inserted into the right atrium via the right femoral vein. Later, we found it possible to avoid a groin incision by cannulating the ascending aorta with a wire-guided, thin-walled 20F arterial cannula equipped with a tapered, pliable dilator (Medtronic DLP, Grand Rapids, MI) and the right atrium via the right femoral vein using a 21F percutaneous Bio-Medicus cannula. However, we abandoned the right parasternal approach for aortic valve surgery due to limited adaptability and wound complications.

Table 2
Details of Surgical Procedures
Among 35 Patients Undergoing Aortic Valve Surgery

Operative details (n = 365)	*n*	%
Incision		
Hemisternotomy	326	89.3
Right parasternal	37	10.1
Right thoracotomy	2	0.0
Cannulation for cardiopulmonary bypass		
Arterial cannulation		
Aorta	307	0.8
Femoral artery	58	15.9
Venous cannulation		
Right atrium/SVC[a]	163	44.7
Femoral vein/SVC	156	42.7
Innominate vein	35	9.6
Innominate + femoral	11	3.0
Cardioplegia		
Antegrade only	162	44.4
Retrograde	6	2.0
Antegrade + retrograde	197	54.0
Procedure		
Aortic valve repair	2	0.5
Aortic valve replacement	363	99.5

[a]Superior vena cava.

Currently, we mainly use an upper mini-sternotomy ($n = 326$, 89.3%), carried into the third or fourth intercostal space on the right (**Fig. 4a**). A Koros sliding coronary artery bypass retractor (Baxter Corp., Chicago, IL) is used for exposure. Unless there is an ascending aortic aneurysm that must be resected, the distal aorta is usually cannulated. Alternatively, the femoral artery can be used for cannulation. Direct venous cannulation is most commonly used via a right-angle 24 fr cannula (Research Medical, Midvale, UT) positioned in the right atrium. Other possibilities for venous cannulation include innominate vein or femoral vein access (**Fig. 4b**) *(22)*. The use of smaller cannula sizes is feasible with vacuum-assisted venous drainage on CPB.

Both combination antegrade and retrograde ($n = 197$, 54.0%) and antegrade only ($n = 162$, 44.4%) cold blood potassium cardioplegia was used in the vast majority of these MIAVR cases. After crossclamping the aorta, antegrade cardioplegia was administered through the aortic root and/or by Spencer cannula into the coronary ostia; additional intermittent doses were given through the coronary ostia as necessary. Retrograde cardioplegia was delivered by a Heartport (Redwood City, CA) transjugular catheter to avoid wound clutter *(23)*. Additional myocardial protection was provided by moderate systemic hypothermia (28°C), which was used in the majority of cases.

Upon completion of either the aortic valve replacement or repair, a ventricular pacing wire was placed on the decompressed right ventricle prior to aortic crossclamp removal. Intracardiac air was evacuated through the aortic root and the left atrium with transesophageal echocardiographic confirmation. After discontinuing CPB and achiev-

Table 3
Intraoperative Details Among 365 Patients Undergoing Minimally Invasive Aortic Valve Surgery

Intraoperative details (n=365)	*n*	*%*
Operative number		
First time	320	87.7
Second time	39	10.7
Third time	5	1.4
Fifth time	1	0.3
Aortic valve repair	2	0.5
Aortic valve replacement	363	99.5
Carpentier Edwards pericardial	174	47.7
St Jude mechanical	109	29.9
Homograft	55	15.1
Hancock	23	6.3
Freestyle	1	0.3
Toronto SPV	1	0.3
Secondary procedures		
Ascending aortic aneurysm repair	17	4.7
One-vessel bypass grafting	4	1.1
Atrial septal defect repair	2	0.5
Ascending aorta endarterectomy	3	0.8
Left ventricular outflow tract repair	1	0.3
Left ventricular myectomy	1	0.3
Sinus valsalva aneurysm repair	1	0.3
Sub-aortic membrane repair	1	0.3
Excision of anterior mediastinal tumor	1	0.3
Closure of patent foramen ovale	1	0.3
Operative duration (min)		
Ischemic (aortic crossclamp)		
Mean ± SD	91.3 ± 40.5	
Median	80	
Cardiopulmonary bypass		
Mean ± SD	124.0 ± 50.5	
Median	112	

ing hemostasis, the incisions were closed. In the parasternal patients, the pectoralis muscles were reapproximated to the sternum. In several cases a Gor-Tex patch (W.L. Gore and Assoc., Inc., Elkton, MD) was used to reinforce the closure. In the mini-sternotomy patients, the sternum was closed with five or six stainless-steel sternal wires. Two mediastinal chest drains were routinely placed through previously placed stab incisions.

Results

Operative Data and Results

For the 365 MIAVR patients, mean aortic crossclamp and total CPB times were 91.3 ± 40.5 and 124.0 ± 50.5 min, respectively. The mean transfusion rate was 2.1 ± 5.1 U per patient. No blood products were transfused in 136 (37.3%) patients, and 39 (10.7%) patients required more than 4 U of packed red blood cells. Fifteen (4.1%) patients were

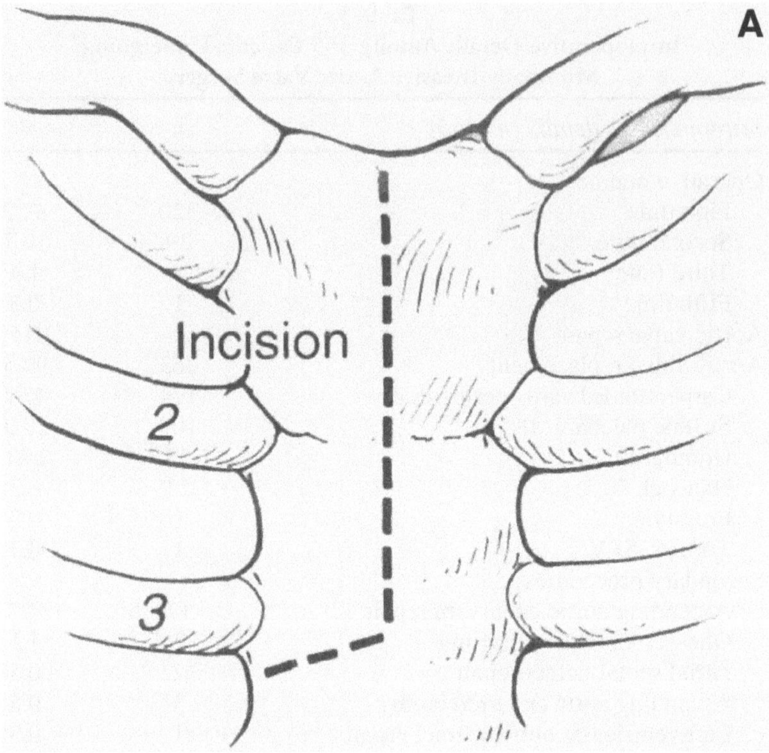

Fig. 4. (**a**) An upper mini-sternotomy consists of a 5–7 cm midline skin incision and a partial upper sternotomy extended to the second or third intercostal space. (**b**) Aortic valve exposure through an upper mini-sternotomy is illustrated. The venous (innominate—right atrial) and aortic cannulae exit from the superior aspect of the incision to aid exposure.

reexplored for bleeding. Fifty-four (14.8%) patients spent more than 48 h in the postoperative intensive care unit.

There were 9 (2.5%) operative deaths from arrhythmia ($n = 3$), stroke ($n = 2$), sepsis ($n = 2$), myocardial infarction ($n = 1$), and respiratory failure ($n = 1$). Early cardiac complications included new atrial fibrillation in 84 (23.0%) patients, conduction block requiring permanent pacemaker implantation in 23 (6.3%) patients, and myocardial infarction in 2 (0.5%) patients. Other significant early complications included strokes ($n =$ 10, 2.7%) and deep sternal infections ($n = 3$, 0.8%). The mean hospital length of stay (LOS) was 7.2±d; 79 (21.6%) patients had less than 5-d LOS and 104 (28.5%) had greater than 7-d LOS. A majority of patients were discharged to home, while 79 (21.6%) were transferred to a rehabilitation facility. Early postoperative data are summarized in Tables 4 and 5.

Late postoperative outcomes include 22 (6.0%) deaths from causes such as cancer, congestive heart failure, systemic infections, and respiratory failure. A total of five (1.4%) reoperative aortic valve replacements have been performed for valve endocarditis ($n = 4$, 1.1%) and scarification after aortic valve repair ($n = 1$, 0.3%). Two (0.5%) required reoperation to repair paravalvular leaks.

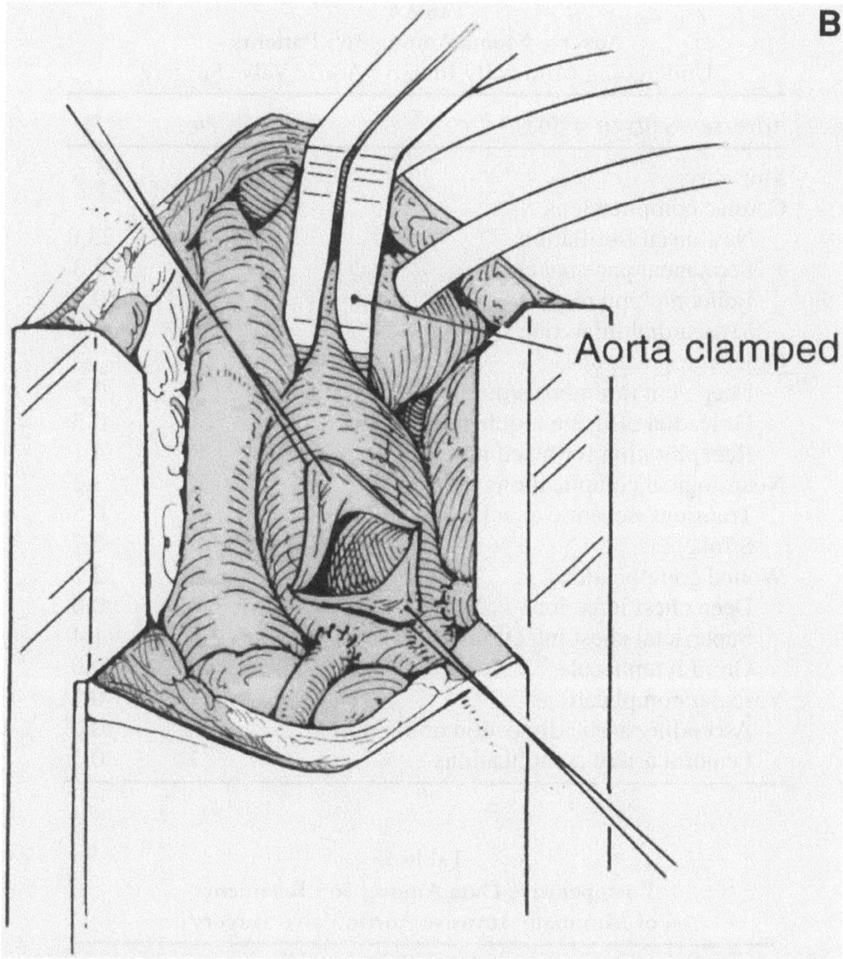

CONCLUSION

Over the past 5 years, minimally invasive aortic valve and root surgery has become feasible in a majority of patients. Currently at the Brigham and Women's Hospital, we use the mini sternotomy in aortic valve replacements and repairs, aortic root procedures, and reoperations. Contraindications to the mini-sternotomy include individual patient characteristics such as chest wall deformities, cardiac malposition, and obesity, concomitant multivessel coronary artery bypass grafting, and autograft aortic valve replacement (Ross procedure). Often, full sternotomy exposure is chosen in elderly patients or those with significant comorbidities to reduce crossclamp times and total operative durations.

The mini-sternotomy, extended into a right intercostal space, has many benefits including good exposure, direct cannulation, and practical conversion to full sternotomy, if necessary. The exposure it provides is familiar to cardiac surgeons and requires few, if any, specialized surgical instruments. With this approach, both internal thoracic arteries are preserved.

Table 4
Adverse Events Among 365 Patients
Undergoing Minimally Invasive Aortic Valve Surgery

Adverse events (n = 365)	*No.*	*%*
Mortality	9	2.5
Cardiac complications		
New atrial fibrillation	84	23.0
Permanent pacemaker	23	6.3
Balloon pump required	1	0.3
Myocardial infarction	2	0.5
Other complications		
Deep vein thrombosis/pulmonary embolism	1	0.3
Pericadial effusion requiring drainage	1	0.3
Reexploration for bleeding	15	4.1
Neurological complications	12	3.3
Transient ischemic attack	2	0.5
Stroke	10	2.7
Wound complications	8	2.2
Deep chest infection	3	0.8
Superficial chest infection	5	1.4
Groin lymphocele	0	0.0
Vascular complications	1	0.3
Ascending aortic dissection or disruption	0	0.0
Femoral artery complications	1	0.3

Table 5
Postoperative Data Among 365 Recipients
of Minimally Invasive Aortic Valve Surgery

Postoperative data	*n*	*%*
Intensive care unit length of stay > 48 h	54	14.8
Hospital length of stay		
Mean (d)	7.2 ± 4.3	
<5 d	79	21.6
>7 d	104	28.5
Red blood cell transfusion		
Mean (U)	2.1 ± 5.1	
None	136	37.3
>4 U	39	10.7
Transfer to rehabilitation facility	79	21.6

The advent of minimally invasive techniques for aortic valve surgery has successfully minimized associated surgical trauma and morbidity while maintaining or improving the surgical efficacy of conventional aortic valve surgery. Undoubtedly, future surgical and technological advances will allow continued improvements in minimally invasive aortic valve surgery techniques.

REFERENCES

1. Harken DE, Soroff HS, Taylor WJ, et al. Partial and complete prostheses in aortic insufficiency. J Thorac Cardiovasc Surg 1960;40:744–762.
2. Starr A. Total mitral replacement: fixation and thrombosis. Surg Forum 1960;11:258–260.
3. Cosgrove DM III, Sabik JF. A minimally invasive approach for aortic valve operations. Ann Thorc Surg 1996;62:596–597.
4. Ammar R, Porat E, Eisenberg DS, Uretzky G. Utility of spiral CT in minimally invasive approach for aortic valve replacement. Eur J Cardio-thorac Surg 1998;14(suppl 1):S130–S133.
5. Aklog L, Adams DH, Couper GS, Gobezie R, Sears S, Cohn LH. Techniques and results of direct access minimally invasive mitral surgery: a paradigm for the future. J Thorac Cardiovasc Surg 1998;116:705–715.
6. Minale C, Reifschneider HJ, Schmitz E, Uckmann FP. Minimally invasive aortic valve replacement without sternotomy. Experience with the first 50 cases. Eur J Cardio-Thorac Surg 1998;14(suppl 1):S126–S129.
7. Cohn LH, Adams DH, Couper GS, Bichell DP. Minimally invasive aortic valve replacement. Semin Thorac Cardiovasc Surg 1997;9:331–336.
8. Bichell DP, Balaguer JM, Aranki SF, et al. Axilloaxillary cardiopulmonary bypass: a practical alternative to femorofemoral bypass. Ann Thorac Surg 1997;64:702–705.
9. Cosgrove DM III, Sabik JF, Navia JL. Minimally invasive valve operations. Ann Thorac Surg 1998;65:1535–1539.
10. Frazier BL, Derrick MJ, Purewal SS, Sowka LR, Johna S. Minimally invasive aortic valve replacement. Eur J Cardio-Thorac Surg 1998;14(suppl 1):S122–S125.
11. Benetti FJ, Mariani MA, Rizzardi JL, Benetti I. Minimally invasive aortic valve replacement. J Thorac Cardiovasc Surg 1997;113:806–807.
12. Colvin SB, Grossi EA, Ribakove G, Galloway AC. Minimally invasive aortic and mitral operation. Oper Tech Thorac Cardiovasc Surg 2000;5(3):212–220.
13. Lytle BW, Cosgrove DM III, Taylor PC, et al. Primary isolated aortic valve replacement. Early and late results. J Thorac Cardiovasc Surg 1989;97:675–694.
14. Bridgewater B, Steyn RS, Ray S, Hooper T. Minimally invasive aortic valve replacement through a transverse sternotomy: a word of caution. Heart 1998;79:605–607.
15. Gundry SR, Shattuck OH, Razzouk AJ, del Rio MJ, Sardari FF, Bailey LL. Facile minimally invasive cardiac surgery via ministernotomy. Ann Thorac Surg 1998;65:1100–1104.
16. Svensson LG. Minimal-access "J" or "j" sternotomy for valvular, aortic, and coronary operations or reoperations. Ann Thorac Surg 1997;64:1501–1503.
17. Tam RKW, Almeida AA. Minimally invasive aortic valve replacement via hemi-sternotomy: a preliminary report. Eur J Cardio-Thorac Surg 1998;14(suppl 1):S134–S137.
18. Byrne JG, Adams DH, Couper GS, Rizzo RJ, Cohn LH, Aranki SF. Minimally invasive aortic root replacement. Heart Surg Forum 1999;2(4):326–329.
19. Cohn LH, Adams DH, Couper GS, et al. Minimally invasive cardiac valve surgery improves patient satisfaction while reducing costs of cardiac valve replacement and repair. Ann Surg 1997;226:421–428.
20. Machler HE, Bergmann P, Anelli-Monti M, et al. Minimally invasive versus conventional aortic valve operations: a prospective study in 120 patients. Ann Thorac Surg 1999;67:1001–1005.
21. Byrne JG, Aranki SF, Couper GS, Adams DH, Allred EN, Cohn LH. Reoperative aortic valve replacement: partial upper hemisternotomy versus conventional full sternotomy. J Thorac Cardiovasc Surg 1999;118:991–997.
22. Zlotnick AY, Gilfeather MS, Adams DH, Cohn LH, Couper GS. Innominate vein cannulation for venous drainage in minimally invasive aortic valve replacement. Ann Thorac Surg 1999;67:864–865.
23. Byrne JG, Hsin MK, Adams DH, et al. Minimally invasive direct access heart valve surgery. J Card Surg 2000;15:21–34.

IV

Minimally Invasive Congenital, Pericardial, and Arrhythmia Surgery

22 Strategies for Reducing Trauma in Congenital Heart Surgery

Redmond P. Burke, MD
and Robert L. Hannan, MD

CONTENTS

INTRODUCTION
SIMPLE CONGENITAL CARDIAC LESIONS
VATS PROCEDURES FOR OTHER EXTRACARDIAC LESIONS
AVOIDING THORACOTOMY FOR PALLIATIVE SHUNTS
ENHANCED OPERATIVE IMAGING AND DOCUMENTATION
ATTEMPTS TO REDUCE INCISIONAL TRAUMA FOR CONGENITAL SURGERY
ALTERNATIVE INCISIONS FOR OTHER CONGENITAL HEART PROCEDURES
EFFORTS TO REDUCE CARDIOPULMONARY BYPASS TRAUMA
ATTEMPS TO REDUCE SURGICAL TRAUMA WITH ROBOTICS
FUSING INTERVENTIONAL CARDIOLOGY AND CARDIAC SURGERY TO REDUCE TRAUMA
HYBRID CLOSURE OF SEPTAL DEFECTS
HYBRID THERAPY FOR PULMONARY ARTERY STENOSIS
CONCLUSION
REFERENCES

INTRODUCTION

Strategies designed specifically to reduce trauma in congenital heart surgery have emerged over the past decade. Parallel advances in endoscopic imaging and cardiopulmonary bypass technology have resulted in new surgical approaches to a variety of congenital heart lesions. The relentless demands for extreme technical precision, speed, and gentleness in congenital heart repairs place profound pressures on these "minimally

From: *Contemporary Cardiology: Minimally Invasive Cardiac Surgery, Second Edition*
Edited by: D. J. Goldstein and M. C. Oz © Humana Press Inc., Totowa, NJ

invasive" techniques, and the surgeons performing them. Consequently, adoption has proceeded at a slow pace and has been limited to straightforward repairs. Advances in interventional cardiology have created striking new opportunities for completely avoiding surgical trauma in patients with simple lesions, and have been adopted at a much more rapid pace. It is possible that combined or hybrid procedures utilizing the technology and skills of both interventional cardiologist and minimally invasive congenital heart surgeon may produce the most important reductions in therapeutic trauma for children with even the most complex forms of congenital heart disease.

SIMPLE CONGENITAL CARDIAC LESIONS

Patent Ductus Arteriosus

Multiple therapeutic options are available for patent ductus arteriosus, the simplest congenital heart lesion. Indeed, thoracotomy or median sternotomy, with ligation or ductal division, has been largely supplanted by transcatheter occlusion techniques. Several limited thoracotomy incisions *(1)*, and more sophisticated video-assisted thoracoscopic surgery (VATS) techniques *(2)*, have been designed to minimize incisional trauma in patients requiring this surgery.

Transcatheter coil occlusion is now a routine outpatient procedure, requiring no incisions, which usually results in complete ductal closure. Residual flow has been reported as a potential limitation requiring repeat procedures *(3)*. Six-month closure rates for the Rashkind device have been reported at 77%, vs a 90% closure rate for Gianturco coils *(4)*. Small femoral vessel size limits the applicability of the transcatheter techniques in premature newborns, and patients with larger ducts (over 4 mm) consistently have had a higher incidence of residual flow. Device migrations, hemolysis, femoral vessel damage, radiation, aortic and pulmonary artery obstructions, and the infectious risk of an intravascular foreign body are other potential complications related to device closure of the patent ductus *(5,6)*.

VATS evolved in response to the striking chest wall morbidity produced by the thoracotomy incision *(7)*. Endoscopic applications in adult general and thoracic surgery soon led to the first pediatric applications. Laborde described a pediatric cardiac VATS procedure for ligation of patent ductus arteriosus (PDA). Using three instrument ports, the duct is dissected with a one-handed cautery technique, and a vascular clip is applied for occlusion. In his first clinical report in 38 patients with patent ductus arteriosus *(2)*, patients ranged from 1.5 to 90 mo in age, and from 2.4 to 25 kg in weight. Successful ductal closure was achieved in every patient. One patient had a permanent recurrent nerve injury, and there were no deaths.

Our technique for VATS occlusion of patent ductus utilizes four thoracostomy incisions, allowing the surgeon to operate with two hands. Routine endotracheal intubation and general anesthesia are sufficient and single-lung ventilation is not necessary. Visualization is achieved with an endoscope (4-mm, 30° angled endoscope [Smith and Nephew, Dyonics, Andover, MA]), and a retractor (Pilling-Weck, Fort Washington, PA). The remaining two ports are used for the endoscopic grasper and cautery, scissors, or clip applier (**Fig. 1**). Under 4× magnification, the surgeon is able to dissect precisely the duct, and apply either vascular clips or intracorporeal ligatures *(10)*. DeCampli described his experience with VATS for patent ductus arteriosus, with no residual flow, recurrent nerve injury, chylothorax, or transfusion in full-term infants and children *(11)*.

VATS for patent ductus arteriosus has also been used effectively in premature newborns *(12)*. In 34 premature newborns weighing 575 g to 2.5 kg, the median procedure

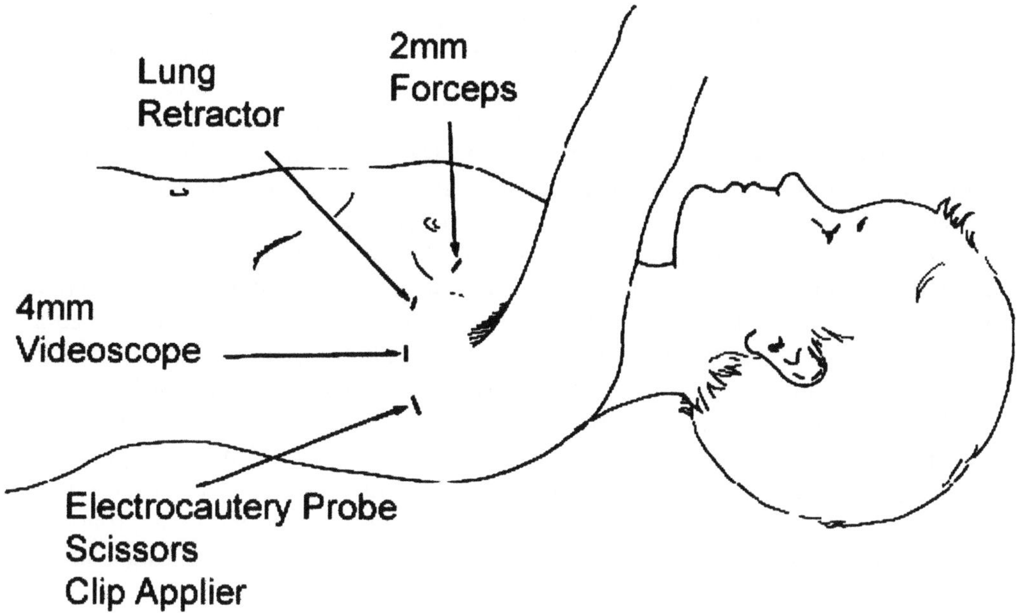

Fig. 1. Instrument positions for VATS PDA ligation.

time was 60 min. Operative mortality was zero, and there was trace residual Doppler flow in two patients. Conversion to thoracotomy was performed in four patients (12%) to improve exposure. Hines et al. described similar results in their group of 21 neonates undergoing VATS PDA interruption *(13)*.

Compared to transcatheter device occlusion techniques, VATS allows highly effective ductal closure with no restrictions based on patient size, hemodynamic condition, or ductal anatomy. VATS does not expose patients to the risks of radiation, device embolization, left pulmonary artery obstruction, aortic obstruction, or the long-term presence of an intravascular foreign body. The learning curve is steep for surgeons lacking endoscopic skills, suggesting that preparation in an animal or simulation laboratory might be beneficial. We are confident that long-term assessment of the VATS technique will show a reduction in the incidence of scoliosis *(7–9)*, postthoracotomy pain syndromes *(14)*, and chest wall deformities *(15)*, described in pediatric patients after posterolateral thoracotomy. Numerous studies demonstrate no convincing differences in cost or efficacy for either transcatheter or surgical closure *(3,16–18)*. The techniques each have strengths and weaknesses, which vary among institutions. At Miami Children's Hospital, we compared the results of VATS and coil occlusion for PDA in a consecutive series of patients and found no significant clinical differences in the techniques. We offer families and referring doctors the option of a VATS approach or transcatheter device, and share the feeling that full thoracotomy for patent ductus can and should almost always be avoided.

Vascular Ring

The first VATS vascular ring division was described in 1993 *(19)*, using the same technique and instrumentation developed for VATS PDA interruption. The left subclavian artery serves as a landmark to initiate endoscopic exposure and dissection of the ring elements. The atretic arch segments, or ligamentum, are identified, ligated proximally and distally, and divided, as in an open approach. In a report comparing VATS vascular ring division to conventional division via thoracotomy *(20)*, VATS was used in eight pediatric patients ranging in age from 40 d to 5.5 yr and in weight from 1.8 to 17.1 kg. Clinical success was achieved in all but one patient, who required reexploration via thoracotomy to divide a residual obstruction created by an undivided ligamentum arteriosum. Complications included transfusion (one patient), and chylothorax (one patient). When compared to a historical control group of patients undergoing vascular ring division via thoracotomy, the VATS patients did not differ in age, weight, intensive care unit or postoperative hospital stay, duration of intubation, or hospital charges.

To date, the authors have performed VATS vascular ring division in 25 patients, ranging in age from 8 d to 5.5 yr. In the past year, procedure times have averaged 2 h. Length of stay has ranged from 1 to 6 d. Conversion to thoracotomy is not considered a complication, but rather, the exercise of good clinical judgment, particularly when the ring is formed by large, patent vessels. In such cases, a 3-cm lateral thoracotomy is used to gain proximal and distal vascular control. There is good evidence that pulmonary function abnormalities will persist in vascular ring patients repaired after the onset of symptoms *(21)*. The decreased chest wall incisional trauma of the VATS approach may justify earlier intervention in these patients with asymptomatic vascular rings, and perhaps improve their long-/term outcomes.

VATS PROCEDURES FOR OTHER EXTRACARDIAC LESIONS

VATS techniques have been used for a variety of other extracardiac congenital lesions and applications. These include pericardial window, epicardial pacemaker insertion, treatment of chylothorax, diaphragm plication *(22)*, interruption of arterial and venous collaterals, and thoracic explorations for esoteric lesions (i.e., absent left pericardium syndrome) *(23)*. Recently, VATS for early treatment of pediatric empyema has been described as a method of decreasing the duration of hospital stay—average postoperative stay was 4.9 d, total stay was 7.3 d *(24)*.

AVOIDING THORACOTOMY FOR PALLIATIVE SHUNTS

Thoracotomy for modified Blalock–Tausig shunt palliation can be avoided in all patients by using a median sternotomy approach *(25)*. It is our opinion that subjecting patients to a thoracotomy incision for palliative shunting is unjustifiable, and patients subjected to bilateral thoracotomies and repeated median sternotomy (frequently seen in patients with pulmonary atresia, ventricular septal defect, and multiple aortopulmonary collaterals) have clearly suffered unnecessary cumulative chest wall trauma. When necessary, staged management can be performed effectively through repeated median sternotomy with minimal risk related to the reoperative sternotomy. Other advantages to the median sternotomy approach for shunts have been well documented and include improved patency, decreased phrenic nerve injury, decreased pulmonary artery stenosis, decreased accidental shunts to the pulmonary vein, better access for conversion to bypass, easier access to the shunt site at reoperation, and decreased chest wall collateral formation in cyanotic patients. Justification for a thoracotomy approach to the modified Blalock–Taussig shunt seems to have been reduced to the expression, "That's the way we've always done it," and should no longer be condoned.

ENHANCED OPERATIVE IMAGING AND DOCUMENTATION

Routine video-assisted procedures for extracardiac lesions led naturally to video-assisted endoscopic applications during open-heart operations *(26)*. We define intraoperative cardioscopy as the use of endoscopic imaging tools during open-heart procedures to facilitate visualization and repair of remote intracardiac structures, and to create visual documentation of cardiac lesions before and after repair. This technique allows surgeons to achieve anatomic visualization without resorting to excessive retraction or extended cardiac incisions. This is a particular advantage when exposure has been limited by the use of small incisions.

Over the past 7 yr at Miami Children's Hospital, this technique has evolved into the routine use of a 4-mm operating endoscope in the operative field as a third eye for the surgical team, exposing remote areas within the ventricles, the ventricular outflow tracts, and the subvalvular apparatus. The pleural spaces are also easily explored with the endoscope. Cardioscopy has been used to facilitate complex valve surgery, ventricular septal defect repair, left ventricular outflow tract resections, placement of septal occlusion devices, and even left ventricular thrombectomy *(27)*.

Video-assisted endoscopic technology also allows collection and storage of digital video and still images, for immediate and future correlation with other imaging modalities (angiography, MRI, and echocardiography). The images can also be digitally stored for long-term reference, allowing surgeons to assess the outcomes of various surgical techniques more accurately, and to prepare for reoperations. We have used routine intraoperative cardioscopy for the past 7 years in 2000 open-heart procedures, with no complications related to the endoscopy *(28)*. Other investigators have described similar experiences with routine intraoperative cardioscopy *(29,30)*.

ATTEMPTS TO REDUCE INCISIONAL TRAUMA FOR CONGENITAL SURGERY

Coincident with our efforts to reduce the use of thoracotomy in congenital heart therapy, publications on alternatives to median sternotomy have proliferated in the thoracic literature. One of the first alternatives to full median sternotomy was reported on the Internet by Levinson *(31)*. In an adult patient, an atrial septal defect was repaired through a lower sternotomy and xiphoid resection, combined with femoral cannulation and fibrillatory arrest. This report was followed by a flurry of alternate incisions.

Thoracotomy

Ironically, despite increasing documentation of the complications of thoracotomy incisions for extracardiac procedures, numerous groups have adopted this incision for simple congenital open-heart repairs. The obvious historical intent of this approach has been to hide the incision under the right breast in female patients. Kappert described a right lateral chest incision and femoral cannulation using port-access equipment (Heartport, Inc, Redwood City, CA). Thirteen adults, from 17 to 61 yr of age, were repaired through 4–8-cm incisions in the fourth intercostal space. Bypass was achieved with femoral cannulation. There was no mortality, and the median hospital stay was 8 d *(32)*. Widespread use of the port-access system has been limited because of complications including aortic dissection related to the aortic cannulae. The large size of these cannulae has also limited the use of port-access technology in the pediatric population, in whom the risk of this approach might be lessened by absence of aortic atherosclerotic lesions.

In India, 37 patients, ranging from 18 to 67 yr in age were approached with a 7-cm right anterior thoracotomy and femoral cannulation, with a centrifugal pump to facilitate cardiac drainage. Aortic clamping was achieved with a special clamp placed through a small midclavicular incision. Hospital stay averaged 4.2 d, and there were no complications or mortality *(33)*. Surgeons in Singapore described a similar technique for atrial septal defects repair via a right anterior thoracotomy with femoral cannulation *(34)*. In Hannover, Germany, three approaches have been compared, including right parasternal incision with central cannulation, anterior submammary mini-incision with femoral arterial and central caval cannulation, and percutaneous cervical cannulation *(35)*. In 24 patients, this technique was used with no neurological complications or mortality, and cosmetic acceptance was described as "high." In Japan, both parasternal and partial sternotomy approaches have been advocated *(36,37)*, and a group in China has also advocated repair of cardiac defects through right lateral thoracotomy *(38)*. In this uncontrolled study of 683 patients, the authors described transecting the sternum when visualization was inadequate, but did not document how often this was necessary. There was no follow-up assessment of chest wall appearance or function to justify the conclusion that lateral thoracotomy is either less invasive than, or cosmetically superior to, median sternotomy.

For numerous reasons, we have not adopted the thoracotomy approach for simple congenital open-heart repairs. In our opinion, the anterior thoracotomy is a cosmetic risk in infants, as the breast tissue is unpredictable in location, and vulnerable to injury and subsequent deformity. In adults, where the incision can be placed to avoid the breast, we counsel patients that the risks of postthoracotomy pain syndrome, breast dysesthesia, femoral vessel cannulation injury, and distance from the operative target outweigh the cosmetic benefit of the submammary incision. Most patients choose a partial lower sternotomy. Cautious observers have rightfully described the many limitations of these variations from established technique for atrial septal defect repair, contending that the only real benefit of a "minimally invasive" approach is cosmetic *(39)*.

Partial Sternotomy

There have been many original descriptions of the partial lower sternotomy for simple congenital heart repairs. Byrne described a series of 59 adult patients repaired through either a right parasternal, submammary, or upper hemisternotomy incision. There was no mortality, and four major complications were seen *(40)*. Del Nido described a similar approach for pediatric atrial septal defect repairs *(41)*. A consecutive series of patients was divided into sternotomy and partial lower sternotomy groups. Within the latter group, patients were cannulated either centrally or femorally. The "minimal access group" experienced no conversions to full sternotomy, no difficulties placing femoral or aortic cannulas, no reexplorations for bleeding, and no significant wound infections. Echo follow-up on 19 of 54 partial sternotomy patients showed no residual atrial shunts. There were no differences between the partial sternotomy group and the full sternotomy group in cardiopulmonary bypass times. There were no remarkable differences between the groups in the incidence of postoperative pericardial effusions, or hospital stay, which averaged 3 d after partial sternotomy, and 4 d after full sternotomy. This experience has now grown *(42)* and been expanded to selected patients with more complex congenital defects *(43)*. Khan also described a lower sternotomy approach sparing the manubrium. Using conventional aortic and bicaval cannulation, with fibrillatory arrest, 115 patients were repaired through a partial sternotomy. Patients had a median hospital stay of 4 d, and there was no mortality *(44)*. There are some data to suggest that the partial lower sternotomy results in less postoperative mediastinal drainage and shorter hospital stays than full sternotomy *(45)*, however, measures of postoperative pain and respiratory mechanics appear to be equal when comparing these two incisions *(46)*.

We share the general impression that a full median sternotomy is neither esthetic nor necessary to expose the atrial septum safely, and have adopted a lower partial sternotomy for atrial septal defect repair. Our limited-incision technique for atrial septal defect repair was designed to utilize standard cardiopulmonary bypass equipment and technique, myocardial protection, neuroprotection (central aortic deairing and superior vena caval drainage), and operative precision. Our rationale for a midline approach is multifactorial: (1) central cannulation avoids femoral vessel injury, (2) midline incision avoids breast tissue and denervation *(47)* and intercostal and phrenic nerve trauma, (3) cardioplegic arrest protects the myocardium and minimizes the risk of air embolism, and (4) rapid conversion to median sternotomy is possible in the event of unexpected anatomy or pathophysiology (such as left superior vena cava, or post-repair pulmonary hypertension and right ventricular dysfunction).

Cardiopulmonary bypass techniques can be modified to facilitate these alternate approaches to median sternotomy. An assisted venous drainage circuit utilizing a constrained vortex cone (Biocone, Medtronics, Minneapolis, MN) allows smaller cannulae to be used without compromising bypass flows *(48)*. Routine carbon dioxide flooding of the operative field at 3 L/min displaces air from the pericardial well and may decrease the risk of air embolism. During longer procedures, sweep flows are increased to avoid increases in circulating carbon dioxide.

ALTERNATIVE INCISIONS FOR OTHER CONGENITAL HEART PROCEDURES

The merits of limited-access incisions in most complex congenital repairs are dubious at best. Strategies to reduce or eliminate circulatory arrest times should supercede concerns about incision size or location. Despite this obvious misplacement of priorities, there have been several reports of complex congenital heart lesions being performed through partial sternotomy incisions. Gundry *(49)* described partial upper and lower sternotomy in a series of 57 pediatric patients, including neonates, for operations including arterial switch, tetralogy of Fallot repair, atrial and ventricular septal defect repair, aortic and mitral valve replacement, and complex arch reconstruction. Using a T incision in the upper or lower sternum, with aortic and atrial cannulation and conventional bypass and myocardial preservation, direct visualization of the heart is achieved and repairs are performed using conventional instrumentation. Potential weaknesses to this approach include the lack of effective chest tube drainage of the mediastinum, prolonged bypass times, the possibility of sternal instability from a T incision, and loss of myocardial protection from rewarming by the chest wall.

At Miami Children's Hospital, we have never used partial sternotomy for complex neonatal surgery. We have used an upper sternotomy routed into the right third interspace for simple aortic lesions, such as subaortic membrane resection (**Fig. 2**). This approach

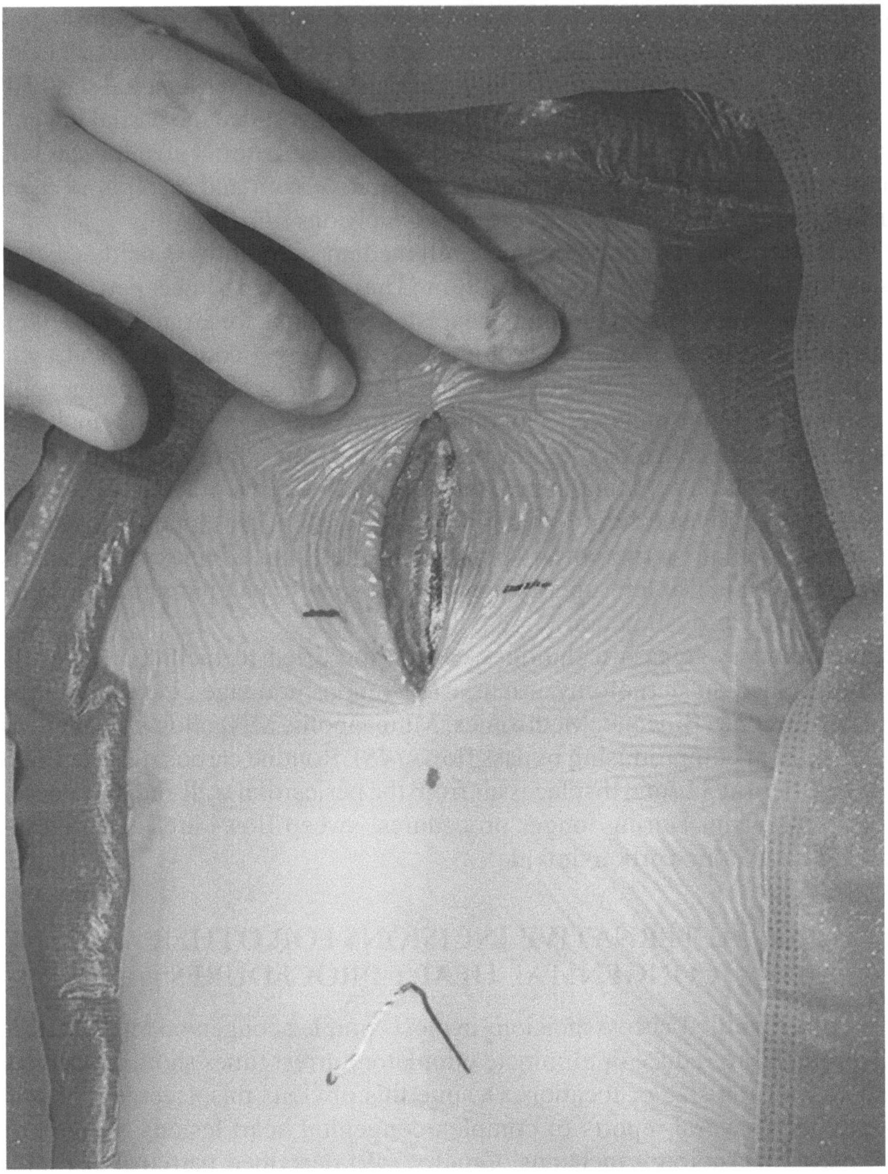

Fig. 2. Operative field during partial sternotomy for subaortic membrane resection.

allows central aortic and venous cannulation and effective deairing. Video-assisted endoscopy improves visualization of the left ventricular outflow tract, and operative precision is not compromised. Partial sternotomy patients tend to have shorter hospital stays to complement their shorter incisions *(50)*.

Alternate incisions for repair of ventricular septal defects have been described, including lower sternotomy and right anterolateral thoracotomy *(38,51,52)*. This approach has not been widely accepted. The disadvantages of these reported techniques for ventricular septal defect repair include: potentially traumatic femoral cannulation, fibrillatory arrest without cardioplegic myocardial protection, loss of precision, highly visible anterior thoracotomy incisions, ventricular incisions to improve exposure, and prolonged operating and bypass times. While these approaches are technically possible, no data are presented to suggest that they are in any way "minimally invasive" or superior to conventional surgical techniques.

An alarming report described a "minimally invasive" approach to right ventricular outflow tract reconstruction *(53)*. The authors chose to avoid repeat sternotomy by using a "left anterior small thoracotomy" with femoral cannulation for bypass, to replace conduits in 4 adolescent patients. No data were presented to support the hypothesis that the technique is less traumatic than a repeat median sternotomy. Given the obvious anatomical tendency for right ventricular-to-pulmonary artery conduits to adhere to the left anterior chest wall, we are concerned that this approach actually increases the risk of conduit entry upon opening the chest.

EFFORTS TO REDUCE CARDIOPULMONARY BYPASS TRAUMA

Research in cardiopulmonary bypass technology, blood conservation, neuroprotection, myocardial protection, inflammation, hypothermia, and acid–base management strategy have constituted the true foundation for minimizing the trauma of congenital heart surgery. We contend that reduction or elimination of circulatory arrest, ischemic arrest, and cardiopulmonary bypass times, while preserving operative precision, constitutes the best ongoing philosophy to further the goal of reducing surgical trauma.

A good example of this philosophy in action is the effort to perform complete single-ventricle palliation for selected patients without any cardiopulmonary bypass. Initial palliation to increase pulmonary blood flow can sometimes be achieved with interventional catheterization. Subsequent bidirectional cavopulmonary anastomosis can be performed without bypass *(54)*, although we strongly believe that maintaining cerebral perfusion by effective superior vena caval drainage is critical. Extracardiac Fontan operations can also be performed without the use of cardiopulmonary bypass *(55)*, by shunting from the inferior vena cava to the common atrium as the extracardiac anastomoses are completed. Patients with more than one source of pulmonary blood flow are perhaps the safest candidates for the off-bypass Fontan procedure. These include patients with bilateral superior vena cava, or with native pulmonary artery flow in addition to their bidirectional cavopulmonary anastomosis. Understanding that obstructed caval blood flow could compromise central nervous system perfusion, we have used these approaches sparingly, and agree with others that careful neurological outcome measurements should form the basis for wider application *(56)*.

Ventricular septal defect repair without cardiopulmonary bypass has been described, although the limitations in precision are cause for concern. Recent studies suggest that some muscular ventricular septal defects might be closed using a device inserted through the right atrium without the need for cardiopulmonary bypass. This technique would allow the use of larger septal occlusion devices, without the risk of vascular trauma from peripheral access, and eliminate the need for cardiopulmonary bypass *(57)*.

ATTEMPTS TO REDUCE SURGICAL TRAUMA WITH ROBOTICS

Building on military applications for robotic battlefield medics, and marketing strategies for personal computers, robotic systems were rapidly developed for cardiac surgery. After a frantic race, voice-activated and computer-assisted systems were used to perform endoscopic coronary artery bypass grafting, mitral valve repair, and atrial septal defect repair.

A truly remote, computer controlled, robotic surgery system (daVinci™ System, Intuitive Surgical, Inc., Mountain View, CA) has been used to perform coronary artery bypass grafting in humans *(58)* (*see* Chapter 31). Robotic arms control the surgical instrumentation and the camera. The surgeon manipulates the instruments through a remote virtual manipulator. These techniques have relied on peripheral access bypass systems (Heartport system, Heartport, Inc., Redwood City, CA), which are simply too large for infant femoral vessels. Adult atrial septal defect repair and mitral valvuloplasty have been performed with varying degrees of robotic assistance *(59–61)*. The other available robotic system uses a voice-controlled robotic arm (Aesop™, Computer Motion, Inc., Goleta, CA) to control a 3-D camera system (Vista system, Vista, Inc., Westborough, MA), and a telemanipulator (Zeus™, Computer Motion, Goleta, CA) for endoscopic suturing *(62)* (*see* Chapter 30).

Purported advantages of these systems include "scaling of the surgeon's hand movements" to increase precision, and filtering to minimize tremor. This may actually be creative marketing of the built-in lag between operator activation and instrument response created by yards of software and hardware between the surgeon and patient. By mounting endoscopic instruments on universal joints that can be advanced through small trocars into the thorax, rotational freedom at the tip of the instruments is improved compared to conventional endoscopic instrumentation; however, in the authors' experience, this capability has never reached that of the human wrist. The virtually complete loss of tactile feedback and the inability to regulate force applied to tissues comprise the two most fundamental weaknesses of the robotic technology.

Pediatric congenital heart applications await resolution of several other limitations in the technology and technique. Current 3-D imaging endoscopes (10-mm) are too large to pass through the infant intercostal space without trauma. Available robotic systems require relatively large (7-mm) ports for instrument insertion. Four such incisions would be as large as a standard median sternotomy in an infant, negating any cosmetic benefit. Furthermore, the pediatric thorax is also too small for adequate separation of the robotic arms controlling the individual instruments.

Current robotic systems were designed to complete very simple anastomotic suture lines, as required for coronary bypass grafting and valve replacement or repair *(60,62,63)*. In training simulators, these anastomoses may require 30 min to finish 10 suture throws *(64)*. A typical repair for tetralogy of Fallot requires approx 100 suture throws, giving us a projected robotic suture time of 300 min. This would produce prohibitively long myocardial ischemic times. It is anticipated that as the instruments are refined and downsized, pediatric applications might be enabled, particularly for simple septal defects. The more daunting technical hurdle will be the absolute necessity for tactile feedback to avoid tissue trauma.

FUSING INTERVENTIONAL CARDIOLOGY AND CARDIAC SURGERY TO REDUCE TRAUMA

A competitive relationship between interventional cardiologists and congenital heart surgeons may hinder the development of less traumatic therapy for congenital heart disease. In contrast, a unified field approach, emphasizing the technological capabilities of both disciplines, might accelerate innovation. To achieve this, we envision a multidisciplinary intervention/surgery/diagnostic theater incorporating all existing therapeutic technology into a single procedure suite.

HYBRID CLOSURE OF SEPTAL DEFECTS

Transcatheter device occlusion for septal defects is evolving at a ferocious pace. Devices and techniques are now available for device closure of atrial *(65)* and ventricular septal defects, patent ductus arteriosus, collateral vessels, and fenestrations. Drawbacks of device occlusion include moderate residual flow rates *(66–68)*; infectious, abrasive, and corrosive risks of persistent intravascular foreign bodies; and vascular trauma related to insertion. Device fractures have been a persistent problem in the mid-term assessments of septal occlusion devices using both Nitinol and stainless steel. To minimize the trauma of using these techniques in our center, surgical backup is provided so that patients found in the laboratory to be unsuitable for device closure can be immediately converted to a surgical approach, sparing the child a second anesthetic, and the family the stress of a failed intervention.

Hybrid procedures are evolving. Building on early cooperative ventures between interventional cardiology and surgery for the management of complex muscular ventricular septal defects *(69)*, a variety of combined procedures have evolved. Video-assisted cardioscopy has been used to guide placement of transcatheter septal occlusion devices *(23)*. Other hybrid procedures include transcatheter closure of extracardiac Fontan fenestrations *(70)* and emergent placements of transcatheter stents for occluded systemic-pulmonary shunts where patients have been stabilized with planned or emergent cardiopulmonary support in the catheterization laboratory *(71)*. A hybrid repair of a pulmonary artery pseudoaneurysm with endovascular stent grafting was recently described *(72)*.

HYBRID THERAPY FOR PULMONARY ARTERY STENOSIS

Hybrid techniques may produce the most effective strategies for managing complex pulmonary artery stenoses. In the operating room, surgical exposure can be used to facilitate transcatheter stent placement. We have developed several variations of this technique at Miami Children's Hospital in the past 2 yr. Most commonly, transcatheter stents have been positioned intraoperatively, on bypass, with video-assisted endoscopic guidance (**Fig. 3**). Conversely, in the catheterization laboratory, angiographically guided stent placement can be facilitated with surgical assistance. Surgeons can place sheaths into central vessels or directly into the right ventricular outflow tract with or without cardiopulmonary bypass. We have recognized several advantages to these hybrid approaches for pulmonary artery angioplasty. Bypass support minimizes hemodynamic instability, central vascular access minimizes peripheral vascular trauma, large stents can be placed in small patients, stents can be removed and repositioned easily and rapidly, and extensive surgical dissection in the hilum can be avoided. Completion angiography allows confirmation of effective surgical and transcatheter interventions, and ensures viable physiology before transfer to the cardiac intensive care unit.

CONCLUSION

Morbidity, mortality, and physiological endpoints continue to form the foundation for therapeutic plans in congenital heart care; however, the potential for emerging technol-

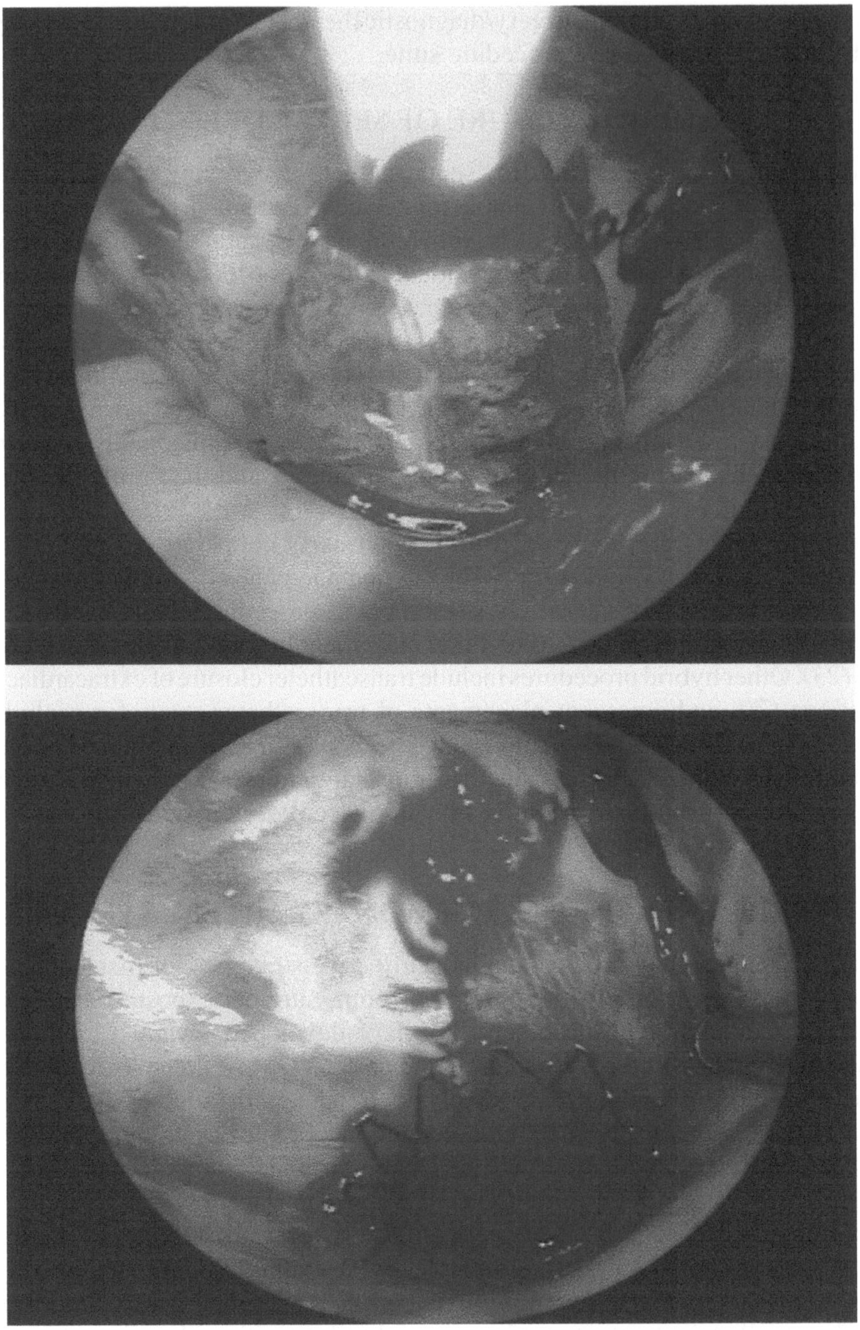

Fig. 3. Video-assisted endoscopic stent implantation. A transcatheter stent is positioned in the left pulmonary artery using endoscopic visualization on cardiopulmonary bypass.

ogy to reduce the trauma of these plans remains tantalizing. We believe that a cumulative measure of trauma to individual patients over time is the best index to develop and maintain the most minimally invasive approach possible at any given time with existing technology. Such a measurement strategy has not yet been realized, but within this technique will lie the justification of our attempts to reduce incision size, procedure times, hospital stay, and the myriad other inadequate measures of our attempts to heal.

REFERENCES

1. Yan D, Xie Q, Zhang Z, Gu C, Kawada S. Surgical treatment of patent ductus arteriosus (PDA) through mini subaxillary extrapleural approach. Ann Thorac Cardiovasc Surg 1999;5(4):233–236.
2. Laborde F, Noirhomme P, Karam J, Batisse A, Bourel P, Saint MO. A new video-assisted thoracoscopic surgical technique for interruption of patient ductus arteriosus in infants and children [see comments]. J Thorac Cardiovasc Surg 1993;105(2):278–280.
3. Hawkins JA, Minich LL, Tani LY, StiMevant JE, Orsmond GS, McGough EC. Cost and efficacy of surgical ligation versus transeatheter coil occlusion of patent ductus arteriosus. J Thorac Cardiovasc Surg 1996;112(6):1634–1638.
4. Janorkar S, Goh T, Wilkinson J. Transcatheter closure of ventricular septal defects using the Rashkind device: initial experience [see comments]. Catheter Cardiovasc Interv 1999;46(l):43–48.
5. Patel HT, Cao QL, Rhodes J, Hijazi ZM. Long-term outcome of transcatheter coil closure of small to large patent ductus arteriosus. Catheter Cardiovasc Interv 1999;47(4):457–461.
6. Duke C, Chan KC. Aortic obstruction caused by device occlusion of patent arterial duct. Heart 1999;82(i):109–111.
7. Van Biezen FC, Bakx PA, De Villeneuve VH, Hop WC. Scoliosis in children after thoracotomy for aortic coarctation. J Bone Joint Surg Am 1993;75(4):514–518.
8. Westfelt JN, Nordwall A. Thoracotomy and scoliosis. Spine 1991;16(9):1124–1125.
9. Wong-Chung J, France J, Gillespie R. Scoliosis caused by rib fusion after thoracotomy for esophageal atresia. Report of a case and review of the literature. Spine 1992;17(7):851–854.
10. Burke RP. Video-assisted thoracoscopic surgery for patent ductus arteriosus. Pediatrics 1994;93(5):823–825.
11. DeCampli WM. Video-assisted thoracic surgical procedures in children. Semin Thorac Cardiovasc Surg 1998;1:61–73.
12. Burke RP, Jacobs JP, Cheng W, Trento A, Fontana GP. Video-assisted thoracoscopic surgery for patent ductus arteriosus in low birth weight neonates and infants. Pediatrics 1999;104(2 pt 1):227–230.
13. Hines MH, Bensky AS, Hammon JW Jr, Pennington DG. Video-assisted thoracoscopic ligation of patent ductus arteriosus: safe and outpatient. Am Thorac Surg 1998;66(3):853–858.
14. Dajczman E, Gordon A, Kreisman H, Wolkove N. Long-term postthoracotomy pain [see comments]. Chest 1991;99(2):270–274.
15. Jaureguizar E, Vazquez J, Murcia J, Diez Pardo JA. Morbid musculoskeletal sequelae of thoracotomy for tracheoesophageal fistula. J Pediatr Surg 1985;20(5):511–514.
16. Galal O, Nehgme R, al Fadley F, et al. The role of surgical ligation of patent ductus arteriosus in the era of the Rashkind device. Ann Thorac Surg 1997;63(2):434–437.
17. Fedderly RT, Beekman RH 3rd, Mosea RS, Bove EL, Lloyd TR. Comparison of hospital charges for closure of patent ductus arteriosus by surgery and by transcatheter coil occlusion. Am J Cardiol 1996;77(9):776–779.
18. Gray DT, Fyler DC, Walker AM, Weinstein MC, Chalmers TC. Clinical outcomes and costs of transcatheter as compared with surgical closure of patent ductus arteriosus. The Patient Ductus Arteriosus Closure Comparative Study Group [see comments]. N Engl J Med 1993;329(21):1517–1523.
19. Burke RP, Chang AC. Video-assisted thoracoscopic division of a vascular ring in an infant: a new operative technique [see comments]. J Card Surg 1993;8(5):537–540.
20. Burke RP, Rosenfeld HM, Wemovsky G, Jonas RA. Video-assisted thoracoscopic vascular ring division in infants and children. J Am Coll Cardiol 1995;25(4):943–947.
21. Marmon LM, Bye MR, Haas JM, Balsara RK, Dunn JM. Vascular rings and slings: long-term follow-up of pulmonary function. J Pediatr Surg 1984;19(6):683–692.
22. Van Smith C, Jacobs JP, Burke RP. Minimally invasive diaphragm placation in an infant. Ann Thorac Surg 1998;65(3):842–844.
23. Burke RP, Wemovsky G, Van Der Velde M, Hansen D, Castaneda AR. Video-assisted thoracoscopic surgery for congenital heart disease. J Thorac Cardiovasc Surg 1995;109(3):499–507; discussion 508.
24. Grewal H, Jackson RJ, Wagner CW, Smith SD. Early video-assisted thoracic surgery in the management of empyema. Pediatrics 1999;103(5):e63.
25. Odim J, Portzky M, Zurakowski D, et al. Sternotomy approach for the modified Blalock-Taussig shunt. Circulation 1995;92(9 suppl):11,256–11,261.

26. Burke RP, Michielon G, Wemovsky G. Video-assisted cardioscopy in congenital heart operations. Ann Thorac Surg 1994;58(3):864–868.
27. Mazza IL, Jacobs JP, Aidousany A, Chang AC, Burke RP. Video-assisted cardioscopy for left ventricular thrombectomy in a child. Ann Thorac Surg 1998;66(l):248–250.
28. Miyaji K, Hannan RL, Ojito J, Dygert JM, White JA, Burke RP. Video-assisted cardioscopy for intraventricular repair in congenital heart disease. Ann Thorac Surg 2000;70(3):730–737.
29. Rao V, Freedom RM, Black MD. Minimally invasive surgery with cardioscopy for congenital heart defects. Ann Thorac Surg 1999;68(5):1742–1745.
30. Miyaji K, Murakami A, Kobayashi J, Suematsu Y, Takamoto S. Transxiphoid approach for intracardiac repair using video-assisted cardioscopy. Ann Thorac Surg 2001;71(5):1716–1718.
31. Levinson M. Heart Surgery Forum 1995. http://www.hsforum.com/heartsurgery/homehsf html.
32. Kappert U, Wagner FM, Gulielmos V, Taha M, Schneider J, Schueler S. Port Access surgery for congenital heart disease. Eur J Cardiothorac Surg 1999;16(suppl 2):S86–S88.
33. Malhotra R, Mishra Y, Sharma KK, Mehta Y, Trehan N. Minimally invasive atrial septal defects repair. Indian Heart J 1999;51(2):193–197.
34. Sim EK, Gob IJ, Grignani RT, Chen XZ, Duranni A. Minimally invasive surgical closure of atrial septal defects via a right anterior thoracotomy. Singapore Med J 1999;40(4):271–272.
35. Cremer JT, Boning A, Anssar MB, et al. Different approaches for minimally invasive closure of atrial septal defects. Ann Thorac Surg 1999;67(6):1648–1652.
36. Murashita T, Hatta E, Miyatake T, Kubota T, Sasaki S, Yasuda K. Partial median sternotomy as a minimal access for the closure of subarterial ventricular septal defect. Feasibility of transpulmonary approach [In Process Citation]. Jpn J Thorac Cardiovasc Surg 1999;47(9):440–444.
37. Sawa Y, Matsuda H. Minimally invasive cardiac surgery—the efficacy of right parasternal approach. Nippon Geka Gakkai Zasshi 1998;99(12):825–830.
38. Liu YL, Zhang HJ, Sun HS, et al. Repair of cardiac defects through a shorter right lateral thoracotomy in children. Ann Thorac Surg 2000;70(3):738–741.
39. Massetti M, Nataf P, Babatasi G, Khayat A. Cosmetic aspects in minimally invasive cardiac surgery. Eur J Cardiothorac Surg 1999;16(suppl 2):S73–S75.
40. Byme JG, Adanis DH, Mitchell ME, Cohn LH. Minimally invasive direct access for repair of atrial septal defect in adults. Am J Cardiol 1999;84(8):919–922.
41. del Nido PJ, Bichell DP. Minimal-access surgery for congenital heart defects. Semin Thorac Cardiovasc Surg 1998;1:75–80.
42. Bichell DP, Geva T, Bacha EA, Mayer JE, Jonas RA, del Nido PJ. Minimal access approach for the repair of atrial septal defect: the initial 135 patients. Ann Thorac Surg 2000;70(l):115–118.
43. Nicholson IA, Bichell DP, Bacha EA, del Nido PJ. Minimal sternotomy approach for congenital heart operations. Ann Thorac Surg 2001;71(2):469–472.
44. Khan JH, McEUiftmey DB, Reddy VM, Hanley FL. A 5-year experience with surgical repair of atrial septal defect employing limited exposure. Cardiol Young 1999;9(6):572–576.
45. Luo W, Chang C, Chen S. Mini sternotomy versus full sternotomy in congenital heart defects: a prospective randomized study. Ann Thorac Surg 2001;71(2):473–475.
46. Laussen PC, Bichell DP, McGowan FX, Zurakowski D, DeMaso DR, del Nido PJ. Postoperative recovery in children after minimum versus full-length sternotomy. Ann Thorac Surg 2000;69(2):591–596.
47. Cherup LL, Siewers RD, Futrell JW. Breast and pectoral muscle maldevelopment after anterolateral and posterolateral thoracotomies in children. Ann Thorac Surg 1986;41(5):492–497.
48. Ojito JW, Hannan RL, Miyaji K, et al. Assisted venous drainage cardiopulmonary bypass in congenital heart surgery. Ann Thorac Surg 2001;71(4):1267–1271.
49. Gundry SR, Shattuck OH, Razzouk AJ, del Rio MJ, Sardari FF, Bailey LL. Facile minimally invasive cardiac surgery via a ministernotomy. Ann Thorac Surg 1998;65(4):1100–1104.
50. Miyaji K, Hannan RL, Ojito JW, White JA, Burke RP. Minimally invasive resection of congenital subaortic stenosis. Ann Thorac Surg 2000;69(4):1273–1275.
51. Lin PJ, Chang CH, Chu IJ, et al. Minimally invasive cardiac surgical techniques in the closure of ventricular septal defect: an alternative approach. Ann Thorac Surg 1998;65(l):165–169.
52. Chu SH, Chou NK, Chou TF, Wang SS. Left anterolateral thoracotomy for simultaneous correction of ventricular septal defect and coarctation of the aorta. Tex Heart Inst J 1994;21(2):158–160.
53. Inianaka K, Takamoto S, Murakami A, Kaneko Y. Minimally invasive extracardiac conduit replacement via a left anterior small thoracotomy. J Thorac Cardiovasc Surg 1999;118(6):1124–1125.

54. Jahangiri M, Keogh B, Shineboume EA, Lincoln C. Should the bidirectional Glenn procedure be performed through a thoracotomy without cardiopulmonary bypass? J Thorac Cardiovasc Surg 1999;118(2):367–368.
55. Burke RP, Jacobs JP, Ashraf MH, Aidousany A, Chang AC. Extracardiac Fontan operation without cardiopulmonary bypass. Ann Thorac Surg 1997;63(4):1175–1177.
56. Jonas RA. Commentary [In Process Citation]. J Thorac Cardiovasc Surg 1999;118(5):957.
57. Amin Z, Gu X, Berry JM, Titus JL, Gidding SS, Rocchini AP. Periventricular closure of ventricular septal defects without cardiopulmonary bypass. Ann Thorac Surg 1999;68(l):149–153.
58. Loulmet D, Carpentier A, d'Attellis N, et al. Endoscopic coronary artery bypass grafting with the aid of robotic assisted instruments [see comments]. J Thorac Cardiovasc Surg 1999;118(l):4–10.
59. Chitwood WR Jr. Video-assisted and robotic mitral valve surgery: toward an endoscopic surgery. Semin Thorac Cardiovasc Surg 1999;11(3):194–205.
60. Reichenspurner H, Boehm D, Reichart B. Minimally invasive mitral valve surgery using three-dimensional video and robotic assistance. Semin Thorac Cardiovasc Surg 1999;11(3):235–243.
61. Falk V, Walther T, Autschbach R, Diegeler A, Battellini R, Mohr FW. Robot-assisted minimally invasive solo mitral valve operation. J Thorac Cardiovasc Surg 1998;115(2):470–471.
62. Reichenspumer H, Damiano RJ, Mack M, et al. Use of the voice-controlled and computer-assisted surgical system ZEUS for endoscopic coronary artery bypass grafting [see comments]. J Thorac Cardiovasc Surg 1999;118(l):11–16.
63. Shennib H, Bastawisy A, McLoughlin J, Moll F. Robotic computer-assisted telemanipulation enhances coronary artery bypass. J Thorac Cardiovasc Surg 1999;117(2):310–313.
64. Gulbins H, Boehm D. 3-D visualization improves the dry-lab coronary anastomosis using the Zeus Robotics System. Heart Surg Forum 1999;4:318–325.
65. Hausdorf G, Schneider M, Franzbach B, Kampmann C, Kargus K, Goeldner B. Transcatheter closure of secundum atrial septal defects with the atrial septal defect occlusion system (ASDOS): initial experience in children. Heart 1996;75(i):83–88.
66. Hekmat K, Mehlhom U, Rainer V. Surgical repair of a large residual atrial septal defect after transcatheter closure. Ann Thorac Surg 1997;63(5):1456–1458.
67. Das GS. Failure of devices used for the closure of atrial septal defects [letter; comment]. J Thorac Cardiovasc Surg 1997;113(2):426–427.
68. Agarwal SK, Ghosh PK, Mittal PK. Failure of devices used for closure of atrial septal defects: mechanisms and management [see comments]. J Thorac Cardiovasc Surg 1996;112(i):21–26.
69. Bridges ND, Perry SB, Keane JF, et al. Preoperative transcatheter closure of congenital muscular ventricular septal defects. N Engl J Med 1991; 324(19):1312–1317.
70. Zahn EM, Chang AC, Burke RP, Jacobs JP. Transcatheter closure of an extracardiac Fontan fenestration. Ann Thorac Surg 1998;66(l):260–262.
71. Zahn EM, Chang AC, Aldousany A, Burke RP. Emergent stent placement for acute Blalock-Taussig shunt obstruction after stage I Norwood surgery [see comments]. Cathet Cardiovasc Diagn 1997;42(2):191–194.
72. Hannan RL, Miyaji K, Burke RP, Zahn EM. Endovascular stent graft treatment of a pulmonary artery pseudoaneurysm. Ann Thorac Surg 2001;71(2):727–729.

23 Thoracoscopic Pericardial Surgery

P. Michael McFadden, MD

CONTENTS

INTRODUCTION
HISTORY
PERICARDIAL ANATOMY AND PHYSIOLOGY
PATIENT SELECTION AND PREPARATION
ANESTHETIC MANAGEMENT
SURGICAL TECHNIQUE
PERICARDIAL EFFUSION AND TAMPONADE
PERICARDIAL CONSTRICTION
PERICARDIAL TUMORS
CONGENITAL PERICARDIAL DEFECTS
PERICARDIAL CYSTS
EPICARDIAL PACEMAKER IMPLANTATION
DIAPHRAGM PACING
SUMMARY
REFERENCES

INTRODUCTION

The pericardium is a unique organ because of the strategic position it occupies within the chest and its close proximity to other vital structures. The pericardium is subject to many of the pathological conditions that affect other organs, such as congenital abnormalities, inflammation, infection, trauma, systemic metabolic disorders, and neoplastic disease. The anatomical and functional effects of these conditions on the pericardium generally result in effusive, restrictive, or constrictive conditions that may compromise cardiac function. In most patients, pericardial disease is asymptomatic, self-limited, and responsive to medical therapy. Symptomatic patients who do not respond to traditional medical therapy or who become physiologically compromised may require surgery. A variety of surgical procedures, requiring subxiphoid, thoracic, and sternal

From: *Contemporary Cardiology: Minimally Invasive Cardiac Surgery, Second Edition*
Edited by: D. J. Goldstein and M. C. Oz © Humana Press Inc., Totowa, NJ

incisions, have been proposed and used effectively to diagnose and treat pericardial diseases and their sequelae. The development of video-assisted thoracoscopy and remarkable advances in endoscopic instrumentation over the last two decades has ushered a paradigm shift from open to minimally invasive approaches to treat pericardial disease.

HISTORY

The first anatomical description of the human pericardium is found in the writings of Hippocrates in the fourth century BC *(1)*. Observations in animals recorded by Galen (AD 131–201) five centuries later first described inflammatory pericarditis and the effects of pericardial effusion and constriction on the movement of the heart. For the next 2000 yr, observations on pericardial disease were limited to postmortem anatomical descriptions of pericarditis, pericardial effusion, adhesions, pericardial constriction, and calcific pericarditis. It was not until the eighteenth century that physicians began describing the physical findings associated with pericardial effusion and constriction such as pain, percussion dullness, enlargement of the cardiac silhouette, and pericardial friction rub. Recognition of the physiological effects of pericardial disease began in the 1800s with observations by Kussmaul and others. Treatment of pericardial effusion by pericardiocenthesis, subxiphoid drainage, and pericardial resection soon followed and ushered in the era of surgical management of pericardial disease *(1–3)*.

Thoracoscopy for the diagnosis and treatment of diseases of the chest found its origins in the early 1900s *(4–7)*. However, most surgeons failed to embrace thoracoscopy at that time because its utility was limited due to rudimentary instrumentation and the absence of endotracheal anesthesia. Despite these limitations, a few entrepreneurial surgeons continued to develop the field of thoracoscopy during the twentieth century *(8–13)*. Thoracotomy, sternotomy, and subxiphoid approaches to manage pericardial disease were adopted by the majority of surgeons with excellent results. The introduction of the double-lumen endobronchial tube in the 1970s made single-lung ventilation possible. This innovation not only enhanced open thoracotomy but also rekindled an interest in thoracoscopy. The subsequent development of video-assisted thoracoscopic instrumentation in the 1980s was a major stimulus for the enthusiastic expansion of thoracoscopy as it is practiced today. Video-assisted thoracoscopy has in many circumstances supplanted open surgical procedures in the diagnosis and treatment of many diseases of the chest and pericardium. Essentially every known malady of the pericardium that has been treated by open pericardial window, pericardiectomy, biopsy, or resection may with proper indication be preferentially managed now by video-assisted thoracoscopy.

PERICARDIAL ANATOMY AND PHYSIOLOGY

The pericardium arises from mesenchymal lacunae that develop between the pleural spaces and the diaphragm in the first trimester of fetal life. Fusion of the lacunae result in the formation of a sac called the pericardium, which encompasses the heart from the diaphragm to the base of great vessels and laterally to the hilum of each lung. The fibrous outer layer of the pericardium is composed of dense collagen tissue. The inner layer is a thin serosal surface that lines the entire pericardial cavity and covers the heart. The serosal surface around the heart is termed the visceral pericardium or epicardium. The parietal pericardium is composed of the fibrous sac and the serosal surface lining it *(14)*.

A neurovascular bundle comprised of the phrenic nerve, the pericardiophrenic artery and vein, and a pericardial fat pad transverses the parietal pericardium bilaterally. Functionally, the pericardium protects and maintains the heart in a stable midthoracic position. It prevents overdistention, torsion, and pendulous motion that may occur with volume overload or change in body position *(15)*. It also serves as a barrier for the spread of infection *(14)*. The inner serosal surface is comprised of cuboidal cells that contain microvilli, which are responsible for both the secretion and absorption of a clear plasmalike fluid *(16)*. The 15–30 mL of pericardial fluid normally found in the pericardial space lubricate the surface and reduce friction to the beating heart. Disease or conditions that alter either the secretion or reabsorption of pericardial fluid may result in pericardial dysfunction and lead to compromised cardiac function.

PATIENT SELECTION AND PREPARATION

Selection of appropriate candidates for a video-assisted thoracoscopic approach for the diagnosis and management of pericardial disease depends on the complexity of the problem to be addressed and the physical condition and limitations of the individual patient *(17)*. In general, the patient must be able to tolerate general anesthesia and contralateral single-lung ventilation. Patients with a single lung, pulmonary hypertension, or advanced interstitial lung disease who are unable to maintain acceptable arterial oxygen saturations, blood pH, and systemic blood pressure due to poor pulmonary reserve are not considered candidates for a thoracoscopic pericardial procedure. The thoracoscopic approach is directed by the type, location, and complexity of the pericardial disease. Inflammatory conditions that cause concomitant pleuropericarditis may result in adhesions that limit access to the pleural space. Likewise, patients with a history of pleurodesis, irradiation, emphysema, or previous thoracoscopy must be selected carefully. Ventilator-dependent patients are generally poor candidates due to their underlying lung disease and inability to sustain single-lung ventilation. The physiological effects of pericardial effusion, constriction or restriction under the conditions of general anesthesia, a lateral decubitus position, and single-lung ventilation must be considered and individualized for each patient.

The thoracoscopic procedure along with its objective, anticipated results, and possible complications are reviewed with the patient preoperatively. If the procedure cannot be successfully accomplished thoracoscopically or should complications arise, the possibility of conversion to open thoracotomy must be included in the consent. The cardiothoracic surgeon must be familiar with intrathoracic anatomy and the pathophysiology of pericardial disease. The surgeon must be thoroughly trained and experienced in thoracoscopic technique and capable of managing emergent surgical complications *(18–20)*.

ANESTHETIC MANAGEMENT

The thoracoscopic approach to the pericardium requires general endotracheal anesthesia. Continuous monitoring of the oxygen saturation and arterial blood pressure is mandatory. Patients with cardiac embarrassment from effusion, tamponade, or constriction may require more invasive central venous or pulmonary arterial monitoring in order to better evaluate and maintain hemodynamic stability. Rebound hypertension can be anticipated following the relief of cardiac tamponade or effusion. The hypertensive response encountered after pericardiectomy for constriction is often short-lived, and hypotension from poor contractility due to developing interstitial myocardial edema may result. Bladder catherization is usually reserved for those patients in whom more difficult hemodynamic management is anticipated or when the duration of the thoracoscopic pericardial procedure is expected to be prolonged.

A double-lumen endobronchial tube is required to allow decompression of the lung on the side of the procedure. Although either a right- or left-sided double-lumen endobronchial tube may be used, a left-sided tube is preferred because of its ease of placement and stability *(21,22)*. Single-lumen endotracheal tubes with bronchial blockers are commonly used in children and patients with small tracheal diameters, in whom the larger-profile double-lumen tubes would be contraindicated *(23)*. We have found the bronchial blocker tubes less reliable, as they frequently dislodge and are difficult to reposition. Proper position and function of the endobronchial tube are essential and are confirmed by auscultation and fiber-optic bronchoscopy before and after turning the patient to the appropriate lateral decubitus position for thoracoscopy. Flexion of the table assists the surgeon by widening the intercostal spaces to facilitate thoracoscopy. A supine position with arm extension is utilized to provide access to either side of the pericardium when more extensive procedures are required, such as bilateral pericardial windows or total pericardiectomy.

Anesthetic agents that delay immediate postoperative extubation are avoided. Significant postoperative pain is rare. If oral analgesics do not suffice, consideration may be given to the use of intercostal nerve blocks or epidural pain catheters. Nonsteroidal anti-inflammatory agents are often beneficial when combined with oral analgesics for postoperative intercostal pain *(17)*.

SURGICAL TECHNIQUE

A video-assisted thoracoscopic approach to the pericardium is performed, with the patient prepared in a lateral decubitus position as for thoracotomy. The lung on the operative side is decompressed and a 2-cm thoracoport incision is made in the fifth or sixth intercostal space in the mid-auxiliary or posterior-axillary line. The pleural space is digitally explored for adhesions and to ensure deflation of the lung. If a coexisting pleural effusion is encountered, it should be aspirated and sent for appropriate studies when indicated. A 15-mm thoracoport is placed through the incision into the pleural space. A 0° thoracoscope with video camera attachment is introduced through the thoracoport and the entire pleural cavity and its contents are thoroughly evaluated. Particular attention should be given to the pericardial anatomy and the location and course of the phrenic nerve and the accompanying pericardiophrenic artery and vein. On the right, the phrenic nerve courses laterally on the vena cava superiorly and traverses the pericardial reflection, which closely approximates the right lung hilum. On the left, the phrenic nerve courses more anteriorly and away from the hilum and reaches the diaphragm just posterior to the pericardial apex. This left-sided anatomical relationship is important, as it allows for both anterior and posterior approaches to the left pericardium (**Fig. 1**). Two additional thoracoport sites are usually necessary to allow for the introduction of instruments to perform the indicated procedure. These sites are best positioned one or two interspaces lateral to the endoscopic camera port and in the anterior-axillary line to avoid "dueling" of equipment and to facilitate operative exposure *(24)* (**Fig. 2**). Thoracoport sites are individualized depending on the anatomy and particular character-

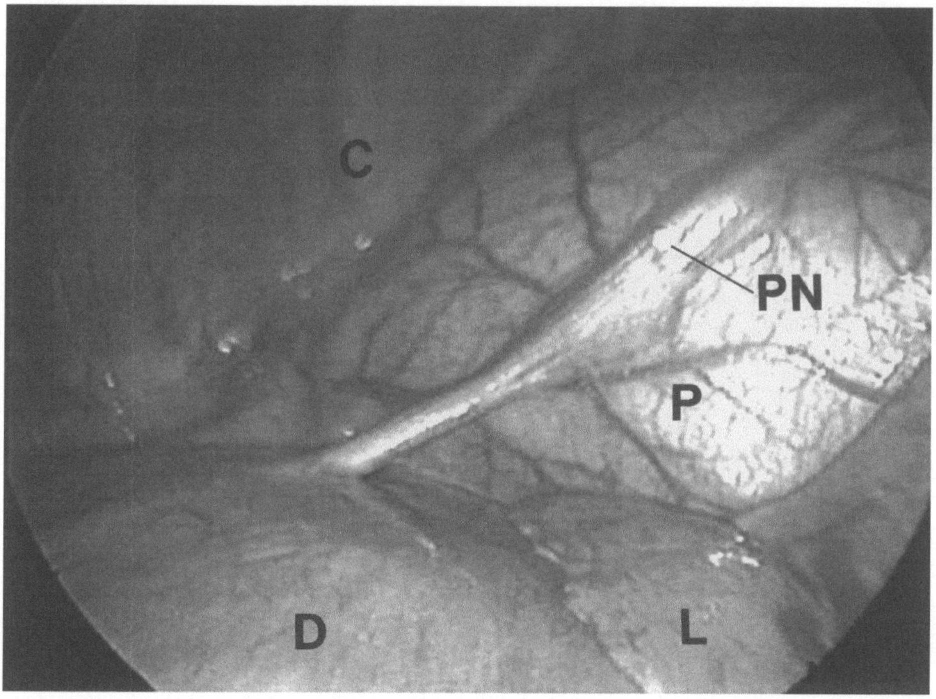

Fig. 1. Thoracosopic exposure of the left pericardium. Note relationship of the phrenic nerve (PN), pericardium (P), chest wall (C), diaphragm (D), and lung (L).

istics of the patient. Video monitors are oriented so that both the surgeon and assistant have good visualization. During the procedure, close attention is given to homeostasis, as the pericardium is a highly vascular structure, particularly in disease. At the termination of the procedure a chest tube is placed posterolateral to the lung through the most inferior incision to provide adequate, dependent postoperative pleural drainage. The remaining thoracoport incisions are closed with absorbable sutures. The patient is extubated in the operating room unless there is an indication for continued ventilatory support. An erect anterior–posterior chest film is obtained in the recovery room to confirm full expansion of the lung and appropriate chest tube position.

PERICARDIAL EFFUSION AND TAMPONADE

An accumulation of fluid within the pericardial sac may result from a variety of benign or malignant conditions. Acute inflammation or systemic conditions that involve the pericardium and alter the balance between secretion and reabsorption of pericardial fluid may result in pericardial effusion. Causes of pericarditis and pericardial effusion include inflammatory, infectious, neoplastic, postsurgical, systemic metabolic, and traumatic etiologies (Table 1).

Acute pericardial effusions are often symptomatic, due either to direct effects of pericardial inflammation and irritation or to the adverse physiological effects of tamponade on cardiac function. Since the pericardium is essentially noncompliant, cardiac compression may occur with relatively small amounts of acute pericardial effusion. The character of the effusion may be serous, serosanguinous, hemorrhagic, or chylous,

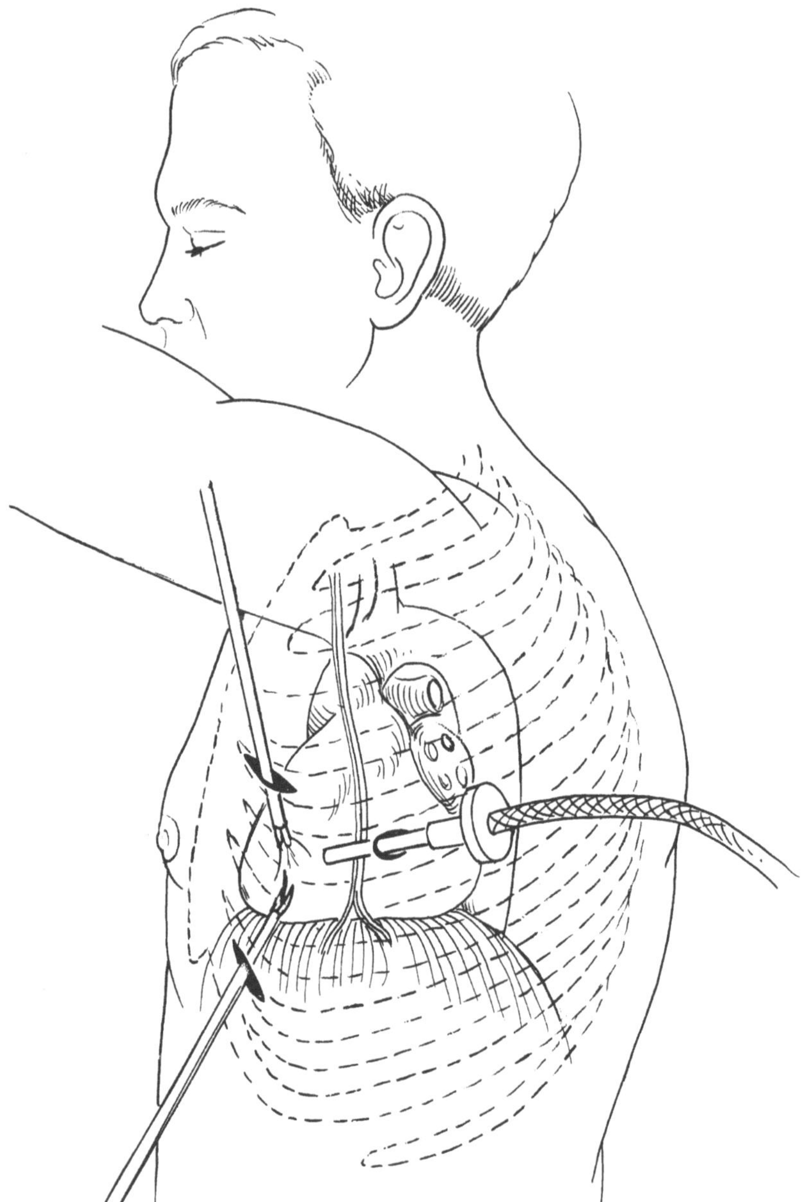

Fig. 2. Video-assisted thoracoscopic approach to the pericardium. Working thoracoports are placed lateral and slightly anterior to video-thoracoscopic camera ports to avoid "dueling" of the instruments during the procedure.

depending on the cause. Initial treatment consists of bed rest, pain control, and pharmacological treatment of the specific etiology, such as administration of anti-inflammatory agents for nonspecific pericarditis, antibiotics for infectious pericarditis, dialysis for uremia, and thyroid replacement for myxedema. Some cases may require pericardiocentesis to determine the cause and treat the effusion. These measures alone are effective in

Table 1
Causes of Pericarditis and Pericardial Effusion

Inflammatory
Acute nonspecific pericarditis
Dressler's syndrome
Infectious
Viral
Bacterial
Tuberculous
Parasitic
Neoplastic
Metastatic carcinoma
Lymphoma/leukemia
Primary pericardial/cardiac malignancy
Postirradiation
Postsurgical
Postpericardiotomy syndrome
Postthoracotomy
Chylopericardium
Hemothorax
Postoperative
Anticoagulation (delayed)
Systemic metabolic
Uremia
Cirrhosis
Amylodosis
Hypothyroidism
Connective tissue disorders
Lupus erythematosis
Rheumatoid arthritis
Rheumatic fever
Traumatic
Penetrating
Blunt

resolving the inflammation and effusion in most patients. However, in cases of acute cardiac tamponade or when accelerated reaccumulation of effusion occurs following pericardiocentesis, rapid and effective drainage is indicated. Effective drainage aids not only in establishing the diagnosis and resolving the symptoms of effusion but also in preventing the recurrence of effusion or the development of late pericardial constriction.

Simple bedside subxiphoid pericardial drainage performed under local anesthesia and sterile preparation is quick and usually effective. This is especially true in the case of cardiac tamponade following open-heart surgery or catheter-induced complications occurring after percutaneous cardiac intervention. Open pericardial window and pericardiectomy also provide excellent pericardial drainage, but they require time for patient mobilization and preparation, thoracotomy, and general anesthesia. These procedures may also be performed thoracoscopically. Thoracoscopic drainage is less morbid than surgical thoracotomy but shares the same constraints as thoracotomy with regard to preparation, mobilization, and general anesthesia. Severely compromised patients benefit from the most expeditious approach to pericardial drainage *(25)*. Thoracoscopic pericardiectomy and pericardial window appear to be best suited for drainage of chronic effusions in hemodynamically stable patients. Visualization of the pericardium is excellent, and wide resection of the pericardium both anterior and posterior to the phrenic nerve on the left is possible. In the presence of a highly vascular pericardium, an endoscopic stapler may be useful to ensure hemostasis when opening or resecting the pericardium.

Thoracoscopic drainage has demonstrated excellent results, with a low incidence of recurrence, morbidity, and mortality *(15)*. Advocates of the procedure report better visualization, avoidance of the morbidity of thoracotomy, and shorter hospitalization. Despite these distinct advantages, long-term survival with video-assisted thoracoscopic pericardiectomy has not been affected *(15,26,27)*. This is likely the result of frequent application of thoracoscopic pericardial resection in patients with malignant effusions, a condition that portends a poor survival. Thoracoscopic pericardiectomy for adherent pericardial constriction has been proposed but has yet to be adopted as a satisfactory alternative to managing this late sequelae of pericardial disease.

PERICARDIAL CONSTRICTION

Pericardial constriction is the result of a chronic constrictive inflammatory process of the pericardium that may lead to significant morbidity. The etiology is usually idiopathic, but other frequent causes are mediastinal irradiation, connective tissue disorders, tuberculosis, neoplastic disease, and trauma *(28,29)*. Since the advent of open-heart surgery in the 1950s, postoperative pericarditis has become another important cause of pericardial constriction *(30)*. Essentially, constriction may result from any process that causes pericarditis. Fibrosis and pericardial thickening constricts the ventricles, impedes diastolic filling, and leads to reduced cardiac output. The process is insidious and the clinical course is that of progressive deterioration. Hemodynamic evidence of impaired diastolic ventricular filling at cardiac catherization along with other supportive studies such as computerized tomography and magnetic resonance imaging are helpful in making the diagnosis. Definitive treatment of pericardial constriction requires pericardiectomy.

Although the technique of thoracoscopic pericardiectomy has advanced, its use is limited to the management of pure effusive pericardial disease or in patients with pericardial constriction who demonstrate a combined effusive–constrictive component *(15,31–34)*. Thoracoscopic pericardiectomy for dense, adhesive pericardial constriction has not been advocated. Adequate exposure for control of possible hemorrhagic complications or for the institution of cardiopulmonary bypass, should it be required, is limited. Thoracoscopic pericardiectomy in the presence of adherent and patent coronary bypass grafts will also be dangerous. Additionally, a thoracoscopic approach is not possible in patients who require concomitant cardiac procedures, such as valve replacement or coronary artery revascularization. For these reasons, median sternotomy remains the approach of choice for pericardial resection in pericardial constriction, as it has demonstrated excellent results, lesser morbidity, and shorter hospital stays while allowing greater flexibility for the performance of concomitant procedures *(35–39)*. In a rather limited number of patients, thoracoscopic pericardiectomy for pericardial constriction may be possible. However, the indications and limitations of this approach for pericardial constriction have yet to be defined.

PERICARDIAL TUMORS

The majority of pericardial neoplasms are metastatic malignancies. The pericardium is involved in approx 8.5% of patients with malignant tumors. The heart is also involved in the majority of patients with pericardial metastases *(1)*. Malignant pericardial effusion and hemopericardium are frequent sequelae of pericardial malignancy and result from lymphatic obstruction or bleeding from the tumor. Carcinoma of the lung and breast are the two malignancies that most frequently involve the pericardium *(40,41)*. Owing to the proximity of these two organs to the pericardium, local extension and lymphatic spread are common routes to pericardial involvement. Melanoma, leukemia, and sarcoma are metastatic tumors that have a particular propensity for hematogenous spread to the pericardium *(1)*. Other tumors, such as malignant thymoma, thymic carcinoma, teratoma, and pleural mesothelioma, which arise in proximity, also often involve the pericardium. The associated pericardial effusion and bulky extent of the metastatic implants often result in cardiac compromise from tamponade or cardiac compression. Therefore, the role of thoracoscopy in pericardial tumor management is often limited to diagnostic biopsy in occult disease or the creation of a pericardial window for drainage of a known symptomatic malignant pericardial effusion.

Primary pericardial malignancies, tumors that arise directly from the pericardium or its associated structures, are very rare. Angiosarcoma constitutes the most common sarcoma of pericardial origin and often involves the right atrium *(42)*. Thoracoscopic biopsy of an angiosarcomatous tumor must be undertaken with caution, as this tumor is highly vascular and prone to hemorrhage. Owing to its extent, vascular nature, and frequent cardiac involvement, thoracoscopic resection of angiosarcoma is usually not possible. Management of these tumors typically requires extensive open surgical resection or even cardiac transplantation *(43,44)*. Primary pericardial mesothelioma is exceedingly rare and comprises only 0.7% of all mesotheliomas *(45)*. Liposarcoma of the pericardial fat and malignant neurogenic tumors of the autonomic or phrenic nerves may also be encountered. If these tumors are small, localized, and not associated with a malignant pericardial or pleural effusion, thoracoscopic resection may be considered.

Benign tumors of the pericardium are also uncommon. However, thoracoscopic resection is the procedure of choice when a benign diagnosis is confirmed and the tumor can be removed technically without compromising the surrounding cardiac, vascular, or neural structures.

CONGENITAL PERICARDIAL DEFECTS

Defects of the pericardium are rare and occur in fetal life as a result of compromised circulation to the developing pleuropericardial membrane. The majority of congenital pericardial defects are found on the left. The diagnosis is usually made serendipitously while the patient is undergoing evaluation for more common symptomatic cardiac disorders. A prominence of the left heart border or pulmonary artery on plain chest film may suggest a pericardial defect (**Fig. 3**). However, computerized axial tomography, cinemagnetic resonance imaging, and cardiac catherization best establish the diagnosis *(46–48)*. Complete absence of the pericardium and defects smaller than 2 cm are usually asymptomatic. However, defects that are large enough to allow partial herniation of the

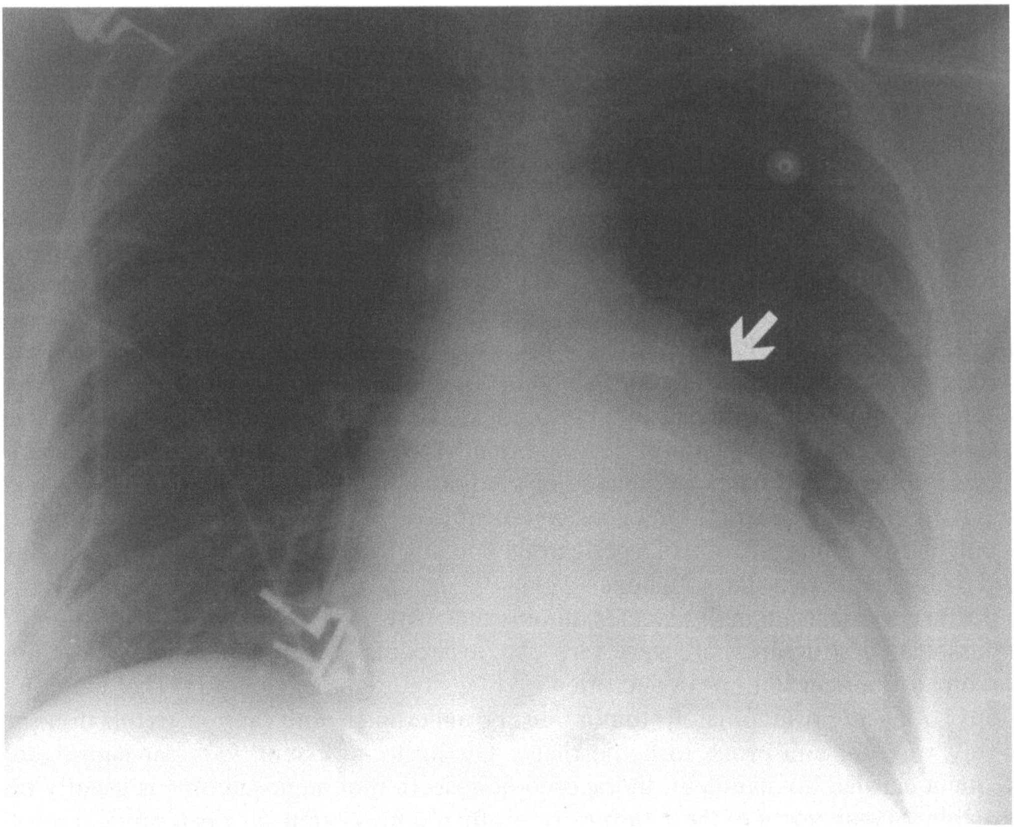

Fig. 3. Preoperative chest roentgenogram showing convex prominence of left heart and border (arrow). From: Risher WH, Rees AP, Ochsner JL, et al. Thoracoscopic resection of pericardium from symptomatic congenital pericardial defect. Reprinted with permission from the Society of Thoracic Surgeons. Annals of Thoracic Surgery 1993;56:1390–1391.

left atrial appendage or a portion of the left ventricle may predispose to cardiac symptoms such as palpitations, dyspnea, syncope, and chest discomfort (**Fig. 4**). Angina has resulted from partial cardiac herniation and dynamic compression of the coronary arteries by the lower border of the pericardial defect *(46)* (**Fig. 5**). Symptomatic pericardial defects require surgical management to alleviate symptoms and prevent complications. Wide thoracoscopic pericardial resection is usually sufficient to relieve constriction and resolve the cardiac compromise. Endostapling of the left atrial appendage base may even be required in some patients with infarction of the atrial appendage or when systemic emboli result from thrombi with the atrial appendage.

PERICARDIAL CYSTS

Pericardial cysts, like pericardial defects, develop in embryonic life. Cysts are derived from mesenchymal origin and may arise either from a diverticulum of the developing pericardium or an abnormal fusion of the pericardial lacunae. Unlike pericardial defects, cysts occur most often on the right and usually do not communicate with the pericardial cavity *(32)*. The radiographic appearance is classically teardrop in shape, due to the frequent location within the anterior costophrenic angle *(49)*. Pericardial cysts are benign and usually unilocular and contain a clear watery fluid. They are found in persons of all

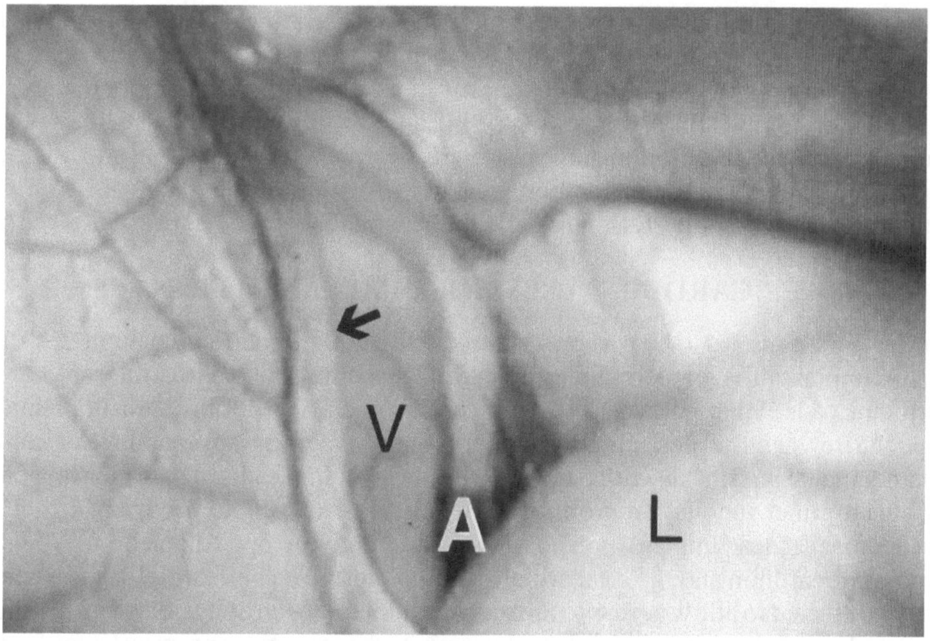

Fig. 4. Thoracoscopic appearance of a congenital left pericardial defect demonstrating partial cardiac herniation (V = ventricle, A = left atrium, L = lung, arrow = pericardial border).

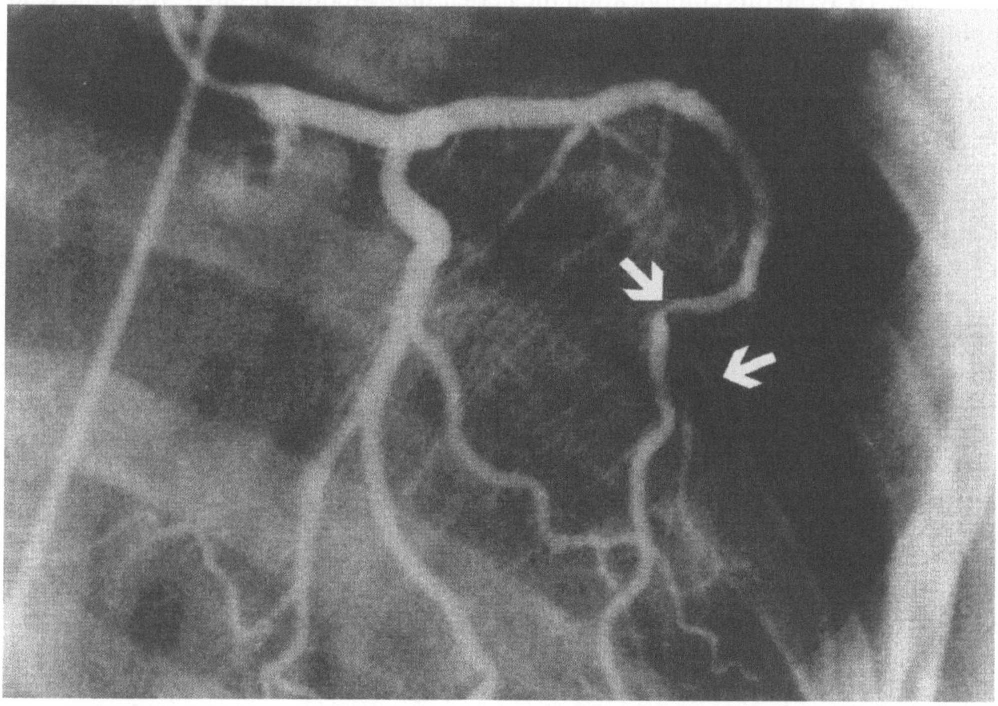

Fig. 5. Migratory coronary obstructions of left anterior descending and diagonal arteries due to impingement of congenital left pericardial defect (arrows). From: Risher WH, Rees AP, Ochsner JL, et al. Thoracoscopic resection of pericardium from symptomatic congenital pericardial defect. Reprinted with permission from the Society of Thoracic Surgeons. Annals of Thoracic Surgery 1993;56:1390–1391.

ages. Radiographic studies are usually diagnostic, but aspiration or resection is indicated if the diagnosis is uncertain or if the cyst is symptomatic.

Most pericardial cysts may be easily approached thoracoscopically, where they may be aspirated or completely resected *(50–53)*. Large or thick-walled cysts may require marsupialization and fulguration of the base with electrocautery or laser *(54,55)*. The cyst fluid and wall are submitted for pathological confirmation of the diagnosis. Complete resection of a symptomatic cyst is important, since recurrence of cysts has been observed *(53)*.

EPICARDIAL PACEMAKER IMPLANTATION

Consideration may also be given to a transpericardial thoracoscopic approach to the heart for implantation of permanent epicardial pacemaker leads or internal cardiac defibrillator pads. Most patients requiring cardiac pacing or defibrillator implantation have adequate venous access and will preferentially undergo transvenous lead implantation under local anesthesia with excellent results *(56)*. In the absence of central venous access due to either venous compromise or preexisting transvenous hardware, a thoracoscopic approach to lead implantation provides an alternative to open thoracotomy *(57–59)*. When the pericardium and the pericardial space are normal, a pericardial window on the left may be created to allow access to the myocardium for electrophysiological testing by the use of a hand-held wand electrode to determine what may be appropriate sites for lead implantation. "Screw-in" bipolar epicardial leads may then be implanted in the areas that demonstrate the best thresholds for capture, sensing, and impedance. Hemostasis must be ensured at the time of lead implantation, as intrapericardial bleeding may lead to tamponade. To avoid this complication the pericardial window through which the leads are placed must be opened widely to allow for pericardial decompression should bleeding occur. The leads are passed medial to the lung in the anterior–superior mediastinum and tunneled transthoracically into a subcutaneous pocket anterior to the pectoralis muscle. The leads are secured to the pectoral fascia to prevent migration and then connected to the pacing pulse generator or defibrillator. If the pericardial space is found to be obliterated and a thin pericardium adherent to the heart is encountered, placement of the leads into the heart may still be possible. Most recently, biventricular pacing therapy has gained acceptance for the treatment of advanced congestive heart failure in patients with prolonged QRS intervals. Because of the difficulties associated with the placement of the coronary sinus lead for capture of the left ventricle, thoracic surgeons are increasingly being asked to position the left ventricular lead on the lateral wall of the heart. This can easily be accomplished with thoracoscopic approaches.

DIAPHRAGM PACING

A discussion of thoracoscopic pericardial surgery would be incomplete without mentioning diaphragmatic pacing, a surgical procedure with limited but important application. Patients with neurological injury or conditions that result in central respiratory paralysis and who require ventilatory support may be candidates for diaphragmatic pacing. Tetraplegia, central sleep apnea, congenital hypoventilation syndrome, and certain brainstem lesions are common causes of central hypoventilation and apnea. An intact phrenic nerve (lower motor neuron) and functional diaphragmatic muscle are necessary requisites for diaphragm pacing *(60)*. The site of phrenic nerve stimulation may be selected anywhere along its cervical or intrathoracic course. Because the majority of these patients have undergone tracheostomy for mechanical ventilation and prevention

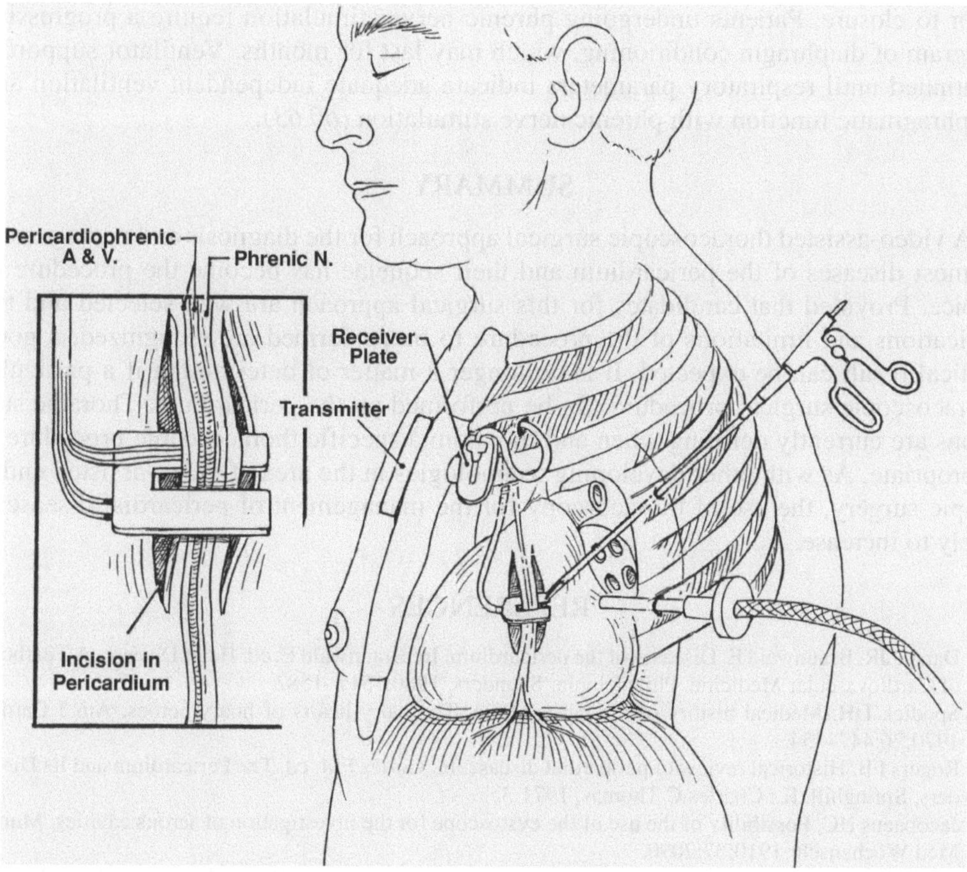

Fig. 6. Illustration of intra-thoracic placement of left phrenic nerve stimulator by video-assisted thoracoscopy.

of aspiration, the once-popular cervical approach to phrenic nerve stimulation has generally been abandoned in order to avoid infection of the implantable hardware and improve patient comfort *(61)*. Median sternotomy, thoracotomy through the anterior second intercostal space or axilla, and paramediastinotomy have each provided excellent exposure to the intrathoracic phrenic nerve. However, a less invasive thoracoscopic approach has recently been advocated, which provides excellent visualization and exposure of the phrenic nerve and application of the pacing electrode *(62)*.

Phrenic nerve stimulation requires successive pulse currents to effect diaphragmatic contraction. A biphasic, alternating, positive and negative current is preferred over a monophasic current because it does not require as much energy and is less likely to cause phrenic nerve injury. Although a variety of devices have been developed for phrenic nerve stimulation, the basic component of each consists of nerve electrode strips, electrode wires, a receiver, and an external stimulator (pacer). Longitudinal windows anterior and posterior to the phrenic nerve are created thoracoscopically, and bipolar strips are applied to either side of the nerve (**Fig. 6**). Because electrocautery poses a potential to nerve injury, the pericardial windows are best created with sharp dissection. Once the strips are secured into position, the electrode wires are tunneled into a subcutaneous position in the anterior chest wall and attached to a receiver. Pacer function is verified prior to closure. Patients undergoing phrenic nerve stimulation require a progressive program of diaphragm conditioning, which may last for months. Ventilator support is continued until respiratory parameters indicate adequate independent ventilation and diaphragmatic function with phrenic nerve stimulation *(60,63)*.

SUMMARY

A video-assisted thoracoscopic surgical approach for the diagnosis and management of most diseases of the pericardium and their sequelae has become the procedure of choice. Provided that candidates for this surgical approach are well selected and the indications and limitations of the procedure to be performed are recognized, a good clinical result can be expected. It is no longer a matter of determining if a particular thoracoscopic surgical procedure can be performed on the pericardium. Thoracic surgeons are currently defining when and in whom a specific thoracoscopic procedure is appropriate. As with other developing technologies in the area of video-assisted endoscopic surgery, the use of thoracoscopy for the management of pericardial disease is likely to increase.

REFERENCES

1. Darsee JR, Braunwald E. Diseases of the pericardium. In: Braunwald E, ed. Heart Disease: A Textbook of Cardiovascular Medicine. Philadelphia: Saunders, 1980:1517–1582.
2. Spodick DH. Medical history of the pericardium. The hairy hearts of hoary heroes. Am J Cardiol 1970;26:447–454.
3. Rogers FB. Historical review of pericardial disease. In: Cortes FM, ed. The Pericardium and Its Disorders. Springhill, IL: Charles C Thomas, 1971:3.
4. Jacobaeus HC. Possibility of the use of the cystoscope for the investigation of serous cavities. Munch Med Wochenschr 1910;57:2090.
5. Jacobaeus HC. Endopheural operations by means of a thoracoscope. Beitr Klin Tuberk 1915;35:1.
6. Jacobaeus HC. The cauterization of adhesions in pneumothorax treatment of tuberculosis. Surg Gynecol Obstet 1921;32:493.
7. Jacobaeus HC. The proactive importance of thoracoscopy in surgery of the chest. Surg Gynecol Obstet 1922;34:209.
8. Fisher J. Instruments for illuminating dark cavities. Phila J Med Phys Sci 1927;14:409.
9. Lloyd MS. Thoracoscopy and biopsy in the diagnosis of pleurisy with effusion. Q Bull Sea View Hosp 1953;14:128.
10. Hatch HB Jr, DeCamp PT. Diagnostic thoracoscopy. Surg Clin North Am 1966;46:1405–1410.
11. Ochsner A Jr, Ochsner A. Cancer of the lung: recognition and management. Surg Clin North Am 1966;46:1411–1425.
12. DeCamp PT, Moseby PW, Scott ML, Hatch HB Jr. Diagnostic thoracoscopy. Ann Thorac Surg 1973;16:79–84.
13. Miller JI, Hatcher CR Jr. Thoracoscopy: a useful tool in the diagnosis of thoracic disease. Ann Thorac Surg 1978;26:68–72.
14. Jones WG II. Pericardial disease. In: Pearson FG, Deslaurier J, Ginsberg RJ, Hiebert CA, McKneally MF, Urschel HC Jr, eds. Thoracic Surgery. New York: Churchill Livingston, 1995:1373–1383.
15. Caccavale RJ. Video-assisted thoracic surgery for pericardial disease. In: Lewis RJ, ed. Video-Assisted Thoracic Surgery. Chest Surg Clin N Am 1993;3:271–281.
16. Elias H, Boyd LJ. Notes on the anatomy, embryology, and histology of the pericardium. II. J NY Med Coll 1960;2:50–75.
17. McFadden PM, Robbins RJ. Thoracoscopic surgery. Surg Clin North Am 1998;78:763–772.
18. McKneally MF. Video-asssited thoracic surgery. Standards and guidelines. In: Lewis RJ, ed. Video-Assisted Thoracic Surgery. Chest Surg Clin N Am 1993;3:345–351.
19. McKneally MF, Lewis RJ, Anderson RJ, et al. Statement of the AATS/STS Joint Committee on Thoracoscopy and Video Assisted Thoracic Surgery. J Thorac Cardiovasc Surg 1992;104:1.

20. McKneally MF, Lewis RJ, Anderson RJ, et al. Statement of the AATS/STS Joint Committee on Thoracoscopy and Video Assisted Thoracic Surgery. Ann Thorac Surg 1992;54:1.
21. Kraenzler EJ, Hearn CJ. Anesthetic considerations for video-assisted thoracic surgery. Semin Thorac Cardiovasc Surg 1993;5:321–326.
22. Weiss SJ, Cheung AT. Anesthesia for thoracoscopic surgery. In: Kaiser LR, Daniel TM, eds. Thoracoscopic Surgery. Boston: Little, Brown, 1993:17–36.
23. Lobe TE. Pediatric thoracoscopy. Semin Thorac Cardiovasc Surg 1993;5:298–302.
24. Landreneau RJ, Hazelrigg SR, Mack MJ, Keenan RJ, Ferson PF. Video-assisted thoracic surgery for diseases within the mediastinum. In: Shields TW, ed. General Thoracic Surgery. Vol. 2, 4th ed., Baltimore: Williams & Wilkins, 1994:1810–1816.
25. Ginsburg RJ. Thoracoscopy: a cautionary note. Ann Thorac Surg 1993;56:801–803.
26. Tuna IC, Danielson GK. Surgical management of pericardial diseases. Cardiol Clin 1990;8:683–696.
27. Piehler JM, Pluth JR, Schaff HV, Danielson GK, Orszulak TA, Puga FJ. Surgical management of effusive pericardial disease. Influence of extent of pericardial resection on clinical course. J Thorac Cardiovasc Surg 1985;90;506–516.
28. Cameron J, Oesterle SN, Baldwin JC, Hancock EW. The etiologic spectrum of constrictive pericarditis. Am Heart J 1987;113:354–360.
29. Fowler NO. Constrictive pericarditis: its history and current status. Clin Cardiol 1995;18:341–350.
30. Copeland JG, Riley JE, Fuller J. Pericardiectomy for effusive constrictive pericarditis after heart transplantation. J Heart Transplant 1986;5:171–172.
31. Krasna M, Fiocco M. Thoracoscopic pericardiectomy. Surg Laparosc Endosc 1995;5:202–204.
32. Ferguson MK. Thoracoscopic management of pericardial disease. Semin Thorac Cardiovasc Surg 1993;5:310–315.
33. Robles R, Pinero A, Lujan JA, et al. Thoracoscopic partial pericardiectomy in the diagnosis and management of pericardial effusion. Surg Endosc 1997;11:253–256.
34. Hazelrigg SR, Mack MJ, Landreneau RJ, Acuff TE, Seifert PE, Auer JE. Thoracoscopic pericardiectomy for effusive pericardial disease. Ann Thorac Surg 1993;56:792–795.
35. Trotter MC, Chung KC, Ochsner JL, McFadden PM. Pericardiectomy for pericardial constriction. Am Surg 1996;62:304–307.
36. Copeland JG, Stinson EB, Griepp RB, Shumway NE. Surgical treatment of chronic constrictive pericarditis using cardiopulmonary bypass. J Thorac Cardiovasc Surg 1975;69:236–238.
37. McCaughan BC, Schaff HV, Pichler JM, et al. Early and late results of pericardiectomy for constrictive pericarditis. J Thorac Cardiovasc Surg 1985;89:340–350.
38. Seifert FC, Miller DC, Oesterle SN, Oyer PE, Stinson EB, Shumway NE. Surgical treatment of constrictive pericarditis: analysis of outcome and diagnostic error. Circulation 1985;72:II264–II273.
39. Tuna IC, Danielson GK. Surgical management of pericardial diseases. Cardiol Clin 1990;8:683–696.
40. Young JM, Goldman IR. Tumor metastases to the heart. Circulation 1954;9:220–229.
41. Onuigbo, WIB. The spread of lung cancer to the heart, pericardium and great vessels. Jpn Heart J 1974;15:234–238.
42. Burke A, Virmani R. Primary cardiac sarcomas. In: Tumors of the Heart and Great Vessels. Atlas of Tumor Pathology, Third series, Fascicle 16. Washington, DC: Armed Forces Institute of Pathology, 1996:127–170.
43. McFadden PM, Ochsner JL. Atrial replacement and tricuspid valve reconstruction after angiosarcoma resection. Ann Thorac Surg 1997;64:1164–1166.
44. Dein JR, Frist WH, Stinson EB, et al. Primary cardiac neoplasms: early and late results of surgical treatment in 42 patients. J Thorac Cardiovasc Surg 1987;93:502–511.
45. Burke A, Virmani R. Malignant mesothelioma of the pericardium. In: Tumors of the Heart and Great Vessels. Atlas of Tumor Pathology, Third series, Fascicle 16. Washington, DC: Armed Forces Institute of Pathology, 1996:181–194.
46. Risher WH, Rees AP, Ochsner JL, McFadden PM. Thoracoscopic resection of pericardium for symptomatic congenital pericardial defect. Ann Thorac Surg 1993;56:1390–1391.
47. Baim RS, MacDonald IL, Wise DJ, Leukei SC. Computed tomography of absent left pericardium. Radiology 1980;135:127–128.
48. Schiavone WA, O'Donnell JK. Congeintal absence of the left portion of parietal pericardium demonstrated by nuclear magnetic response inaging. Am J Cardiol 1985;55:1439–1440.
49. Ochsner JL, Ochsner SF. Congenital cysts of the mediastinum: 20-year experience with 42 cases. Ann Surg 1966;163:909–920.

50. Mack MJ, Aronoff RJ, Acuff TE, Douthit MB, Bowman RT, Ryan WH. Present role of thoracoscopy in the diagnosis and treatment of diseases of the chest. Ann Thorac Surg 1992;54:403–409.
51. Michel JL, Revillon Y, Montupet P, Sauvat F, Sarnacki S, Sayegh N, N-Fekete C. Thoracoscopic treatment of mediastinal cysts in children. J Pediatr Surg 1998;33:1745–1748.
52. Horita K, Sakao Y, Itoh T. Excision of recurrant pericardial cyst using video-assisted thoracic surgery. Chest 1998;114:1203–1204.
53. Satur CM, Hsin MK, Dussek JE. Giant pericardial cysts. Ann Thorac Surg 1996;61:208–210.
54. Lewis RJ, Caccavale RJ, Sisler GE. Imaged thoracoscopic surgery: a new thoracic technique for resection of mediastinal cysts. Ann Thorac Surg 1992;53:318–320.
55. Naunheim KS, Andrus CH. Thoracoscopic drainage and resection of giant mediastinal cyst. Ann Thorac Surg 1993;55:156–158.
56. Mack MJ, Acuff TE, Ryan WH. Implantable cardioverter defibrillator: the role of thoracoscopy. Ann Thorac Surg 1993;56:739–740.
57. Robles R, Pinero A, Lujan JA, Parrilla P. Thoracoscopic implantation of an epicardial pacemaker. Br J Surg 1996;83:400.
58. Furrer M, Fuhrer J, Altermatt HJ, et al. VATS-guided epicardial pacemaker implantation. Hand-sutured fixation of atrioventricular leads in an experimental setting. Surg Endosc 1997;11:1167–1170.
59. Obadia JF, Kirkorian G, Rescigno G, el Farra M, Chassignoelle JF, Touboul P. Thoracoscopic approach to implantable cardioverter defibrillator patch electrode implantation. Pacing Clin Electrophysiol 1996;19:955–959.
60. Elefteriades JA, Quin JA. Diaphragm pacing. Chest Surg Clin N Am 1998;8:331–357.
61. Weese-Mayer DE, Morrow AS, Brouillette RT, Ilbawi MN, Hunt CE. Diaphragm pacing in infants and children: a life-table analysis of implanted components. Am Rev Respir Dis 1989;139:974–979.
62. Nye JD, Brown WT. Phrenic nerve stimulator. In WT Brown, ed. Atlas of Video-Assisted Thoracic Surgery. Philadelphia: Saunders, 1994:274–276.
63. Chervin RD, Guilleminault C. Diaphragm pacing for respiratory insufficiency. J Clin Neurophysiol 1997;14:369–377.

24 Less Invasive Surgical Treatment of Atrial Fibrillation

Mathew R. Williams, MD
and Michael Argenziano, MD

Contents

Introduction
Enabling Technology
Hypothermic Ablation
Hyperthermic Ablation
Radiofrequency
Microwave
Laser
Ultrasound
Nonthermal Ablation
Conclusions
References

INTRODUCTION

Atrial fibrillation (AF) remains the most prevalent arrhythmia, with as many as 2.2 million cases in the United States alone *(1)*, and it accounts for over 3.1 million office visits a year *(2)*. Despite often being labeled as a benign rhythm, AF plays a role in as many as 15% of all strokes *(3)* and is associated with an increased odds ratio for death (1.5 in men and 1.9 in women) *(4)*. In general, AF is rarely treated successfully by the medical community, with the mainstay of therapy being aimed at ventricular rate control and anticoagulation. New understanding of AF mechanisms combined with technological advances have led to a resurgence of anatomically based curative treatment of AF in both the catheter-based and the surgical arenas.

From: *Contemporary Cardiology: Minimally Invasive Cardiac Surgery, Second Edition*
Edited by: D. J. Goldstein and M. C. Oz © Humana Press Inc., Totowa, NJ

Surgical treatment of AF began in 1980 with the introduction of the left atrial isolation procedure *(5)*, which was successful at restoring sinus rhythm in the right atrium with subsequent conversion of both a normal ventricular response and improved hemodynamics. This approach was abandoned because the left atrium continued to fibrillate and thus the theoretical risk for stasis of blood in the fibrillating left atrium persisted, with a subsequent stroke risk. In 1985 Guiradon introduced the corridor procedure that created an isolated discrete pathway—a corridor—between the sinoatrial node and the atrioventricular node to restore a normal rate *(6)*. This procedure did not receive much acceptance due to both limited success and the fact that both atria continued to fibrillate with unaltered hemodynamics. In 1986 Cox performed his first clinical attempt at treating AF with the atrial transection procedure, which was initially promising but ultimately failed *(7)*. This failure lead Dr. Cox and his colleagues to better characterize the electrophysiological basis for AF *(8)*, which eventually resulted in the introduction of the Maze Procedure *(9)*. Based on clinical results, the procedure underwent revisions to become the Cox-Maze III procedure *(10)*, regarded today as the gold standard surgical treatment for AF.

The Maze III has been applied by Dr. Cox and others *(11,12)* with success rates as high as 98%, though not all groups have been able to duplicate these results *(13)*. Despite excellent results, the procedure has not been applied widely. Reasons for this reluctance are multifactorial but include the invasive nature of the procedure with the need for cardiopulmonary bypass, multiple atriotomies with their associated bleeding risk, and the complex basis of the procedure. These concerns as well as new understandings of AF mechanisms have spawned attempts at less invasive surgical cure of AF. In assessing any new curative treatment of AF it is important that the determination of a successful procedure be well defined. In particular, a procedure to cure AF should not only achieve sinus rhythm but also restore atrial contractility with its associated improvement in hemodynamics and decreased incidence of thromboembolic complications. Finally, a less invasive cure must also address the problems with previous approaches with an acceptable success rate.

The transition to a less invasive approach for curing AF will involve using alternative modalities in lieu of the "cut and sew" technique to create lesions and will ideally be applied from the epicardial surface on the beating heart. It will also undergo modification to be applied through smaller incisions, perhaps with the aid of thoracoscopic or robotic devices. Finally, while subject to much debate, there will likely be an alteration of the lesion set to simplify it from the Maze III. This chapter will discuss the current and forthcoming devices, approaches, and lesion sets that will facilitate the transition of AF surgery to a minimally invasive cure.

ENABLING TECHNOLOGY

In an effort to reduce bleeding, reduce operative time, and ultimately perform ablations from the epicardial surface, multiple technologies have been created to ablate atrial tissue. These technologies can be broken into three categories: hypothermic sources, hyperthermic sources, and nonthermal sources (Table 1). These energy sources can be applied from either the epicardium or the endocardium, and each approach is associated with very different physics.

Surgical approaches from the endocardium generally are on the arrested and opened heart, and successful ablation is easier to accomplish due to the lack of the convective heating or cooling effects of flowing blood. The primary impeding factors to ablating tissue are conductive and convective thermal alterations from ambient air, body tempera-

Table 1
Energy Sources for Atrial Ablation

Mechanism	*Energy Source*	*Company*	*FDA Approval Status*
Hypothermic			
	Cryo	EndoCare, Cryocath, Frigitronics	Treatment of arrhythmias
Hyperthermic			
	Radiofrequency		
	Unipolar	Boston Scientific	Soft tissue ablation
	Bipolar	Atricure	Soft tissue ablation
	Irrigated	Medtronic, Osypka	Pending
	Microwave	AFx	Cardiac ablation
	Laser	Cardiofocus/Edwards	Cardiac ablation
	USG	Spectrasonics, Epicor	Experimental
Nonthermal			
	Chemical	Microheart	Experimental

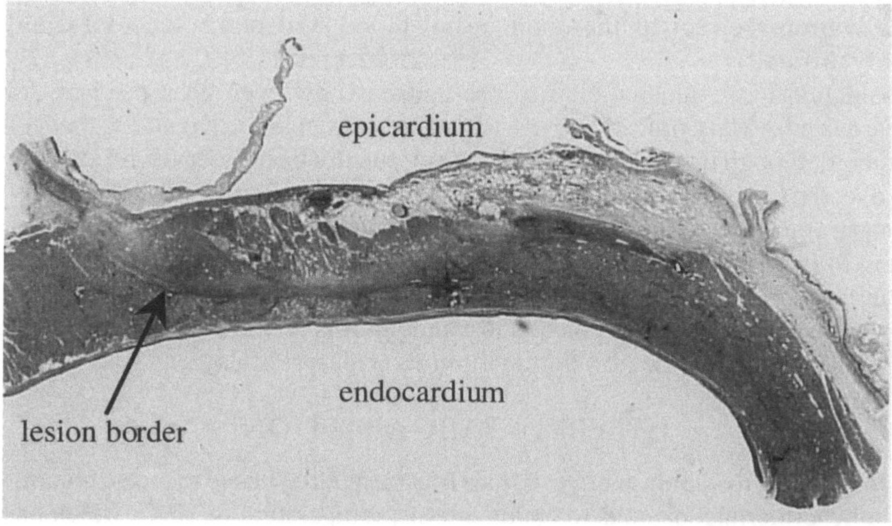

Fig. 1. Trichrome slide of canine atrial tissue obtained 4 wk after unipolar RF ablation. The lesion created is dome-shaped and relatively wide, though it falls short of transmural near the endocardium.

ture, tissue thickness, and perhaps remaining stagnant blood in the atrium, but these are generally easily overcome. Other impeding factors include the degree of contact at the tissue–device interface, intrinsic tissue thermal conductivity (which can be affected by increased deposition of fat or fibrosis in the myocardium), and acquired tissue thermal conductivity alterations such as char formation.

Surgical approaches from the epicardium result in very different ablative physics, since the goal of these lesions is to perform them on the beating heart. In this setting, the flowing blood inside the heart acts as a near-infinite thermal sink, making it difficult to achieve appropriate ablating temperatures at the endocardium while keeping the epicardial temperatures in a safe range (**Fig. 1**). Other limiting factors include the thermal insulation and added thickness from epicardial fat, conduction to surrounding structures, and limited exposure. In some cases the addition of all these factors can make epicardial ablation impossible.

HYPOTHERMIC ABLATION

Cryoablation has the longest history of surgical atrial ablation and is an important component in Dr. Cox's Maze procedures. Cryo is currently the only source that has an arrhythmia-specific indication from the Food and Drug Administration (FDA) in the United States. Cryoablation involves three stages: freeze/thaw, hemorrhagic and inflammatory, and replacement fibrosis *(14)*. The mechanism of cell injury involves mitochondrial and other organelle destruction from ice crystal formation during the first stage and further damage from edema with subsequent necrosis during the second stage. For successful ablation to occur, the tissue must reach at least –55°C for 2 min, and in some cases repeat ablations must be performed. Other methods of optimizing ablation include increasing the probe size, increasing the ablation time, increasing the number of freeze/thaw cycles, increasing the tank pressure, or changing the gas to allow colder temperatures to be reached. Current modifications have been aimed at creating flexible linear probes for use in epicardial and endocardial ablation. At this time there is a lack of evidence to demonstrate the feasibility of epicardial cryoablation, though it is expected that the warming effect of the endocardial blood will make successful ablation extremely difficult.

Cryoablation has extensive clinical use and has now even been used by some to complete an entire Maze procedure *(15)*. In general, cyroablation has an excellent clinical safety record, though its use in AF surgery has typically been reserved for creating spot lesions over the tricuspid and mitral valve annuli. This practice has resulted in a few cases of coronary artery stenosis, though this is a rare complication *(16)*.

Owing to its generally safe record and arrhythmia-specific indication, cryoablation will continue to play a role in endocardial ablation. Its future in minimally invasive approaches has yet to be determined, and although it is an attractive energy source, its bulky nature and limited flexibility may limit its widespread use.

HYPERTHERMIC ABLATION

The majority of available energy sources rely on heating tissue to create ablation. The goal of a hyperthermic lesion is to obtain a tissue temperature of 50°C, which has been shown to cause irreversible loss of cellular excitability *(17)*. It is important, however, to ensure that the tissue does not achieve temperatures of above 100°C, since that will cause water to boil with a risk for cavitation or potential wall disruption. The mechanism for cell injury is not entirely understood but likely results from injury to the sarcolemmal membrane with subsequent calcium overload of the cytosol.

The available hyperthermic sources span the electromagnetic spectrum from the massive radiofrequency waves to fine near-infrared laser. Each behaves differently in terms of tissue penetration and the mechanism by which heat is produced, but ultimately the end result is simply to heat the tissue to the point of cell death.

RADIOFREQUENCY

Radiofrequency (RF) ablation has been available for many years, though it has not been used extensively by surgeons until recently. RF is the source most familiar to

Table 2
Comparison of Different Types of Radiofrequency

Type	*Advantages*	*Disadvantages*
Unipolar		
	Most flexible	Poor epicardial
	Generally safe	Comparitvely longer lesion times
	Good clinical history	Possibility for collateral injury
	Less expensive	Some char formation
	Long lesions	Inefficient
Irrigated		
	More efficient	Less flexible
	Good clinical history	Nonspecific ablation parameters
	Less expensive	? Epicardial
	Prevents char formation	Possibility for collateral injury
		Irrigation required
Bipolar		
	Most efficient	No flexibility
	No collateral injury	Little clinical use
	Effective from epicardium	More expensive
	Feedback mechanism	

cardiologists performing catheter-based arrhythmia treatments. RF is essentially unmodulated alternating current at 500–1000 kHz, which is not dissimilar to conventional electrocautery. The frequency of RF is so rapid that it is unable to capture cardiac tissue and thus there are not problems with stimulating the heart or inducing fibrillation. The mechanism of heat generation with RF is termed resistive or ohmic heating. Essentially, the RF energy is emitted from the probe over a very small area and thus has a high current density. This high current encounters the tissue, which acts as a resistor, and heat is generated. The true resistive heating occurs only around 1 mm deep into the tissue and the remainder of ablation occurs via conductive heating from the area of resistive heating. This results in a relatively inefficient heating process, yet it provides for well-controlled and generally safe ablation. In reality these lesions rarely take more than 1 min to create. Although there are multiple modifications of RF, there are three general methods: unipolar, bipolar, and irrigated. Each has its own relative advantages and disadvantages (Table 2).

Unipolar ablation relies on grounding pads to act as the other pole and is the simplest way to apply the energy. With unipolar ablation, the energy is focused at the ablating surface (highest current density) and disperses throughout the body to exit the ground. This is the slowest and most inefficient of the RF modalities but is also the most controlled method. It can be applied using two different methods: energy control and temperature control. Energy control regulates the amount of power delivered and does not monitor the temperature. Temperature control relies on setting a goal temperature and the RF energy is regulated such that an appropriate power is provided to maintain the goal temperature. The current unipolar surgical device uses temperature-control ablation. The ideal goal temperature is not entirely clear. For endocardial ablation, experimental data have demonstrated reliable and effective ablation if ablation is performed for 60 s at 70°C. However, because there is greater variability in humans (particularly those with multiple pathologies), we and many others use 80°C for 60 s. It is also important to note that the hottest temperature will actually be achieved just below the surface. As a result, the goal temperature is usually a few degrees cooler than the hottest tissue temperature and therefore the goal temperature should never be set at more than 95°C to avoid potential tissue disruption. Ablations must be performed for at least 60 s, because a steady state is not achieved until 40–50 s of energy application.

The use of standard RF from the epicardial surface is unfortunately not as simple as from the endocardium. Because the primary method of ablation with RF is through conductive heating, it is more prone to energy losses from other variables. In the case of epicardial ablation, the convective cooling of the endocardial blood makes transmural ablation nearly impossible in tissue greater thicker than 4 mm, though the flow dynamics are probably more important than tissue thickness. This is particularly true if epicardial fat is present, because the fat serves as an excellent insulator of RF energy. In general, epicardial RF lesions will become wide but will fall just short of transmurality on the endocardial side (**Fig. 1**). It is important to note, as will be discussed later, that lesions may not need to be transmural in order to be electrically effective.

Some of the inefficiencies of unipolar ablation can be overcome by irrigating the active electrode with a saline solution. Irrigated or "cooled tip" RF ablation improves efficiency by various means. The cooling effect on the surface of the tissue actually drives the focus (hottest point) of energy deeper into the tissue, providing for both faster and deeper ablation. The irrigation also prevents the accumulation of char on the ablating surface, as can occur with standard unipolar ablation. This char can serve as an insulator and prevent the creation of an optimal lesion. With irrigated designs (**Fig. 2**), it is important that the entire ablating element be uniformly irrigated and thus longer or flexible devices are more difficult to create.

With both irrigated and standard RF, the energy disperses from a single element and there is the possibility to ablate adjacent noncardiac tissue such as the esophagus. Adjacent damage is generally avoided provided appropriate ablation parameters are followed.

Bipolar RF is another modality that has the ability to make very fast and discrete lesions. This modality relies simply on having a pole on each side of the tissue to be ablated. This focuses all of the energy between the two poles, and lesions can be made in less than 10 s. The current bipolar product also has impedance sensors that detect when transmural ablation has occurred. The bipolar application coupled to the sensing mechanism provides for reliable transmural and electrophysiologically effective lesions. These lesions can also be created from the epicardium, provided the lesion is in an area of the heart that can be opposed to itself or one of the poles can be inserted into the heart through a purse string. Since both poles must be perfectly opposed to each other, there is very limited flexibility with the device.

MICROWAVE

Microwave energy has been used successfully in Europe and recently became available in the United States. Microwave ablation can be performed at either 915 or 2450 MHz, which are the frequencies allowed by the Federal Communications Commission (FCC) for medical microwave use. The current device uses 2450 MHz and works through dielectric heating. Essentially, the microwave causes oscillation of dipoles (which happen to be water molecules), producing kinetic energy and resulting heat generation. Not all of the ablation occurs through dielectric effects, and there is a component of conductive heating.

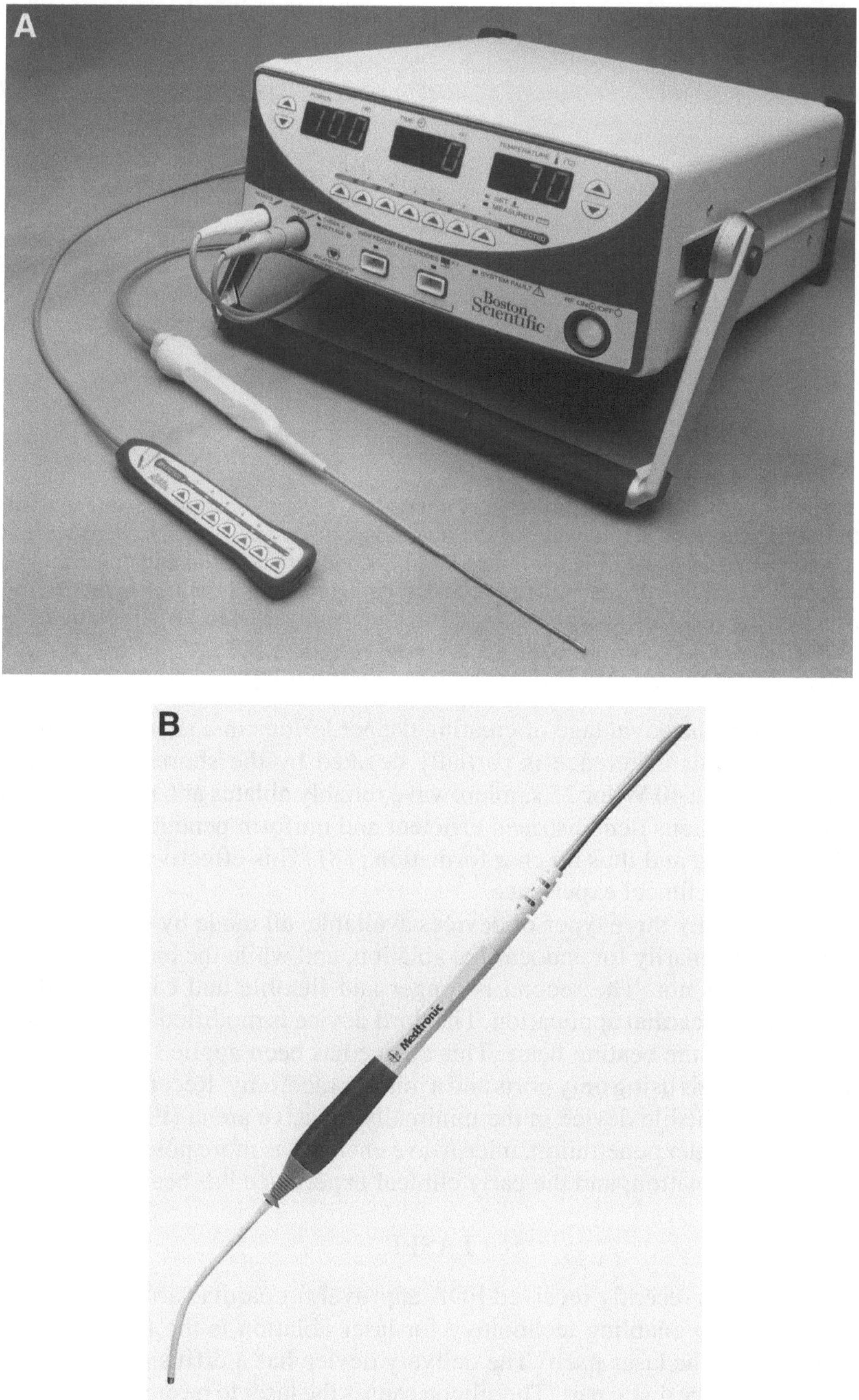

Fig. 2. Example of radiofrequency ablation systems. **(A)** The Cobra Ablation system, a unipolar, mutiple-element device that allows creation of linear RF lesions up to 9 cm in length. (Courtesy EPT, San Jose, CA.) **(B)** The Cardioblate system, a unipolar, irrigated design. The tip is continuously irrigated and the device is used like a pen to slowly draw the lesion. (Courtesy Medtronic Corp., Minneapolis, MN.)

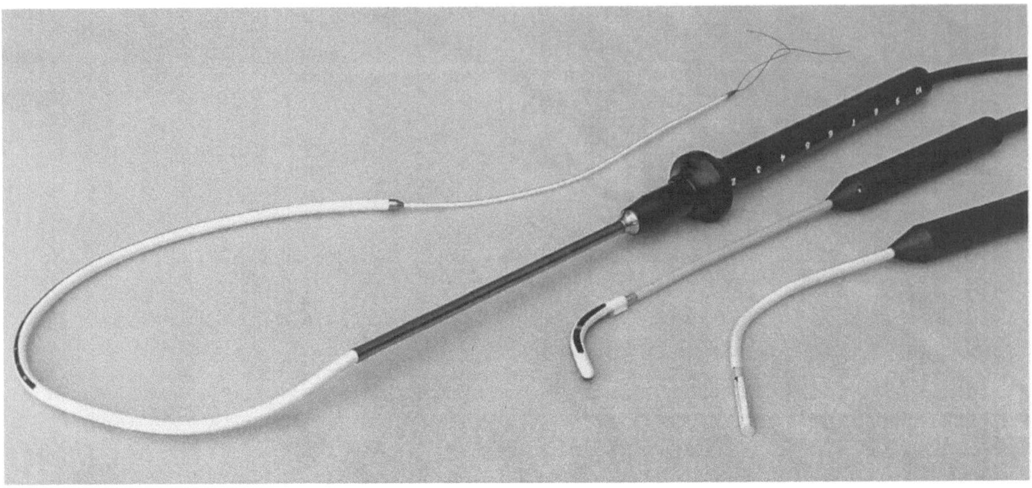

Fig. 3. Example of the microwave ablation system. (*Top*) Flex 10 device: the antennae sit within a sheath that is placed on the outside of the heart. The device can be placed using minimally invasive approaches. (*Middle*) Flex 4 device: used for both endocardial and epicardial ablation. Consists of a linear and malleable unidirectional ablating element 4 cm in length. (*Bottom*) Flex 2 device: a rigid 2-cm-long ablating device used predominantly in endocardial ablation. (Courtesy AFx, Fremont, CA.)

Microwave has the advantage of creating deeper lesions in a shorter amount of time than RF, though this difference is partially negated by the shorter lesion length. In benchtop work using 40 W for 25 s, microwave reliably ablates at 6 mm depth. Thermal profiles of these lesions demonstrated efficient and uniform penetration depth without areas of overheating and thus no char formation *(18)*. This effectiveness has been corroborated by good clinical experience.

There are currently three types of devices available, all made by the same company. One is intended primarily for endocardial ablation, and while the handle is flexible, the ablating element is not. The second is longer and flexible and can be used for both epicardial and endocardial application. The third device is modified for minimally invasive application on the beating heart. This device has been applied successfully in our laboratory on animals using only ports and a minithoracotomy. Recent clinical work also shows it to be a valuable device in the minimally invasive arena (**Fig. 3**).

Because of its better penetration, microwave energy has more potential to be successful for epicardial ablation, and the early clinical experience has been promising.

LASER

Laser energy has recently received FDA approval for cardiac ablation in the United States. The primary enabling technology for laser ablation is the fiber-optic delivery device rather than the laser itself. The delivery device has a diffusing tip that contains silicon particles in the distal part. The silicon causes the laser to be emitted perpendicular to the fiber direction. A gold foil is then placed halfway around the circumference of the diffusing tip, which reflects the energy back in the other direction. The end result is unidirectional linear ablation of 2–5 cm with a flexible configuration. The mechanism of laser ablation is wavelength-dependent but works predominantly by inducing a harmonic

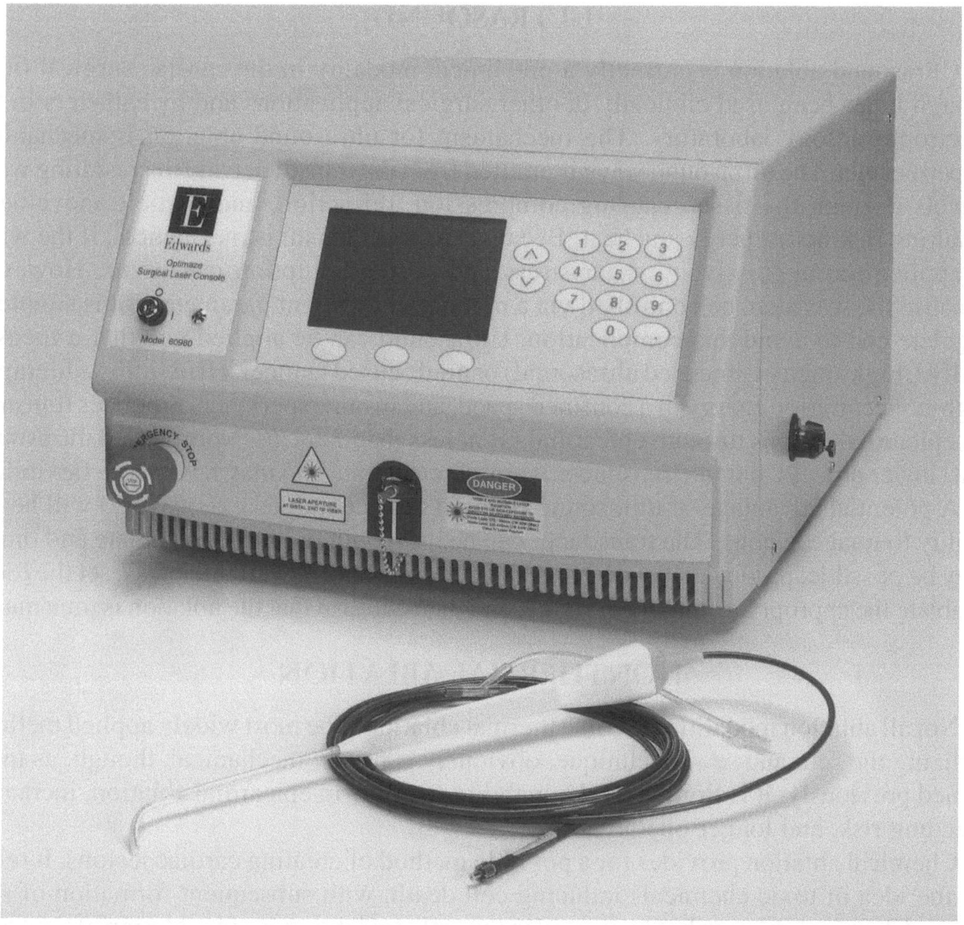

Fig. 4. The Optimaze Ablation System. The device consists of a 980-nm diode laser and a diffusing-tip hand piece that permits linear ablation up to 5 cm in length. (Courtesy Edwards Lifesciences, Irvine, CA.)

oscillation in water molecules, with resulting kinetic energy and heat generation. The currently used wavelength for cardiac ablation utilizes a 980-nm diode laser. This wavelength was chosen because of its good penetration of cardiac tissue with minimal pigment absorption. This wavelength reliably ablates tissue with absorption of actual laser energy as deep as 4 mm into the tissue, with further ablation occurring via conductive heating mechanisms. The amount of heat absorbed by the tissue and the ablation depth can be altered by changing the power and/or the wavelength of the laser, and this may be advantageous in optimizing epicardial ablation, especially through epicardial fat. Preliminary work in animals with epicardial ablation is very promising, though more data are required prior to reaching any conclusions.

In preclinical work in our laboratory we have been able to create 100% transmural lesions in canines from an endocardial approach. These lesions were found to be electrophysiologically effective when subjected to pacing *(19)*. This technology has now been applied clinically, with encouraging early results. With the current clinical device, lesions are created in 36 s for a length of 5 cm (**Fig. 4**).

ULTRASOUND

Ultrasound ablation is currently a preclinical modality in the cardiac surgical field, though it has been used clinically in other surgical applications and by catheters in the electrophysiology laboratory. The mechanism for ultrasound ablation is mechanical hyperthermia. The ultrasound wave is emitted from the transducer and the resulting wave travels through the tissue causing compression, refraction, and particle movement, resulting in kinetic energy and heat. Because the mechanism is mechanical, if the wave is applied too aggressively, shear stress and tissue disruption can occur. However, because the wave can be controlled via a number of different parameters, it is simple to regulate and to avoid this complication. Ultrasound can be applied in either a focused (HIFU, high-intensity focused ultrasound) or nonfocused manner. HIFU allows for rapid, high-concentration energy in a confined space, and in our experience, produces transmural epicardial lesions through epicardial fat in less than 2 s *(20)*. Nonfocused ultrasound is a slower process, but the transducer is simpler to create and may have more flexibility.

A potential advantage of ultrasound (though not yet studied extensively) will be the ability to image lesions. The transducer can be used both to image and ablate and thus it may be possible, particularly with HIFU, to determine atrial wall thickness, set the focus to ablate the appropriate amount of tissue, and then confirm that the ablation is transmural.

NONTHERMAL ABLATION

Not all ablation modalities involve thermal ablation. The most widely applied method, utilizing the "cut and sew" technique, obviously is purely mechanical, though, as mentioned previously, it is limited by the inability to perform epicardial ablation, increased bleeding risk, and longer operative time.

Chemical ablation provides for a possible method of creating cardiac lesions. It relies on the idea of toxic chemicals inducing cell death, with subsequent formation of scar tissue. Chemical ablation has been used in the catheter laboratory for ablation of ventricular arrhythmias by infusing alcohol selectively into a coronary artery that feeds the arrhythmogenic area *(21)*. This principle could not be used in the atria due to the widely varied and collateralized blood supply. Thus, for atrial ablation the toxic chemicals must be placed directly into the atrial wall. Our attempts at doing this with a needle have been variably successful, and it has been difficult to localize the ablation. Utilization of needle-free jet injection technology has overcome this problem and allows well-controlled and very rapid transmural ablation in a linear fashion. The needle-free technology essentially propels the chemical out a small orifice at a high velocity, resulting in penetration of the epicardium. If the correct pressure parameters are used, the chemical jet rapidly loses its velocity upon entering the tissue, distributes relatively evenly throughout the atrial wall, and creates a transmural lesion. While much of these data are still preliminary, we have been able to perform linear transmural ablation from the epicardium in animals, and have found these to be electrophysiologically effective. Ethanol was used as the chemical and the ablation time per each lesion (2-cm length) was a fraction of a second. Further work, primarily in survival models, is required to determine if chemical ablation will be a useful modality, but it has several advantages because it does not depend on thermal mechanisms, ablates regardless of tissue type (i.e., is not hindered by epicardial fat), and is a relatively inexpensive technology.

MINIMALLY INVASIVE APPROACHES AND LESION SETS FOR SURGICAL TREATMENT OF AF

As with all surgery, calling a procedure "minimally invasive" can be a subjective matter. The same is true for surgical treatment of atrial fibrillation. Many authors have described techniques and approaches, all of which are in a sense less invasive ways of treating AF, compared to the traditional technique of the Maze III. When evaluating such techniques, it is important to understand that a less invasive technique may also be a less effective technique. In terms of AF surgery, a less invasive operation may simply involve utilizing one of the above-described energy sources to create Maze III lesions or to reduce the number of lesions. Taken to an extreme, it might involve creating fewer lesions, with an alternative energy source, on the beating heart with endoscopic techniques.

Many authors have presented clinical data with alternative energy modalities, with generally similar results. This includes authors performing the lesions outlined by the Maze III using an alternative energy source. There are two recent publications in which authors have substituted radiofrequency energy for "cut and sew" lesions and essentially followed the lesions described by Dr. Cox's Maze III. Both of these groups used an irrigated-design catheter for the ablations. One of the reports is a randomized study comparing the addition of the AF procedure to no AF procedure in patients having concurrent mitral valve surgery. The study found that the group having the RF–Maze III in addition to mitral valve surgery had an 80% success in achieving sinus rhythm compared to 27% in those having only mitral valve surgery *(22)*. The other study involved 122 patients and achieved a success of 78.5% in obtaining sinus rhythm *(23)*.

More recently, many investigators have been limiting their approaches to the left atrium, driven largely by data suggesting that focal sources of automaticity originate in the pulmonary veins *(24)* and that microrotors of reentry anchor themselves near the pulmonary veins and produce fibrillatory conduction *(25)*. Thus, isolating the pulmonary veins and the posterior left atrium may be sufficient to cure AF. There are many different lesion sets proposed to achieve this isolation (**Fig. 5**), and at the present time there is no way of determining which, if any, is superior. There are multiple active debates as to which lesions if any are absolutely necessary, though all agree that the pulmonary veins must be addressed in some manner. The predominant controversies include the necessity for the mitral valve lesion and the necessity of removing or isolating the left atrial appendage. The mitral annular lesion is felt by Dr. Cox to be absolutely necessary to control atrial fibrillation, while others feel the lesion is important only to prevent a left atrial flutter, which can be addressed by other lesions such as the one used to remove left atrial appendage. Ideally this lesion will not be necessary, as it will be a difficult lesion to perform on the beating heart from the epicardial surface, since it will require ablating directly over the circumflex artery and coronary sinus. However, if the lesion is found to be necessary, it may require either placement of a device in the atrium through a purse string or the assistance of our interventional cardiology colleagues. The left atrial appendage is felt by some to play a role in the origin and initiation of AF, though this is not a commonly held view. Its importance likely relies in the fact that most documented intracardiac thrombi in patients with AF are found in the left atrial appendage. For this reason, removing or at least anatomically excluding the left atrial appendage may reduce the stroke rate even if the patient remains in AF. It may be in the future that an ideal lesion

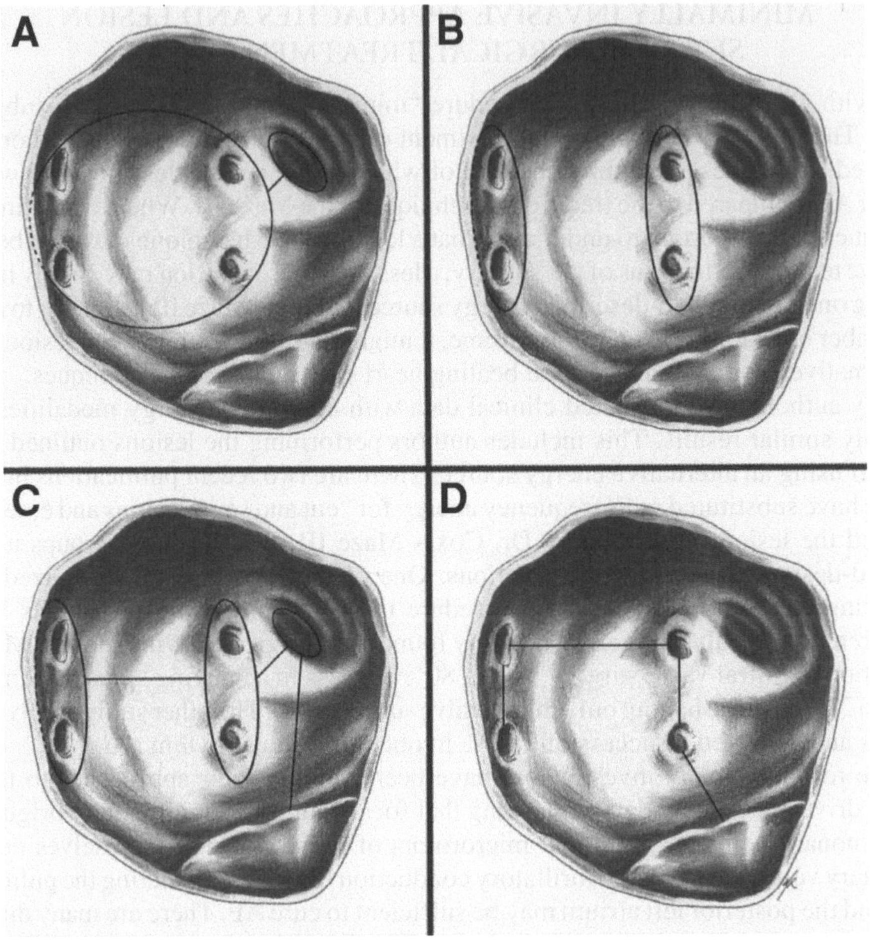

Fig. 5. Examples of some of the advocated left atrial lesion sets. (**A**) The lesion set currently advocated by our group. It involves complete encirclement of the posterior left atrium containing all the pulmonary veins. The left atrial appendage is also either removed or electrically and anatomically isolated. A lesion is then made from the pulmonary vein lesion to the left atrial appendage lesion. This lesion set can easily be accomplished from the epicardium with minimal dissection. (**B**) The initial procedure described by Melo, in which only the left and right veins are isolated. This approach has a theoretical advantage in that the posterior left atrium is preserved to contribute to left atrial contractility. This approach can also be performed from the epicardium. (**C**) The approach advocated by Benussi. Part of this lesion set is currently performed from the epicardium and part from the endocardium. The left atrial appendage is also addressed. A lesion in also performed to the mitral valve annulus, which may be difficult from the epicardial surface. (**D**) The approach advocated by Knaut and several other European investigators. This lesion set has been termed the "7." In most groups' experience the left atrial appendage is not addressed, though it can be easily accomplished if desired. This lesion set is interesting in that it does not actually isolate the pulmonary veins but probably disrupts microrotors of reentry. This lesion set shares similar success with those that actually isolate the pulmonary veins. A lesion to the mitral annulus is required and thus epicardial performance is limited.

set will be patient-specific, based on intraoperative variables that are as yet poorly understood. Another possibility will be a multispecialty approach in which the cardiac surgeon creates the left-sided lesions and, if unsuccessful, the cardiologist follows up by creating right-sided lesions.

The clinical results of left-sided-only ablations are varied, but again the definition of success is different in each series. Some centers require bi-atrial contraction before success is achieved, whereas others rely solely on electrophysiological data. These approaches have been performed predominantly with RF energy, though microwave, cryo, and "cut and sew" techniques have also been utilized *(26–30)*. The reported success rates in these studies vary between 70% and 90%, with most centers reporting rates between 75% and 80%. Comparison among these studies is rather difficult due to variations in lesion sets, baseline patient characteristics, energy sources, and the type and number of concomitant procedures. The great majority of the patients in all of these studies had concurrent mitral valve surgery. This is promising for the success of a limited left atrial procedure for a couple of reasons. First, it is likely that patients with mitral valve disease will be more difficult to treat due to concurrent atrial pathology and the general state of health of the patients. Additionally, the results for left atrial procedures during mitral valve surgery are quite similar to the largest reported series of Maze III patients during concurrent mitral valve surgery, with a success rate of 76% *(31)*, suggesting that a full Maze III may not be of additional benefit.

While the results of these studies are extremely promising, the success of surgical treatment of AF will rely on the ability to create lesions from the epicardium and to that end there have been several investigators pursing this goal. On the clinical side there is growing experience with epicardial ablation, though most investigators have too little experience to report meaningful results. The two largest series of epicardial ablation have been with RF, and both still utilized cardiopulmonary bypass. They demonstrated success rates of 76.9% and 95%, though the latter also utilized right atrial lesions *(32,33)*. Another series of isolated pulmonary vein ablation on the beating heart without mitral valve surgery had extremely promising results, suggesting that limited procedures may be even more successful in patients without valvular disease *(34)*. There have been anecdotal reports of successful beating-heart epicardial microwave and bipolar RF ablations, though at this time there have been no published series.

The epicardial field has advanced more on the preclinical front and there should be more widespread clinical application in the upcoming year. In our laboratory, we have achieved 100% electrical isolation of the posterior left atrium (containing all pulmonary veins) in a beating-heart canine model. This approach utilized a specialized microwave device and was performed using a 3-cm thoracotomy and three thoracoscopy ports in the left chest that allowed removal of the left atrial appendage with a stapling device *(35)*. We have also developed a totally endoscopic version of this operation, using robotic technology, which we have performed in a few patients with lone AF.

Another important issue that has come out of epicardial ablation is the question of whether lesions need to be transmural to be effective. Most surgeons feel a lesion must be transmural to be effective, and indeed this is probably a reasonable goal. However, there is increasing data from both surgical and catheter-based investigations suggesting that lesions may not need to be transmural to be effective. Perhaps, then, discussions about lesion quality should be based on electrophysiological effectiveness rather than just transmurality. In reality, most (though not all) transmural lesions are electrophysiologically effective, but many nontransmural lesions are also effective *(35,36)*. The reasons for this are uncertain but may be related to the lesion width. It may also be that simply inducing a conduction delay may be sufficient to prevent or disrupt maintenance of AF.

CONCLUSIONS

Surgical treatment of AF has received renewed attention. This is due partly to the realization that AF is a morbid arrhythmia and one that is poorly managed by traditional medical therapy. Interest in these procedures has been further fueled by the development of new energy sources, minimally invasive techniques, and an understanding of AF mechanisms. The future of the field has yet to be realized but ultimately will involve a procedure on the beating heart from the epicardial surface utilizing endoscopic techniques. Indeed, surgical treatment for AF may provide a definitive cure for many of the thousands of patients with AF and at the same time represent the first cardiac operation that may be performed as an outpatient procedure.

REFERENCES

1. Feinberg WM, Blackshear JL, Laupacis A, Kronmal R, Hart RG. Prevalence, age distribution, and gender of patients with atrial fibrillation; analysis and implications. Arch Intern Med 1995;155:469–473.
2. Stafford RS, Singer DE. National patterns of warfarin use in atrial fibrillation. Arch Intern Med 1996;156:2537–2541.
3. American Heart Association. 1998 Heart and Stroke Statistical Update. American Heart Association, 1997.
4. Gasjewski J, Singer RB. Mortality in an insured population with atrial fibrillation. JAMA 1981;245:1540–1544.
5. Williams JM, Ungerleider RM, Logland GK, et al. Left atrial isolation: new technique for the treatment of supraventricular arrhythmias. J Thorac Cardiovasc Surg 1980;80:373–380.
6. Guiradon GM, Campbell CS, Jones DL, et al. Combined sino-atrial node atrio-ventircular node isolation: a surgical alternative to His bundle ablation in patients with atrial fibrillation. Circulation 1985;72:III–220.
7. Cox JL, Schuessler RB, Boineau JP. The development of the maze procedure for the treatment of atrial fibrillation. Sem Thorac Cardiovasc Surg 2000;12:2–14.
8. Cox JL, Canavan TE, Schuessler RB, et al. The surgical tretment of atrial fibrillation: II. Intraoperative electrophysiologic mapping and description of the electrophysiologic basis of atrial flutter and atrial fibrillation. J Thorac Cardiovasc Surg 1991;101:406–426.
9. Cox JL. The surgical treatment of atrial fibrillation: IV. Surgical Technique. J Thorac Cardiovasc Surg 1991;101:584–592.
10. Cox JL, Jaquiss RD, Schuessler RB, et al. Modification of the maze procedure for atrial flutter and fibrillation. II. Surgical technique of the Maze III procedure. J Thorac Cardiovasc Surg 1995;110:485–495.
11. Cox JL, Schuessler RB, Lappas, DG, et al. An 8-1/2 year clinical experience with surgery for atrial fibrillation. Ann Surg 1996;224:267–275.
12. McCarthy PM, Gillinov AM, Castle L, Chung M, Cosgrove D. The Cox-Maze Procedure: the Cleveland Clinic experience. Semin Thorac Cardiovasc Surg 2000;12:25–29.
13. Kosakai Y. Treatment of atrial fibrillation using the Maze Procedure: the Japanese experience. Semin Thorac Cardiovasc Surg 2000;12:44–52.
14. Lustgarten DL, Keane D, Ruskin J. Cryothermal ablation: mechanism of tissue injury and current experience in the treatment of tachyarrhythmias. Prog Cardiovasc Dis 1999;41:481–498.
15. Cox JL, Ad N, Palazzzo T, et al. Current status of the Maze Procedure for the treatment of atrial fibrillation. Semin Thorac Cardiovasc Surg 2000;12:15–19.
16. Holman WL, Ikeshita M, Ungerleider RM, Smith PK, Ideker RE, Cox JL. Cryosurgery for cardiac arrhythmias: acute and chronic effects on coronary arteries. Am J Cardiol 1983;51:149–155.
17. Nath S, Lynch C, Whayne JG, Haines DE. Cellular electrophysiological effects of hyperthermia on isolated guinea pig papillary muscle. Implications for catheter ablation. Circulation 1993;88:1826–1831.
18. Williams MR, Knaut M, Berube D, Oz MC. Application of microwave energy in cardiac tissue ablation: from *in vitro* analyses to clinical use. Ann Thorac Surg 2002;74:1500–1505.

19. Williams MR, Casher J, Klein KA, et al. Linear atrial ablation using laser energy. Submitted.
20. Williams MR, Kourpanidis S, Casher J, et al. Epicardial atrial ablation with high intensity focused ultrasound on the beating heart. Circulation 2001;104(17):II-409.
21. Weismuller P, Mayer U, Richter P, et al. Chemical ablation by subendocardial injection of ethanol via catheter—preliminary results in the pig heart. Eur Heart J 1991;12(11):1234–1239.
22. Khargi K, Deneke T, Haardt H, et al. Saline-irrigated, cooled-tip radiofrequency ablation is an effective technique to perform the maze procedure. Ann Thorac Surg 2001;72:S1090–S1095.
23. Sie HT, Beukema WP, Misier AR, et al. Radiofrequency modified Maze in patients with atrial fibrillation undergoing concomitant cardiac surgery. J Thorac Cardiovasc Surg 2001;122:249–256.
24. Haissaguerre M, Jais P, Shah DC, et al. Spontaneous initiation of atrial fibrillation by ectopic beats originating in the pulmonary veins. N Engl J Med 1998;339:659–666.
25. Jalife J, Berenfeld O, Skanes A, Mandapati R. Mechanisms of atrial fibrillation: mother rotors or multiple daughter wavelets, or both? J Cardiovasc Electrophysiol 1998;9:S2–S12.
26. Sueda T, Nagata H, Shikata H, et al. Simple left atrial procedure for chronic atrial fibrillation associated with mitral valve disease. Ann Thorac Surg 1996;62:1796–1800.
27. Graffigna A, Pagani F, Minzioni G, Salerno J, Vigano M. Left atrial isolation associated with mitral valve operations. Ann Thorac Surg 1992;54:1093–1097.
28. Kottkamp H, Kindricks G, Hammel D, et al. Intraoperative radiofrequency ablation of chronic atrial fibrillation: a left atrial curative approach by elimination of anatomic "anchor" reentrant circuits. J Cardiovasc Electrophysiol 1999;10:772–780.
29. Williams MR, Stewart JR, Bolling SF, et al. Surgical treatment of atrial fibrillation using radiofrequency energy. Ann Thorac Surg 2001;71:1939–1944.
30. Knaut M, Spitzer SG, Karolyi L, et al. Intraoperative microwave ablation for curative treatment of atrial fibrillation in open heart surgery—the MICRO-STAF and MICRO-PASS pilot trial. Microwave application in surgical treatment of atrial fibrillation. Microwave application for the treatment of atrial fibrillation in bypass-surgery. Thorac Cardiovasc Surg 1999;47(S3):379–384.
31. Kosakai Y. Treatment of atrial fibrillation using the Maze Procedure: the Japanese experience. Semin Thorac Cardiovasc Surg 2000;12:44–52.
32. Benussi S, Pappone C, Nascimbene S, et al. A simple way to treat chronic atrial fibrillation during mitral vavle surgery: the epicardial radiofrequency approach. Eur J Cardiothorac Surg 2000;17:524–529.
33. Raman JS, Seevanayagam S, Storer M, Power JM. Combined endocardial and epicardial radiofrequency ablation of right and left atria in the treatment of atrial fibrillation. Ann Thorac Surg 2001;72:S1096–S1099.
34. Williams MR, Garrido M, Casher JM, et al. A minimally invasive beating heart approach to pulmonary vein isolation for the treatment of atrial fibrillation. Proceedings of the Cardiovascular Therapeutics and Technologies Meeting, Miami Beach, FL, 2001.
35. Taylor GW, Walcott GP, Hall JA, et al. High-resolution and histologic examination of long radiofrequency lesions in canine atria. J Cardiovasc Electrophysiol 1999;10:1467–1477.
36. Williams MR, JA Sanchez, Barbone A, et al. Simultaneous endocardial contact activation mapping and beating heart epicardial radiofrequency pulmonary vein isolation. Circulation 2000;102(18): II-443–II-444.

V

Miscellaneous Aspects of Minimally Invasive Cardiac Surgery

25 The Economic Impact of Minimally Invasive Cardiac Surgery

Aftab R. Kherani, MD, *Elizabeth H. Burton,* BA, *and Mehmet C. Oz,* MD

CONTENTS

INTRODUCTION
MINIMALLY INVASIVE VALVE SURGERY
MINIMALLY INVASIVE CORONARY ARTERY BYPASS GRAFTING
CONCLUSIONS
REFERENCES

INTRODUCTION

As the focus of cardiac surgery moves from simple mortality endpoints to more quality-of-life metrics, the importance of minimally invasive surgery has grown. Yet to assess the true value that these innovations bring to people, we must determine the cost efficacy of the technology. Proponents of this technology claim that these advanced technologies translate to decreased cost and decreased morbidity. Numerous studies have been conducted in an attempt to clarify this issue.

MINIMALLY INVASIVE VALVE SURGERY

In 1997, Cohn and colleagues described their experience with minimally invasive valve procedures at Brigham and Women's Hospital. Their study included a comparison of charges associated with minimally invasive techniques and traditional sternotomy. They found that the former was associated with approx 20% lower hospital charges. Additionally, these patients returned to work nearly 2 wk earlier, translating to further economic benefit on a societal scale. Their pain medication requirement was less, and they returned to normal activity in less than half the time *(1)*.

From: *Contemporary Cardiology: Minimally Invasive Cardiac Surgery, Second Edition*
Edited by: D. J. Goldstein and M. C. Oz © Humana Press Inc., Totowa, NJ

Cosgrove and colleagues recently compared their minimally invasive valve experience to the traditional median sternotomy approach at the Cleveland Clinic Foundation. They compared their observations of the first 40 patients to undergo aortic valve procedures via a right parasternal incision with 40 patients who underwent the standard median sternotomy. They found that postoperative length of stay was 5.8 ± 3.0 d compared to 7.8 ± 6.5 d, $p < 0.001$. This, in part, contributed to a 19% reduction in direct costs. This group similarly examined mitral valve procedures. Here, no statistical significance was seen in postoperative length of stay, while direct costs were 7% lower for the minimally invasive group *(2)*.

Comparisons among the various types of minimally invasive procedures have also been made. Early data suggest that port-access valve surgery via a small anterior thoracotomy is associated with statistically significantly longer operating room time. The difference was nearly 2 h, theoretically adding an extra $1500 to $3000 in cost per case. The charges associated with the disposable Endo CPB System further adds to the cost difference between the two methods *(3)*. Inferences can certainly be made with data from this study as well as the others described; however, to address definitively the economic question surrounding different approaches to valve procedures requires a prospective, controlled, randomized studying comparing the various minimally invasive approaches to each other as well as to the traditional median sternotomy. Cost should be among the variables analyzed.

MINIMALLY INVASIVE CORONARY ARTERY BYPASS GRAFTING

In recent years, several groups have compared minimally invasive direct coronary artery bypass grafting (MIDCABG) and full sternotomy off-pump methods (OPCAB) to traditional on-pump coronary artery bypass grafting (CABG). One factor studied by many of these institutions is how costs compare. The issue of cost in this area is of great interest especially in the United States, where Medicare alone spends roughly $4 billion annually on coronary artery bypass grafting procedures *(4)*. In this field, there does exist a prospective randomized study examining the economic outcome of off-pump coronary artery bypass surgery. This research is from the United Kingdom and involves 200 patients undergoing first-time coronary artery bypass grafting prospectively randomized to either conventional CABG or off-pump surgery. Pre- and intraoperative variables were similar between the two groups. This study observed a significant difference ($p < 0.001$) in cost, defined as the sum of charges involving operating equipment, bed occupancy, and transfusion requirement, between the two groups. The hospital costs of the on- and off-pump groups were $3731.6 ± $1169.7 and $2615.1 ± $953.6, respectively. The increased cost reflects increased morbidity seen in the group undergoing conventional treatment *(5)*.

In the United States, several retrospective studies exist. One such study examined MIDCABG, OPCAB, and conventional CABG costs. This study demonstrated hospital costs of $15,000, $17,000, and $19,000, respectively. This represents a statistically significant difference between the conventional and less invasive techniques *(6)*. In addition to an apparent cost advantage, a multicenter trial involving several Veterans Affairs hospitals demonstrated significant improvement in terms of risk-adjusted morbidity and mortality (0.52 vs 0.56 multivariable odds ratios for off-pump and on-pump, respectively) *(7)*.

A German study examined cost of conventional CABG, MIDCABG, OPCAB, and Port-Access™ CABG (PACABG) *(8)*. Compared to total cost of traditional CABG ($16,230, n = 60), OPCAB ($14,060, n = 5), and MIDCAB ($14,050, n = 5) were associated with lower cost, but PACABG ($17,230, n = 5) was more expensive. This study was hampered by its nonrandomized design, small sample size, and lack of data on cost as it pertains to duration of rehabilitation and length of time away from work. Also lacking long-term follow-up data was Magovern's retrospective comparison between MIDCABG ($n = 60$) and traditional CABG ($n = 55$) *(9)*. The former group had a decreased incidence of transfusion, shorter intubation time, and lower estimated hospital costs ($11,200 ± $3100 vs $15,600 ± $4200, $p < 0.001$). The decreased morbidity and cost enjoyed by MIDCABG patients were particularly evident in high-risk patients. The advantages experienced in the short run by the MIDCABG group, however, were balanced by the fact that at 6 mo, five patients in this group had recurrent ischemia in the left anterior descending artery distribution, mostly due to anastomotic stricture. The costs associated with treating these patients were not included in this analysis.

The morbidity and cost advantages observed in high-risk patients in the Magovern study were the focus of Del Rizzo's study, which compared safety and cost-effectiveness of MIDCABG in high-risk (HR) and low-risk (LR) patient populations *(10)*. HR patients were significantly older than their LR counterparts (72.2 ± 11.6 yr vs 63.3 ± 9.7 yr, $p = 0.006$); HR patients also were significantly ($p < 0.05$) more likely to be female, have a history of stroke, chronic obstructive pulmonary diseases (COPD), peripheral vascular disease, prior cardiac surgery, congestive heart failure, and require urgent operation. HR patients revascularized via MIDCABG enjoyed a 50% cost saving over traditional CABG patients. However, the costs associated with the latter group were not actual cost data; rather, they were determined from a cost regression model based on Ontario Ministry of Health funding. Professional fees, capital depreciation, and long-term follow-up of these patients were not considered in this study.

There are data that lend support to Del Rizzo's findings. One study out of the University of Pittsburgh found an average savings of $8375 ($p < 0.0001$) enjoyed by MIDCABG patients over CABG patients *(11)*. Doty and colleagues further compared MIDCABG to stenting, percutaneous transluminal angioplasty (PTCA), and conventional CABG (for single-vessel disease) *(12)*. Costs associated with the MIDCABG procedure were lower than for conventional CABG and stenting but greater than for PTCA.

Additional support for the utilization of minimally invasive techniques can be found in certain subsets of the patient population. Boyd and colleagues demonstrated differences in several areas in their retrospective review of their OPCAB experience in elderly (age greater than 70) patients supporting the utilization of off-pump surgery in this population. They observed significant differences ($p < 0.05$) between patients undergoing off-pump and on-pump procedures in mean hospital stay (6.3 ± 1.8 d vs 7.7 ± 3.9 d), average intensive care unit stay (24.0 ± 10.9 h vs 36.6 ± 33.5 h), and morbidity (in terms of postoperative atrial fibrillation or low-output syndrome). The cost associated with off-pump cases also was significantly lower at $6702 ± $1047 compared to $7784 ± $2846 ($p < 0.05$) *(13)*. The Christiana Hospital (Medical Center of Delaware) similarly observed that in this same patient population, postoperative length of stay was significantly lower in their MIDCABG group compared to their CABG group (6.09 vs 8.39 d, $p = 0.013$). Interestingly, the same group observed a significantly higher postoperative length of stay in their MIDCABG group compared to their CABG group among their patients under the age of 70 *(14)* (Table 1).

Table 1

The most recent study of the elderly was performed retrospectively on octogenarians undergoing either OPCAB or conventional CABG *(15)*. There was no statistically significant survival difference between the two groups. OPCAB patients enjoyed advantages in terms of perioperative stroke (0% OPCAB vs 7.1% CABG, $p = 0.04$), prolonged

Table 1
Summary of Retrospective Conventional vs Minimally Invasive Coronary Artery Bypass Graft Studies

CABG Cost and LOS	*Cost ($)*		*LOS (d)*		
	On-pump	*Off-pump*	*On-pump*	*Off-pump*	*p*
Minneapolis Heart Institute *(8)*	19,000	17,000	—	—	<0.05
Canada (Multicentered) *(10)*[a]	7784 ± 2846	6702 ± 1047	7.7 ± 3.9	6.3 ± 1.8	<0.05
Christiana Hospital *(11)*[a]	—	—	6.09	8.39	0.013

[a]Patient population age > 70.

ventilation (1.7% OPCAB vs 11.8% CABG, $p = 0.02$), and transfusion rate (33% OPCAB vs 70.4% CABG, $p < 0.001$). A shorter hospital stay (6.3 d OPCAB vs 11.5 d CABG, $p < 0.001$) translated to cost savings for the OPCAB group ($9,363 OPCAB vs $12,312 CABG, $p < 0.001$).

During January and February of 2000, 52 on-pump CABGs and 42 off-pump CABGs were performed at New York Presbyterian Hospital–Columbia. A retrospective review of this small sample of patients showed off-pump total costs to be significantly different than on-pump total costs ($p = 0.015$). On average, off-pump cases cost approx $22,000 less than on-pump cases. The average postoperative length of stay was 13 d ± 20.4 vs 7.8 ± 7 for off-pump ($p = 0.078$). We further broke our patient population into subgroups based on age (<70 and ≥70), gender, and number of grafts (three or four). In this subanalysis, significant cost differences between on-pump and off-pump cases (the former being associated with higher costs) in our <70 patients and our male patients were observed. With regard to postoperative length of stay, we saw a significant difference only in our male patients, again in favor of the off-pump method (Table 2).

In our patient pool, as would be expected, a handful of patients had protracted hospital stays. Thus, we also analyzed our data eliminating outliers that fell beyond two standard deviations (Table 3). Again, significant cost differences favoring the off-pump method among all patients as well as our <70 and male subgroups were observed. Additionally, our subgroups of three and four grafts now demonstrated significant difference. Regarding length of stay, again only our male subgroup demonstrated a significant difference. Overall, our data favor the less invasive off-pump procedure; however, since the data are derived from a nonrandomized population, we could control for the severity of illness in the two cohorts.

In our review of the literature, there is some evidence favoring off-pump surgery from prospective studies. For instance, Lee and colleagues performed a case-controlled study comparing outcomes and costs associated with 100 consecutive patients undergoing OPCAB procedures and those associated with 100 contemporary matched conventional CABG patients. Three important demographic differences existed between the two groups. First, on-pump cases averaged 3.8 ± 1.0 grafts, significantly higher than the 3.1 ± 1.0 grafts for the off-pump cases ($p < 0.001$). Second, all renal-failure patients who were dialysis-dependent underwent the OPCAB procedure. Finally, five times as many conventional CABG patients were undergoing reoperation (10% vs 2%, $p = 0.03$). This being said, this group had numerous findings seemingly favoring the off-pump technique. They

Table 2
The Columbia Experience, January–February 2000

Columbia CABG Data, January–February 2000 (On vs Off)		*Total cost ($)*			*Postoperative Length of Stay (d)*		
		On-pump	*Off-pump*	*p*	*On-pump*	*Off-pump*	*p*
Total experience (n = 57 vs 48)		52,130.58 ± 59,504.19	30,530.98 ± 25,569.50	0.015	13.00 ± 20.38	7.85 ± 6.95	0.078
Age	< 70 (n = 29 vs 34)	61,041.69 ± 75,027.96	30,489.94 ± 29,690.93	0.047	15.76 ± 26.74	7.74 ± 7.80	0.13
	≥ 70 (n = 28 vs 14)	42,902.25 ± 36,505.63	30,630.64 ± 11,222.10	0.11	10.00 ± 9.51	8.14 ± 4.47	0.40
Gender	Female (n = 8 vs 13)	70,526.75 ± 94.242.89	45,483.85 ± 44,274.41	0.50	22.63 ± 41.05	11.85 ± 11.52	0.49
	Male (n = 49 vs 35)	49,127.12 ± 52,630.89	24,977.06 ± 9731.11	0.0028	11.43 ± 14.85	6.37 ± 3.40	0.025
No. of grafts	3 vessels (n = 18 vs 25)	34,472.11 ± 8657.36	32,455.60 ± 23,571.65	0.70	7.61 ± 2.23	7.76 ± 3.95	0.88
	4 vessels (n = 21 vs 9)	60,438.05 ± 70,719.38	36,473.89 ± 43,016.12	0.27	14.33 ± 19.56	10.67 ± 13.71	0.56

Table 3
The Columbia Experience, Excluding Outliers Beyond Two Standard Deviations

Columbia CABG Data, January–February 2000 (On vs Off)		*Total cost ($)*			*Postoperative Length of Stay (d)*		
		On-pump	*Off-pump*	*p*	*On-pump*	*Off-pump*	*p*
Total experience (n = 54 vs 46)		39,558.85 ± 21,897.53	25,641.87 ± 9684.39	0.00007	8.78 ± 7.068	6.72 ± 3.35	0.060
Age	< 70 (n = 27 vs 32)	41,894.04 ± 22,799.72	23,459.28 ± 8195.99	0.0004	9.11 ± 8.84	6.094 ± 2.57	0.097
	≥ 70 (n = 27 vs 14)	37,223.67 ± 21,125.66	30,630.64 ± 11,222.10	0.20	8.44± 4.85	8.14 ± 4.47	0.84
Gender	Female (n = 7 vs 11)	37,380.71 ± 10,385.24	27,757.18 ± 9675.37	0.072	8.14 ± 3.13	7.82 ± 3.09	0.83
	Male (n = 47 vs 35)	39,883.26 ± 23,185.61	24,977.06 ± 9731.11	0.00019	8.87 ± 7.50	6.37 ± 3.40	0.047
No. of grafts	3 vessels (n = 18 vs 25)	34,472.11 ± 8657.36	28,171.50 ± 10,049.51	0.036	7.61 ± 2.23	7.21 ± 2.89	0.61
	4 vessels (n = 20 vs 8)	46,635.35 ± 32,451.20	22,197.25 ± 4274.10	0.0035	10.70 ± 10.53	6.13 ± 1.64	0.73

observed a significantly reduced postoperative length of stay (6.1 ± 2.5 d vs 7.1 ± 3.3 d, $p = 0.003$) and a 29% lower variable direct cost per case ($p < 0.001$) *(16)*. Selection biases likely play a role in this prospective study.

When addressing the outstanding economic question of the costs of minimally invasive cardiac surgery, the majority of data are found in nonrandomized studies done at various institutions throughout the United States, Canada, and Europe. Many of these studies suggest that minimally invasive cardiac procedures hold various advantages over conventional surgery in terms of cost and morbidity. However, recent prospective data do not definitively support these findings. In 2001, the University of Utah published its OPCAB experiences and showed no significant difference in terms of complication rate, length of hospital stay, and hospital costs. Costs were comparable aggregately and when divided into surgical, intensive care, and ward-care costs *(17)*.

CONCLUSIONS

To summarize, there is no clear answer to whether minimally invasive cardiac surgery confers a significant cost benefit over traditional methods. This technology, which is ever changing, is still in its infancy. For instance, robotic surgery shows promise in ASD repair, mitral valve repair, and even coronary artery bypass grafting. It will be some time before we will know how long-term savings through improved outcomes may justify the substantial fixed costs associated with acquiring and learning this new technology.

Today, we lack the support of controlled, randomized studies to compare the two accurately with regard to the bottom line. This is the first issue that must be addressed. To this end, there is promising new research on the horizon. The Octopus Study from Europe is comprised of two multicenter randomized clinical trials *(18)*. The first is known as the OctoStent trial and compares the medical effectiveness of intracoronary stent placement with off-pump coronary bypass grafting. The second, termed the OctoPump trial, looks at neurological status following on- and off-pump bypass grafting. Secondary endpoints for both trials will be cost-effectiveness.

Our institution is in the midst of a Comparative On and Off Pump (COOP) CABG trial. The trial is a prospective, randomized pilot study designed to examine costs and mortality and morbidity for on-pump vs off-pump patients as well as determine whether neurocognitive differences exist between the two groups. Neurocognitive function is evaluated with simple neurocognitive tests that are administered preoperatively and then again at 1 wk, 1 mo, and 6 mo postoperatively. The tests are blindly scored and will help determine if the deleterious effects of the cardiopulmonary bypass system translate into any significant neurocognitive differences.

Preliminary data from our COOP CABG study is in line with the other current prospective data available. With approximately half of the total patients enrolled ($n = 45$), initial cost analysis shows no significant difference between on- and off-pump procedures. Specifically, current COOP CABG cost data show on-pump costs of \$30,716 ± \$11,071 vs \$30,299 ± \$11,597 for off-pump procedures (p = ns). Although these data suggest little difference in overall costs, they do reveal a significantly lower utilization of operating-room resources for the off-pump group. These data raise interesting questions about cost differences between the on- and off-pump groups. We hope that our completed randomized study will clearly delineate how the two procedures compare from an economic perspective *(19)*.

The results of these trials will help define what niche minimally invasive cardiac surgeries will fill. However, when comparing them to conventional procedures, results such as duration of time away from work postoperatively must be noted to get an accurate sense of cost-effectiveness on a societal scale. Upcoming randomized controlled studies will evaluate and probably validate the utilization of minimally invasive surgery for patients with certain comorbidities that may not tolerate cardiopulmonary bypass well. As minimally invasive technologies mature, assessment of cost-efficacy may become the major driving force to adoption of these procedures.

REFERENCES

1. Cohn LH, Adams DH, Couper GS, et al. minimally invasive cardiac valve surgery improves patient satisfaction while reducing costs of cardiac valve replacement and repair. Ann Surg 1997;226:421–428.
2. Cosgrove DM, Sabik JF, Navia JL. Minimally invasive bypass operations. Ann Thorac Surg 1998;65:1535–1539.
3. Arom KV, Emery RW, Kshettry VR, Jancy PA. Comparison between Port-Access and less invasive valve surgery. Ann Thorac Surg 1999;68:1525–1528.
4. Subramanian S, Liu C-F, Cromwell J, Thestrup-Nielsen S. Preoperative correlates of the cost of coronary artery bypass surgery: comparison of results from three hospitals. Am J Med Qual 2001;16:87–91.
5. Ascione R, Lloyd CT, Underwood MJ, Lotto AA, Pitsis AA, Angelini GD. Economic outcome of off-pump coronary artery bypass surgery: a prospective randomized study. Ann Thorac Surg 1999;68:2237–2242.
6. Arom KV, Emery RW, Flavin TF, Petersen RJ. Cost effectiveness of minimally invasive coronary artery bypass surgery. Ann Thorac Surg 1999;68:1562–1566.
7. Plomondon ME, Cleveland JC Jr, Ludwig ST, et al. Off puimp coronary artery bypass is associated with improved risk-adjusted outcomes. Ann Thorac Surg 2001;72:114–119.
8. Reichenspurner H, Boehm D, Detter C, Schiller W, Reichart B. Economic evaluations of different minimally invasive procedures for the treatment of coronary artery disease. Eur J Cardiothorac Surg 1999;16(suppl 2):S76–S79.
9. Magovern JA, Benckart DH, Landreneau RJ, Sakert T, Magovern GJ Jr. Morbidity, cost, and six-month outcome of minimally invasive direct coronary artery bypass grafting. Ann Thorac Surg 1998;66:1224–1229.
10. Del Rizzo DF, Boyd WD, Novick RJ, McCkenzie FN, Desai ND, Menkis AH. Safety and cost-effectiveness of MIDCABG in high-risk CABG patients. Ann Thorac Surg 1998;66:1002–1007.
11. Zenati M, Domit TM, Saul M, et al. Resource utilization for minimally invasive direct and standard coronary artery bypass grafting. Ann Thorac Surg 1997;63:S84–S87.
12. Doty JR, Fonger JD, Nicholson CF, Sussman MS, Salomon NW. Cost analysis of current therapies for limited coronary artery revascularization. Circulation 1997;96(suppl II):II16–II20.
13. Boyd WD, Desai ND, Del Rizzo DF, Novick RJ, McCkenzie N, Menkis AH. Off pump surgery decreases postoperative complications and resource utilization in the elderly. Ann Thorac Surg 1999;68:1490–1493.
14. Lemole GM, Choudri AF, Oz MC, Goldstein DJ, Gianguzzi R, Nguyen HC. Economic impact o fless invasive cardiac operations. In: Oz MC, Goldstein DJ, eds. Contemporary Cardiology: Minimally Invasive Cardiac Surgery. Totwa, NJ: Humana Press, 1998.
15. Hoff SJ, Ball SK, Coltharp WH, Glasfford DM. Lea JW 4th, Petracek MR. Coronary artery bypass in patients 80 years and over: is off pump the operation of choice? Ann Thorac Surg 2002;74:S1340–S1343.
16. Lee JH, Abdelhady K, Capdeville M. Clinical outcomes and resource usage in 100 consecutive patients after off-pump coronary bypass procedures. Surgery 2000;128:548–555.
17. Bull DA, Neumayer LA, Stringham JC, Meldrum P, Affleck DG, Karwande SV. Coronary artery bypass grafting with cardiopulmonary bypass versus off-pump coronary bypass grafting: does eliminating the pump reduce morbidity and cost? Ann Thorac Surg 2001;71:170–173.
18. van Dijk D, Nierich AP, Eefting FD, et al. The Octopus study: rationale and design of two randomized trials on medical effectiveness, safety, and cost-effectiveness of bypass surgery on the beating ehart. Control Clin Trials 2000;21:595–609.
19. Gelijns A, Gupta L, Kherani A, Burton E, Oz MC. Comparative on and off-pump CABg pilot trial. Unpublished data.

26 Minimally Invasive Cardiac Surgery

Quality-of-Life Issues

Giulio Pompilio, MD, PHD,
Francesco Alamanni, MD, *and Paolo Biglioli,* MD

CONTENTS

INTRODUCTION
QUALITY OF LIFE AND MINIMALLY INVASIVE CARDIAC SURGERY: DOES IT REALLY MATTER?
MINIMALLY INVASIVE CARDIAC SURGERY AND QUALITY-OF-LIFE: MEASUREMENT TOOLS
MINIMALLY INVASIVE CARDIAC SURGERY AND QUALITY-OF-LIFE ISSUES: LITERATURE REVIEW
INSTITUTIONAL EXPERIENCE
CONCLUSIONS
REFERENCES

INTRODUCTION

Since 1948, when the Word Health Organization defined health not only as the absence of disease, but also as the presence of physical, social, and mental well-being, studies on the quality of life (QoL) in medicine have become increasingly important in daily clinical practice and in medical research. The term "quality of life" refers to the physical, psychological, and social aspects of an individual's health, aspects that should be considered as a separate entity as they are closely related to the personal experience, expectations, hopes, and impressions the patient has concerning his or her own health *(1)*.

This is therefore a complex subject and any attempt to conceive of indices with which to measure QoL, thus adopting a "scientific" approach, must inevitably take into account its analytical, personal, and empirical nature. Essentially, the only reliable control of QoL studies is the individual. To identify the general aim of a study on the quality of life in the medical field, Testa and Simonson *(1)* proposed the following definition: "measure-

From: *Contemporary Cardiology: Minimally Invasive Cardiac Surgery, Second Edition*
Edited by: D. J. Goldstein and M. C. Oz © Humana Press Inc., Totowa, NJ

ment of the quality of life should address, that is, cover, each objective and subjective component (symptom, condition or social role) that is important to members of the patient population and susceptible to being affected positively or negatively by interventions."

Despite the objective difficulty of the analysis, in various branches of medicine, studies on QoL have increased exponentially, not least in cardiac surgery, especially over the last 5 yr. In this chapter we analyze the impact QoL has had on minimally invasive cardiac surgery (MICS), probably the most important innovation in cardiac surgery in recent years.

It is not easy to give a brief definition of MICS, as there is considerable literature on various surgical strategies and interventions described under this "umbrella" term. Generally, MICS involves cardiac surgery techniques and strategies that together reduce surgical trauma as much as possible and that increase patient acceptance of, and satisfaction with, the operation. This said, it seems obvious that MICS is something that is closely linked to the QoL.

However, a review of the literature dedicated to QoL in MICS does not exactly reflect this point of view. From 1995 to the present day, the PubMed database has listed more than 180 articles that discuss various aspects of MICS; of these, only five (less than 3%) address issues related to QoL.

QUALITY OF LIFE AND MINIMALLY INVASIVE CARDIAC SURGERY: DOES IT REALLY MATTER?

It is therefore opportune to ask which aspects of MICS concern QoL. QoL is, in fact, a generic term that encompasses the total well-being of the person, including functional capacity, symptoms, and the patient's perception of well-being *(2)*. The concept of "minimally invasive" should theoretically imply benefits derived from reduced surgical trauma. The hope of using MICS approaches is that patients benefit by having less postoperative physical discomfort, earlier return to physical fitness, and expedited resumption of their normal daily activities. Patients are also expected to be more satisfied with the operation from a cosmetic point of view than patients who have had conventional techniques.

Moreover, MICS may also reduce the impact of surgery on the patient's psychological status. It is well known that the patient's emotional status (anxiety, depression, self-control) plays an important role on the QoL of heart surgery patients. Theoretically, variables related to the patient's psychology, such as resuming a normal family, social, and sexual life and getting back to work, may benefit in the early and long-term period from a minimally invasive approach.

Furthermore, the interesting hypothesis that various factors linked to QoL may influence the "quod vitam et valitudinem" long-term prognosis of heart surgery patients has been recently suggested. Hertz *(3)* and Rumsfeld *(4)* have carried out elegant studies on the impact of preoperative QoL on long-term survival (5 yr) of patients who had had coronary artery bypass (CAB). Their interesting conclusions were in agreement: conditions linked to low QoL before surgery are an independent risk factor for long-term survival. It would therefore be useful, for instance, to establish if variables that are theoretically linked to the techniques of minimally invasive surgery, such as long-term patient satisfaction with the operation, in terms of physical and psychological well-being, can significantly improve the prognosis of those patients in whom preoperative indices suggest an unfavorable impact of QoL on life expectancy. This factor may then lead the surgeon to consider minimally invasive techniques.

It is clearly not easy to provide definitive answers to such complex questions. This is because randomized and prospective studies are needed on traditional surgical techniques and because of the many different types of surgery described as MICS. We strongly believe, however, that any surgeon practicing minimally invasive cardiac surgery should be cognizant and sensitive to QoL issues.

Recent studies have attempted to answer the many questions raised. Before reviewing the pertinent literature, it is necessary to briefly consider the instruments used in cardiac surgery to analyze QoL.

MINIMALLY INVASIVE CARDIAC SURGERY AND QUALITY OF LIFE: MEASUREMENT TOOLS

QoL cannot be measured directly, but rather through a series of items in a questionnaire that are awarded a numerical score. Various questionnaires have been used to measure QoL in heart surgery. Table 1 reports the main studies and questionnaires used to date in cardiac surgery. It is immediately evident that there are many methods for assessing QoL. Each author clearly used the questionnaires he or she believed most appropriate to the aim of the study. It is just as obvious that there is no questionnaire that is universally accepted as measuring the main issues of QoL in cardiac surgery. However, from a careful review of the methods used, it appears that a combination of certain questionnaires could adequately cover the majority of issues inherent to the QoL in a prospective study on minimally invasive cardiac surgery.

Physical Activity Score

The Physical Activity Score (PAS) represents one dimension of an angina-specific questionnaire *(5)*, the Angina Pectoris Quality of Life questionnaire, which contains six questions, for the self-estimation of physical abilities and limitations. Each response is graded from 1 to 6 and the mean value for all six questions is calculated. The higher the total value, the greater is the degree of disability.

The PAS is a useful instrument for quantifying the benefits of MICS in postoperative recovery, with special reference to the resumption of normal daily activities. In the long term, it can be used to measure and compare the degree of physical well-being achieved after MICS and conventional surgery. It should be noted that the questionnaire indirectly also refers to the clinical, situation of the patient as the reappearance of, for example, angina, or a worsening of the patient's New York Heart Association (NYHA) class, is directly reflected in their degree of physical activity and therefore in their QoL.

Nottingham Health Profile

The Nottingham Health Profile (NHP) is divided in two parts *(6)*. Part I consists of 38 statements that convey limitations of activity or aspects of distress in six dimensions: physical mobility, pain, sleep, energy, social isolation, and emotional reactions. Patients are required to indicate by a yes/no answer which of the problems they are experiencing at the time they complete the questionnaire. A score ranging from 0 to 100 can be calculated for each dimension of this part of the profile; the higher the score, the greater the limitations in the activity or the distressing social and emotional problems. Parts II lists the seven aspects of life that are found to be most affected by a person's state of health: occupation, ability to perform jobs around the house, social life, home relationships, sexual life, hobbies, and holidays; a yes/no answer indicates which areas are affected by the respondent's present state of health.

Table 1
Main Studies and Questionnaires Used to Date in Cardiac Surgery[a]

Reference	*Type of procedure*	*Questionnaire*	*Type of QL study*
Chocron S et al.: Ann Thorac Surg 1996	CAB, valve or combined procedures	NHP	Comparative study, outcome and QL
Nielsen D et al.: Crit Care Med 1997	Miscellaneous	NHP	QL in complicated patients
Sjöland H et al.: J Hyperten 1997	CAB	PAS, NHP, PGWBI	Hypertensive patients
Hlatky MA et al.: N Engl J Med 1997	CAB and PTCA	Duke ASI, RAND MHI	Comparative study
Shapira OM et al.: Chest 1997	Valve surgery	Duke MOS	Elderly patients
Westin L et al.: J Int Med 1997	CAB and PTCA	Self-made	Comparative study
Soklano JA et al.: Ann Surg 1998	CAB	Euro QL	Octogenarians
Fruitman DS, et al.: Ann Thorac Surg 1999	CAB, AVR, MVR, and combined	SAQ, RAND SF-36	Octogenarians
Rumsfeld JS et al.: JAMA 1999	CAB	SF-36	Long-term outcome and prognosis
Herlitz J et al.: 1999	CAB	PAS, NHP, PGWBI	Long-term outcome and prognosis
Sjöland H et al.: J Int Med 1999	CAB	PAS, NHP, PGWBI	Gender influence
Yun KL, et al.: Ann Thorac Surg 1999	CAB, valve or combined procedures	HSQ	Time-related QL
Smith HJ et al.: Heart 2000	CAB	QLI, SF-36, QLMI, SEIQL	Comparative study

[a]NHP=Nottingham Health Profile; PAS=Physical Activity Score; PGWBI=Physiological General Well-Being Index; Duke ASI=Duke University Activity Status Index; RAND MHI=RAND Mental Health Inventory; Duke MOS=Duke University Medical Outcomes Study; HSQ=Health Status Questionnaire; Euro QL-Euro Quality of Life Questionnaire; SF36=Short Form 36; QLI=Quality of Life Index-Cardiac Version; QLMI=Quality of Life after Myocardial Infarction Questionnaire; SEIQL=Schedule for the Evaluation of Individual Quality of Life.

The NHP partially completes the PAS for those aspects related to the resumption of physical activity after the operation. Part I concerns aspects of QoL that often deteriorate in the postoperative period of conventional surgery, mainly concerned with the patient's physical and mental well-being, as, for example, the normal rhythms of sleeping and waking or the degree of anxiety. MICS might, we believe, have a positive influence on these variables, compared to conventional surgery. Part II is useful to assess the markers that indicate the patient has returned to normal social and family life, and therefore to assess the long-term benefits of MICS on the QoL of the patient who has had surgery.

The Psychological General Well-Being Index

The Psychological General Well-Being Index (PGWBI) contains 22 questions, dealing with six sections of well-being: anxiety, depressed mood, vitality, general health, self-control, and well-being *(7)*. The response format is graded from 1 to 6 (total score range 22–132), with the highest value corresponding to superior well-being.

The PGWBI completes both parts of the NHP. The emphasis on the state of well-being may be of interest for patients who have MICS, especially because of the beneficial influence this type of surgery has on the level of patient satisfaction and acceptance of surgery.

MINIMALLY INVASIVE CARDIAC SURGERY AND QUALITY-OF-LIFE ISSUES: LITERATURE REVIEW

The impact of minimally invasive cardiac surgery on QoL has received little attention in the literature. Table 2 highlights the principal articles covering the subject.

Pain

The Leipzig group has addressed the problem of quantifying postoperative pain after MICS and comparing it with that after conventional surgery in two studies. Walther and colleagues *(8)* carried out a prospective study on 338 patients who had had a coronary bypass, aortic, and/or mitral valve replacement with both the minimally invasive method and with conventional surgery using median sternotomy. The MICS techniques used were left anterior minithoracotomy with beating heart (minimally invasive direct coronary artery bypass or MIDCAB) (*see* Chapter 9); right lateral minithoracotomy using CPB and endoaortic clamping of the aorta to replace the mitral valve (*see* Chapters 19 and 20), and partial sternotomy with the usual CPB arrangement for aortic valve replacement (*see* Chapter 21).

The assessment of postoperative pain was made using a standard "pain questionnaire," which provides information on the intensity of the pain, the nature of the pain, where it is, how it changes over time, how it changes with physical activity, and the most effective doses of the most efficient painkillers. Two different scoring tests were used: a verbal rating scale, which allows differentiation between no pain, mild pain, moderate pain, severe pain, and unbearable pain; and a visual analog scale, which quantifies pain on a scale from 1 (no pain) to 10 (the worst pain the patient has ever experienced).

The level of postoperative pain diminishes in all patients during the first postoperative week, with no difference between MICS and conventional patients in their use of painkillers. Recipients of the MIDCAB operation and those who underwent minimally invasive approaches to the mitral valve benefited from less pain after postoperative d 3 than those who have had conventional sternotomy, which causes pain and tension in the back muscles for some time. Interestingly, however, patients who underwent the MIDCAB

Table 2
Principal Recent Papers[a]

Reference	*Type of procedure*	*Questionnaire*	*Type of QoL study*
Massetti M et al.: Eur J Cardiothorc Surg 1999	Miscellaneous MICS	Home-made	Cosmetic aspects
Grossi EA et al.: Eur J Cardiothorac Surg 1999	MIDCAB	DASI	Pain, stress response, QL
Walther T et al.: Ann Thorac Surg 1999	Miscellaneous MICS	Pain Q, NHP	Pain and QL
Biglioli P et al.: Ann Thorac Surg 1999	MIDCAB	PAS, PGWBI	QL
Diegeler A et al.: Heart Surg Forum 2000	MIDCAB	HNP	Pain, QL

[a]QL=Quality of Life; MIDCAB=minimally invasive coronary bypass grafting; Pain Q=pain questionnaire; DASI=Duke Activity Status Index; NHP=Nottingham Health Profile; PAS=Physical Activity Score; PGWBI=Psychological General Well-being Index.

operation experienced more severe incisional pain for 48 h after the operation, making local anesthetic and/or epidural catheter useful in relieving pain.

These results are confirmed elsewhere by the same authors *(9)* in a case series that included only patients who underwent a MIDCAB. The difference in the postoperative levels of pain was close to reaching statistical significance until postoperative d 7. In this study, using a modified version of the NHP questionnaire, they also assessed the aspects of QoL that are linked directly to postoperative pain (degree of limitation of mobility and physical activity by pain). They observed a net improvement in MIDCAB patients in resuming their normal physical activities after the operation compared to those who had had conventional surgery. These results were confirmed 3 mo after surgery.

Cosmetic Issues

The cosmetic effects of a midline thoracic scar may have a negative impact on patients' self-concepts and therefore on their QoL. Massetti et al. *(10)* investigated the long-term cosmetic impact of MICS in a series of 56 young female patients who, in a 17-yr time span, underwent atrial septal defect closure through a right anterolateral thoracotomy. Patients completed a multiple-choice questionnaire focusing on self-evaluation of the esthetic result and its psychological influence. In particular, the patients were asked about their impression regarding: (1) the volume and the symmetry of the breasts; (2) a description of the quality (color, dimension, and visibility) of the scar; (3) their feelings about the scar when dressings were removed, appearance in a bathing suit, playing sports, buying bras, and during intimate relations with partners; and (4) their satisfaction or dissatisfaction resulting from surgery.

The answers of the questionnaires suggested that the patient's subjective impressions are at least commensurate with the objective findings. More than 90% of the patients self-evaluated the cosmetic result of the operation as excellent or good. Regarding the psychological influence of the surgical scar, absence of troubles as described in point 3 are found in more than 80% of patients. Hence, the minimally invasive approach to atrial septal defect through small right thoracotomy appears to have a positive long-term impact on patients' QoL. The inferences of the authors were that, once surgeons perfected the surgical techniques, the challenge remained to reduce the impact of the cosmetic blemish that median sternotomy may leave on the patient's chest.

Quality of Life

The Leipzig group *(8,9)* assessed QoL in patients undergoing MICS using a modification of the Nottingham Health Questionnaire. The latter consisted of the inclusion of one possible positive answer in each category. Different aspects of QoL were analyzed, including mobility, social status, level of activities, emotional state, and sleeping disorders. Changes in QoL were evaluated preoperatively, early in the postoperative period, and during interviews at 3 mo postoperatively.

When considering miscellaneous MICS patients (different MICS approaches in coronary and valve diseases), the authors *(8)* were not able to assess at 3 mo relevant differences in postoperative QoL for MICS in comparison with conventional surgery. On the other hand, using the same QoL measurements, if MIDCAB patients only are considered *(9)*, a statistically improved outcome regarding QoL aspects such as mobility, and a trend toward less limitations in terms of activities and sleep, were observed. No differences between surgical groups could be evaluated regarding emotional and social aspects.

Grossi and colleagues *(11)* evaluated QoL in port-access (PA) vs standard sternotomy coronary bypass patients (STD). The Duke Activity Status Index questionnaire was administered to patients preoperatively and at the end of postoperative wk 1, 2, 4, and 8. This questionnaire measured return to normal functional activity in terms of 12 common activities of daily living, including the patient's ability to walk, climb stairs, work around the house, and perform related activities. In addition, as an indication of rapidity of recovery, patients were asked to rate their health compared to the preoperative level at the same postoperative time periods.

A significantly higher percentage of PA patients compared with STD patients were able to walk one or two blocks at 1 wk, climb stairs at 1 and 2 wk, and engage in moderate recreational activity and heavy housework at 8 wk. The PA group reported a significantly higher percentage of return to preoperative activity level than did the STD group.

CENTRO CARDIOLOGICO MONZINO IRCCS EXPERIENCE

Patients and Methods

Between March 1995 and March 2001, 108 patients underwent MIDCAB at our institution. Mean age was 59 ± 9.7 yr, 72 (66.6%) were male, 37 (34.2%) had unstable angina, 48 (44.4%) had a history of hypertension, 7 (6.4%) had insulin-dependent diabetes mellitus, 9 (8.3%) had chronic renal failure, 3 (2.7%) had a previous stroke, 3 (2.7%) had a previous transient ischemic attack, 43 (39.8%) had a previous remote myocardial infarct (>3 mo), 17 (15.7%) had a recent myocardial infarct (<3 mo), and 21 (19.4%) had previously undergone a percutaneous intervention.

All patients completed three self-administered questionnaires for the evaluation of their quality of life, including the Nottingham Health Profile (Parts 1 and 2), the Physical Activity Score, and the Psychological General Well-Being Index questionnaires before

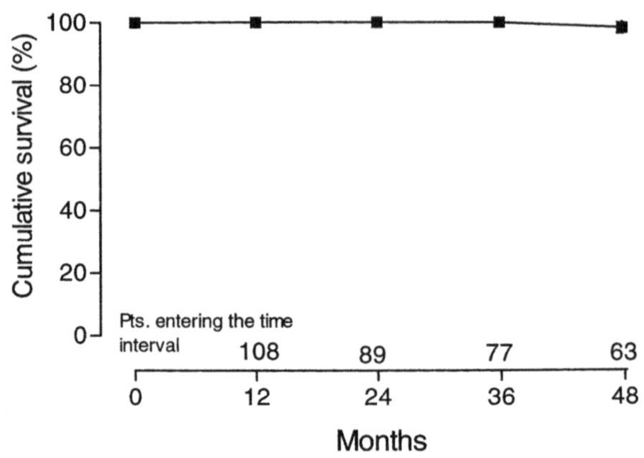

Fig. 1. Kaplan-Meyer survival 48 mo after MIDCAB.

surgery. The same questionnaires were then mailed to patients 6 ($n = 108$) and 12 ($n = 108$) mo after surgery *(12)*. At 48 mo (n = 63 pts.) postoperatively, QoL information was obtained by direct interview. All the questionnaires were validated carefully and tested for reliability.

Clinical follow-up information, available for 100% of the patients, was obtained every year postoperatively by means of mailed questionnaires and at the fourth postoperative year by direct examination of the patient. The date of the last inquiry was between January and April 2001. The following clinical endpoints were collected for each patient: (1) survival; (2) acute myocardial infarction-free survival; (3) angina-free survival; (4) redo-free survival; (5) PTCA-free survival; (6) PTCA to LAD-free survival. Survival rates of the entire patient population were determined by Kaplan–Meier survival analysis, and the estimated survival proportions are reported ± the standard error of the estimates.

Early Results

All patients underwent MIDCAB through a left anterior thoracotomy and in all cases a LIMA-to-LAD anastomosis was performed on a beating heart; no conversions to sternotomy were performed. No perioperative deaths occurred. Two patients (1.8%) showed suffered a perioperative myocardial infarction, without hemodynamic deterioration. Four patients (3.7%) underwent reoperation for bleeding. The mean ventilatory support time and the mean ICU stay were 7 ± 7.4 h and 15 ± 10 h, respectively, while postoperative length of stay was 5.4 ± 1.5 d.

Late Results

Average follow-up was 39 ± 13.4 mo (median 41). Survival and survival-free estimates of the patient population are reported in **Figs. 1, 2,** and **3**; of note, 4-yr survival was 98% ± 1.8%, redo-free survival was 97% ± 0.9%, acute myocardial infarction-free survival was 95% ± 1.9%, and angina-free survival was 90% ± 4.4%.

Measurement of Quality of Life

The Physical Activity Score improved significantly after the operation, with improvements of 26.8% and 34.2% at 12 and 48 mo, respectively (Table 3). The same behavior was shared by the Psychological General Well-Being Index, which improved 25.6% and

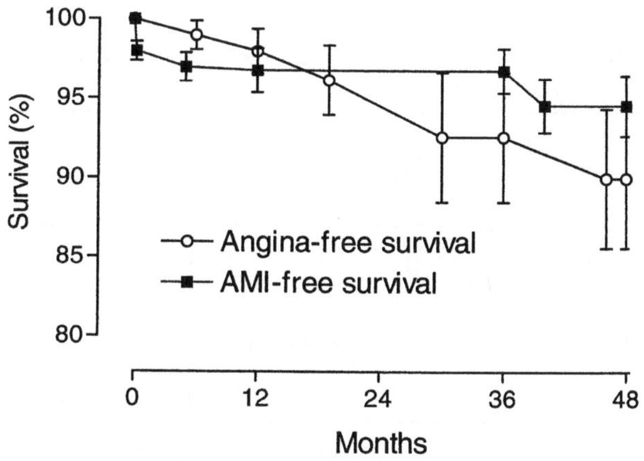

Fig. 2. Freedom from angina and acute myocardial infarction (AMI) 48 mo after MIDCAB.

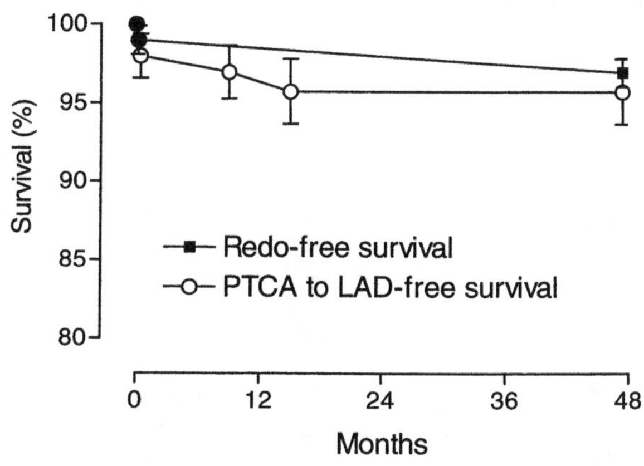

Fig. 3. Freedom from reoperation, percutaneous coronary angioplasty (PTCA) to the left anteriordescending coronary artery (LAD), 48 mo after MIDCAB.

Table 3
Average Physical Activity Scores Before and After MIDCAB[a]

	All patients population (n = 108)		
	Before surgery	*12 mo after surgery*	
Average score	4.3 ± 0.8 [4.5]	3.1 ± 0.7 [3.3]*	
% change		–27.9%	
	Patients who reached 48 mo follow-up interval (n = 63)		
	Before surgery	*12 mo after surgery*	*48 mo after surgery*
Average score	4.1 ± 1.2 [4.4]	3.0 ± 1.1 [3.1]*	2.83 ± 1.3 [3.4]*
% change		–26.8%	–31%

[a]Scores are reported as mean ± s.d. [median in brackets]. * = $p < 0.01$ vs before surgery. Negative % change values indicate an improvement.

Table 4
Average Total Scores for the Psychological General Well-Being Index Before and After MIDCABG[a]

	All patients population (n = 108)		
	Before surgery	*12 mo after surgery*	
Average score	82.9 ± 8.9 [82.0]	103.5 ± 7.3 [104.0]*	
% change		+24.8%	
	Patients who reached 48 mo follow-up interval (n = 63)		
	Before surgery	*12 mo after surgery*	*48 mo after surgery*
Average score	83.1 ± 8.4 [81.5]	104.4 ± 9.1 [104]*	111.6 ± 6.8 [102.5]*
% change		+25.6%	+34.2%

[a]Scores are reported as mean ± s.d. [median in brackets].
* = p <0.01 vs before surgery. Positive % change values indicate an improvement.

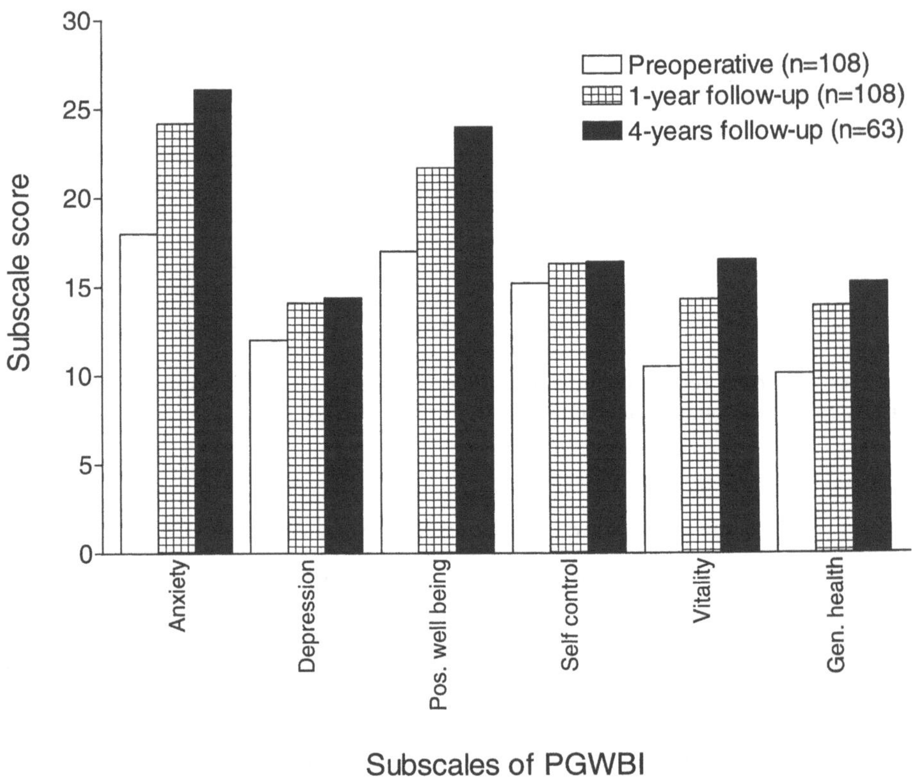

Fig. 4. Bar graph of the six different domains of the Psychological General Well-Being Index (PGWBI) as assessed before, 1 yr, and 4 yr after MIDCAB.

26.2% at 12 and 48 mo, respectively (Table 4). The analysis of the six different subscales of the test revealed further improvements at 12 and 48 mo in anxiety, positive well-being, vitality, and general health domains (**Fig. 4**). Improvements seem to be reached in all

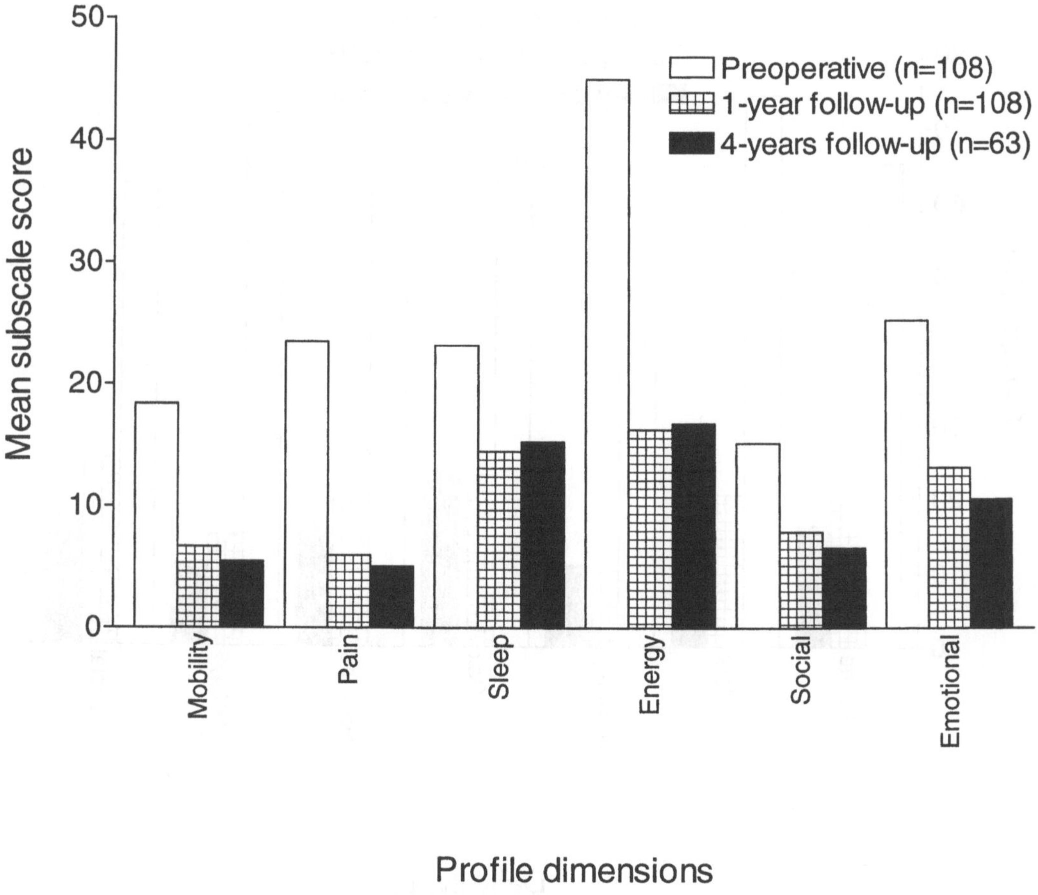

Fig. 5. Bar graph of the six different domains of the Notthingham Health Profile (NHP) Part I as assessed before, 1 yr, and 4 yr after MIDCAB.

subscales. In particular, the positive well-being and the vitality scales show a favorable trend from 12 to 48 mo postoperatively.

Figure 5 reports the average scores of Part 1 of the Nottingham Health Profile, with lower scores indicating better health status. One year after surgery there were important improvements in all the dimensions of this score. A further improvement when comparing 1- and 4-yr results was seen mainly in mobility, social, and emotional subscales.

With regard to Part 2 of the Nottingham Health Profile (**Fig. 6**), the percentage of patients who were experiencing problems in daily living was also markedly improved 1 yr after surgery. At 4 yr, further improvements were observed in home, work recovery, hobbies, and social life in general, indicating a long-term benefit of MIDCAB in daily living.

CONCLUSIONS

Despite the difficulty of analyzing a subject so closely related to varying subjective and social conditions, our data and the literature indicate that MICS seems to have a positive impact on the QoL of heart surgery patients. The concept of QoL after surgery, however, cannot disregard clinical results (both in short postoperative and long-term periods), as the primary expectation of surgery lies in its outcome. Results of MICS are

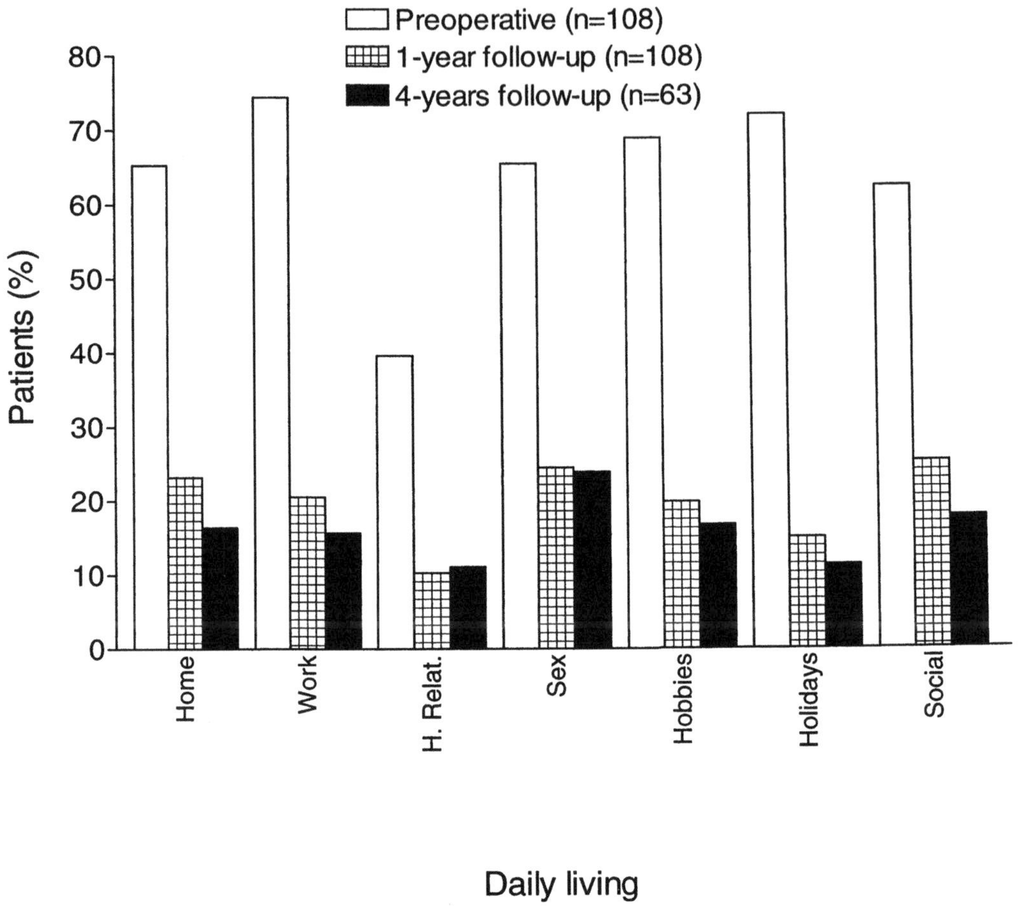

Fig. 6. Bar graph of the seven different domains of the Notthingham Health Profile (NHP) Part II as assessed before, 1 yr, and 4 yr after MIDCAB.

now accepted as satisfactory in terms of mortality and morbidity *(8–13)*; patients can therefore enjoy further advantages in terms of QoL because of lower levels of invasiveness and surgical trauma.

Although the available data are still preliminary, MICS seems to have a good effect on both the physical and psychological aspects of the patient's status. Our findings indicate that 4 yr after MIDCAB, patients experience a constant improvement in physical and psychological well-being and social quality of life.

Specific questionnaires are required to measure QoL in MICS rather than the various tested generic and disease-specific questionnaires for QoL available in heart surgery literature. Condition-specific questionnaires (QL questionnaires and functional-living indexes for MICS) and situation-specific ones (trial-specific modules and checklists) able to strengthen reliability and validity of studies dedicated to QoL in MICS *(13)* are needed. These questionnaires would supply useful additional information for the selection of those patients who may better benefit from a mini-invasive approach (depending on sex, age, social position, etc.).

On the other hand, many questions remain unanswered. First, the effective long-term superiority of MICS to improve QoL (or graft patency or survival) needs further confirmation. Second, long-term prognosis of MICS patients has to be analyzed and compared to conventional techniques with prospective studies to identify those patients whose QoL may have a negative impact on life expectancy. These data are not available today because of the young age of clinical trials in MICS; it is hoped that they will become known as the follow-up period increases. Finally, there is the need to prospectively match many of the interventions labeled as MICS for their impact on QoL, especially in cases of different approaches to the same pathology (for instance mini-sternotomy vs mini-thoracotomy for the revascularization of LAD coronary artery). It is possible that some surgical interventions described as "minimally invasive" do not provide any real benefit in terms of QoL. Once again, such a selection can be carried out as the survey and follow-up period is extended.

It has been said that "in addition to relieving clinical symptoms and prolonging survival, a primary objective of any health care intervention is the enhancement of quality of life and wellbeing" *(14)*. There is a well-founded hope that minimally invasive heart surgery has the potential to meet this laudable objective.

REFERENCES

1. Testa MA, Simonson DC. Current concepts: assessment of quality-of-life outcomes. N Engl J Med 1996;334(13):835–840.
2. Stewart AL, Ware JE. Measuring functioning and well being—the Medical Outcomes Study approach. Durham, NC: Duke University, 1992;1–449.
3. Herlitz J, Wiklund I, Caidahl K, et al. Determinants of an impaired quality of life five years after coronary artery bypass surgery. Heart 1999;81:342–346.
4. Rumsfeld JS, Mc Whinney S, McCarthy M, et al. Health-related quality of life as a predictor of mortality following coronary artery bypass graft surgery. JAMA 1999;281:1298–1303.
5. Wilson A, Wiklund I, Lahtl T, Wahl M. A summary index for the assessment of quality of life in angina pectoris. J Clin Epidemiol 1991;44:981–988.
6. Hunt S, Wiklund I. Cross-cultural variation in the weighting of health statements: a comparison of English and Swedish valuations. Health Policy 1987;8:227–235.
7. Dupuy H. The Psychological General Well-being (PGWB) Index. In: Wenger NK, Mattson ME, Furberg CD, Elison J, eds. Assessment of Quality of Life in Clinical Trials of Cardiovascular Therapies. Greenwich, CT: Le Jacq Publishers, 1985:170–183.
8. Walther T, Falk V, Metz S, Diegeler A, Battellini R, Autschbach R, Mohr FW. Pain and quality of life after minimally invasive versus conventional cardiac surgery. Ann Thorac Surg 1999;67:1643–1647.
9. Diegeler A, Walther T, Metz S, et al. Comparison of MIDCAB versus conventional CAB surgery regarding pain and quality of life. Heart Surg Forum 1999;2(4):290–296.
10. Massetti M, Nataf P, Babatasi G, Khayat A. Cosmetic aspects in minimally invasive cardiac surgery. Eur J Cardiothorac Surg 1999;16(suppl 2):S73–S75.
11. Grossi EA, Zakow PK, Ribakove G, et al. Comparison of postoperative pain, stress response, and quality of life in port access vs. standard sternotomy coronary bypass patients. Eur J Cardiothorac Surg 1999;16(suppl 2):S39–S42.
12. Biglioli P, Antona C, Alamanni F, et al. Minimally invasive direct coronary artery bypass grafting: mid-term results and quality of life. Ann Thorac Surg 2000;70(2):456–460.
13. Osoba D. Guidelines for measuring health-related quality of life in clinical trials. In: Staquet MJ, Hays RD, Fayers P, eds. Quality of Life Assessment in Clinical Trials. Methods and Practice. Oxford Univ Press, 1998:19–35.
14. Berzon RA. Understanding and using health-related quality of life instruments within clinical research studies. In: Staquet MJ, Hays RD, Fayers P, eds. Quality of Life Assessment in Clinical Trials. Methods and Practice. Oxford Univ Press, 1998:1–15.

27 Experimental Percutaneous Mitral Valve Repair

Juan P. Umaña, MD *and Peter Fitzgerald,* MD

CONTENTS

INTRODUCTION
MANAGEMENT OF MITRAL REGURGITATION
THE EDGE-TO-EDGE TECHNIQUE
DEVELOPMENT OF AN OFF-PUMP MITRAL VALVE REPAIR
FUTURE TRENDS
REFERENCES

The dogmas of the quiet past are inadequate for the stormy present. The occasion is piled high with difficulty, and we must rise with the occasion.... We must think anew and act anew—Abraham Lincoln

INTRODUCTION

Over the past few years we have witnessed an impressive increase in the number of percutaneous cardiac procedures, in parallel with the development of new technology. Drug-impregnated stents implanted in the coronary circulation promise significant decreases in restenosis rates. Covered endovascular stent-grafts are being used successfully to treat descending thoracic aortic aneurysms and dissections, significantly lessening the morbidity and mortality of surgical intervention, and ongoing trials are evaluating the safety and efficacy of percutaneous device closure of atrial septal defects.

Contrary to other cardiovascular structures, the mitral valve (MV) is less appealing for percutaneous intervention, owing to its location (difficult access and risk of embolism) and the complexity of its subvalvular apparatus. The concept of intervening on the mitral valve without the use of cardiopulmonary bypass was introduced by Harken and Bailey in 1948 with the use of closed mitral commissurotomy for mitral stenosis. More recently, Reyes et al. compared percutaneous balloon valvuloplasty to open surgical commissuro-

From: *Contemporary Cardiology: Minimally Invasive Cardiac Surgery, Second Edition*
Edited by: D. J. Goldstein and M. C. Oz © Humana Press Inc., Totowa, NJ

tomy *(1,2)* and found on long-term follow-up that durability was better for the percutaneous procedure, while there was no difference in the incidence of embolic complications. Application of similar technologies to repair incompetent mitral valves has only recently been entertained, with improved understanding of the pathophysiology of mitral regurgitation and the subvalvular apparatus.

MANAGEMENT OF MITRAL REGURGITATION

The mitral valve and its subvalvular apparatus play a crucial role in maintaining left ventricular geometry and optimizing the mechanical efficiency of the left ventricle (LV). An intact subvalvular apparatus helps maintain the ellipsoid shape of the LV, decreasing wall stress at end-systole and preserving a normal ratio of wall thickness to ventricular diameter *(3)*. As a consequence, treatment of mitral regurgitation (MR) should aim to preserve this mechanism while using autologous materials to avoid thromboembolic complications. Mitral valve repair methods developed by Carpentier et al. have been used successfully for the last three decades with excellent reproducibility and 98% freedom from reoperation at 10 yr *(4)*. These techniques preserve ventricular function, are associated with lower mortality rates, and have fewer thromboembolic complications when compared to MV replacement *(5–7)*.

Optimal timing for operation in mitral regurgitation remains controversial owing to the very nature of the condition, which progresses insidiously due to loading conditions causing left ventricular function to appear normal on echocardiogram until late in the disease process. As a consequence, patients are referred for surgery when compensatory mechanisms have been overrun and poor prognostic indicators are present, i.e., decreased ejection fraction (<60%), increased end-systolic dimension (≥45 mm), and pulmonary hypertension *(8–12)*. This delayed referral pattern is in part based on evidence that medically treated patients with severe MR who are in New York Heart Association (NYHA) Class I or II have a 5-yr survival rate in excess of 85%, which is only slightly lower than the survival rate in an age-matched population *(13)*. Another factor leading to untimely referral is the reluctance on the part of cardiologists to send asymptomatic patients for "open-heart surgery," with its attendant morbidity and mortality.

Some of these referral biases could be overcome with the development of a minimally invasive method of valve repair that would allow cardiac surgeons to perform a less morbid procedure early in the course of mitral regurgitation, perhaps altering the natural history of the disease. A subset of patients who would benefit from a percutaneous or closed approach are those with ischemic mitral regurgitation due to inferior/lateral wall myocardial ischemia. This patient population is particularly challenging, as the addition of mitral repair to routine myocardial revascularization can increase operative mortality to 10–15%. Nonetheless, studies suggest that long-term prognosis for these patients is better if revascularization is accompanied by repair of the mitral valve. An off-pump or "closed-heart" technique would facilitate addressing the valve in these situations, decreasing operative mortality/morbidity and improving long-term outcome. In more advanced cases, where pulmonary hypertension has developed and ventricular function is depressed, the benefits of avoiding cardiopulmonary bypass altogether are self-evident.

THE EDGE-TO-EDGE TECHNIQUE

The idea of minimally invasive cardiac surgery emerged around 1995, when surgeons began to realize the benefits of smaller incisions and shorter cardiopulmonary bypass times. An improved understanding of the pathophysiology of cardiopulmonary bypass, its deleterious effects on neurocognitive function, and its proinflammatory effect was followed by a resurrection of off-pump coronary bypass operations. With it, methods were developed to perform coronary revascularization and valve surgery thoracoscopically and with the help of robotics *(14)*. Nevertheless, conventional mitral valve repair techniques can only be performed on cardiopulmonary bypass, and although potentially amenable to a totally endoscopic approach, an off-pump approach would not be feasible in most circumstances. Alfieri et al. in 1998 reported their experience using a simplified method of mitral valve repair in 121 patients, which consisted of suturing the prolapsing portion of the diseased leaflet to the corresponding free edge of the opposing leaflet (**Fig. 1**). In their earlier series, 93% of patients had a concomitant ring annuloplasty, except for those patients with restricted leaflet motion or small annuli *(15)*. Short-term results were impressive, with an overall survival of 92 ± 3.1% at 6 yr, 95 ± 4.8% freedom from reoperation, and no instances of mitral stenosis. In a recent update *(16)*, the same group corroborated their results with a mean follow-up of 2 yr (range, 1 mo to 7 yr). Operative mortality was 0.7%, and actuarial survival at 5 yr was 94% ± 3%. Freedom from reoperation was significantly better when a ring was used concomitantly with the leaflet suture (92% vs 72%). Although the numbers are impressive, most patients who had an edge-to-edge repair without a ring had extensive calcification of the posterior annulus, which in itself compromises durability of any type of repair.

Umaña et al. in 1998 published the Columbia experience using the edge-to-edge technique ("bow-tie" repair) in 10 patients with ischemic regurgitation. The bow-tie repair was used as an adjunct to ring annuloplasty in cases in which mitral valve replacement was felt to have resulted in unacceptably high morbidity or mortality due to poor left ventricular function. Mitral regurgitation was significantly reduced from 4+ to 1+ on average, and left ventricular ejection fraction improved from 33% ± 13% to 45% ± 11% ($p = 0.016$) prior to discharge *(17)*. Mean follow-up was 337 d (range 85–554 d), and reoperation rate was 40%, all in patients with underlying structural leaflet pathology or papillary muscle rupture. A particularly interesting observation was the significant improvement in ejection fraction seen in this small patient cohort. We hypothesized that the bow-tie stitch could have an "anchoring" effect on the dysfunctional posterior papillary muscle, therefore decreasing paradoxical motion of the posterolateral segment and improving overall ventricular function. To test this hypothesis we used an ovine model of ischemic mitral regurgitation, and studied the effect of the bow-tie repair on ventricular geometry, degree of regurgitation, and mitral annular function *(18)*. Animals were infarcted by surgically ligating the obtuse marginal branches 2 and 3 of the circumflex coronary artery, which leads to posterior papillary muscle tethering and development of chronic regurgitation as described by Llaneras et al. *(19)*. Using three-dimensional sonomicrometry array localization (3D-SAL), the mitral valve annulus, papillary muscles, and ventricular long and short axes were studied in three different conditions: baseline (with existing regurgitation), during snaring of posterior mitral suture annuloplasty (deVega type), and during snaring of the bow-tie stitch.

We found that both techniques achieved similar control of regurgitation (3+ to 1+; $p < 0.05$) (**Fig. 2**). Mitral annular contractility defined as [(maximum area – minimum area)/maximum area] × 100, was significantly impaired by conventional posterior annuloplasty, while it did not change with the bow-tie repair (**Fig. 3**). To determine changes in ventricular geometry and ventriculo-mitral interaction, we measured the distance from the valvular plane to the tips and bases of the papillary muscles, as well as

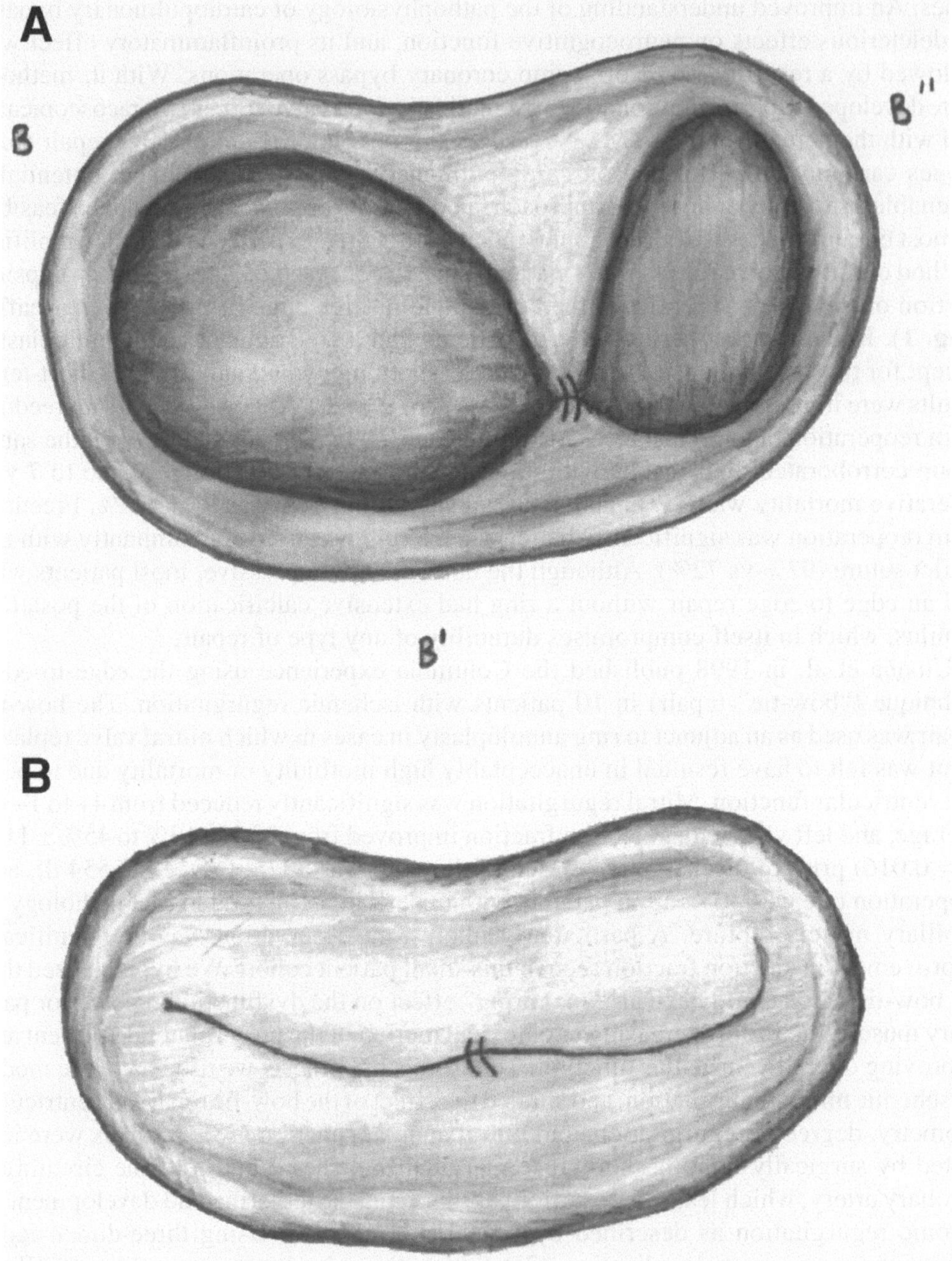

Fig. 1. "Bow-tie" repair—Atrial view. (**A**) Diastole. (**B**) Systole.

between papillary muscle bases throughout the cardiac cycle (**Fig. 4**). It was of interest to find that the edge-to-edge repair led to an increase in distance from the base of the papillary muscles to the plane of the valve. On the other hand, the distance between the bases of the papillary muscles decreased with the use of the bow-tie repair. These findings suggest that this simple repair may cause an accentuation of the elliptical shape of the ventricle even after an ischemic insult. This, in turn, may improve hemodynamic performance and facilitate ventricular remodeling, as the wall tension of the left ventricle decreases.

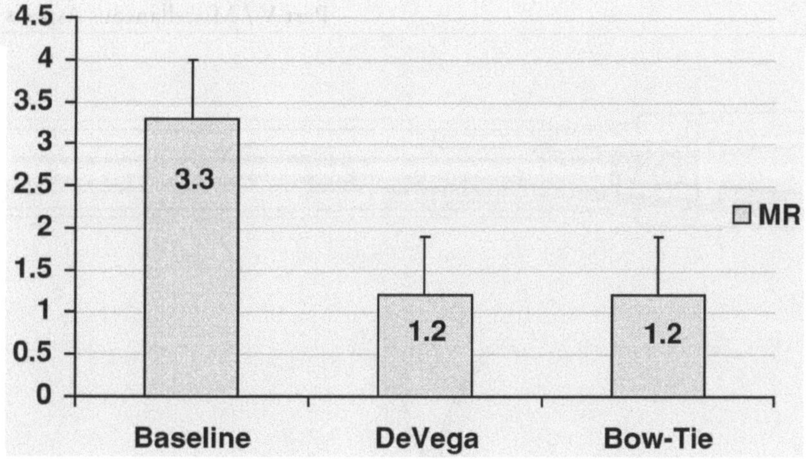

Fig. 2. Degree of mitral regurgitation.

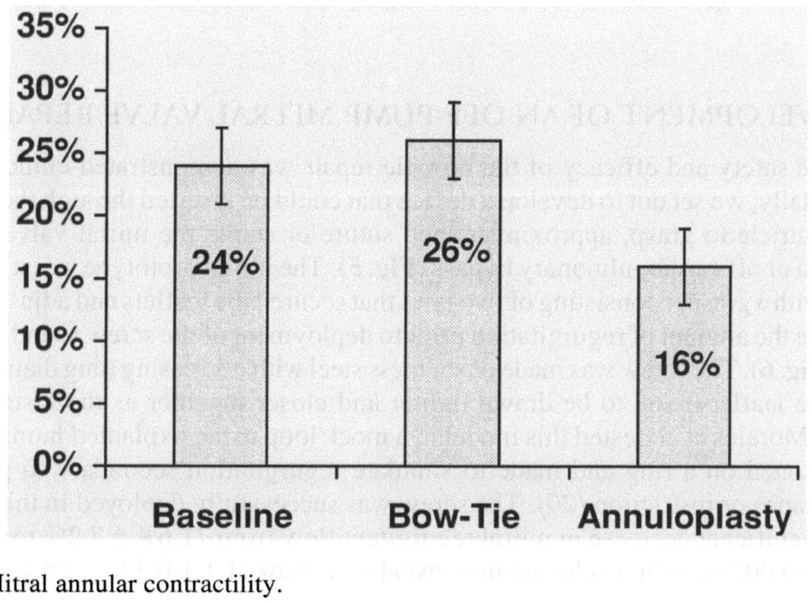

Fig. 3. Mitral annular contractility.

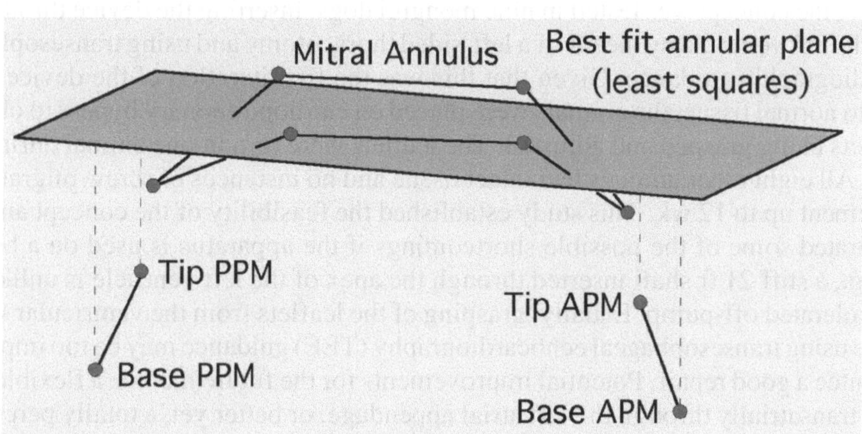

Fig. 4. Ventricular geometry—measurements. PPM, posterior papillary muscle; APM, anterior papillary muscle.

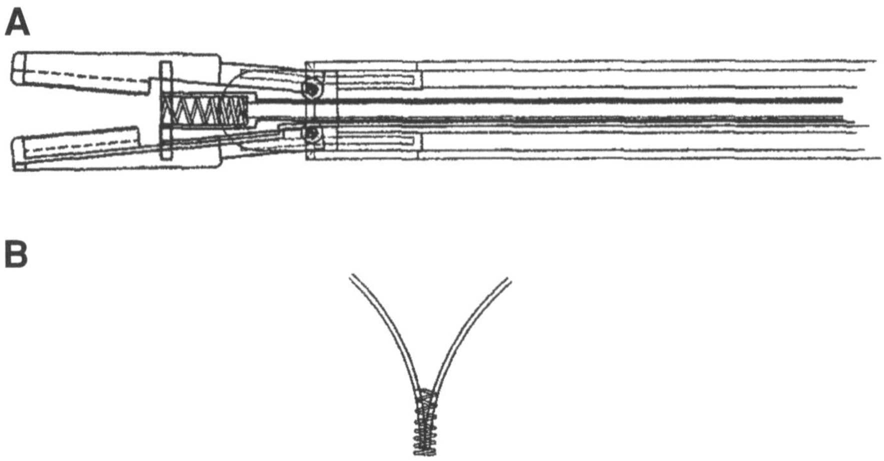

Fig. 5. Coil-fastening device. (**A**) Grasper and undeployed coil. (**B**) Coil fastener holding leaflets together.

DEVELOPMENT OF AN OFF-PUMP MITRAL VALVE REPAIR

Once the safety and efficacy of the bow-tie repair was demonstrated clinically and experimentally, we set out to develop a device that could be inserted through the apex of the left ventricle to grasp, approximate, and suture or staple the mitral valve leaflets together, on or off cardiopulmonary bypass (**Fig. 5**). The initial prototype was a stainless steel tool with a grasper consisting of two jaws that secured the leaflets and adjusted them to minimize the amount of regurgitation prior to deployment of the screw found between the jaws (**Fig. 6**). The screw was made of stainless steel with decreasing rung diameter that allowed the leaflet tissue to be drawn tighter and closer together as the fastener was advanced. Morales et al. tested this model in a mock loop using explanted human mitral valves mounted on a ring and made to simulate regurgitation secondary to posterior leaflet prolapse or restriction *(20)*. The screw was successfully deployed in this model, finding a significant decrease in mitral regurgitant flow from 71.6% ± 7.2% to 34.4% ± 17.3% ($p = 0.0025$), with no change in transvalvular flow (1.1 ± 0.3 to 1.2 ± 0.4 L/min; $p = 0.7$).

In vivo, the concept was tested in nine mongrel dogs, inserting the device through the apex of the left ventricle by means of a left-sided thoracotomy and using transesophageal echocardiographic guidance. Given that this was the first iteration of the device being applied to normal tissue, the animals were placed on cardiopulmonary bypass to observe the leaflets being grasped and adjusted. The leaflets were torn in one animal during this process. All eight other animals had intact tissue and no instances of screw migration or dislodgement up to 12 wk. This study established the feasibility of the concept and also demonstrated some of the possible shortcomings if the apparatus is used on a beating heart, e.g., a stiff 21 fr shaft inserted through the apex of the left ventricle is unlikely to be well tolerated off-pump. Equally, grasping of the leaflets from the ventricular side of the valve using transesophageal echocardiography (TEE) guidance may be too imprecise to guarantee a good repair. Potential improvements for the future include a flexible shaft inserted transatrially through the left atrial appendage, or better yet, a totally percutaneous intravenous version introduced transeptally into the left atrium. The instrument can

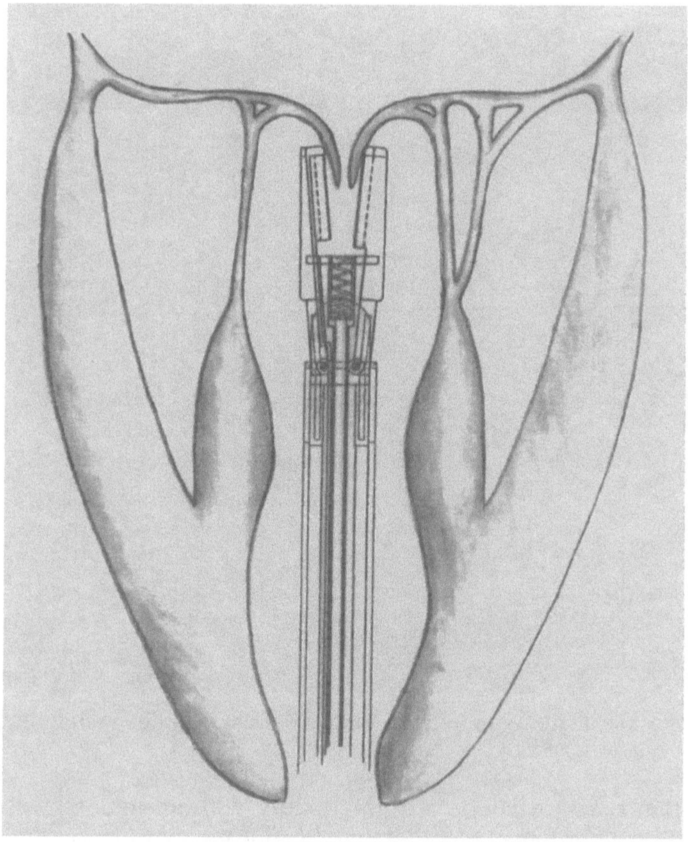

Fig. 6. Grasper—fastener device in place.

then be placed across the plane of the annulus, apposing and immobilizing the leaflets temporarily while the staple, screw, or suture is applied. Alfieri et al. recently reported experience with a similar device that is introduced through the left atrial appendage and uses suction to immobilize the leaflets while a central suture is applied. An integrated knot pusher and cutter is subsequently used to secure the stitch. This technique was reportedly successful in eight beating-heart sheep models, and the authors postulate that it may be applicable to the treatment of ischemic regurgitation in conjunction with revascularization procedures or mitral regurgitation in the setting of heart failure.

Although the bow-tie repair may be beneficial in ischemic mitral regurgitation, we doubt that it will be effective in cases of regurgitation secondary to annular dilatation, where the effective area of coaptation is severely reduced. This cohort of patients requires an annular reduction procedure in order to restore the normal mitral leaflet area-to-mitral valve orifice ratio of 2.5:1 *(21)*. Recently, Timek and colleagues *(22)* determined that certain echocardiographic predictors help in assigning patients who will benefit from annular reduction procedures. Measurements in the four-chamber view relating to the coaptation distance from the annular plane may separate those patients better suited for repair vs replacement. Specifically, a distance less than 4–5 mm may indicate pure annular dilation with little chordal apparatus abnormalities that may be efficiently corrected by ring annuloplasty. Bolling and colleagues have treated functional mitral regur-

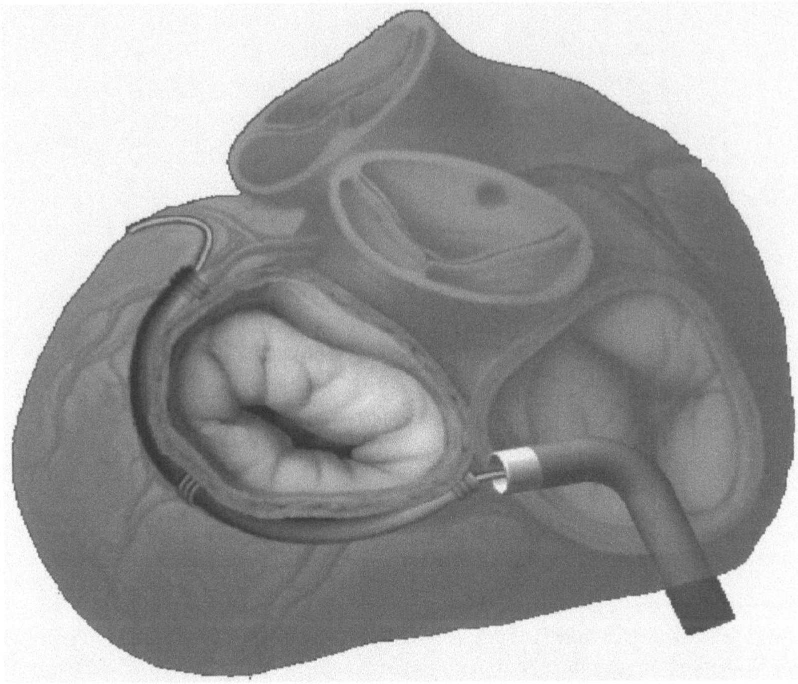

Fig. 7. Coronary sinus anatomy in relation to mitral valve annulus with tightening rod *in situ*.

gitation in patients with dilated cardiomyopathy with an undersized, complete, rigid annuloplasty ring. They have observed that, in addition to unloading the ventricle, there is "acute" remodeling of the base of the heart, with restoration of the ellipsoid shape of the left ventricular cavity *(21)*. Alternate strategies to reduce annular dimensions in cardiomyopathic patients have been proposed by Buchanan and co-workers, who hypothesized that an external banding procedure could reduce mitral regurgitation. They showed that by positioning a tightening external circumferential band, annular morphology could be changed and regurgitation improved in a mongrel dog model.

In the mid- to late 1990s others began to use routine cannulation and navigation of the coronary venous system for *in situ* bypass and drug delivery, which raised the possibility of intervening on certain adjacent structures such as the pericardium and mitral valve. The coronary venous anatomy approaches most regions of the myocardium without significant valvular obstruction or presence of atherosclerotic disease. Although these venous conduits can be variable in their exact location and drainage pattern, the coronary sinus, as it courses the AV grove to the great cardiac vein, is fairly predictable. In this location, it circumnavigates a large portion of the outside of the mitral valve annulus (**Fig. 7**). Using this conduit for the placement of a device, either percutaneously or surgically, may provide a way to grip the annulus of the mitral valve and change its geometry. Such a change could, in theory, help reduce mitral regurgitation in certain pathological conditions. In congestive cardiomyopathy, the anterior, lateral, and posterior segments of the annulus are at risk for dilatation. A mechanical rod that can be placed into the coronary sinus extending to the great cardiac vein could be adjusted and "crimped" from the vein, to tighten these three segments of the annulus. A percutaneous tightening rod has been prototyped and delivered percutaneously through the internal jugular vein.

It has been placed into the coronary sinus and advanced into the great cardiac vein, near the transition of the anterior interventricular vein but not extending into the interventricular groove (**Fig. 7**). The transition to the great cardiac vein can, in some instances, run close to (and often cross over) the circumflex artery. This region needs to be avoided in order not to transmit compression onto adjacent arterial structures. Navigation and placement of such a device can be guided fluoroscopically with the use of routine cath lab equipment. It is important to use transcutaneous echocardiography to characterize and assess mechanical manipulation of the annulus—specifically, understanding the impact on leaflet coaptation and reduction of mitral regurgitation as the device is tightened. If this device favorably affects the anatomy and regurgitant volume, then disconnection can be accomplished and the partial annuloplasty ring left in place permanently. Based on chronic evaluation of many animal studies, there is no need for anticoagulation, as endothelium completely covers the device at 30 d. Additionally, no erosion or migration of the device has been observed long term. Initial human feasibility studies are presently underway to determine if certain patient subsets plagued with large amounts of mitral regurgitation as part of their congestive heart failure constellation can be improved either permanently or as a bridge to definitive surgical correction.

FUTURE TRENDS

Although these techniques may represent the future of mitral valve repair, use of either one alone is unlikely to yield results comparable to conventional methods such as "the French correction." We postulate that at this stage in the development of this technology, the best way to address valvular as well as subvalvular dysfunction, is by using *both* techniques in combination. This could be done with an intravenous device placed in the right atrium for insertion of the transcoronary sinus apparatus, which could then be inserted transeptally across the mitral to apply an edge-to-edge suture.

REFERENCES

1. Reyes VP, Raju BS, Wynne J, et al. Percutaneous balloon valvuloplasty compared with open surgical commissurotomy for mitral stenosis. N Engl J Med 1994;331:961–967.
2. Carabello BA, Crawford FA. Therapy for mitral stenosis comes full circle. N Engl J Med 1994;331:1014–1015.
3. David TE, Armstrong S, Sun Z. Left ventricular function after mitral valve surgery. J Heart Valve Dis 1995;4(suppl 2):S175–S180.
4. Carpentier A. Cardiac valve surgery—the "French correction." J Thorac Cardiovasc Surg 1983;86:323–337.
5. Yun KL, Miller DC. Mitral valve repair versus replacement. Cardiol Clin 1991;9:315–327.
6. Gillinov AM, Cosgrove DM, Lytle BW, et al. Reoperation for failure of mitral valve repair. J Thorac Cardiovasc Surg 1997;113:467–475.
7. Gillinov AM, Cosgrove DM, Blackstone EH, et al. Durability of mitral valve repair for degenerative disease. J Thorac Cardiovasc Surg 1998;116:734–743.
8. Enriquez-Sarano M, Tajik AJ, Schaff HV, Orszulak TA, Bailey KR, Frye RL. Echocardiographic prediction of survival after surgical correction of organic mitral regurgitation. Circulation 1994;90:830–837.
9. Zile MR, Gaasch WH, Carroll JD, Levine HJ. Chronic mitral regurgitation: predictive value of preoperative echocardiographic indexes of left ventricular function and wall stress. J Am Coll Cardiol 1984;3:235–242.
10. Wisenbaugh T, Skudicky D, Sareli P. Prediction of outcome after valve replacement for rheumatic mitral regurgitation in the era of chordal preservation. Circulation 1994;89:191–197.
11. Crawford MH, Souchek J, Oprian CA, et al. Determinants of survival and left ventricular performance after mitral valve replacement: Department of Veterans Affairs Cooperative Study on Valvular Heart Disease. Circulation 1990;81:1173–1181.

12. Hochreiter C, Niles N, Devereux RB, Kligfield P, Borer JS. Mitral regurgitation: relationship of noninvasive descriptors of right and left ventricular performance to clinical and hemodynamic findings and to prognosis in medically and surgically treated patients. Circulation 1986;73:900–912.
13. Ross J.The timing of surgery for severe mitral regurgitation. N Engl J Med 1996;335:1456–1458.
14. Felger JE, Chitwood RW, Nifong W, Holbert D. Evolution of mitral valve surgery: toward a totally endoscopic approach. Ann Thorac Surg 2001;72:1203–1209.
15. Maisano F, Torraca L, Oppizzi M, et al. The edge-to-edge technique: a simplified method to correct mitral insufficiency. Eur J Cardiothorac Surg 1998;13:240–246.
16. Alfieri O, Maisano F, De Bonis M, et al. The double-orifice technique in mitral valve repair: a simple solution for complex problems. J Thorac Cardiovasc Surg 2001;122:674–681.
17. Umaña JP, Salehizadeh B, DeRose JJ, et al. "Bow-tie" mitral valve repair: an adjuvant technique for ischemic mitral regurgitation. Ann Thorac Surg 1998;66:1640–1646.
18. Umaña JP, DeRose JJ, Choudhri A, et al. "Bow-tie" mitral valve repair successfully addresses subvalvular dysfunction in ischemic mitral regurgitation. Surg Forum 1997;48:279–280.
19. Llaneras MR, Nance ML, Streicher JT, et al. Large animal model of ischemic mitral regurgitation. Ann Thorac Surg 1994;57:432–439.
20. Morales DLS, Madigan JD, Coudhri AF, et al. Development of an off bypass mitral valve repair. Heart Surg Forum 1999;2:115–120.
21. Bolling SF, Smolens IA, Pagani FD. Surgical alternatives for heart failure. J Heart Lung Transplant 2001;20:729–733.
22. Timek TA, Dagum P, Lai DT, et al. Pathogenesis of mitral regurgitation in tachycardia-induced cardiomyopathy. Circulation 2001;104(suppl I):I-47–I-53.

28 Alternative Anastomotic Techniques

David A. D'Alessandro, MD
and Mehmet C. Oz, MD

Contents

Introduction
Mechanical Anastomotic Systems
Vascular Connectors
Symmetry ™ Bypass System
Automatic Anastomotic Device
One Shot System
Heartflo™
GraftConnector
Ventrica
Vasconnect
Anastomotic Adhesives
BioGlue
Laser Welding
Robotic Surgery
Conclusion
References

INTRODUCTION

Technical advances in percutaneous techniques for coronary artery disease have lessened the need for surgical revascularization. Although the superior patency rates achieved by surgical approaches are widely recognized, the morbidity associated with surgery limits the overall outcome. For this reason, surgeons have continued to refine techniques to minimize morbidity. Examples include the development of minimally invasive direct coronary artery bypass (MIDCAB), off-pump coronary artery bypass (OPCAB), and, most recently, robotics. This evolution in cardiac therapies represents the focus of this book.

From: *Contemporary Cardiology: Minimally Invasive Cardiac Surgery, Second Edition*
Edited by: D. J. Goldstein and M. C. Oz © Humana Press Inc., Totowa, NJ

Current methods of surgical graft anastomoses necessitate time-consuming hand-sewn techniques and generous exposure. Many investigators believe that the future of coronary bypass surgery will involve increased use of robotics and minimalist approaches. Various alternative means to traditional suturing have been proposed and tested to achieve patent, hemostatic anastomoses. These include use of lasers, glues, clips, and mechanical devices. These strategies have been used by themselves or in combination to improve or advance the art and technique of coronary revascularization surgery and are the focus of this chapter.

The technologies described herein may provide the following potential benefits:

1. They may reduce operative time and time spent on cardiopulmonary bypass (CPB).
2. They may improve the quality of coronary anastomoses while limiting intersurgeon disparity.
3. They may reduce the need for aortic manipulations.
4. They may minimize needed operative exposure.
5. They may create superior vascular connections translating into improved long-term outcomes.

In order to achieve these goals and to become commercially successful, these technologies must meet all the following requirements:

1. They must demonstrate reproducible results regardless of both surgeon and patient variability.
2. They must demonstrate long-term patency results equivalent or superior to those of suture techniques.
3. They must create hemostatic anastomoses.
4. They must not add exorbitant cost.

The remainder of this chapter will describe the evolution of the various anastomotic strategies and the more prominent emerging commercial systems. One should evaluate each technology based on its theoretic ability to achieve the above-stated benefits while meeting these requirements.

MECHANICAL ANASTOMOTIC SYSTEMS

The surgical stapler is perhaps the most widely used tool for mechanical anastomoses. All staplers have the same principal design. A pusher system advances a U-shaped wire through two or more objects to be joined and into an anvil that bends the wire in some fashion to secure them. Over 200 years ago, the French literature reported the use of a stapler for large-vessel repair *(1)*. While staples became commonplace in other industries, they did not gain surgical notoriety until much later.

Humer Hültl, a Hungarian surgeon, pioneered surgical stapling, introducing a gastrointestinal stapler that he used in a series of gastrectomies in 1906 *(2)*. Von Brücke later introduced a device that placed individual staples in 1935 *(3)*. Another Hungarian group was among the first to develop a vascular anastomotic stapler, as presented by Bikfalvi and Dubecz in 1953 *(4)*. Intended for larger (6–8-mm) vessels, this device joined everted vessels using U-shaped silver clasps. While this represented a technical milestone, it was not immediately applicable to small vessel anastomoses.

About this time, a Russian group of engineers and surgeons was refining a similar but more sophisticated device. Established in 1952, the Soviet Scientific Research Institute for Experimental Surgical Apparatus and Instruments brought together multiple disci-

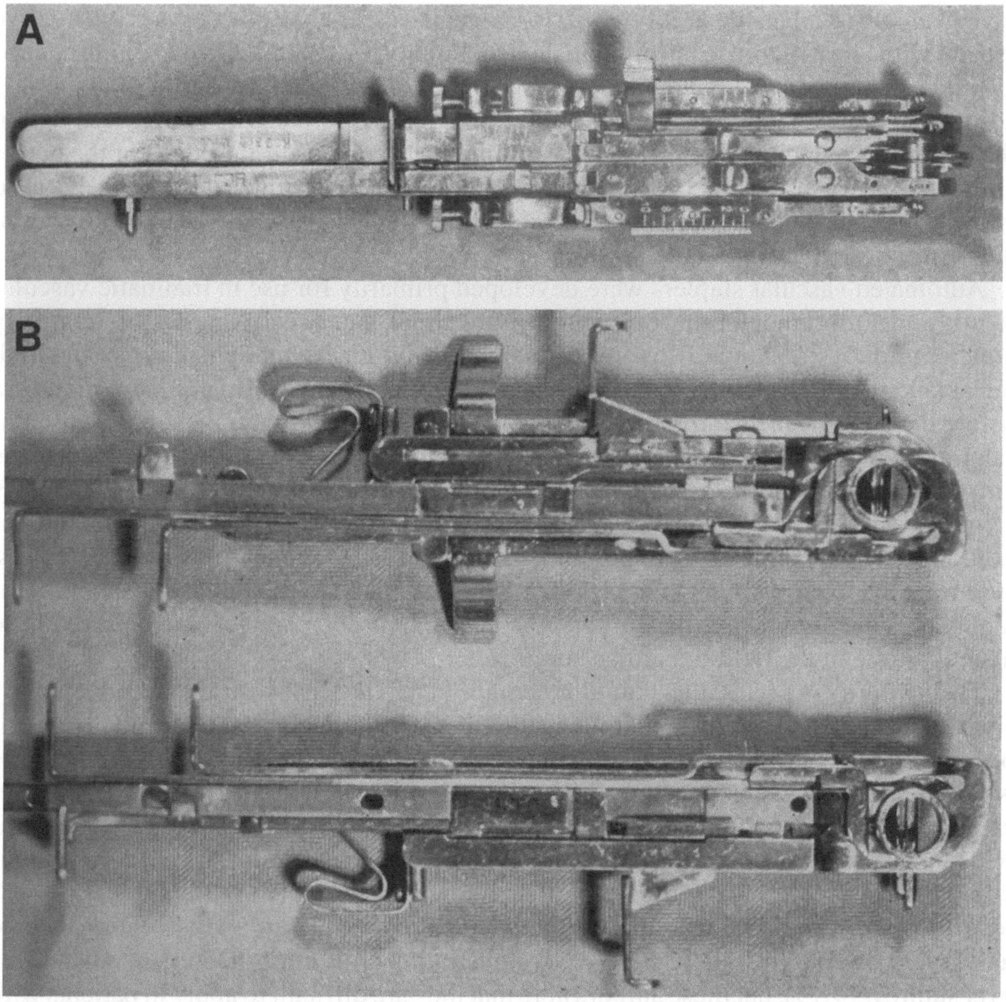

Fig. 1. Androsov stapling device pictured assembled and in component halves (Reprinted with permission from *Surgery*.)

plines to develop a vascular stapler based on the work done by Gudov beginning in 1941 *(5)*. Resulting from this collaboration, in 1956, Androsov described the use of an automated, circular stapling device for joining damaged blood vessels in an end-to-end fashion *(6)*. In contrast to previous designs, this device joined vessels from 1.3 to 15 mm in diameter using U-shaped clips constructed of tantalum wire (**Fig. 1**). These early investigators appreciated the importance of intimal apposition and the advantage of avoiding an intimal foreign body. Nevertheless, their device, although elaborate, was cumbersome and costly *(7)*, and it never achieved commercial success.

In 1958, Inokuchi, a Japanese surgeon, described a simplified apparatus employing the same principles *(8)*. He further compared the stapled anastomosis with current suture technique, demonstrating reduced early thrombogenicity and improved late histological characteristics of the automated anastomoses. Also in 1958, Vogelfanger and Beattie reported a similarly simplified Canadian stapler *(9)*. A U.S. version was later developed with disposable staple inserts to simplify operative use *(10)*. This device was intended to give general surgeons the ability to perform small-vessel anastomoses and even nerve repairs with an easy-to-use, affordable device. Finally, in 1960, Takaro *(11)* introduced a simple stapling device that he used to anastomose Dacron interposition grafts to dog aortas. This anastomotic system was unique in that the Dacron graft was stapled within the lumen of the recipient vessel, thus avoiding the need to evert the edges of the native artery. While Takaro's device showed foresight into the difficulty of everting diseased vessels, his experimental work demonstrated these stapled anastomoses to be inferior in quality to those that were hand-sewn.

Automated vascular staplers were developed primarily for use in traumatic vascular injury and limb amputation, offering a more rapid and precise repair of relatively nondiseased vessels. Some also foresaw their use in the emerging field of organ and limb transplantation, in which rapid reestablishment of blood flow was paramount in the era before the establishment of preservation techniques. Enthusiasm for these early vascular stapling devices was in part fueled by the results achieved with hand-sewn methods in the era of catgut- or braided silk-sutured anastomoses and prior to the widespread availability of magnification. Subsequent advances in microvascular technique, loupe magnification, and suture materials such as polypropylene lessened the benefit of vascular staplers. Additionally, hand-sewn techniques were more adaptable to the diseased vessels commonly encountered in vascular surgery. As a result, vascular staplers have played little historical role in the field of cardiac surgery.

The modern era of vascular stapling perhaps began in 1992 with the introduction by Kirsch and colleagues of an arcuate-legged clip *(12)*. These clips were originally developed for use in neurosurgical vascular anastomoses, but the benefits of this technology, which created vascular connections with minimal endothelial injury, were widely recognized. The VCS Auto Suture device (US Surgical Corp., Norwalk, CT) is a later-generation clip dispenser. This device places titanium arcuate-legged clips, which come in four different sizes and can dispense 25 clips in quick succession (**Fig. 2**). Nataf et al. *(13)* reported their experience with these clips in 10 patients undergoing conventional coronary artery bypass grafting (CABG). Nonpenetrating clips have theoretical advantages over sutures *(14,15)*, but these authors note that they are difficult to apply in patients with calcified coronaries. Calcifications complicate vessel edge eversion, thus compromising anastomotic integrity. Despite the availability of this device, few surgeons have adopted these stapling techniques, and the current role of this technology in cardiac surgery is limited.

VASCULAR CONNECTORS

Concurrent with the development of stapling devices, intra- and extraluminal coupling and stent devices were also under development. In 1900, Payr reported the use of an intraluminal, absorbable magnesium ring for vascular end-to-end coupling *(16)*. A decade later, Lespinasse and colleagues *(17)* published their development of a magnesium ring anastomosis that provided vascular coupling without the presence of an endothelial foreign body. Nakayama et al. *(18)* later described the clinical use of a tantalum ring anastomotic system for coupling small (1.5–4-mm) arteries in either end-to-end or end-to-side fashion.

Blakemore and Lord *(19)* introduced a Vitallium-alloy cannulae system for performing vein interposition arterial anastomoses. These authors targeted their system for the repair of wartime extremity injuries, where rapid restoration of blood flow is vital for limb salvage. They reported a 90% patency rate when bridging femoral artery defects in dogs.

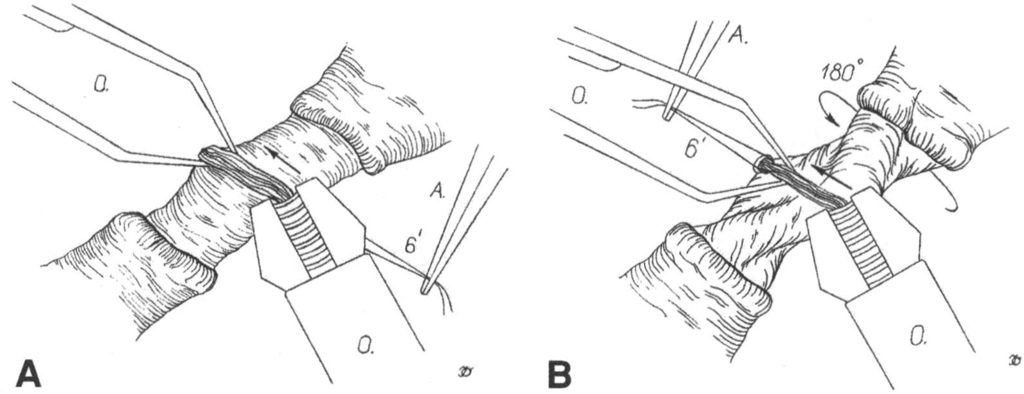

Fig. 2. Technique for performing a stapled microvascular anastomosis is illustrated. **(A)** Everting forceps are used to stabilize the vessels while clips are applied form right to left. **(B)** The vessels are rotated 180 degrees and the posterior walls are similarly joined. (Reprinted with permission from the *Annals of Thoracic Surgery*.)

Inspired by this work and others, Carter and Roth *(20)* later reported their experience with polyethylene rings for use in nonsutured anastomoses of the left internal mammary artery to the circumflex coronary artery in dogs. These authors achieved an 83%, 2-mo patency rate. The main advantage of their technique was speed, as they could perform these anastomoses in less than 3 min, a marked improvement over standard suture technique.

In 1960, Rohman and others *(21)* described the use of a tantalum ring for internal mammary-to-coronary anastomoses in dogs, achieving 18-mo graft patency in some animals. Several others demonstrated experimental success with ringed or ring-pin systems *(22–24)*. Lemole *(25)* recently described a collar-and-punch method designed to facilitate end-to-side or side-to-side anastomoses. This system allows the creation of an anastomosis without the need to occlude blood flow in the native vessel. A sleeve-and-collar combination attached to the graft vessel is sutured to the target vessel prior to making an arteriotomy. Once secured, a punch system is employed to create the arteriotomy and thus complete the anastomosis. This system seems particularly suited for off-pump coronary artery bypass (OPCAB) procedures, in which temporary occlusion of coronary flow may be detrimental. It awaits commercial development.

As with vascular staplers, historical interest in these and other anastomotic systems waned concurrent with improvements in hand-sewn techniques. Early devices were often cumbersome and hampered by intolerable thrombosis rates, despite sometimes achieving long-term successes. More recent adaptations have had difficulty gaining acceptance and commercial success in an arena dominated by standardized suture techniques with proven efficacy and durability. Current anastomotic devices combine stapling and intraluminal stent technology to perform assisted or total automated anastomoses. The leading designs in or approaching the marketplace will be described subsequently. The present impetus driving these automated anastomotic systems is the need to perform vascular connections using minimal exposure, with a thrust toward total endoscopic approaches. While perhaps none of these devices has achieved this goal, as a group they represent a necessary step in the evolution of minimal-access surgery. Clinical experience with these and future designs will lead to technological refinements necessary for a total endoscopic anastomotic tool.

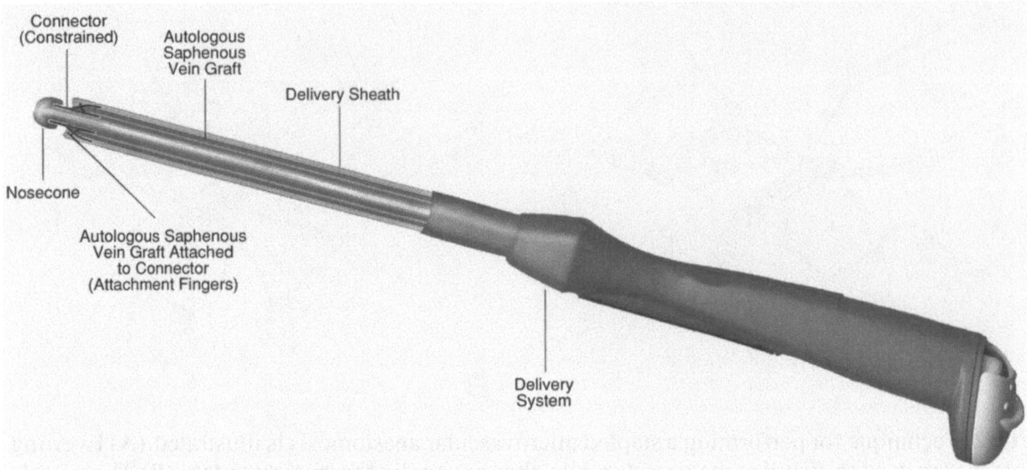

Fig. 3. Schematic of the Symmetry™ Bypass System deliver system with a loaded vein graft. (Printed with permission from St. Jude Medical, Inc.)

SYMMETRY™ BYPASS SYSTEM

The St. Jude Medical Anastomotic Technology Group (Minneapolis, MN) has invested considerably in systems designed for creating both proximal aortosaphenous and distal coronary anastomoses. Among these, the Symmetry™ Bypass System, Aortic Connector, is currently the only U.S. Food and Drug Administration (FDA)-approved and commercially available automated device for proximal anastomoses. This device facilitates the creation of a sutureless anastomosis via a Nitinol, self-expanding connector. When using this system, the operator places the harvested saphenous vein conduit in the delivery system (**Fig. 3**). One of four stent sizes is selected. The vein is guided into the delivery system and the ends everted over the connector hooks. An aortic cutter is next used to make a clean, circular aortotomy, essential for proper stent deployment and hemostasis. Finally, the graft is delivered and a 90° stented anastomosis is performed in seconds, completing the process (**Fig. 4**). The obvious advantage of this and other similar devices is their ability to perform aortic anastomosis without the need for clamping, a maneuver that has been associated with atheroemboli and stroke *(26)*. Eckstein et al. *(27)* reported the first clinical series using this device in 20 consecutive patients undergoing OPCAB. This device is currently gaining popularity among surgeons in the United States, but its efficacy and effects on postoperative neurological morbidity remain to be established. In the current era of cost containment, the cost of this device may prove too high for many clinicians.

Currently, St. Jude is developing a stented system for sutureless side-to-side coronary anastomoses designed for use with saphenous vein conduits. This delivery system employs a balloon expandable intraluminal stainless steel stent that facilitates a hemostatic anastomosis in less than 3 min. Eckstein et al. *(28)* recently reported the first clinical use of this anastomotic device. This system awaits FDA approval.

Fig. 4. (*Right*) Cartoon depicting the Symmetry™ Bypass System's cut then connect sequence to a complete anastomosis. (Printed with permission from St. Jude Medical, Inc.).

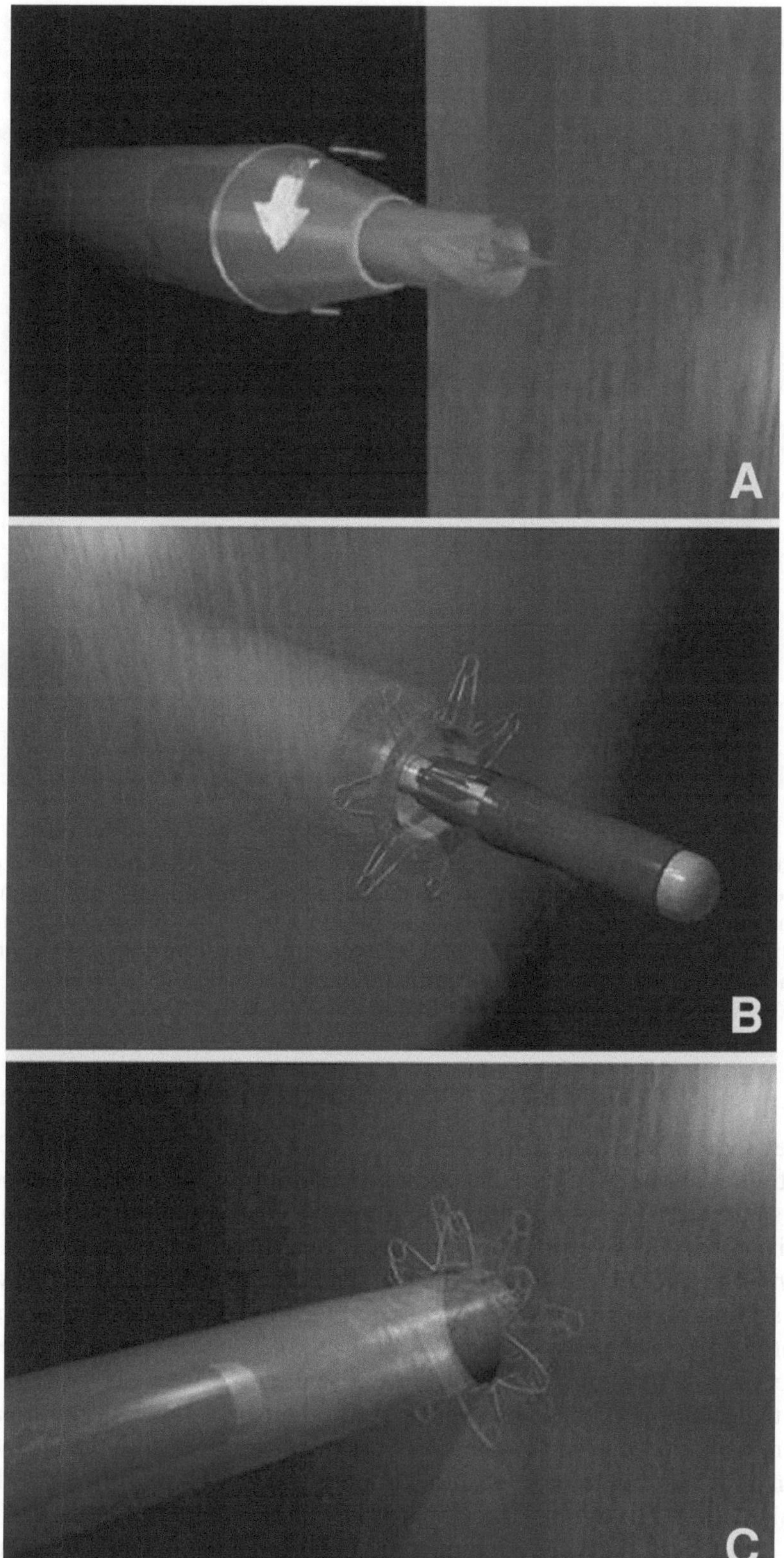
A
B
C

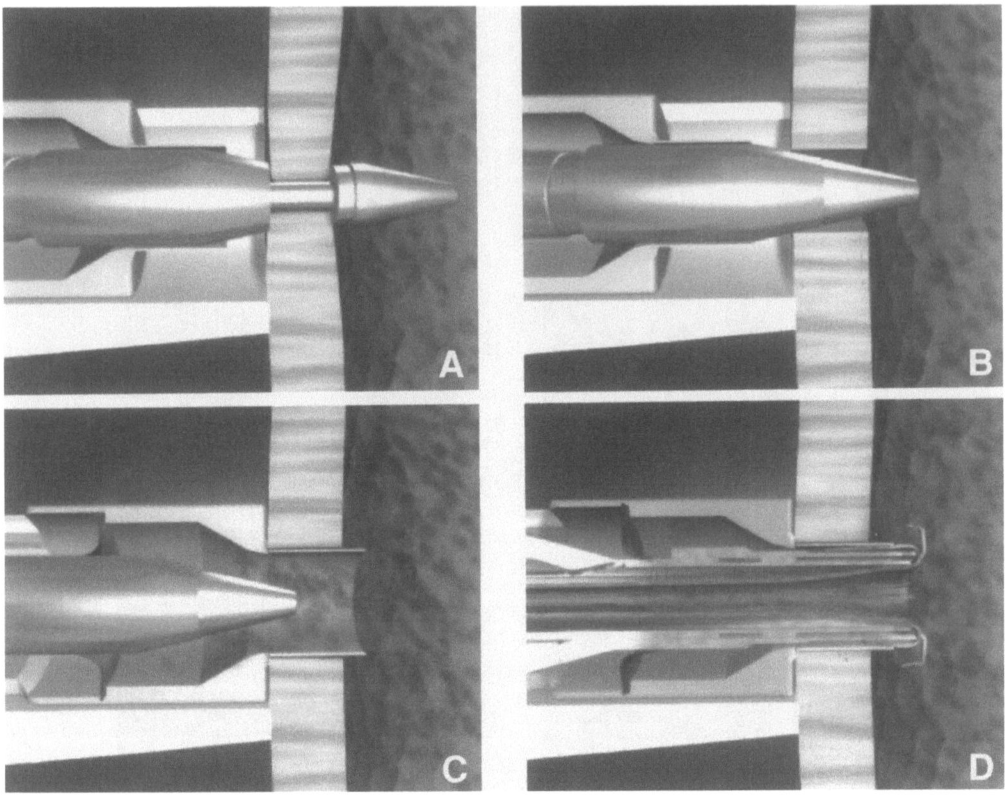

Fig. 5. Cartoon depicting Ethicon's Automatic Anastomotic Device deployment sequence. **(A)** Punching device creates a 3.2 mm hole in the unclamped aortic wall. **(B)** Aortic punch is withdrawn and an internal sealing ring prevents aortic backflow. **(C)** The delivery system is advanced into the aortic lumen. **(D)** Mounted vein graft is delivered into the aortic lumen. Once in place (not shown), inner pins partially penetrate the aortic intima while outer pins stabilize the graft to the adventitia. (Printed with permission from Ethicon, Inc.)

AUTOMATIC ANASTOMOTIC DEVICE

Marketed by Ethicon, Inc. (Summerset, NJ), the Automtic Anastomotic Device is a Nitinol extraluminal stent system that combines aortotomy and aortosaphenous anastomosis in a single step. Use of this device requires previous mounting of the conduit vein on the delivery system, everting the vein edges over the distal pins. Next, a punching device is inserted through the delivery handle, creating an aortotomy, and is withdrawn through a sealing ring that prevents excessive bleeding. The loaded vein graft is then inserted through the aortotomy and deployed (**Fig. 5**). The self-expanding Nitinol stent system creates a hemostatic, intima-to-intima seal. Once the vein graft is loaded, a maneuver that can be performed by support staff on the back table, the entire aortotomy and delivery maneuver can be completed in less than 2 min. As with the St. Jude device, this system does not require aortic side clamping and can be performed with minimal aortic manipulation. The unique aspect of this device is a delivery system that creates an aortotomy and places the vein conduit in a single maneuver. Once the aortotomy is created, the applicator is never removed from the aorta. This will facilitate placement of

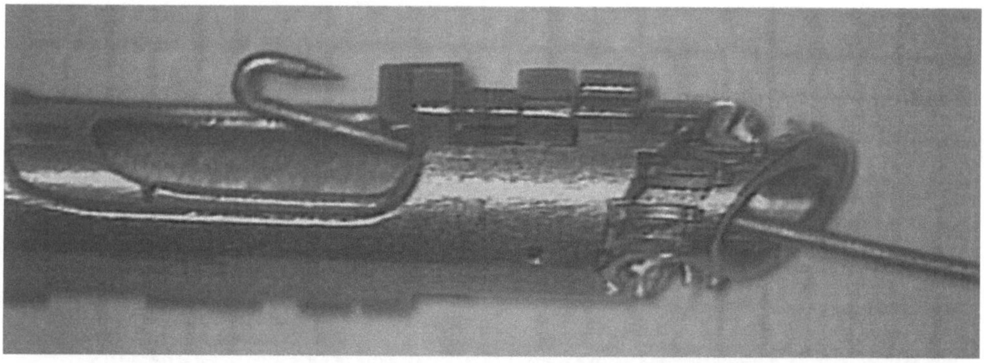

Fig. 6. Close-up of the one-shot anastomotic stapler. The graft vessel is hooked and pulled through the clip housing. The vessel end is then everted across the anvil and secured over the ends of the clips. The loaded cartridge is next placed in the firing handle and deployed. (Reprinted with permission from the *Journal of Thoracic and Cardiovascular Surgery.*)

veins from a distance. Calafiore et al. *(29)* reported limited clinical experience with the first generation of this device, with promising results. They noted several limitations that will be addressed in later versions.

ONE SHOT SYSTEM

Developed by United States Surgical Corporation (Norwalk, CT), the One Shot System places 10 or 12 evenly spaced titanium clips to everted and approximated endothelium. The system utilizes arcuate-legged titanium clips which are nonpenetrating and which autoregulate closing pressure depending on the thickness of interposed tissue. The application device instantaneously applies a ring of clips that are both hemostatic and equivalent to conventional sutures with respect to tensile and burst strengths. The system can be used to create both proximal and distal anastomoses in either an end-to-side or end-to-end fashion. The donor graft is positioned through a disposable cartridge housing and the edges are everted over the distal clips (**Fig. 6**). The donor graft is then positioned on the target site at a 45° angle and the clips are fired simultaneously, creating an anastomosis with direct intimal apposition and an uninterrupted endothelium. Disposable cartridges are equipped with variable clip sizes ranging from 10 to 12 in number and can be used on target vessels less than 2 mm in diameter.

This device has been tested extensively in animal models and in cadaveric studies and more recently in a clinical trial creating arteriovenous access fistulas *(30)*. Heijmen et al. *(31)* reported their experience with a device prototype creating distal anastomoses in a porcine OPCAB model, noting several shortcomings. While the One Shot device received FDA marketing approval in 1997, technical difficulties have prevented its commercial use in cardiac surgery. US Surgical recently suspended research and development of the One Shot System due to ongoing design concerns.

HEARTFLO™

Developed by Perclose/ Abbott Labs (Redwood, CA), the Heartflo™ device simultaneously deploys 10 interrupted 7-0 polypropylene sutures (**Figs. 7** and **8**). Once placed, the sutures are then hand-tied in the conventional fashion. This device can facilitate both

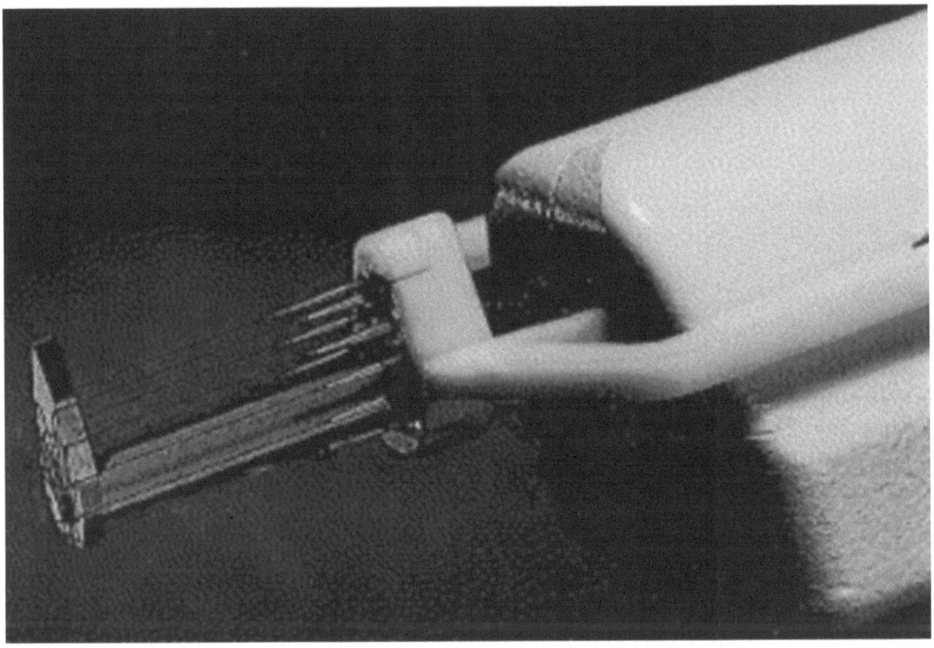

Fig. 7. The Heartflo automated anastomotic device. (Reprinted with permission from the *Annals of Thoracic Surgery*.)

side-to-side and end-to-side anastomoses. Tozzi and co-workers *(32)* demonstrated superior anastomotic properties using the Heartflo system compared to running sutured anastomoses. Shennib et al. *(33)* described their initial experience with this device in a porcine model, performing IMA-to-LAD anastomoses in a side-to-side fashion. While the authors found this prototype design cumbersome and time-consuming to operate, they noted that the next-generation Heartflo addresses these limitations and is modified for use in the total endoscopic setting.

GRAFTCONNECTOR

Developed by Jomed International AB (Helsinborg, Sweden), the GraftConnector™ is a Nitinol-stented anastomosis system that combines polytetrafluorethylene (PTFE) and vascular conduits, and facilitates a sutureless anastomosis. This system, designed for target site, end-to-side anastomoses, requires a four-step delivery sequence (**Fig. 9**). Solem et al. *(34)* evaluated this device in an animal OPCAB model and showed similar patency rates and shorter anastomotic times when compared to standard surgical technique. More recently, Tozzi and colleagues *(35)* presented 6-mo animal data that documented increased anastomotic diameters and conduit blood flow when using this device, compared to running suture technique. Furthermore, these authors demonstrated this device's ease of use, requiring less manual dexterity than hand-sewing methods, an important requirement of any system with applicability in minimally invasive cardiac surgery. These studies, however, compare GraftConnector anastomoses with hand-sewn anastomoses in an OPCAB animal model without the use of a cardiac stabilizer. Although this experimental design highlights the ease of use of this system, one may question the precision of hand sewing in such a scenario and therefore its clinical relevance. While this

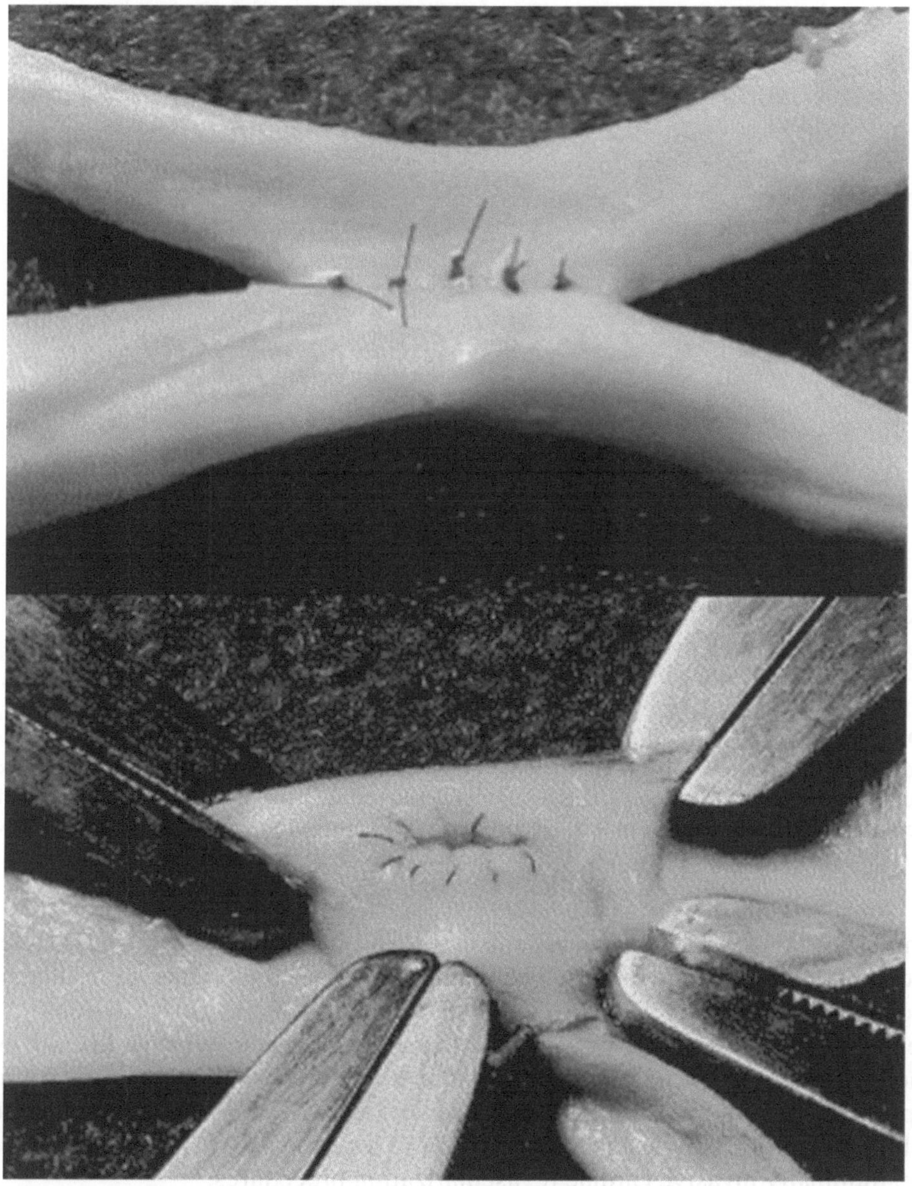

Fig. 8. External and internal views of the automated anastomosis. (Reprinted with permission from the *Annals of Thoracic Surgery*.)

system is intriguing and deserving of further study, it has not been evaluated in the clinical arena and remains in the development phase.

VENTRICA

The Magnetic Vascular Positioner (MVP™), developed by Ventrica®, Inc. (Freemont, CA), represents one of the more novel approaches to alternative anastomoses. Introduced in 2001 *(36)*, this system utilizes the self-aligning and self-sealing characteristics of magnetic attraction to achieve rapid, hemostatic vascular connections. The MVP system

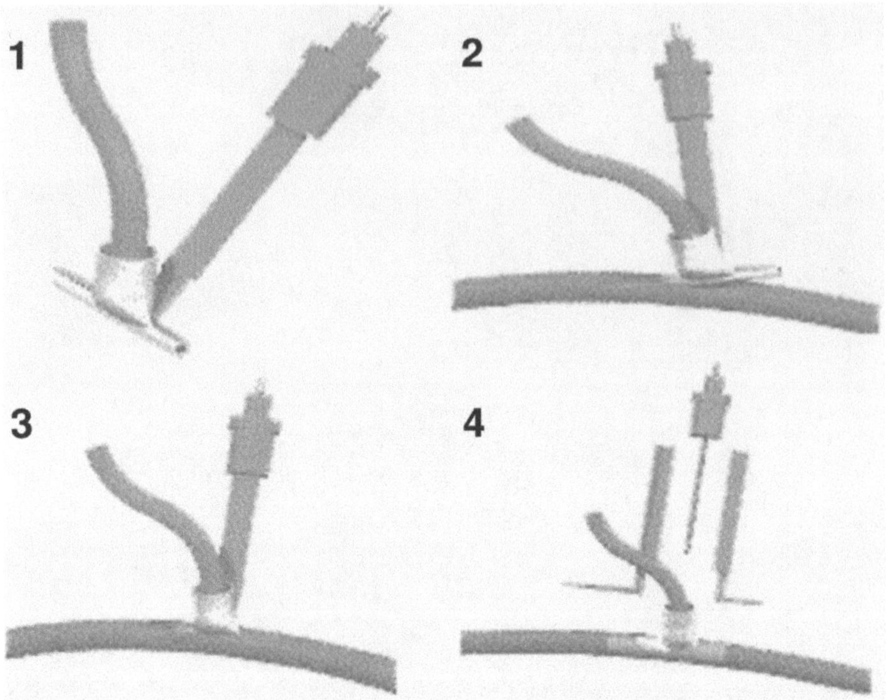

Fig. 9. Schematic of the GraftConnector (GC) anastomotic sequence. (1) The graft vessel is positioned in the sidearm of the GC. (2–3) An arteriotomy is created and the stent-system is inserted into the target artery. (4) The device is deployed and the stented graft self-expands to secure and complete the anastomosis. (Reprinted with permission from the *Annals of Thoracic Surgery*.)

accomplishes this by a delivery mechanism that inserts elliptical magnetic couplers in both conduit and recipient vessels. The magnets are joined to create an instantaneous anastomosis (**Figs. 10** and **11**).

Ventrica is concurrently developing the MagnePort™ system, which utilizes the same technology to provide proximal aortic vascular connections without the need for aortic clamping. These systems await FDA approval and are currently undergoing preclinical and clinical testing. Their design simplicity, however, seems particularly well suited for future, minimally invasive cardiac revascularization procedures.

VASCONNECT

Coalescent Surgical, Inc. (Sunnyvale, CA), has developed another unique and innovative concept for vascular anastomoses. Their nitinol U-Clip Device combines the speed and versatility of Nitinol with the flexibility of hand-sewing technique. This system consists of a self-closing Nitinol wire attached to a needle delivery member (**Fig. 12**). Once detached, the Nitinol clip assumes its preformed shape, approximating tissue similar to suture but obviating knot tying. The U-Clip device was evaluated in a bovine model by Hill et al. *(37)* and proved effective for use in an OPCAB model. These authors point out that such a device, which allows rapid deployment of interrupted clips using conventional sewing technique, may prove superior to continuous suture technique, as it allows anastomotic expansion. The simplified anastomotic technique that this system provides also seems well suited for minimally invasive and robotic-assisted approaches.

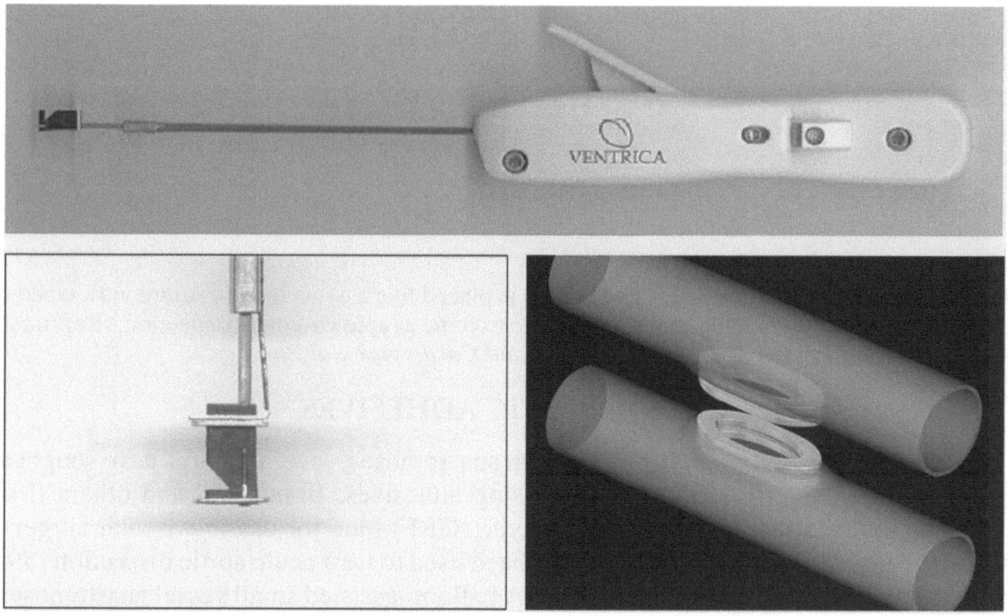

Fig. 10. Delivery system with close up and schematic of the magnetic connection. (Printed with permission form Ventrica, Inc.)

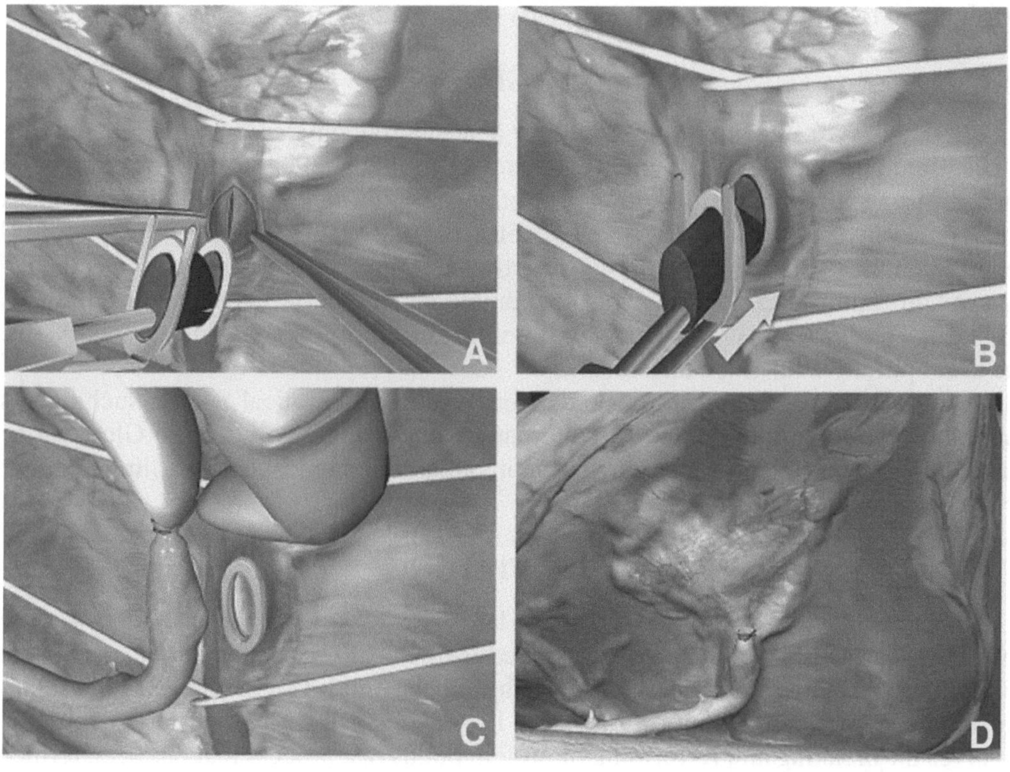

Fig. 11. (**A**) The MVP™ is inserted into standard arteriotomy. (**B**) The MVP™ delivery device is activated to create the anastomotic port. (**C**) The identically prepared graft is approximated to the artery. (**D**) A virtually instantaneous anastomotic connection is created. (Printed with permission form Ventrica, Inc.)

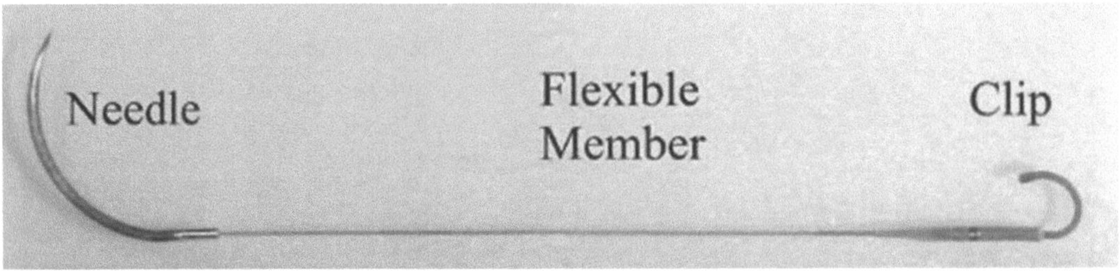

Fig. 12. The Nitinol U-Clip device. The U-Clip is placed like a conventional suture via a tapered needle and utilizes nitinol alloy shape memory to execute a rapid vascular connection. (Reprinted with permission form the *Journal of Thoracic and Cardiovascular Surgery.*)

ANASTOMOTIC ADHESIVES

Recognizing the limitations of hand-sewn anastomoses, several groups have sought a sutureless alternative to joining vessels using adhesives. Braunwald and others first developed the gelatin–resorcin–formaldehyde (GRF) glue for use in vascular surgery *(38)*. Since its development, GRF glue has been used to treat acute aortic dissection *(39)* and more recently has been applied to PTCA balloon-assisted small vessel anastomoses *(40)*. Application of other biological glues such as cyanoacrylates *(41)*, fibrin glues *(42)*, and urethane polymers has been reported with similar results. While a glued anastomosis has theoretic advantages, several limitations have stymied their clinical adoption. These include concerns over tissue toxicity, lack of flexibility, inadequate tensile strength, intraluminal thrombosis, and pseudo-aneurysm formation.

BIOGLUE

BioGlue (CryoLife, Inc., Marietta, GA) is a gluteraldehyde compound containing concentrated bovine serum albumin. Once mixed in the applicator tip, this compound forms a strong adhesive with a setting time of under 2 min. The glue is biologically inert and is under investigation for treatment of aortic dissection. Gundry and colleagues *(43)* reported on the use of this glue for constructing coronary anastomoses with a catheter-assisted procedure (**Fig. 13**). They further demonstrated long-term patency in 2 animals (10 mo and 1 yr) without evidence of intraluminal thrombosis or anastomotic aneurysms, the usual pitfalls with glued anastomoses.

While totally glued anastomoses have yet to become a clinical reality, such agents might become important adjuncts to alternative anastomotic approaches. Glue can be easily applied via catheters and may prove invaluable in hemostasis in a limited endoscopic surgical field.

LASER WELDING

Jain and Gorisch first reported the use of lasers for vascular repair in 1979 *(44)*. The following year, Morris and Carter *(45)* described use of the CO2 laser for microanastomoses. Since that time, a myriad of energy sources have been employed in both vascular repair and in anastomotic construction *(46–48)*. The mechanism by which lasers function involves the breaking and re-forming of protein bonds in a process that has been termed "welding." The theoretical advantages of laser-assisted anastomoses are speed, their ability to grow, the minimal foreign body reaction, and improved long-term patency.

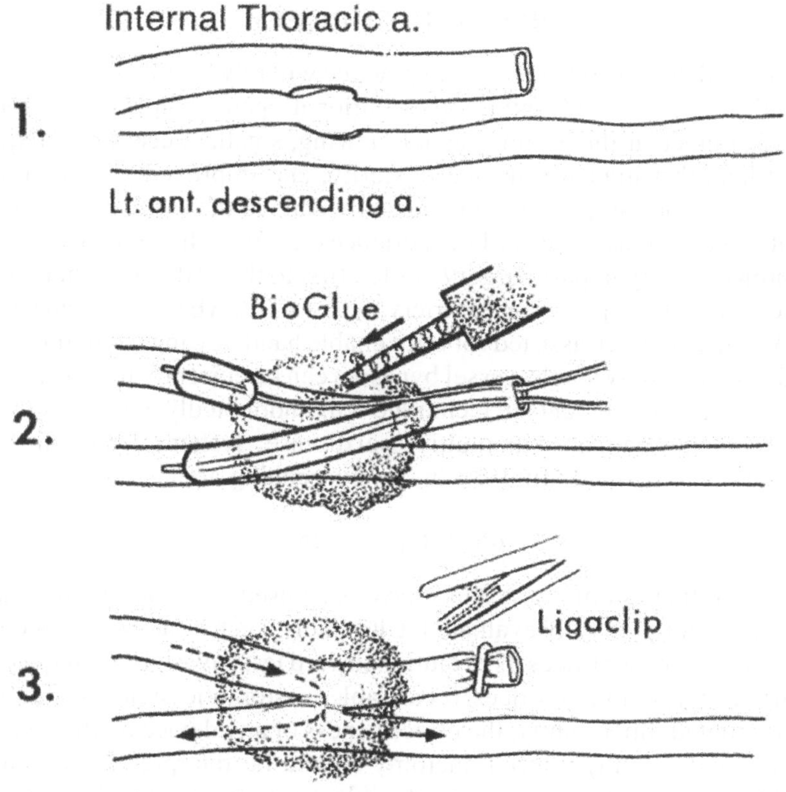

Fig. 13. Schematic of BioGlue anastomosis. (1) Graft and target vessels are approximated and arteriotomies are performed. (2) Balloon catheters are placed as shown and BioGlue is applied and allowed to set for 2 min. (3) Catheters are removed restoring flow and the distal graft vessel is clipped completing the anastomosis. (Reprinted with permission form the *Journal of Thoracic and Cardiovascular Surgery.*)

Critics have raised concern over the long-term potential for anastomotic disruption or aneurysm formation when applying laser techniques to larger vessels *(49)*. Nakata and co-workers *(50)*, however, demonstrated CO_2 laser anastomotic bursting pressures equivalent to that of standard suture anastomoses without propensity for aneurysm formation in rabbit carotid arteries. They further demonstrated reduced long-term intimal hyperplasia, suggesting a role for lasers in coronary bypass surgery.

The efficiency of laser welding has since been improved by the addition of dye solders *(51–53)* to the vessel surface, which increases the absorbance of the laser light and thus increases heat deposition. Utilizing this effect, Maitz and colleagues *(54)* adapted the original Payr technique, substituting a protein tube for the absorbable magnesium ring, and successfully performed sutureless anastomoses.

Although these techniques have been utilized in clinical microvascular surgery applications, they have not gained widespread acceptance in cardiovascular surgery. This is perhaps due to ongoing concern over the short- and long-term durability of these anastomoses in a setting where sudden disruption could be catastrophic. Furthermore, the laser energy sources are cumbersome and necessitate the use of protective eyewear. Lastly, laser-assisted anastomoses are difficult to perform in a limited surgical field.

ROBOTIC SURGERY

Many believe that the future of surgical practice will rely heavily on robotics. Robotic equipment affords several advantages to traditional open or laparoscopic procedures. These include binocular three-dimensional viewing, smaller access port requirements, movement filters that improve manual dexterity, and improved vision from multiple camera angles. Robotic surgery has only recently entered the cardiac surgical arena, but several centers have amassed an early experience *(55–58)*. The trend toward minimally invasive coronary artery bypass surgery has led first to the MIDCAB, then the OPCAB, and now the total endoscopic coronary artery bypass (TECAB), which can be performed off-pump. While computer-assisted robotics enable hand-sewing technique, exposure is limited and generally only single-vessel bypasses can be currently performed. Improved instrumentation and refinements in technique will undoubtedly extend the reach of this technology to include patients with multivessel disease. Systems that facilitate the anastomotic process will certainly find use in this burgeoning arena.

CONCLUSION

Automated graft anastomotic systems have been used successfully, but their overall effectiveness has not been fully evaluated. Ultimately, such systems will become necessary as cardiac surgery continues its evolution toward less invasive techniques. As investigators and industry continue the quest for a usable anastomotic device, several challenges must be surmounted. Importantly, the effectiveness of any device on the research bench or in animals with healthy arterial anatomy should be interpreted with caution. For clinical utility, a device must create reproducible anastomoses in varied target site locations and on diseased, calcified vessels that are characteristic in this patient population. The prevailing anastomotic technology may become as fundamental to coronary surgery as polypropylene has been over the past several decades. This financial incentive will drive these technologies and reshape the field of coronary bypass surgery.

REFERENCES

1. Carrel A. Results of transplantation of blood vessels, organs, and limbs. JAMA 1908;51:1662.
2. Cooper P, Christie SG. Develpoment of the surgical stapler with emphasis on vascular anastomosis. Trans N Y Acad Sci 1963;25:365–377.
3. Von Brücke H, Über ein neuartiges chirurgisches Nähinstrument. Zentralbl Chir 1935;62:1684–1686.
4. Bikfalvi A, Dubecz S. Observations in animal experiments with mechanized vessel suture. J Int Chir 1953;5:481–495.
5. Mallina RF, Miller TR, Cooper P, Christie SG. Surgical stapling. Sci Am 1962;207:48–56.
6. Androsov PI. New method of surgical treatment of blood vessel lesions. AMA Arch Surg 1956;73:902–920.
7. Miller TR, Corso PF, Mallina RF. Preliminary evaluation of the Adrosov stapling device for the circular suture of blood vessels. Surgery 1962;51:216–219.
8. Inokuchi. A new tyope of vessel-suturing apparatus. AMA Arch Surg 1958;77:954–957.
9. Vogelfanger IJ, Beattie WG. A concept of automation in vascular surgery: a preliminary report on a mechanical instrument for arterial anastomosis. Can J Surg 1958;1:262–265.
10. Mallina RF. The technical aspects of the vascular stapler. Trans N Y Acad Sci 1963;253–264.
11. Takaro T. A simple stapling device for the anastomosis of blood vessels. J Thorac Cardiovasc Surg 1960;40:673–684.
12. Kirsch WM, Zhu YH, Hardesty RA, Chapolini R. A new method for microvascular anastomosis. Am Surg 1992;58:722–727.
13. Nataf P, Kirsch W, Hill AC, et al. Nonpenetrating clips for the coronary anastomosis. Ann Thorac Surg 1997;63:S135–S137.

14. Boeckx WD, Darius O, van den hof B, van Holder C. Scanning electron microscope analysis of the stapled microvascular anastomosis in the rabbit. Ann Thorac Surg 1997;63:S128–S134.
15. Zeebregts CJ, van den Dungen JJ, Kalicharan D, Cromheecke M, van der Want J, van Schilfgaarde R. Nonpenetrating vascular clips for small-caliber anastomosis. Microsurgery 2000;20:131–138.
16. Payr E. Beitrage zur Technique der Blutgefass- und Nervennaht nebst Mittheilungen über die Verwendung eines resorbirbaren Metalles in de Chirurgie. Arch Klin Chir 1900;62:67–93.
17. Lespinasse VD, Fisher GC, Eisenstaedt J. A practical mechanical method of end-to-end anastomosis of blood-vessels. JAMA 1910;55:1785–1790.
18. Nakayama K, Tamiya T, Yamamoto K, Akimoto S. A simple new apparatus for small vessel anastomosis (free autograft of the signmoid included). Surgery 1962;52:918–931.
19. Blakemore AH, Lord JW. A nonsuture method of blood vessel anastomosis. JAMA 1945;127:685–691.
20. Carter EL, Roth EJ. Direct nonsuture coronary artery anastomosis in the dog. Ann Surg 1958;148:212–218.
21. Rohman M, Goetz RH, Dee R. Double coronary artery-internal mammary tantalum ring technique. Surg Forum 1960;11:236–237.
22. Carton CA, Kessler LA, Seidenberg B, Hurwitt ES. Experimental studies in the surgery of small blood vessels. Nonsuture anastomosis of arteries and veins using flanged ring prosthesis and plastic adhesive. Surg Forum 1960;11:238–239.
23. Ratan RS, Leon M, Lovette JB, Levowitz BS, Magovern GJ, Kent EM. Modified nonsuture anastomosis of coronary artery and internal mammary artery in dogs. Surg Forum 1960;11:239–241.
24. Holt GP, Lewis FJ. A new technique of end-to-end anastomosis of small arteries. Surg Forum 1960;11:242–243.
25. Lemole GM. Procedure for bypassing an occlusion in a blood vessel. US Patent 5,893,369. 1999 Apr 13.
26. Sylivris S, Levi C, Matalanis G, et al. Pattern and significance of cerebral microemboli during coronary artery bypass grafting. Ann Thorac Surg 1998;66:1674–1678.
27. Eckstein FS, Bonilla LF, Englberger L, et al. Minimizing aortic manipulation during OPCAB using the Symmetry Aortic Connector System for proximal vein graft anastomoses. Ann Thorac Surg 2001;72:S995–S998.
28. Eckstein FS, Bonilla LF, Meyer B, et al. Sutureless mechanical anastomosis of a saphenous vein graft to a coronary artery with a new connector device. Lancet 2001;357:931–932.
29. Calafiore AM, Bar-El Y, Vitolla G, et al. Early clinical experience with a new surtureless anastomotic device for proximal anastomosis of the saphenous vein to the aorta. J Thorac Cardiovasc Surg 2001;121:854–858.
30. Nataf P, Hinchliffe P, Manzo S, et al. Facilitated vascular anastomoses: The one-shot device. Ann Thorac Surg 1998;66:1041–1044.
31. Heijmen RH, Hinchliffe P, Borst C, et al. A novel one-shot anastomotic stapler prototype for the coronary bypass grafting on the beating heart: feasibility on the pig. J Thorac Cardiovasc Surg 1999;117:117–125.
32. Tozzi P, Hayoz D, Ruchat P, et al. Animal model to compare the effects of suture technique on cross-sectional compliance on end-to-side anastomoses. Eur J Cardiothorac Surg 2001;19:477–481.
33. Shennib H, Korkola SJ, Bousette N, Giaid A. An automated interrupted suturing device for coronary artery bypass grafting: automated coronary anastomosis. Ann Thorac Surg 2000;70:1046–1048.
34. Solem JO, Boumzebra D, Al-Buraiki J, Nakeeb S, Rafeh W, Al-Halees Z. Evaluation of a new device for quick sutureless coronary artery anastomosis in surviving sheep. Eur J Cardiothorac Surg 2000;17:312–318.
35. Tozzi P, Solem JO, Boumzebra D, et al. Is the GraftConnector a valid alternative to running suture in end-to-side coronary artery anastomoses? Ann Thorac Surg 2001;72:S999–S1003.
36. Presentation. Advanced Cardiac Techniques Meeting. New York, NY. May 2001.
37. Hill AC, Maroney TP, Virmani R. Facilitated coronary anastomosis using a nitinol U-Clip device: bovine model. J Thorac Cardiovasc Surg 2001;121:859–870.
38. Braunwald NS, Gay W, Tatooles CJ. Evaluation of cross-linked gelatin as a tissue adhesive and hemostatic agent: an experimental study. Surgery 1966;59:1024–1030.
39. Bachet J, Goudot B, Teodori G, et al. Surgery of type A acute aortic dissection with gelatin-resorcin-formol biological glue: a twelve-year experience. J Cardiovasc Surg 1990;31:263–273.
40. Oiwa H, Takamoto S, Murakami A, Tanaka O, Furuse A. Experimental study of small arterial anastomosis with gelatin-resorcon-formaldehyde glue and collagen sheet. Artif Organs 2001;25(4):281–291.
41. Takenaka H. Sutureless anastomosis of blood vessels using cyanoacrylate adhesives. Jpn J Surg 1992;22:46.

42. Dowbak GM, Rohrich RJ, Robinson JB, Peden E. Effectiveness of a new non-thrombogenic bio-adhesive in microvascular anastomoses. J Reconstruct Microsurg 1994;10(6):383–386.
43. Gundry SR, Black K, Izutani H. Sutureless coronary artery bypass with biologic glued anastomoses: preliminary in vivo and in vitro results. J Thorac Cardiovasc Surg 2000;120:473–477.
44. Jain KK, Gorisch W. Repair of small blood vessels with the neodynium-YAG laser: a preliminary report. Surgery 1979;85:684–688.
45. Morris JR, Carter M. Laser assisted microvascular anastomosis (LAMA) (abstr). Orthopedic Research Society. Las Vegas, NV, 1980.
46. Gomes OM, Macruz Z, Armelin E, Aerbini EJ. Vascular anastomosis by argon laser beam. Texas Heart Instit J 1983;10:145–149.
47. Frazier OH, Painvin GA, Morris JR, Thomsen S, Neblett CR. Laser-assisted microvascular anastomosis: angiographic and anatomopathologic studies on growing microvascular anastomoses: preliminary report. Surgery 1985;97:585–589.
48. Lewis WJ, Uribe A. Contact diode laser microvascular anastomosis. Laryngoscope 1993;103:850–853.
49. Quigley MR, Bailes JE, Kwaan HC, Cerullo LJ, Brown JT. Aneurysm formation following low power CO_2 laser-assisted vascular anastomosis. Neurosurgery 1986;18:292–299.
50. Nakata S, Campbell CD, Pick R, Replogle RL. End-to-side and end-to-end vascular anastomoses with a carbon dioxide laser. J Thorac Cardiovasc Surg 1989;98:57–62.
51. Reali UM, Gelli R, Giannotti V, Gori F, Pratesi R, Pini R. Experimental diode laser-assisted microvascular anastomosis. J Reconstr Microsurg 1993;9:203–210.
52. Oz MC, Johnson JP, Parangi S, et al. Tissue soldering by use of indocyanine green dye-enhanced fibrinogen with near infrared diode laser. J Vasc Surg 1990;11:718–725.
53. Chuck RS, Oz MC, Delohery TM, et al. Dye-enhanced laser tissue welding. Lasers Surg Med 1989;9:471–477.
54. Maitz PKM, Tricket RI, Dekker P, et al. Sutureless microvascular anastomoses by a biodegradable laser-activated solid protein solder. Plastic Reconstr Surg 1999;104:1726–1731.
55. Falk V, Diegeler A, Walther T, et al. Total endoscopic coronary artery bypass grafting. Eur J Cardiothorac Surg 2000;17:38–45.
56. Falk V, Autschbach R, Walther T, Diegeler A, Chitwood WR, Mohr FW. Computer enhanced mitral valve surgery—towards a total endoscopic procedure. Sem Thorac Surg 1999;11:244–249.
57. Reuchenspurner H, Damiano RJ, Mack M, et al. Use of the voice-controlled and computer-assisted surgical system Zeus for endoscopic coronary artery bypass grafting. J Thorac Cardiovasc Surg 1999;118:11–16.
58. Mohr FW, Falk V, Diegeler A, et al. Computer-enhanced "robotic" cardiac surgery: experience in 148 patients. J Thorac Cardiovasc Surg 2001;121(5)842–853.

29 Making Cardiopulmonary Bypass Less Invasive

James R. Beck, CCP, *Linda B. Mongero,* CCP, *and A. Kenneth Litzie*

Contents

Introduction
Major Milestones in ECC Development
Paradigm Constraint: What Is ECC?
Disconnect Between Knowledge and Practice
Setting for Paradigm Shift
Extracorporeal Circuit Components
Clinical Application: Closed Extracorporeal Circuits
Safety and Efficacy: Closed ECCs
Summary
References

INTRODUCTION

Most physicians believe that cardiopulmonary bypass (CPB) is the most invasive aspect of open-heart surgery. Modification of current CPB circuits to reduce the trauma induced by these systems is a rational approach to improving clinical results, and recent developments have reinforced the value of these changes. Of all the characteristics of CPB circuits, problems associated with less-than-optimal postoperative patient outcomes fall into two general areas: (1) the nonendothelial foreign surface area (NEFSA) causing the systemic inflammatory response syndrome (SIRS) *(1,2)*; and (2) a constellation of extracorporeal circuit (ECC) characteristics (size, hemodilution, emboli production, etc.), causally related to a number of deleterious postoperative patient sequelae *(3–9)*.

MAJOR MILESTONES IN ECC DEVELOPMENT

Membrane oxygenators and myocardial preservation are the most significant recent achievements in ECC. These two technological innovations have afforded countless

From: *Contemporary Cardiology: Minimally Invasive Cardiac Surgery, Second Edition*
Edited by: D. J. Goldstein and M. C. Oz © Humana Press Inc., Totowa, NJ

cardiac surgical patients the opportunity to avoid key hematological dyscrasias that affect the major organ systems.

Chemical treatments for the NEFSA of the ECC have also become available recently. The goal of surface modification is to present a more uniform surface for blood contact in an attempt to moderate the pathological inflammatory response *(10–12)*. Although their chemistries differ greatly, each approach appears to afford some degree of diminution of some indices of cellular- or plasma-protein-mediated stimulation of SIRS secondary to contact with NEFSAs. The maximal expression of the benefits of these "biocompatible" surface treatments, as assessed by sensitive hematological activation markers, is thought to be masked by the multifold contribution of other traditional ECC technologies and practices. There is now good evidence that the very nature of cardiopulmonary bypass technology may be the most fundamental and principal contributor to postbypass patient morbidity.

PARADIGM CONSTRAINT: WHAT IS ECC?

The current technology and practice of cardiopulmonary bypass routinely conjures up an image similar to the one on the right in **Fig. 1**. Extracorporeal circulation for support of the cardiac surgical patient is inextricably associated with the image of a 700-kg machine, 30 m of plastic tubing, and a host of discrete extracorporeal components.

Given the voluminous literature documenting patient morbidity attributable to this traditional technology, it is curious to note that developments in ECC over the last 15 yr have continued to be constrained within the physical and functional paradigms embodied in that old technology. Commodity-type products of differing shapes, sizes, colors, with a panoply of user-configured ports, connections, and conveniences have dominated the new-product offerings available to clinicians. The focus of ECC development over these years appears to have been user-oriented rather than patient-oriented, suggesting a somewhat fatalistic belief that the morbidity associated with traditional CPB has reached a tolerable plateau. The acceptability of patient morbidity attributable to traditional CPB justifying the absence of meaningful developments in extracorporeal equipment has, in recent years, been challenged with the advent of off-pump coronary artery bypass (OPCAB) procedures, as described throughout this book.

DISCONNECT BETWEEN KNOWLEDGE AND PRACTICE

Compounding the complicated landscape of moderating perfusion outcomes are time-honored patient management practices that have been shown to contribute to patient morbidity. The tolerance of deleterious patient outcomes directly attributable to ECC components and techniques is perhaps best exemplified by the continuing use of traditional cardiotomy suction techniques. The impact on patient outcome indices (e.g., SIRS, coagulation disorders, neurobehavioral deficits) that results from the practice of directly returning shed blood from the surgical wound has been clearly documented in numerous scientific publications *(5,7–9,12–17)*. The use of cardiotomy suction, and more importantly cardiotomy-based reservoirs, exposes patients to two of the most damaging aspects of ECC design, a massive blood–air interface and abundant silica/silicon antifoam agents *(18–21)*.

Other examples of tolerance for characteristics of traditional ECC that are causally related to increasing patient morbidity and cost of care are hemodilution and homologous

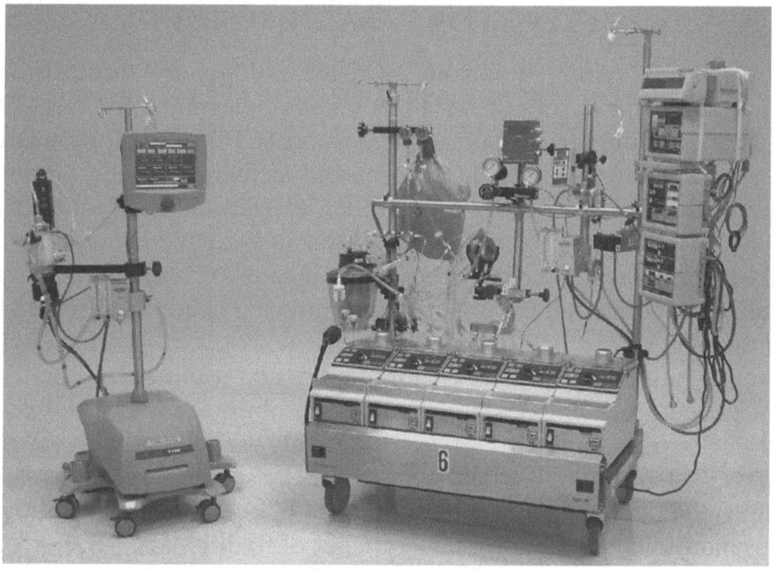

Fig. 1. New and traditional cardiopulmonary bypass circuit.

blood use. In light of the consensus of scientific opinion regarding the physiological desirability of obtaining and maintaining higher perioperative hemoglobin and hematocrit levels in cardiac surgical patients *(3,5,22–26)* and a similar consensus of opinion regarding the morbidity and cost impact of allogenic blood use, 20–40% reductions in baseline hematocrit levels are still routine during cardiac surgery.

Several technologies have emerged over the past several decades that attempt to moderate these hemodilutional effects. Autologous blood processing techniques and ultrafiltration technologies have emerged based on the clinical need to moderate the excessive hemodilutional volume characteristic of contemporary CPB techniques. There are over 240 studies investigating the use of ultrafiltration in routine CPB. Recent commercial popularity for assisted venous drainage technologies, most notably vacuum-assisted venous return (VAVD), have allowed modification of traditional ECC components in an attempt to reduce the hemodilutional effect *(27–34)*. Although the application of assisted drainage was originally driven by the need for smaller cannulae in light of port-access and minimally invasive surgical techniques, a modest 20–30% reduction in hemodilutional volume can be realized in the most aggressive applications. The unfortunate by-product of this technology has been the increased physical size of ECC components designed for assisted-return applications. Increased volume capacity has subsequently increased the NEFSA of the ECC.

Preoperative blood conservation strategies abound, each in its own way attempting to compensate for the significant hemodilutional impact of traditional ECCs on oxygen-carrying capacity (anemia), bleeding diathesis (thrombocytopenia), and systemic edema (hypoproteinemia). The uses of aprotinin, preoperative autologous blood donation, erythropoietin therapy, preoperative acute normovolemic hemodilution, and platelet-rich plasmapheresis have both advocates and detractors in the medical literature *(35–40)*. The absence of compelling and ubiquitous support for many such preoperative strategies account for their irregular presence in local, regional, or national standards of care.

SETTING FOR PARADIGM SHIFT

The inherent shortcomings of existing ECC technology, and the associated patient morbidity, has spurred the development of new technologies and techniques. One attempt to avoid the pathophysiological responses to traditional CPB technology was to eliminate it completely by reviving and popularizing an old technique, operating on a "beating heart," albeit with new and enabling technologies (retractors, immobilizers, apical positioners) *(41–44)*. Though seemingly an ideal solution to CPB morbidity, persistent questions about the therapeutic equivalence and technical challenges of beating-heart revascularization as compared to surgery on the arrested heart have limited the growth of this technique.

From the recognition that mechanical circulatory and respiratory support of the cardiac surgical patient is an adjunct to the surgeon's ability to perform a complete and effective surgical repair, some different embodiments of minimally invasive cardiopulmonary bypass systems have been developed. These systems offer the same level of circulatory and respiratory support as traditional CPB, but without subjecting patients to the numerous morbidity-producing characteristics of traditional CPB. For example, the CORx System technology (CardioVention, Inc., Santa Clara, CA) was developed specifically to address the four most significant and best-documented features of traditional CPB technology that are causally related to various forms of postoperative patient morbidity. Those four areas are listed in Table 1.

With the creation of these improved, minimally invasive extracorporeal circuits, a "hybrid" procedure has evolved that enables surgeons and anesthesiologists to provide to their patients many of the benefits of OPCAB procedures (e.g., no aortic crossclamp, no global myocardial ischemia) without the hemodynamic instability, volume loading and hemodilution, extensive vasopressor support, and expensive disposable instrumentation typical of most OPCAB procedures. This hybrid procedure is described as a "pump-assisted beating-heart," and is rapidly growing in popularity. Early clinical results support expectations of improved postoperative patient outcomes. Future and current studies in the areas of SIRS, hemoglobin levels, plasma protein levels, and coagulation will help illuminate the mechanisms of these observed improvements.

EXTRACORPOREAL CIRCUIT COMPONENTS

The principal components of "minimally invasive" ECCs vary somewhat among manufacturers. Some manufacturers have simply interconnected their existing ECC components with shorter pieces of tubing and renamed the assemblage a minimal or low-prime ECC. One exception to this approach is the CORx System. This device was newly designed specifically to address the objectives of a minimally invasive ECC. This new concept in ECC integrates three primary, and traditionally separate and discrete components, of a typical CPB circuit into a single, ultra-low NEFSA and hemodilutional component. The three components combined in the integrated oxygenation system (IOS™) are the venous reservoir (venous air-handling chamber), the blood pump (centrifugal), and the blood oxygenator (**Fig. 2**).

ECC Components—Venous Air Removal

A traditional venous reservoir serves two primary purposes: to remove air that inadvertently enters the venous drainage line and to store blood in the ECC. Unfortunately, the perception that a traditional venous reservoir completely removes all air in the venous

Table 1
Traditional CPB Characteristics Causally Related to Post-operative Patient Morbidity

Large non-endothelial foreign surface area
Large extracorporeal and hemodilutional volume
Large obligatory direct blood-gas interface
Large eluting silicon-oil / silica particle antifoam agent

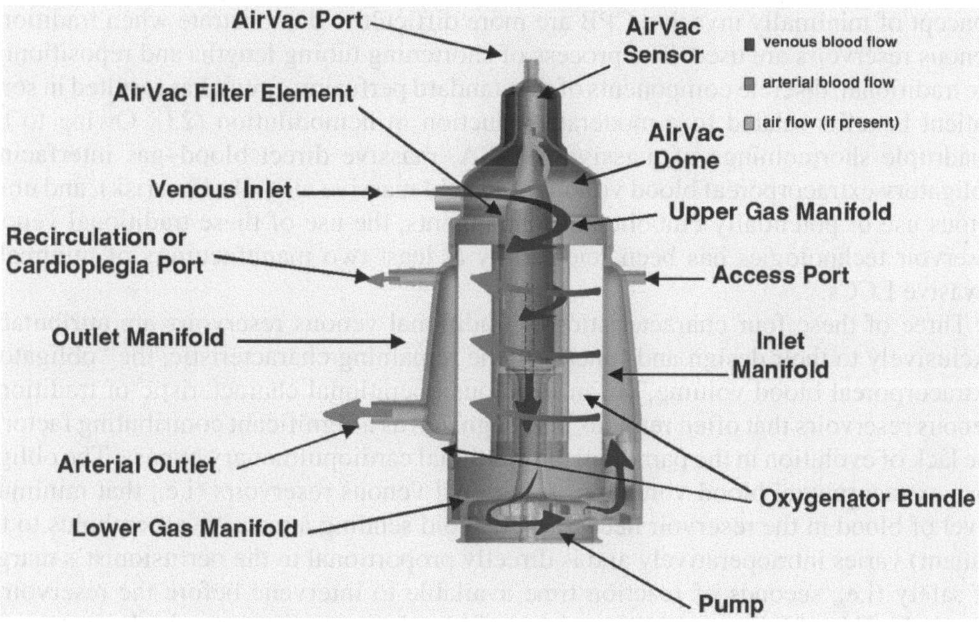

Fig. 2. Components of the CORx IOS.

blood is incorrect *(45)*. In fact, nearly all instances of air down the venous line are associated with embolic high-intensity signals in the patient's cerebral circulation. Equally unfortunate is the fact that the process of removing some of the air in venous blood in traditional CPB circuits actually adds a measurably significant dose of lipoidal and particulate microemboli by a largely unacknowledged, but well-documented, characteristic of the "antifoam" agent that is present in the majority of venous reservoirs *(18,19,21)*. Most of the minimally invasive ECC circuits available in the United States and Europe rely on the passive air-removal characteristics of an oxygenator, a traditional venous reservoir, and/or an arterial line filter. One device on the market in both the United States and in Europe uses a newly developed, active air-removal system that can serve as an adjunct to any inherent passive capabilities of an oxygenator or arterial-line filter.

This new active air-removal technology has been integrated into CardioVention's CORx™ System. It substitutes the passive and chemical antifoam technologies described above with an active air-removal system (AirVac™) that utilizes electronics to sense air in venous blood and trigger its removal before coming into contact with the integrated centrifugal pump (**Fig. 2**). This active air-removal mechanism is a significant step in ECC technology for at least three reasons: (1) it does not rely on the decades-old technology of chemical defoaming, with its inherent cerebral embolic characteristics; (2) it does not rely on the passive air-removal characteristics of membrane oxygenators and arterial line filters; and (3) in contrast to many other "closed" circuits, active venous air removal evacuates venous air before it contacts the centrifugal blood pump, where large air bubbles can be atomized into countless gaseous microemboli that cannot be removed by traditional defoaming technologies.

ECC Components—Venous Reservoir

Many of the improvements in patient outcome measurements promised by the new concept of minimally invasive CPB are more difficult to demonstrate when traditional venous reservoirs are used. The process of shortening tubing lengths and repositioning the traditional, discrete components of the standard perfusion circuit has resulted in some patient benefits related to a moderate reduction in hemodilution *(23)*. Owing to the quadruple shortcomings of massive NEFSA, massive direct blood–gas interfacing, obligatory extracorporeal blood volume (to avoid massive air embolism risk), and ubiquitous use of potentially embolic antifoam agents, the use of these traditional venous reservoir technologies has been rejected by at least two manufacturers of minimally invasive ECCs.

Three of these four characteristics of traditional venous reservoirs are attributable exclusively to their design and function. The remaining characteristic, the "obligatory extracorporeal blood volume," is an insidious operational characteristic of traditional venous reservoirs that often remains unrecognized as a significant contributing factor to the lack of evolution in the paradigm of traditional cardiopulmonary bypass. The obligatory extracorporeal blood volume of traditional venous reservoirs (i.e., that minimum level of blood in the reservoir necessary to avoid sending a massive air embolus to the patient) varies intraoperatively and is directly proportional to the perfusionist's margin of safety (i.e., seconds of reaction time available to intervene before the reservoir is emptied). This obligatory minimum level of blood is necessary even in the instance of systemic hypovolemia or poor venous return.

In the newest generation of minimally invasive systems, alternatives to traditional venous reservoirs include approaches such as the "elective venous blood reservoir" (**Fig. 3**).

The use of closed blood bags as elective venous blood reservoirs is characterized by the fact that they:

1. Are elective, not obligatory
2. Have no mandatory minimum extracorporeal blood volume requirement for safe use
3. Contain no chemical antifoam agents that can embolize
4. Have no direct blood-gas interface

ECC Components—Centrifugal Pump

Centrifugal pumps are the pumps of choice for the minimally invasive ECC movement. They can be tethered to a location closer to the patient than is possible for a roller pump, they are both pre- and after-load sensitive, and they are incapable of pumping a massive air embolism to the patient under catastrophic circumstances. A unique and functionally significant step in the revolution that describes the departure from traditional cardiopulmonary bypass is the integration of the centrifugal pump into a single, multifunctional component. The only integrated centrifugal pump at this time is the CORx IOS device (**Fig. 4**). The centrifugal pump in this device, and other closed-loop

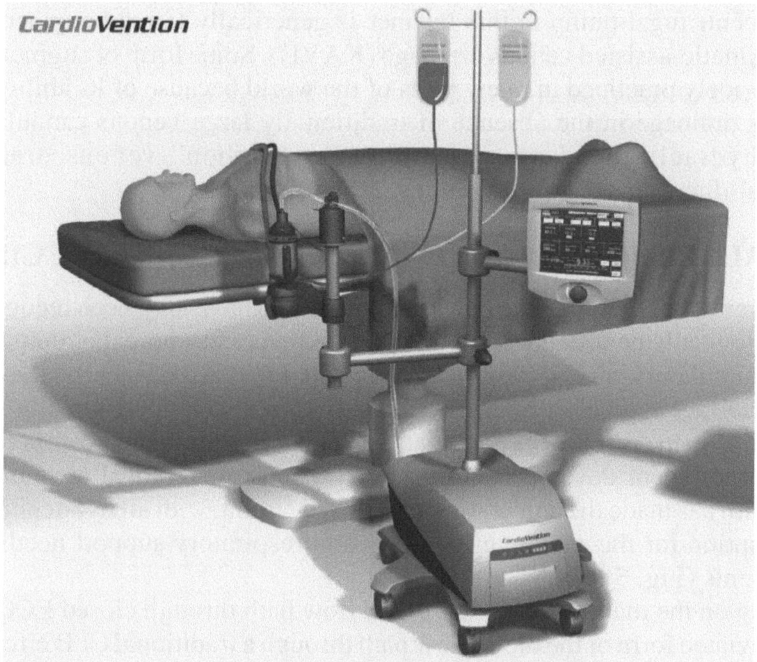

Fig. 3. Elective (nonobligatory) venous reservoir.

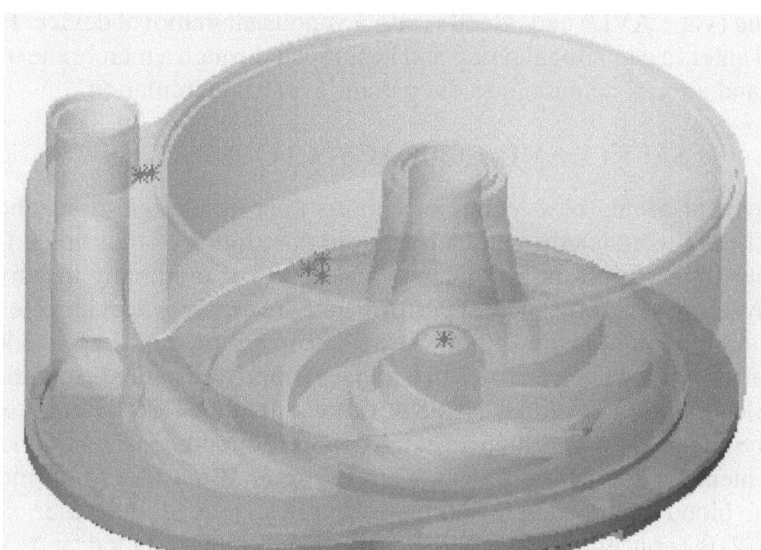

Fig. 4. Integrated centrifugal pump.

ECC systems, serves two purposes. First, it is the means by which a pressure gradient is formed between the venous cannula and the ECC to achieve right heart decompression (i.e., control venous drainage). The same pump also serves as the "arterial" pump, and propels venous blood through the oxygenator where carbon dioxide and oxygen transfer occur.

Use of a centrifugal pump in this manner is generically termed augmented venous drainage or kinetic-assisted venous drainage (KAVD). Some form of augmented venous drainage is widely practiced in many parts of the world because of its ability to accomplish venous drainage in the absence of traditionally large venous cannulae, gravity-generated hydraulic head pressure to power "siphon" venous drainage, and large-internal-diameter venous drain lines.

CLINICAL APPLICATION: CLOSED EXTRACORPOREAL CIRCUITS

Closed circuits (i.e., not open to the atmospheric air) have long been recognized as the most physiologically beneficial and technically safe extracorporeal circuits with which to perform circulatory and/or respiratory support *(46)*. Avoidance of the continuous blood-gas interface typical of open circuits is believed to reduce numerous indices of SIRS, as well as help preserve the coagulation mechanism for better postoperative hemostasis *(11)*. The recent development of active venous air-removal technologies (e.g., CORx AirVac) has made the application of a closed circuit, with all its attendant benefits, a practical option for the routine circulatory and respiratory support needs of cardiac surgical patients (**Fig. 5**).

Depending on the manufacturer, the blood flow path through closed ECC systems is just an abbreviated form of the blood flow path through a traditional CPB circuit with one or more of the notable qualitative and quantitative differences defined in Table 1. With few exceptions, blood flow through closed ECC systems follows the following sequence: venous blood is aspirated from the right heart through the venous cannula, flows down the venous line (via KAVD) and, ideally, into a venous air-removal device. From there, venous blood enters a centrifugal pump and is pumped through a membrane oxygenator, arterial line, and arterial cannula into the patient's arterial circulation.

SAFETY AND EFFICACY: CLOSED ECCS

The deployment of any new technology raises appropriate questions about patient safety and efficacy. Challenging the decades-old paradigms of traditional CPB raises these questions to the forefront. In this new generation of minimally invasive, closed-circuit ECC systems, several aspects of performance are nearly self-evident (e.g., oxygen transfer, carbon dioxide transfer, blood flow rate capability, etc.) Less evident are the design and performance characteristics that argue to improved patient outcome measurements (e.g., hemodilutional volume, NEFSA, venous air-removal efficiency, etc.). Issues germane to the adequacy with which an extracorporeal circuit satisfies a patient's metabolic requirement for the delivery of oxygen in a circuit that does not unnecessarily traumatize the blood include: (1) the ability of the ECC to load molecular oxygen onto hemoglobin; (2) the concentration of hemoglobin in the patient's blood; and (3) the blood flow rate necessary to deliver adequate volumes of oxygenated blood to the patient's tissues. New mini-systems (e.g., CORx) that do not create the same magnitude of clinically significant levels of hemodilution (anemia) as traditional CPB systems do (**Fig. 6**) are able to transfer at least equivalent volumes of oxygen as those traditional systems, and under many circumstances, even more. Of added interest is that, secondary to the more normal levels of hemoglobin in the "minisystem," the nonphysiologically high pO_2 levels of traditional CPB are not needed to ensure adequate oxygen transfer. Attributable to the routinely higher concentrations of hemoglobin afforded by minisystems, the resulting proportionately higher oxygen-carrying capacity of the patient's blood requires a notably

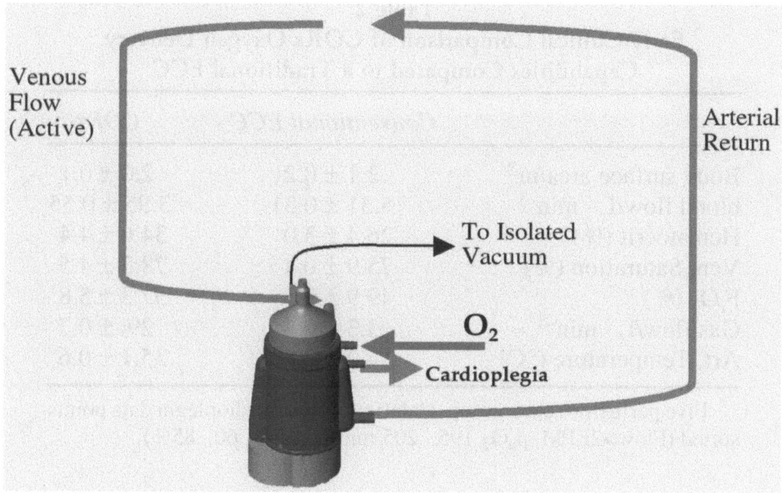

Fig. 5. CORx "closed" A/V loop circuit.

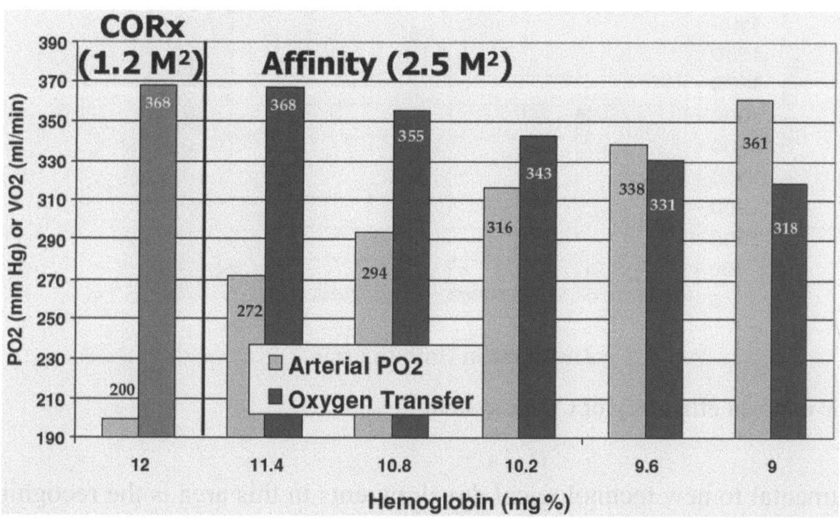

Fig. 6. Comparison of oxygen transfer and corresponding pO_2 of CORx and Medtronic affinity oxygenators.

lower extracorporeal blood flow rate (Table 2), and thus a greatly reduced number of times the patient's blood volume is required to be circulated through the ECC. A reduced number of passes through the ECC results not only in a reduction of the NEFSA-to-blood contact ratio, but does so without sacrificing total patient perfusion as reflected by venous oxyhemoglobin saturation.

Unique among all of these considerations is the most recently recognized requirement for these very small, closed, minimally invasive ECC systems—venous air removal. Some of these circuits rely on historical and somewhat ambiguous assumptions about the reliability of physical characteristics of static circuit components (e.g., oxygenator, centrifugal pump, etc.) to remove air. Others have developed new technology to address this need.

Table 2
Early Clinical Comparison of CORx Oxygen Delivery Capabilities Compared to a Traditional ECC

	Conventional ECC	*CORx*
Body surface area/m^2	2.1 ± 0.2	2.0 ± 0.1
blood flow/L · min^{-1}	5.31 ± 0.31	3.95 ± 0.55
Hematocrit (%)	26.4 ± 3.0	34.6 ± 4.4
Ven. Saturation (%)	75.9 ± 0.4	78.3 ± 4.5
F_iO_2 (%)	49.9 ± 9.5	57.3 ± 5.8
Gas flow/L · min^{-1}	3.3 ± 0.4	29. ± 0.7
Art. Temperature (°C)	34.2 ± 2.6	35.1 ± 0.6

Five perfusions each group. Calafiore blood cardioplegia data points sorted (Flow>2LPM, p_aO_2 195...205 mmHg, S_vO_2 60...85%).

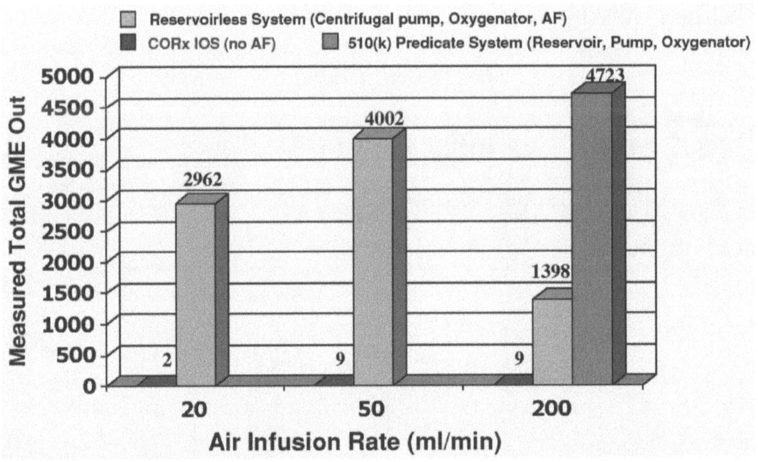

Fig. 7. Air-removal efficiency of CORx system.

Fundamental to new technological developments in this area is the recognition that under certain circumstances, all extracorporeal circuits (large, small, open, closed) have the ability to transform macro-air into micro-air (<100 μm), and, furthermore, have the ability to pass this micro-air past all currently known levels of safety to the patient's arterial system. Traditional ECC design has relied on large extracorporeal, volume-dependent, discrete devices to provide a sometimes unjustified level of confidence to the clinician *(45,47,48)*. Venous reservoirs with large-surface-area filter screens treated with silica-based antifoam agents in conjunction with membrane oxygenators and equally large-volume arterial line filters comprise the primary line of traditional defense. Of the minimally invasive ECC systems, some rely on an oxygenator or arterial filter, to the exclusion of any venous air-removal technology, to protect the patient from gaseous microemboli. Another ECC (CORx System) augments these more traditional means by actively removing air from the venous blood before it comes into contact with the centrifugal pump. Because all mechanical systems have design parameter limitations, operation of these systems within the manufacturer-defined limits is essential. Under those conditions, the newest venous air-removal technology (CORx AirVac) provides a comparable, if not superior, method of ECC air elimination. **Figure 7** illustrates the air-

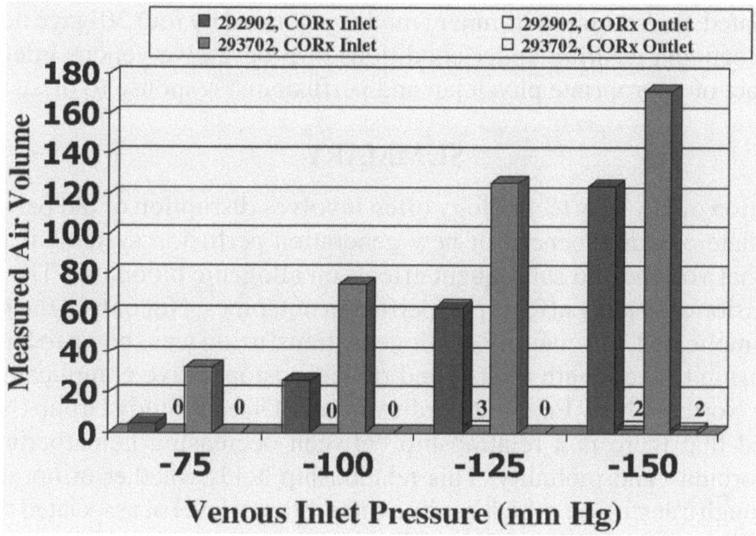

Fig. 8. CORx air entrainment removal model illustrated with two venous cannula, a 29×29 fr and a 29 × 37 fr two-stage cannula at increasing levels of venous outlet resistance.

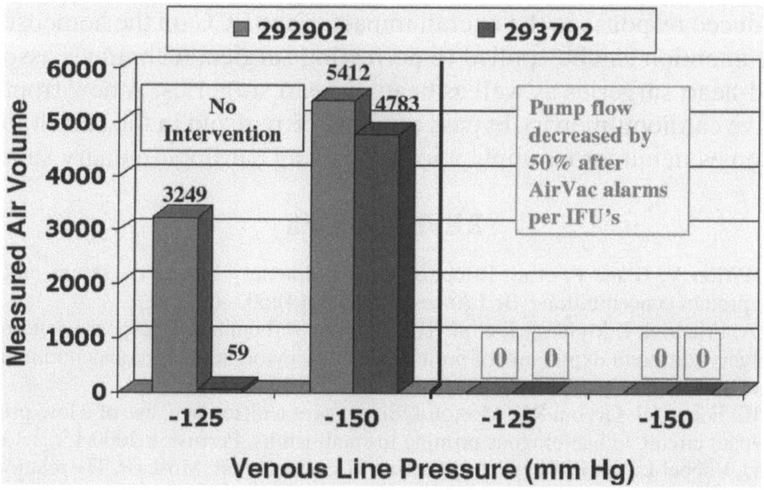

Fig. 9. Effect of perfusionist intervention in the incidence of air detection in extreme entrainment model CORx GME output.

removal efficiency of the CORx system compared to two common ECC configurations. Even at clinically significant air infusion rates of 200 mL/min, the CORx AirVac technology demonstrates favorable air-handling capabilities.

Although air injection is a commonly used benchmark in device comparison, a more realistic clinical model is that of air entrainment through a venous aspiration model. This technique more closely simulates air entrained through a leaking venous cannula purse string or compromised right atrial integrity. **Figure 8** illustrates the ability of this same device to handle air entrained in this manner.

As the only active venous air-removal technology on the market thus far, a worst-case experiment challenge creates a baseline performance record to which other future technologies will be compared. **Figure 9** illustrates the ability of the CORx System to remove air in a simulated, micro-air environment model generated by four 30-gage needles in the near-venous cannula position under conditions of progressive venous inlet resistance, and the impact of appropriate physician and perfusionist response to these conditions.

SUMMARY

The adoption of any new technology often involves disruption of old paradigms. The most immediate outcome benefit of new-generation perfusion systems is the reduced hemodilutional volume and subsequent effects on allogenic blood use. The use of allogenic transfusion adversely affects postperfusion outcomes. Not only is the incidence of transfusion implicated, the quantity of allogenic transfusion was shown to have a significant relationship to the length of stay and rate of postoperative complications *(49)*. In addition, the Northern New England Cardiovascular Disease Study Group (NNECDSG) demonstrated that there is a relationship between decreasing hematocrit values and increased morbidity and mortality. This relationship holds whether or not correction is achieved through transfusion, which has its own additional level of associated risk and cost.

Quantifiable benefits are also realized through the immediate reduction in direct costs associated with the procurement and administration of blood products. Table 3 summarizes some of the potential benefits of reduced hemodilution seen by the application of these technologies.

With a reduced response to the overall impact of the ECC on the homeostatic mechanisms, more attention can be applied to perfecting surgical techniques associated with both stopped-heart surgeries as well as beating-heart surgeries. A new frontier in minimally invasive cardiopulmonary bypass can now be realized in the search for improved patient outcomes in numerous applications requiring cardiopulmonary support.

REFERENCES

1. Aouifi A, Piriou V, Blanc P, et al. Effect of cardiopulmonary bypass on serum procalcitonin and C-reactive protein concentrations. Br J Anaesth 1999;83(4):602–607.
2. Sablotzki A, Friedrich I, Muhling J, et al. The systemic inflammatory response syndrome following cardiac surgery: different expression of proinflammatory cytokines and procalcitonin in patients with and without multiorgan dysfunctions. Perfusion 2002;17(2):103–109.
3. Cormack JE, Forest RJ, Groom RC, Morton J. Size makes a difference: use of a low-prime cardiopulmonary bypass circuit and autologous priming in small adults. Perfusion 2000;15(2):129–135.
4. Aukerman J, Voepel-Lewis T, Riegger LQ, Siewert M, Shayevitz JR, Mosca R. The relationship between extracorporeal circuit prime, albumin, and postoperative weight gain in children. J Cardiothorac Vasc Anesth 1998;12(4):408–414.
5. Balachandran S, Cross MH, Karthikeyan S, Mulpur A, Hansbro SD, Hobson P. Retrograde autologous priming of the cardiopulmonary bypass circuit reduces blood transfusion after coronary artery surgery. Ann Thorac Surg 2002;73(6):1912–1918.
6. Cromer MJ, Wolk DR. A minimal priming technique that allows for a higher circulating hemoglobin on cardiopulmonary bypass. Perfusion 1998;13(5):311–313.
7. Brooker RF, Brown WR, Moody DM, et al. Cardiotomy suction: a major source of brain lipid emboli during cardiopulmonary bypass. Ann Thorac Surg 1998;65(6):1651–1655.
8. Taggart DP, Westaby S. Neurological and cognitive disorders after coronary artery bypass grafting. Curr Opin Cardiol 2001;16(5):271–276.
9. Spanier T, Tector K, Schwartz G, et al. Endotoxin in pooled pericardial blood contributes to the systemic inflammatory response during cardiac surgery. Perfusion 2000;15(5):427–431.
10. Heyer EJ, Lee KS, Manspeizer HE, et al. Heparin-bonded cardiopulmonary bypass circuits reduce cognitive dysfunction. J Cardiothorac Vasc Anesth 2002;16:37–42.

Table 3
Expected Clinical Value of CORx Technology of Reduced ECC Hemodilution

CORx feature	*Primary benefits*	*Operational benefit*	*Possible clinical benefit*	*Possible cost benefit*
			Reduction of all ransfusion-related morbidity	Reduction in total cost-of-care vis-à-vis additional treatments
			Reduced rate of transfusion-related febrile response	Reduction in total cost-of-cared vis-à-vis additional time in ICU
			Reduced rate of transfusion reaction	Reduction in total cost of care vis-à-vis additional time in ICU
	Higher hemoglobin	Better intraoperative gas exchange	Reduced rate of and allogenic transfusion	Reduction in total cost-of-care vis-à-vis additional treatments
Reduced Hemodilution (Minimal to no dilution)	Higher platelet count	None	Reduced post-operative blood loss and blood product transfusion	Reduction in total cost-of-care vis-à-vis additional time in ICU
	Higher total protein and colloid osmotic pressure	More stable intravascular volume and viscosity	Less post-op pulmonary edema	Reduction in total cost-of-care vis-à-vis less ventilator time and ICU time
			Less post-op systemic edema and weight gain	Reduction in total cost-of-care vis-à-vis less ICU time

11. Nishida H, Aomi S, Tomizawa Y, et al. Comparative study of biocompatibility between the open circuit and closed circuit in cardiopulmonary bypass. Artif Organs 1999;23(6):547–551.
12. Aldea GS, Soltow LO, Chandler WL, et al. Limitation of thrombin generation, platelet activation, and inflammation by elimination of cardiotomy suction in patients undergoing coronary artery bypass grafting treated with heparin-bonded circuits. J Thorac Cardiovasc Surg 2002;123(4):742–755.
13. Mueller XM, Tevaearai HT, Horisberger J, Augstburger M, Boone Y, von Segesser LK. Smart suction device for less blood trauma: a comparison with Cell Saver. Eur J Cardiothorac Surg 2001;19(4):507–511.
14. Anderson RE, Hansson LO, Liska J, Settergren G, Vaage J. The effect of cardiotomy suction on the brain injury marker S100beta after cardiopulmonary bypass. Ann Thorac Surg 2000;69(3):847–850.
15. Chung JH, Gikakis N, Rao AK, Drake TA, Colman RW, Edmunds LH Jr. Pericardial blood activates the extrinsic coagulation pathway during clinical cardiopulmonary bypass. Circulation 1996;93(11):2014–2018.
16. Kincaid EH, Jones TJ, Stump DA, et al. Processing scavenged blood with a cell saver reduces cerebral lipid microembolization. Ann Thorac Surg 2000;70(4):1296–1300.
17. Jones DR, Hill RC, Hollingsed MJ, et al. Use of heparin-coated cardiopulmonary bypass. Ann Thorac Surg 1993;56(3):566–568.
18. Challa VR, Moody DM, Troost BT. Brain embolic phenomena associated with cardiopulmonary bypass. J Neurol Sci 1993;117(1-2):224–231.
19. Suchil BL, Hernandez RN, Hurtado J, Orsornio Vargas AR. [Antifoaming agent microembolism in patients undergoing extracorporeal circulation. Its frequency in post mortem material and its pathogenic potential in vitro]. Rev Esp Cardiol 1992;45(9):578–583.
20. Orenstein JM, Sato N, Aaron B, Buchholz B, Bloom S. Microemboli observed in deaths following cardiopulmonary bypass surgery: silicone antifoam agents and polyvinyl chloride tubing as sources of emboli. Hum Pathol 1982;13(12):1082–1090.
21. Plasse HM, Spencer FC, Mittleman M, Frost JO. Unilateral sudden loss of hearing: an unusual complication of cardiac operation. J Thorac Cardiovasc Surg 1980;79(6):822–826.
22. Kmiecik SA, Stammers AH, Petterson CM, et al. The effect of volume replacement on serum protein concentration during cardiopulmonary bypass. J Extra Corpor Technol 2001;33(4):227–232.
23. McCusker K, Vijay V, DeBois W, Helm R, Sisto D. MAST system: a new condensed cardiopulmonary bypass circuit for adult cardiac surgery. Perfusion 2001;16(6):447–452.
24. Nakanishi K, Shichijo T, Shinkawa Y, et al. Usefulness of vacuum-assisted cardiopulmonary bypass circuit for pediatric open-heart surgery in reducing homologous blood transfusion. Eur J Cardiothorac Surg 2001;20(2):233–238.
25. Rousou JA, Engelman RM, Flack JE III, Deaton DW, Garb JL, Owen SG. The "primeless pump": a novel technique for intraoperative blood conservation. Cardiovasc Surg 1999;7(2):228–235.
26. Rosengart TK, DeBois W, O'Hara M, et al. Retrograde autologous priming for cardiopulmonary bypass: a safe and effective means of decreasing hemodilution and transfusion requirements. J Thorac Cardiovasc Surg 1998;115(2):426–438.
27. Willcox TW. Vacuum-assisted venous drainage: to air or not to air, that is the question. Has the bubble burst? J Extra Corpor Technol 2002;34(1):24–28.
28. Bevilacqua S, Matteucci S, Ferrarini M, et al. Biochemical evaluation of vacuum-assisted venous drainage: a randomized, prospective study. Perfusion 2002;17(1):57–61.
29. Mueller XM, Tevaearai HT, Horisberger J, Augstburger M, Burki M, von Segesser LK. Vacuum assisted venous drainage does not increase trauma to blood cells. ASAIO J 2001;47(6):651–654.
30. Mathews RK, Sistino JJ. In-vitro evaluation of the hemolytic effects of augmented venous drainage. J Extra Corpor Technol 2001;33(1):15–18.
31. Berryessa R, Wiencek R, Jacobson J, Hollingshead D, Farmer K, Cahill G. Vacuum-assisted venous return in pediatric cardiopulmonary bypass. Perfusion 2000;15(1):63–67.
32. Ogella DA. Advances in perfusion technology—an overview. J Indian Med Assoc 1999;97(10): 436–437, 441.
33. Munster K, Andersen U, Mikkelsen J, Pettersson G. Vacuum assisted venous drainage (VAVD). Perfusion 1999;14(6):419–423.
34. Lau CL, Posther KE, Stephenson GR, et al. Mini-circuit cardiopulmonary bypass with vacuum assisted venous drainage: feasibility of an asanguineous prime in the neonate. Perfusion 1999;14(5):389–396.
35. Groom RC. High or low hematocrits during cardiopulmonary bypass for patients undergoing coronary artery bypass graft surgery? An evidence-based approach to the question. Perfusion 2002;17(2):99–102.
36. Cross MH. Autotransfusion in cardiac surgery. Perfusion 2001;16(5):391–400.

37. Tempe DK, Banerjee A, Virmani S, et al. Comparison of the effects of a cell saver and low-dose aprotinin on blood loss and homologous blood usage in patients undergoing valve surgery. J Cardiothorac Vasc Anesth 2001;15(3):326–330.
38. Ruel MA, Rubens FD. Non-pharmacological strategies for blood conservation in cardiac surgery. Can J Anaesth 2001;48(4 suppl):S13–S23.
39. Iguchi A, Tanaka S. Preoperative autologous blood donation and plateletpheresis in patients undergoing elective cardiac operations—factors that influence the need for homologous blood transfusion. Jpn Circ J 1997;61(3):236–240.
40. Christenson JT, Reuse J, Badel P, Nowicki B, Simonet F, Schmuziger M. Autologous platelet sequestration in patients undergoing coronary artery bypass grafting. Eur J Cardiothorac Surg 1996;10(12):1083–1089.
41. Do QB, Goyer C, Chavanon O, Couture P, Denault A, Cartier R. Hemodynamic changes during off-pump CABG surgery. Eur J Cardiothorac Surg 2002;21(3):385–390.
42. Hernandez F, Cohn WE, Baribeau YR, et al. In-hospital outcomes of off-pump versus on-pump coronary artery bypass procedures: a multicenter experience. Ann Thorac Surg 2001;72(5):1528–1533.
43. Hart JC, Puskas JD, Sabik JF III. Off-pump coronary revascularization: current state of the art. Semin Thorac Cardiovasc Surg 2002;14(1):70–81.
44. Kim KB, Lim C, Lee C, et al. Off-pump coronary artery bypass may decrease the patency of saphenous vein grafts. Ann Thorac Surg 2001;72(3):S1033–S1037.
45. Jones TJ, Deal DD, Vernon JC, Blackburn N, Stump DA. How effective are cardiopulmonary bypass circuits at removing gaseous microemboli? J Extra Corpor Technol 2002;34(1):34–39.
46. Mongero LB, Sistino JJ, Beck J, Smith CR. Current perfusion techniques for repair of giant cerebral aneurysms using deep hypothermia and circulatory arrest. J Extra Corpor Technol 1994;26:13–17.
47. Kurusz M. Gaseous microemboli: sources, causes, and clinical considerations. Med Instrum 1985;19(2):73–76.
48. Butler BD. Biophysical aspects of gas bubbles in blood. Med Instrum 1985;19(2):59–62.
49. Shapira OM, Aldea GS, Treanor PR, et al. Reduction of allogeneic blood transfusions after open heart operations by lowering cardiopulmonary bypass prime volume. Ann Thorac Surg 1998;65(3):724–730.

VI Robotic Surgery

30 Robotics and Telemanipulation

The Zeus™ System

Hersh S. Maniar, MD, *Sunil M. Prasad,* MD, *and Ralph J. Damiano, Jr.,* MD

Contents

Background
Advantages of Robotic Systems
Clinical Results
Robotic Training
Future Directions
References

BACKGROUND

Endoscopic technology has been employed in various surgical specialities to decrease the morbidity of operations and hasten patient recovery *(1–3)*. These procedures are performed through small ports, with visualization achieved by using an endoscopic camera. Unfortunately, there has been little success with endoscopic techniques in the field of cardiac surgery. Despite numerous attempts over the past decade, manual endoscopic cardiac surgery has proven to be impossible, owing in great part to the limitations of conventional endoscopic instrumentation.

Traditional endoscopic instruments magnify a surgeon's tremor. Given their longer length, even the slightest operator tremor becomes amplified. Involuntary tremor, a hindrance when performing routine procedures with conventional endoscopy, becomes prohibitive with the microsurgery required during cardiac procedures. The ports required for endoscopic instruments also limit the surgeon's range of motion by producing fixed pivot points at their insertion sites in the chest wall. The resulting "fulcrum effect" requires a surgeon to move the handle of an endoscopic instrument in the reverse direction that he or she intends the instrument tip to travel. These counterintuitive movements

From: *Contemporary Cardiology: Minimally Invasive Cardiac Surgery, Second Edition*
Edited by: D. J. Goldstein and M. C. Oz © Humana Press Inc., Totowa, NJ

make it difficult to judge accurately the deflection of the instrument tip for prescribed movements of the instrument handles.

Operative visibility in minimally invasive surgery is also challenging. Endoscopes provide only a two-dimensional image, instead of the traditional three-dimensional visibility surgeons have in open procedures. Adapting to the loss of depth perception can be a difficult transition. In addition, the viewing angle from an endoscope is often misaligned with respect to the instrumentation. This creates a visuomotor incompatibility and increases the level of procedural difficulty *(4,5)*. Given the combination of impaired visibility and reduced dexterity, it is not surprising that few endoscopic applications have been incorporated into microsurgical disciplines.

Robotic surgical systems represent an enabling technology for the development of endoscopic, minimally invasive cardiac surgery. These systems provide several mechanisms to overcome the inherent difficulties of conventional endoscopy for the performance of microsurgery. The two robotic systems currently in use are the Zeus™ system, developed by Computer Motion (Goleta, CA) and the DaVinci™ system developed by Intuitive Surgical (Mountain View, CA). The latter is described in the following chapter. Each system is commercially available and has been used clinically in both general and cardiac surgery. This chapter focuses on the Zeus robotic system and its applications in the field of cardiac surgery.

Computer Motion initially introduced a voice-controlled robotic arm (Aesop™) to position and hold an endoscopic camera in 1994. This robotic arm is mounted on the operating table and responds to over 20 simple voice commands (**Fig. 1**). Aesop eliminates the need for a dedicated camera holder, and the surgeon-controlled camera avoids potential miscommunications between surgeon and assistant. The arm remains motionless unless directed, providing a more stable visual field than a hand-held camera. This feature is particularly important for microsurgery. Kavoussi et al. have shown that a robotic camera arm more effectively manipulated and controlled the video endoscope than a human assistant during laparoscopic procedures *(6)*. Overall efficiency, including repositioning and cleaning of the endoscopic camera, was improved three- to fivefold when a robotic arm was used. The robotic system has been found to be more stable and precise than a manually guided camera assistance *(7)*. The Aesop robotic arm has established an excellent record of performance and has now been used to assist in over 125,000 clinical procedures, including both coronary and valvular surgery *(8)*.

The Zeus Robotic Microsurgical System was developed and first introduced into clinical use in 1998 *(9)*. Designed as a telemanipulator, the surgeon's movements are digitized and filtered by a signal processor, before being relayed to the robotic arms for the completion of a given movement. The Zeus system has three primary components: (1) an interface console, where the surgeon sits and manipulates instrument handles; (2) a signal processor, where the motions are filtered and scaled; and (3) two effector robotic arms that are mounted on the operating room table. The arms are designed to hold instruments similar in length to conventional endoscopic instruments, with custom-made instrument tips that are freely interchangeable between the robotic arms (**Figs. 2** and **3**).

Two instrument handles designed to replicate standard microsurgical instruments are attached to the surgeon console. The instrument handles can be interchanged depending on the surgeon's preference. Housed within the console, a 16-in. video monitor displays the operative field. The surgeon remains seated, with the endoscopic image placed directly in front, at eye level, and close to the hands. This ergonomic configuration replaces the often awkward postioning required in laparoscopic procedures. Overall surgical

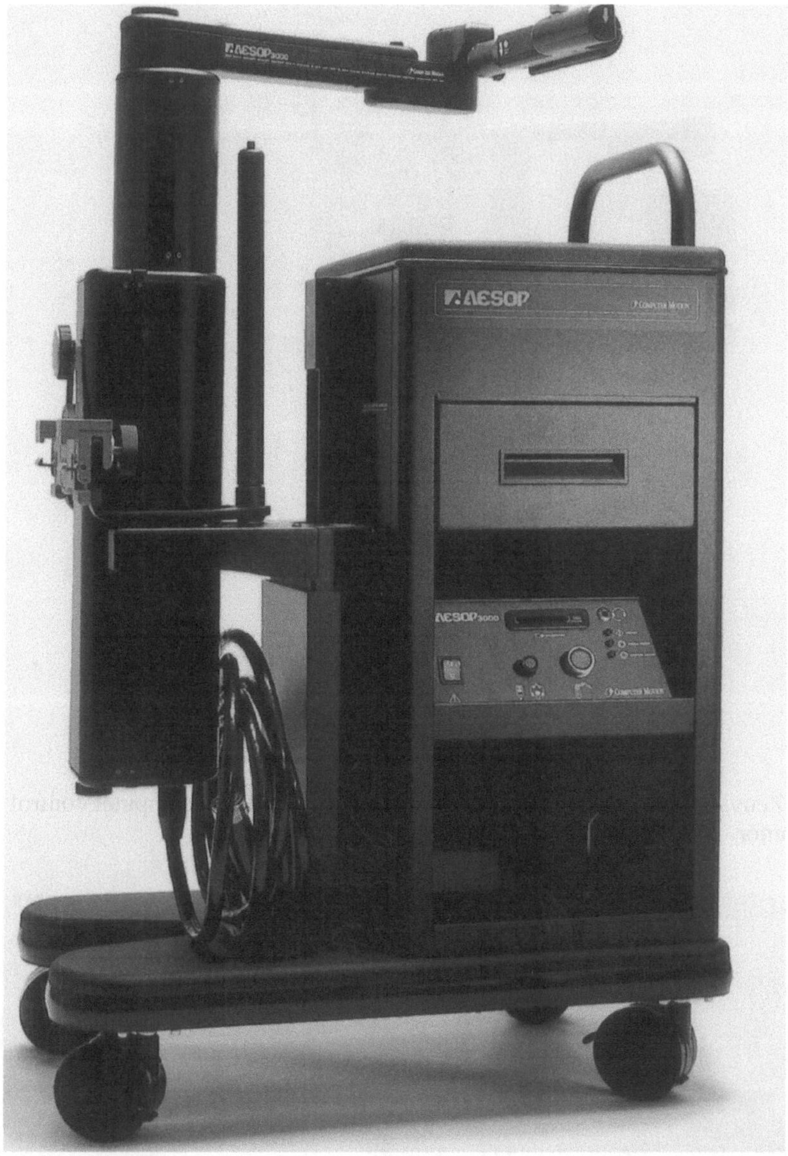

Fig. 1. The Aesop robotic arm. It can be mounted to the operating table and accommodates most conventional endoscopes.

performance has been shown to improve with this surgeon–instrument positioning *(10)*. A second display beneath the video monitor functions as a touch screen to provide control of instrument type, motion scaling, and the performance characteristics of the instrument end-effectors.

ADVANTAGES OF ROBOTIC SYSTEMS

The principal advantage of robotic assistance is the incorporation of a signal processor between the surgeon's hands and the instrument tips. By converting the surgeon's movements into a digital signal, his or her motions are processed to help compensate for the

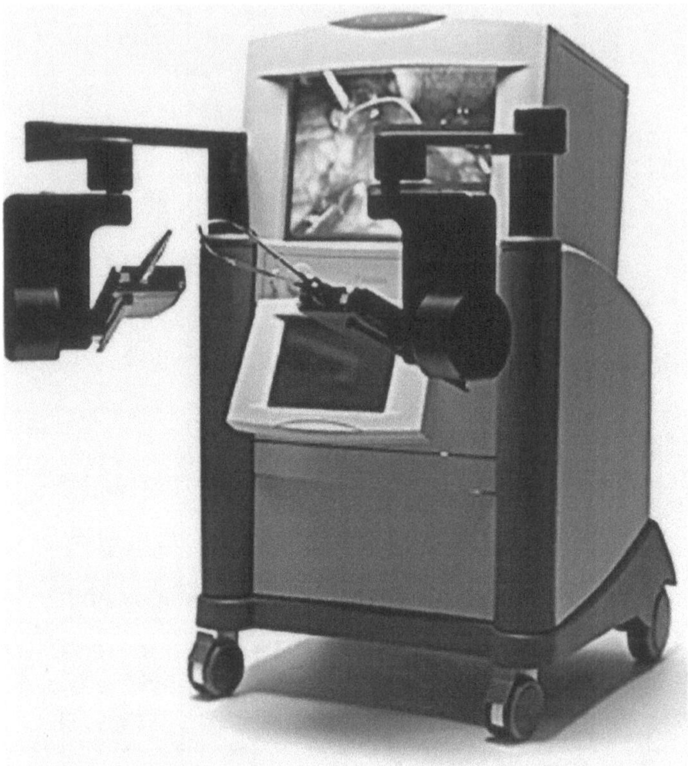

Fig. 2. The Zeus surgical console consists of instrument handles, a computer control system, and a video monitor.

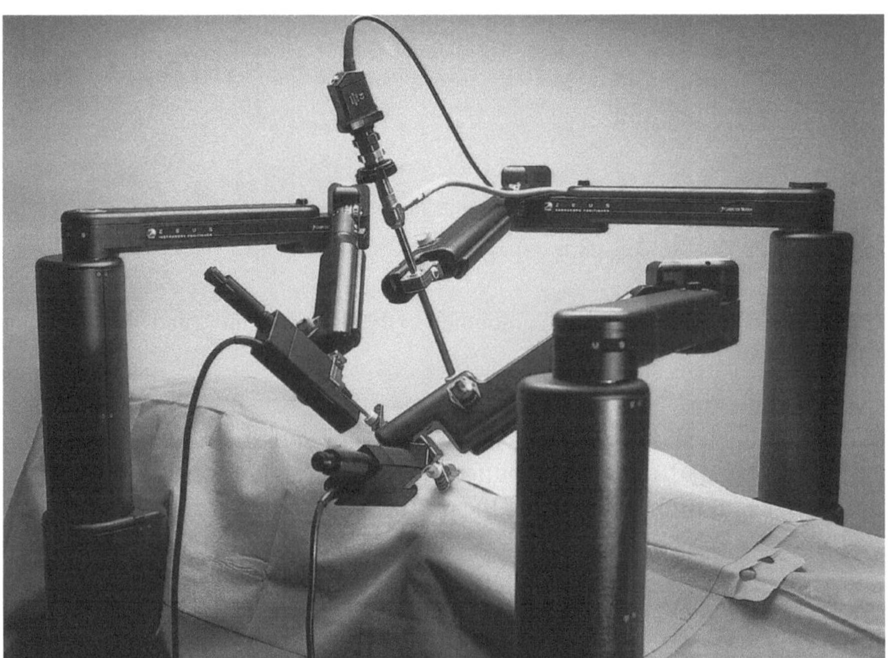

Fig. 3. The Zeus robotic arms are shown here attached to the operating room table.

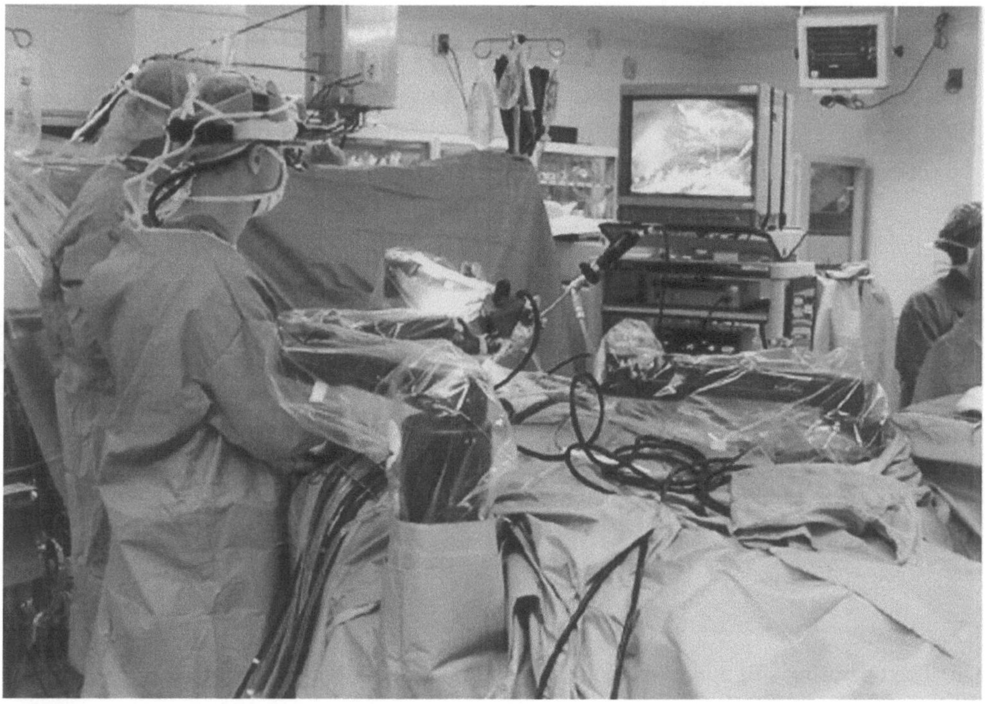

Fig. 4. The surgical team is positioned at the operating table and the robotic arms are positioned to minimize intrusions into the surgical working space.

shortcomings of conventional endoscopy. Tremor, a small-amplitude, high-frequency signal, can be filtered by the digital processor and effectively eliminated. To further improve surgical precision, the system provides for motion scaling. This allows gross movements at the console to be translated into fine movements by the robotic instruments at the operative site. For example, a 5-mm movement at the console, scaled at a ratio of 5 to 1, yields a 1-mm movement at the instrument tip. The Zeus system permits variable degrees of motion scaling (from 1:1 to 10:1), depending on surgeon preference, and can be increased in concert with the magnification. This "scaled telepresence" allows a surgeon to operate comfortably on extremely small structures. Work in our laboratory has shown that motion scaling plays a potentially greater role than tremor filtration in enhancing surgical precision with robotics *(11)*.

The degree of instrument rotation is also enhanced by the computer system. Zeus can increase instrument pronation and supination as needed, eliminating the rotational constraints of conventional endoscopy. Finally, computer-assisted instrumentation can remove the counterintuitive movements (fulcrum effect) required during manipulation of traditional endoscopic instruments. The digital processor automatically translates the surgeon's movements such that the robotic arms and instrument tips directly follow the movements of the instrument handles at the surgeon console.

The final components of the Zeus system are the robotic arms, which are mounted to the operating table. The three arms (two instruments and one camera) are lightweight (20 kg) and independent, allowing for flexibility in arm and port positions. The surgical assistant and the remainder of the surgical team are positioned in close proximity to the robotic arms (**Fig. 4**), while the surgeon is seated away from the table at the Zeus console

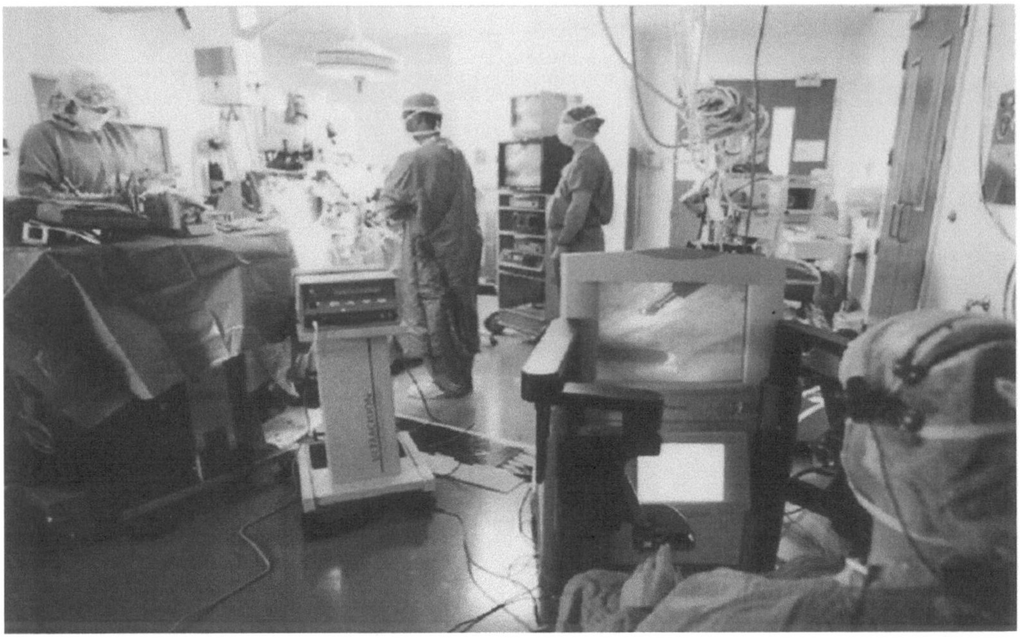

Fig. 5. The operating surgeon is seated at the Zeus surgical interface console.

(**Fig. 5**). If needed, the arms can be repositioned to accommodate the workspace requirements of the operative team.

The endoscopic instruments used in the Zeus system are custom-designed by Scanlan International. More than 20 different end effectors are offered, including needle drivers, ring forceps, tissue graspers, and microscissors (**Fig. 6**). The instruments are between 3 and 5 mm in diameter and are easily inserted through 5-mm ports. These instruments are smaller than conventional endoscopic instruments, are reusable, and can be conventionally sterilized. They can be interchanged freely within seconds during the operative case. The time required to set up the Zeus system has routinely been less than 20 min *(12)*.

CLINICAL RESULTS

The Zeus system has now been used in over 400 cases at 48 centers worldwide. This section describes the clinical results that have been reported with this system.

Coronary Artery Surgery

The Zeus system was first used clinically by Dr. Reichenspurner in Munich in September 1998 *(9)*. In his initial report, two patients with isolated left anterior descending (LAD) coronary artery disease underwent endoscopic harvesting of the left internal thoracic artery (LITA), followed by a small parasternal incision. The incision allowed for manual assistance and facilitation of the coronary anastomoses. The time required for LITA harvesting was 83 ± 110 min, and anastomotic time for both patients was 42 and 40 min. Both patients had uneventful postoperative recoveries, and follow-up revealed no evidence of recurrent angina.

A total of 25 patients with single- and multivessel disease have since undergone robotically assisted coronary artery bypass grafting (CABG) by Reichenspurner and his

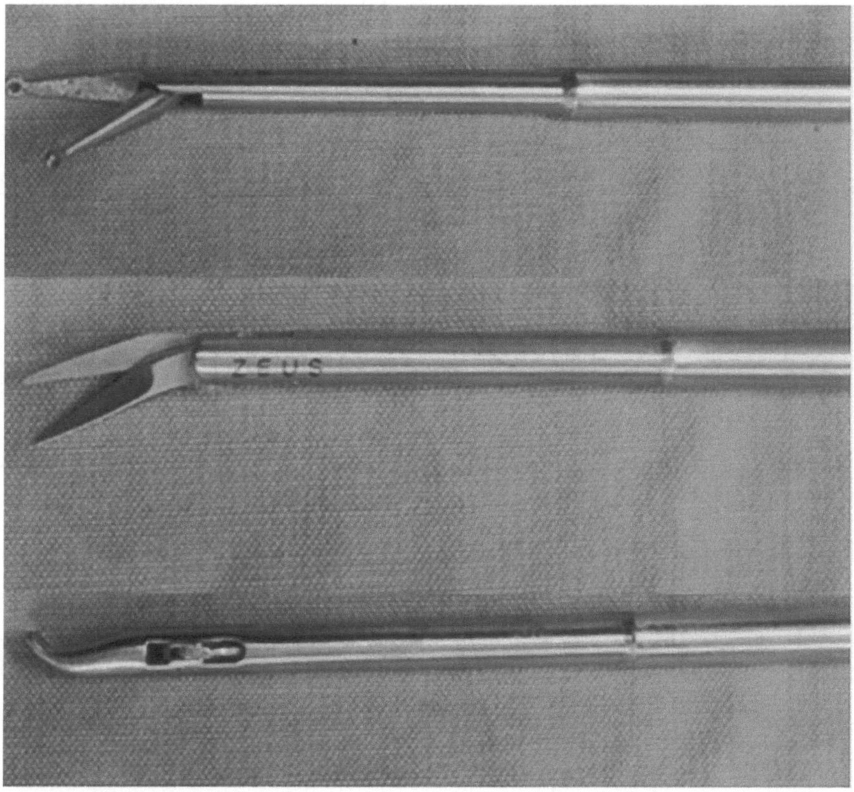

Fig. 6. The Zeus microsurgical instruments: curved needle driver (external diameter 3.9 mm), 15° Potts scissors, ring-tipped internal thoracic artery forceps.

group *(13)*. The initial 13 patients underwent a standard median sternotomy and implementation of cardiopulmonary bypass. Seventeen anastomoses were performed endoscopically in this group, including both LITA-to-LAD ($n = 13$), RITA-to-OM ($n = 2$), and saphenous vein graft to diagonal targets ($n = 2$). The next six patients underwent CABG (LITA-to-LAD) on the beating heart with a sternotomy approach. Continuing forward in a stepwise progression, four of the remaining six patients underwent a beating-heart approach using a limited paramedian incision (2–5 cm) for exposure.

In the entire clinical series, only two cases were converted to a manual anastomosis. Among the off-pump coronary artery bypass patients, the average anastomotic time was 29 min (range 19–50 min) and total operative time averaged 4.9 h (range 4.0–7.5 h). LITA preparation time averaged 55 min. One patient developed postoperative pneumonia requiring prolonged ventilation, but all other patients recovered uneventfully from surgery and were discharged after a median of 10.0 d (range 4–17 d). All patients underwent control angiography 7–9 d after surgery. All anastomoses sutured using the Zeus system were patent, without evidence of a stenosis greater than 50%. Twenty-three of the 25 patients have had postoperative follow-up at 3 mo, and all patients were free from angina, with both mortality and reintervention rates of 0%.

In the United States, the first robotically assisted cardiac surgical procedure was performed by Damiano and his group at Penn State University in December 1998 *(12)*. The U.S. Food and Drug Administration (FDA) approved a prospective single-center

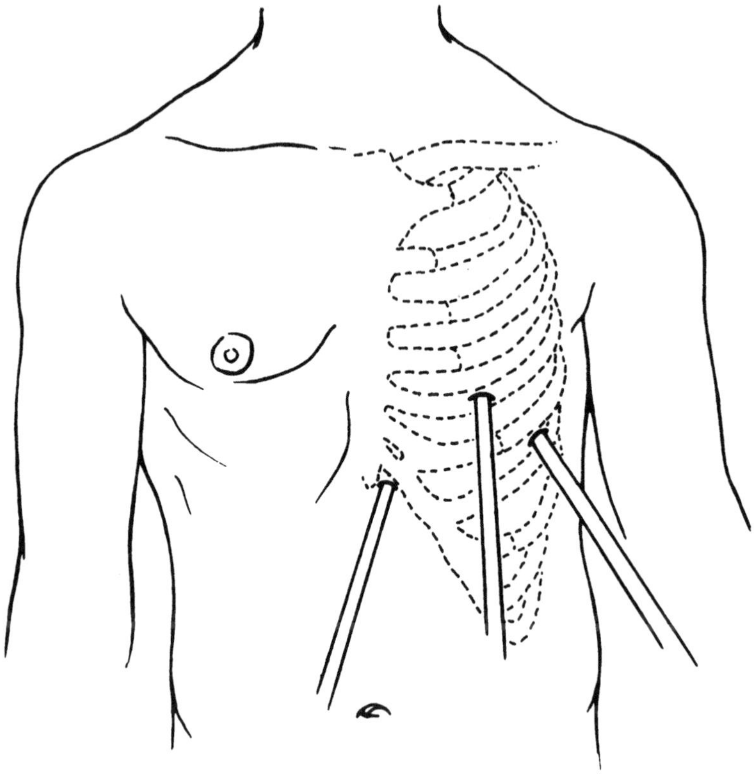

Fig. 7. The left and right instrument ports are positioned subxiphoid and in the seventh intercostal space in the anterior axillary line, respectively. The camera port is positioned in the fifth intercostal space at the mid-clavicular line.

clinical trial to evaluate the efficacy and safety of robotically assisted endoscopic CABG. Nineteen patients underwent a robotically assisted endoscopic anastomosis of the LITA to the LAD. Primary outcome measurements were device-related complications and graft patency at 6–8 wk.

All anastomoses were performed endoscopically through three instrument ports (**Fig. 7**). A 0° endoscope was attached to the Aesop voice-controlled robotic arm. A continuous end-to-side anastomosis was performed with a specially designed 7-cm, double-armed, 7-0 Gore-Tex suture (WL Gore & Assoc., Flagstaff, AZ), and graft flows were assessed using an ultrasonic flow probe and flow meter (Transonic Systems Inc., Ithaca, NY). As this study was approved only for a single-vessel bypass, all other grafts were completed manually prior to the robotic anastomosis.

The robotic system required an average setup time of 16 ± 1 min. There were no intraoperative complications related to port placement and no mechanical failures of the robotic system. The time required to perform the endoscopic LITA-to-LAD anastomosis was 22.5 ± 1.2 min (range 15–31 min), and the last 5 anastomoses were each performed in less than 20 min. All anastomoses were performed successfully, and no repair stitches were required. Eighty-nine percent (17/19) of the grafts measured were patent and had excellent diastolic flow by ultrasound. Average graft flow was 38 ± 5 mL/min. Two of the grafts had inadequate flow and were reconstructed manually. The average length of the stay in the ICU was 1.1 ± 1 d, and the average hospital stay was 4.1 ± 0.4 d.

There has been 100% late follow-up with an average follow-up of 17 ± 4.2 mo *(14)*. At the time, there were no late complications, and all patients were in New York Heart Association Class I. Eight weeks after surgery, graft patency was assessed by coronary angiography. This revealed all grafts to be patent, with TIMI 1 flow and no graft with a stenosis of greater than 50%.

In Canada, Boyd has accumulated a significant experience with endoscopic IMA harvesting using the Zeus system and has the largest series of totally closed endoscopic coronary bypass grafting among all Zeus clinical sites. Boyd and associates have also proceeded in a stepwise fashion toward robotically assisted coronary surgery. Initially, his group prospectively investigated the use of the Aesop robotic arm during ITA harvest *(15)*. In 55 consecutive patients, ITAs were harvested endoscopically using three 5-mm incisions and a 30° endoscope. Anastomoses were initially completed manually through a limited thoracotomy. The average harvest time was 57.4 ± 22.8 min. Robotic camera assistance significantly reduced the number of endoscopic cleanings and was felt to facilitate the more difficult dissections. The Aesop arm responded reliably to greater than 95% of verbal commands, and there was 100% patency in the 14 patients who underwent postoperative angiography.

Subsequently *(16)*, the Harmonic scalpel (Ethicon Endo-Surgery, Cincinnati, OH) was adapted to a Zeus robotic arm and 19 patients underwent LITA harvest using a robotically controlled harmonic scalpel with computer-assisted video control (Aesop). In three patients, the Zeus system was also additionally used for RITA harvest. The investigators concluded that the Zeus system could safely be used for bilateral ITA harvesting even when anterior–posterior working space was limited. The advantages of the robot controlled endoscope included greater exposure, superior image quality, and a consistent quality of assistance, improving video dexterity and lessening surgeon fatigue.

Boyd's group has used the Zeus system for beating-heart coronary anastomoses in 12 patients undergoing single-vessel CABG through a limited thoracotomy. The anastomotic times for the ITA-to-LAD were 80 ± 27 min. No repair sutures were required, and average graft flows were 38 ± 24 mL/min. Follow-up angiography has been performed in all patients. All anastomoses were patent at an average of 1.4 ± 0.8 d postoperatively, and 10 of 12 were of Fitzgibbons grade A.

Boyd has since performed a closed-chest, totally endoscopic, beating-heart CABG on 6 patients using the Zeus robotic system *(17)*. The first totally endoscopic beating-heart case was on September 1999. Using a 0° endoscope, Aesop, and warm carbon dioxide gas insufflation, sufficient working space and visibility were established within the mediastinum. For three patients, a specially designed sternal elevator was required to increase anteroposterior intrathoracic space. With the patients in a right lateral decubitus position, trocars were inserted in the third, fifth, and seventh interspaces along the mid to anterior axillary lines. The Zeus robotic arms were mounted on the operating table (**Fig. 8**). In preparation for the beating-heart anastomosis, an articulating endo-stabilizer (Computer Motion, Goleta, CA) was inserted through a port in the second interspace at the anterior axillary line for LAD stabilization.

In this clinical series, anastomotic times varied between 40 and 74 min (mean 55.8 min). All anastomoses had acceptable flows (mean 28.3 mL/min, range 12–46 mL/min), and no patients required conversion from the robotic technique. Median operative time for the procedure was 6 h (range 4.5–7.5 h). Patients were intubated for an average of 8.5 h (range 0–23 h) postoperatively. All but one patient was discharged from the ICU on the first postoperative day. Postoperatively, all patients underwent coronary angiography before

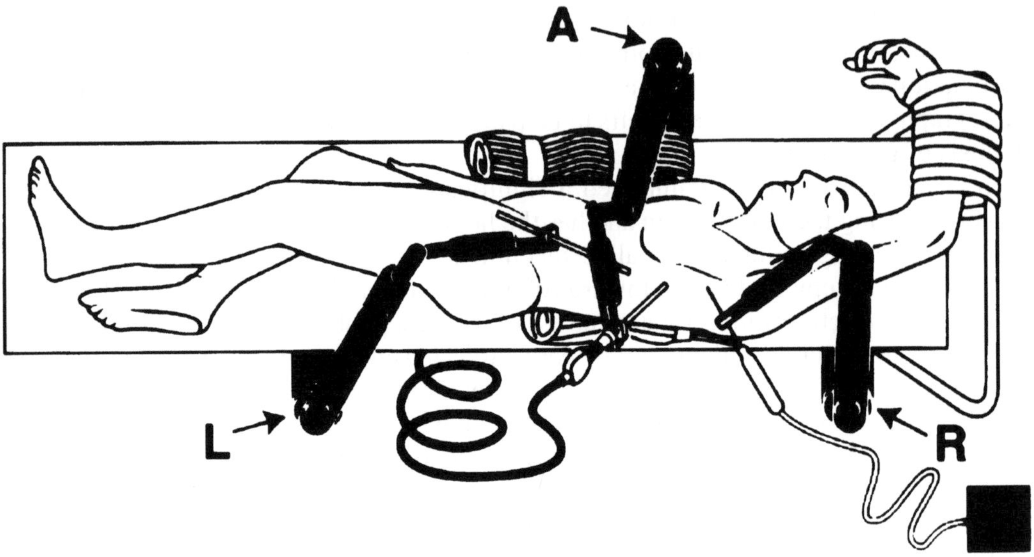

Fig. 8. The patient is positioned in the 30° right lateral decubitus position. The right and left robotic arms are mounted on the left side of the table opposite the patient's head and at the mid-thigh level. The Aesop arm is mounted on the right side of the operating table.

hospital discharge, and five of six grafts were found to be patent. One had a 50% stenosis in the region of the distal snare site. Hospital average length of stay was 4.0 ± 0.9 d. All patients were free from angina, had returned to work, and had normal exercise capacity at a mean follow-up of 145.3 ± 29.6 d.

In summary, the U.S., Canadian, and European experiences have demonstrated the capabilities of robotic assistance for enabling endoscopic CABG. Currently, a prospective, randomized multicenter trial is underway. The objectives of this trial are to assess the safety and effectiveness of the Zeus Robotic Surgical system when used to perform an anastomosis of the LITA to the LAD. Patients are to be randomized to either robotically assisted or traditional CABG. All patients will undergo predischarge angiography to assess LITA-to-LAD patency. This study will be the first randomized trial of robotic cardiac surgery and represents an important step toward validating the use of computer-assisted surgery in coronary bypass grafting.

Valve Surgery

The first steps in minimally invasive valve surgery involved the use of smaller incisions than the traditional median sternotomy but remained direct-vision procedures. Surgeons found that these incisions provided adequate exposure and reported encouraging results, with low mortality and complication rates *(18,19)*. These minimally invasive procedures were often performed with Heartport Port-Access™ (Redwood, CA) technology. This endovascular cardiopulmonary bypass system was usually inserted via the femoral vessels and, as a result, removed the perfusion tubing from the thoracic incision *(20)*.

Chitwood et al. have progressively increased the role of computer assistance for both mitral valve repair and replacement *(21,22)*. Using a three-dimensional head-mounted video display and an Aesop-controlled endoscope, this group has performed computer-assisted surgery for major portions of valvular surgery in 110 patients. In their series, operative mortality was reported at 0.9%. Although aortic crossclamp times were longer than for conventional sternotomy patients, there were fewer reported complications. The surgeon-controlled camera tracking was found to be more intuitive. Technically, the video assistance was particularly advantageous for providing stable lighting and vibration-free viewing of the subvalvular apparatus. These benefits have quickly helped transition this team and others from video-assisted surgery toward video-directed mitral procedures in which almost all of the procedure is performed under endoscopic vision *(23)*. Details of this experience are reported in Chapter 19.

Reichenspurner et al. reported a similar series of 50 patients who underwent mitral valve operations with Port-Access technology and 3-D video assistance, the last 20 patients using the Aesop robotic arm *(23)*. Using a right submammary incision (4–7 cm) and a three-dimensional endoscopic camera, the surgeon was able to see the operative site through both the incision and the endoscopic picture displayed inside his helmet without moving his head. The endoscopic picture was most useful in viewing the subvalvular apparatus and checking the position of sutures and knots. In this series there was no mortality, and at 3 mo follow-up, 85% of patients were in NYHA Class I.

Investigators have now begun to incorporate the Zeus system into mitral valve procedures. As part of a FDA-approved Phase I clinical trial, Grossi has recently reported a case of posterior leaflet prolapse in a 50-yr-old man that was reconstructed with the use of the Zeus telemanipulator *(24)*. Using a right anterior 6-cm thoracotomy, the valve repair required 3 h 2 min of cardiopulmonary bypass, and robotic instrumentation was used for a total of 69 min. Postoperative echocardiography revealed only trace mitral regurgitation, and the patient was discharged on postoperative d 3. Aesop was felt to have afforded superior visualization, allowing for improved teaching and operating-room integration. The investigators have also reported successful completion of a mitral valve replacement using a 3-cm "service entrance" and Port-Access cardiopulmonary bypass in a canine model *(25)*. The procedure was performed using an interrupted-suture technique. After the procedure, normal prosthetic valve function was found in all animals.

Aesop and Zeus have also been used in other cardiac procedures, including atrial septal defect repair and patent ductus arteriosus ligation and pericardiectomy for effusive pericardial disease *(26–28)*. These procedures have principally incorporated the techniques of minimally invasive valvular surgery, including Port-Access™ cardiopulmonary bypass and small "service incisions." These reports are encouraging and indicate the potential applicability for robotics in various types of cardiac surgery. As a first-generation robotic system, Zeus has enabled several cardiac procedures. As these systems improve, their utility in both current and future procedures should continue to expand.

ROBOTIC TRAINING

Before attempting to use a robotic system clinically, it is critical that surgeons undergo extensive training to gain familiarity with both the endoscopic approach and to learn the nuances of the robotic system. There is a definite learning curve with robotic systems, even for simple skill drills. The robotic systems, however, can be easily learned by those with and without prior endoscopic experience *(29)*. The current recommended training regimen includes 80–100 h of practice in inanimate models, live animals, and cadavers. It is recommended that centers without prior robotic experience begin their clinical cases through a full sternotomy. This provides a safety margin for the patient and allows the surgical team to become familiar with robotically assisted endoscopic surgery. Endoscopic experience should be increased gradually by requiring centers first to perform a series of robotically assisted endoscopic ITA harvests, after which the surgeon completes the coronary anastomosis by hand. After the surgical team gains experience and becomes comfortable with the endoscopic ITA takedown, the surgeon can proceed to robotically assisted anastomoses. Eventually, the sternotomy and left thoracotomy can be abandoned, proceeding to a total endoscopic procedure.

FUTURE DIRECTIONS

Although there has been tremendous progress in the development of robotically assisted cardiac surgery over the last several years, there still are many challenges ahead that must be overcome in order to widen the applicability of these techniques and to demonstrate their clinical value. At present, these operations are often lengthy, technically difficult, and applicable only to carefully selected patients. However, as with the introduction of laparoscopy in general surgery, the accumulation of surgical experience with this sophisticated instrumentation in a closed-chest environment will, over time, improve operative choreography, resulting in shorter operating times and easier procedures. The development of parallel technologies to facilitate the anastomoses, improve operative exposure and working space, and assist in port placement will result in significant advances in the field.

One of the most significant challenges that face surgeons embarking on endoscopic procedures is the determination of optimal port placement. Both surgical experience and likely the use of computer guidance should facilitate this in the future. Using computerized tomography and magnetic resonance imaging, preliminary efforts toward the development of a three-dimensional virtual cardiac surgical planning platform has been initiated for use with totally endoscopic cardiac surgery *(30)*. It also is expected that improved microsurgical instruments will help facilitate these procedures. Computer Motion is planning on introducing a Microwrist™. This will add an articulating joint close to the instrument tip or end-effector (**Fig. 9**). This extra degree of freedom should simplify the performance of complex maneuvers in this environment.

The real significance of robotically assisted cardiac surgery lies in the resulting integration of computers into the operating room. This will affect three principal areas: surgeon control, intraoperative imaging, and information access. Future improvements in the digital–manual interface will continue to enhance a surgeon's technical ability with these systems. Endoscopic procedures will become more feasible as computers become more powerful and less expensive. Technological improvements in the robotic systems should bring us closer to a more ideal microsurgical system over the next decade. This ideal system would include fully replicated master kinematics, a full range of end-effectors, effective and simple site delivery, tactile feedback, superb three-dimensional optics, and data fusion capability to allow for computer- and image-guided surgery.

With further enhancements, it is likely that we will be able to preprogram simple surgical maneuvers to assist in suturing and the performance of an anastomosis. These systems may eventually "learn" surgical techniques with the use of neural networks. This will not only allow present procedures to be performed less invasively, it will also enable surgeons to perform a wide range of procedures that heretofore have been impossible because of the inherent physical shortcomings of human beings.

Computers will also revolutionize intraoperative imaging. The future will see the introduction of image-guided cardiac surgery. Surgeons will be able to manipulate images

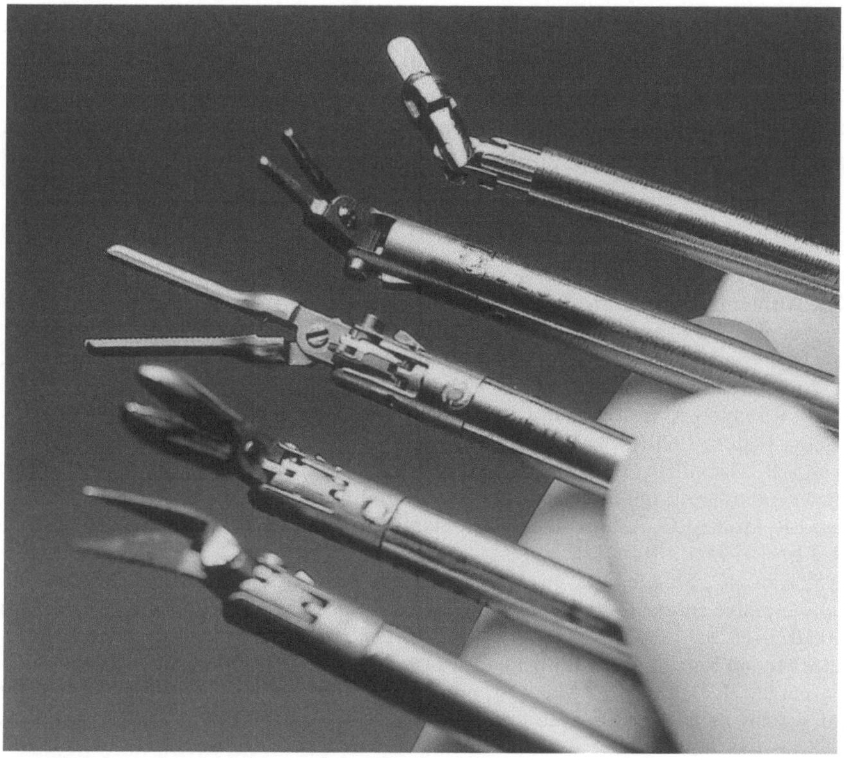

Fig. 9. The Zeus Microwrist instruments provide "wrist" articulation and an additional degree of freedom. (Reprinted with permission of Computer Motion; photograph by Bobbi Bennett.)

intraoperatively and view digital echocardiograms, angiograms, CT, and MRI scans directly on the video monitor. If needed, these images will be superimposed directly on the operative field. Fused with endoscopic pictures, surgeons may be able to define intracardiac and extracardiac anatomy precisely without direct visualization, perhaps one day guiding percutaneous access to intracardiac structures. Manipulation of our digital visual interface may also make it possible to operate on a beating heart while working in "virtual stillness." The movement of the robotic camera and instruments can be synchronized with every heartbeat, effectively canceling cardiac motion and increasing surgical precision. A prototype already has been developed by industry and may become available in the near future.

Finally, there will be improvements in information access. In the operating room, networked video monitors will provide access to the hospital information system and ancillary services (i.e., radiology, cardiac catheterization laboratory, and echocardiography), as well as to local area networks, the Internet, and the hospital library. This technology will allow for experts throughout the world to assist their colleagues via high-speed video links.

As surgeons, our challenge will be not to let ourselves be defined by the size of our incisions. We must become cardiac interventionists, performing a wide range of percutaneous interventions on various intrathoracic structures. Our understanding of the three-dimensional anatomy of the chest and surgical training make us ideally suited to perform these procedures and handle potential complications. It is likely that we will play a key role in the future of gene therapy, angiogenesis, arrhythmia ablation, and other areas not traditionally thought to be the domain of the surgeon. The era of computer-assisted surgery has begun and promises to be one of the dramatic advances in our capability as cardiac surgeons. Robotics and computer assistance has the potential to transform both our operating rooms and our specialty as we enter the new millennium.

REFERENCES

1. Rosen M, Ponsky J. Minimally invasive surgery. Endoscopy 2001;33(4):358–366.
2. Vilos GA, Alshimmiri MM. Cost-benefit analysis of laparoscopic versus laparotomy salpingo-oophorectomy for benign tubo-ovarian disease. J Am Assoc Gynecol Laparosc 1995;2(3):299–303.
3. Seifman BD, Wolf JS Jr. Technical advances in laparoscopy: hand assistance retractors, and the pneumodissector. J Endourol 2000;14(10):921–928.
4. Hanna GB, Cuschieri A. Influence of the optical axis-to-target view angle on endoscopic task performance. Surg Endosc 1999;13(4):371–375.
5. Cresswell AB, Macmillan AI, Hanna GB, et al. Methods for improving performance under reverse alignment conditions during endoscopic surgery. Surg Endosc 1999;13(6):591–594.
6. Kavoussi LR, Moore RG, Adams JB, et al. Comparison of robotic versus human laparoscopic camera control. J Urol 1995;6:2134–2136.
7. Geis WP, Kim HC, McAfee PC, et al. Synergistic benefits of combined technologies in complex, minimally invasive surgical procedures: clinical experience and educational processes. Surg Endosc 1996;10:1025–1028.
8. Computer Motion Report. Santa Barbara, CA, June 2000.
9. Reichenspurner H, Damiano R, Mack M, et al. Use of the voice-controlled and computer-assisted surgical system Zeus™ endoscopic coronary artery bypass grafting. J Thorac Cardiovasc Surg 1999;118:11–16.
10. Hanna GB, Shimi SM, Cuschieri A. Task performance in endoscopic surgery is influenced by location of the image display. Ann Surg 1998;227(4):481–484.
11. Prasad SM, Maniar HS, Klingensmith ME, et al. Prospective randomized evaluation of robotic versus laparoscopic surgical training: advantages of computer-assisted surgery. 2002 American College of Surgeons. San Francisco, CA.
12. Damiano RJ Jr, Ehrman WJ, Ducko CT, et al. Initial United States clinical trial of robotically assisted endoscopic coronary artery bypass grafting. J Thorac Cardiovasc Surg 2000;119(1):77–82.
13. Boehm DH, Reichenspurner H, Detter C, et al. Clinical use of a computer-enhanced surgical robotic system for endoscopic coronary artery bypass grafting on the beating heart. Thorac Cardiovasc Surg 2000;48(4):198–202.
14. Prasad SM, Ducko CT, Stephenson ER, et al. Prospective clinical trial of robotically assisted endoscopic coronary grafting with 1-year follow-up. Ann Surg 2001;233(6):725–732.
15. Boyd WD, Kiaii B, Novick RJ, et al. RAVECAB: improving outcome in off-pump minimal access surgery with robotic assistance and video enhancement. Can J Surg 2001;44(1):45–50.
16. Kiai B, Boyd WD, Rayman R, et al. Robot-assisted computer enhanced closed-chest coronary surgery: preliminary experience using a harmonic scalpel® and ZEUS™. Heart Surg Forum 2000;3(3):194–197.
17. Boyd WD, Rayman R, Desai ND, et al. Closed-chest coronary artery bypass grafting on the beating heart with the use of a computer-enhanced surgical robotic system. J Thorac Cardiovasc Surg 2000;120(4):807–809.
18. Cosgrove DM, Sabik JF, Navia JL. Minimally invasive valve surgery. Ann Thorac Surg 1998;65:1535–1538.
19. Navia JL, Cosgrove DM. Minimally invasive mitral valve operations. Ann Thorac Surg 1996;62:1542–1544.
20. Grossi, EA, La Pietra A, Galloway AC, et al. Videoscopic mitral valve repair and replacement using the port-access technique. Adv Card Surg 2001;13:77–88.
21. Chitwood WR Jr, Nifong LW. Minimally invasive videoscopic mitral valve surgery: the current role of surgical robotics. J Card Surg 2000;15(1):61–75.
22. Chitwood WR Jr. Video-assisted and robotic mitral valve surgery: toward an endoscopic surgery. Semin Thorac Cardiovasc Surg 1999;11(3):194–205.
23. Reichenspurner H, Boehm DH, Gulbins H, et al. Three-dimensional video and robot-assisted port-access mitral valve operation. Ann Thorac Surg 2000;69:1176–1182.
24. Grossi EA, LaPietra A, Applebaum RM, et al. Case report of robotic instrument-enhanced mitral valve surgery. J Thorac Cardiovasc Surg 2000;120(6):1169–1171.

25. La Pietra A, Grossi EA, Derivaux CC, et al. Robotic-assisted instruments enhance minimally invasive mitral valve surgery. Ann Thorac Surg 2000;70:835–838.
26. Luison F, Boyd WD. Three-dimensional video-assisted thoracoscopic pericardiectomy. Ann Thorac Surg 2000;70(6):2137–2138.
27. Torracca L, Ismeno G, Alfieri O. Totally endoscopic atrial septal defect closure using robotic techniques: report of two cases. Ital Heart J 2000;1(10);698–701.
28. Laborde F, Folliguet T, Da Cruz E, et al. Video surgical technique for interruption of patent ductus arteriosus in children and neonates. Pediatr Pulmonol 1997;suppl 16:177–179.
29. Prasad SM, Maniar HM, Damiano RJ Jr, et al. The effects of robotic assistance on learning curves for basic laparoscopic drills. Am J Surg 2002;183:702–707.
30. Chiu AM, Dey D, Drangova M, et al. 3-D image guidance for minimally invasive robotic coronary artery bypass. Heart Surg Forum 2000;3(3):224–231.

31 Robotics and Telemanipulation

The da Vinci™ System

Volkmar Falk, MD, PHD,
Thomas Walther, MD, PHD,
and Friedrich W. Mohr, MD, PHD

CONTENTS

HISTORICAL BACKGROUND AND BASIC PRINCIPLES OF TELEMANIPULATION
THE DA VINCI™ SYSTEM: TECHNOLOGY
EXPERIMENTAL AND CLINICAL EXPERIENCE
DISCUSSION
REFERENCES

HISTORICAL BACKGROUND AND BASIC PRINCIPLES OF TELEMANIPULATION

Telemanipulation systems are a class of robotics that enable the operator to work remotely by a computerized human–machine interface. The first teleoperated devices were built in 1890 by Nicola Tesla, an ingenious inventor who also developed the induction motor and AC power transmission. The concept of teleoperation describes a form of control in which the human directly guides and causes each increment of motion of the manipulator. In the 1950s telemanipulators were used mainly to handle toxic waste. In these early systems, the master and manipulator were kinematically (geometrically) identical. The joints of the manipulator followed that of the master through the same trajectory, representing master and manipulator motions as joint coordinates. Since these systems were purely mechanically linked, the scale between the master and the manipulator was fixed. The first electronically augmented telemanipulator was developed by Goertz *(1)*. Instead of a pure mechanical linkage, motors and sensors connected the master and the manipulator unit. With the availability of computers, online calculation

From: *Contemporary Cardiology: Minimally Invasive Cardiac Surgery, Second Edition*
Edited by: D. J. Goldstein and M. C. Oz © Humana Press Inc., Totowa, NJ

Table 1
Limitations of Conventional Endoscopic Instruments—Comparison to Computer Enhanced Instrumentation Systems

	Endoscopic Instruments	*Telemanipulator*
Degress of freedom	4	4–6
Tremor filter	No	Yes
Motion transmission	Fixed, depending on the ratio of internal/external shaft length	1:1 to 5:1
Hand–eye alignment	Poor	Natural
Fulcrum effect	Reversed mothio	Not an issue
Force ratio (handle/tip)	Large/abnormal/not linear	Programming/linear
Indexing	Not possible	Possible
Ergonomics	Unfavorable	Favorable

of cartesian coordinate transformations became possible. This marked the onset of telemanipulation systems with different kinematic designs for the master and the manipulator. The first six-axis manipulator for human bi-directional telemanipulation was built by Bejczy and Salisbury and included force feedback through motors on the hand controller *(2)*. Since then, a variety of "computer-enhanced" telemanipulation systems have been developed for remote handling in hazardous environments or confined spaces. Most designs follow the anthropomorphic principle, providing a humanlike range of motion for the manipulator joints. Accordingly, the joints of a serial link manipulator can be viewed as shoulder, elbow, and wrist joints.

The introduction of endoscopic techniques in the 1980s heralded the birth of minimally invasive surgery. The use of trocars decreased the surgical trauma associated with large conventional incisions, but at the cost of a substantial loss in dexterity, altered hand–eye coordination, and a limited range of motion (Table 1) *(3,4)*. Interestingly, the development of surgical telemanipulators was not driven by the shortcomings of endoscopic instruments but rather by the idea of remote care of trauma patients *(5)*. An intuitive telemanipulator system that would allow distant surgeons to treat injured patients remotely was thought to potentially improve the outcome from severe injuries. As a result, a prototype telepresence surgery system (SRI) with bimanual force-reflective manipulators with four degrees of freedom (DOF), interchangeable surgical instruments, and stereoscopic video input was developed and used remotely to close arteriotomies and to repair lacerations of internal organs *(6,7)*. In parallel, the German Research Institute in Karlsruhe developed the first 6-DOF telemanipulator (Advanced Robot and Telemanipulator System for Minimally Invasive Surgery, ARTEMIS), which was designed primarily to improve dexterity during laparoscopic procedures and was used to perform experimental cholecystectomies *(8,9)*. The potential for combining the complementary abilities of humans and machines for surgical interventions has been outlined by Taylor (Table 2) *(3,4)*.

THE DA VINCI™ SYSTEM: TECHNOLOGY

Two telemanipulation systems are currently commercially available, the Zeus™ (Computer Motion, Goleta, CA; *see* Chapter 30) and the da Vinci™ system (Intuitive Surgical, Mountain View, CA). The da Vinci technology is based on the early SRI concept. The

Table 2
Complementary Skills of Human Operator and Robotic Devices (Modified from Taylor *[3,4]*)

	Strengths	*Limitations*
Humans	Strong hand–eye alignment	Tremor
	Excellent dexterity	Fatigue
	Flexible	Manipulation and dexterity limited outside natural scale
	Adaptive	Limited geometric accuracy
	Able to use qualitative date	Does not use quantitative data naturally
	Easy to Instruct	Susceptible to radiation, infection
	Able to learn	
	Integrates extensive and diverse information	
Robots	Good geometric accuracy	Poor judgment
	Untiring and stable	Difficult to instruct
	Precisely calibrated forces	Low bandwidth
	Various design options	Limited ability to perform complex control and hand–eye tasks
	Works in hazardous environment	
	Can incorporate various sensors into control laws	

system consists of two major components, a master console and a cart-mounted manipulator. The console houses the display system, the master handles, the user interface, and the electronic controller (**Fig. 1**) *(10–13)*. The master handles are serial link manipulators that act both as high-resolution input devices, reading the position, orientation, and grip commands from the surgeon, and as haptic displays, transmitting forces and torques to the surgeon in response to various measured and synthetic force cues (bi-directional). The masters are gravity-compensated to minimize fatigue of the operator. The image of the surgical site is transmitted to the surgeon through a high-resolution stereo display (two separate optical channels with a maximum resolution of 2.0 mrad/line pair). The system projects the image of the surgical site atop the surgeon's hands (via mirrored overlay optics), while the controller transforms the spatial motion of the tools into the camera frame of reference. In this way the system provides natural hand–eye coordination (**Fig. 2**). Motion scaling allows for various ratios for master and manipulator motions. By activating a foot switch, the operator is able to temporarily uncouple and reposition the masters in the working field while the instrument tips remain stationary (indexing). A tremor filter is used to minimize involuntary motions. The camera is also controlled by the master handles. By activating a foot switch, the masters control motion of the scope in four axes (rotational, insertion, two translational). A variety of scopes is available (0°, 30°, small, and wide-angled view). By selecting the scope at the console, the masters are automatically realigned according to the chosen scope angle.

The patient-side cart consists of two instrument manipulators and a central camera manipulator (**Fig. 3**). The camera manipulator has 4 DoF and holds the endoscope. The multiple-use end-effectors attach interchangeably to the two instrument manipulators, which feature an automated instrument recognition system. The manipulator provides 3 DoF (insertion and translation in two planes), while the end-effectors add another 3 DoF

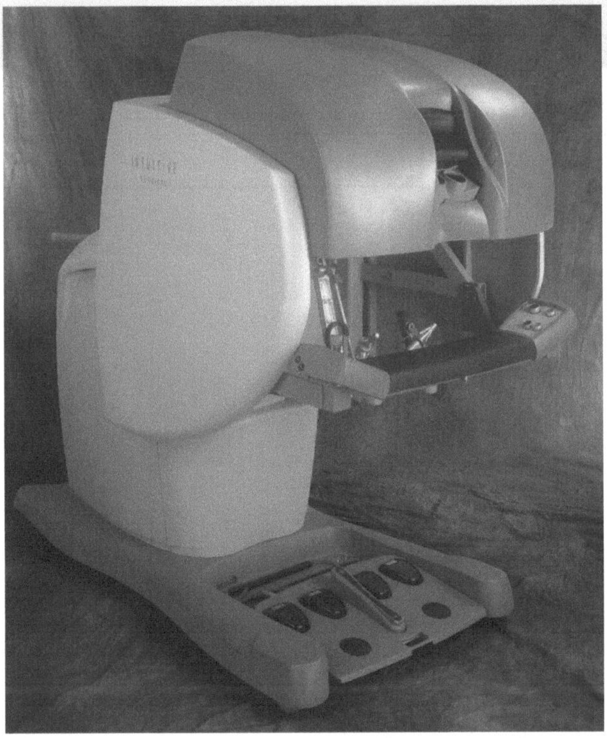

Fig. 1. Da Vinci surgical telemanipulation system: surgeon's console.

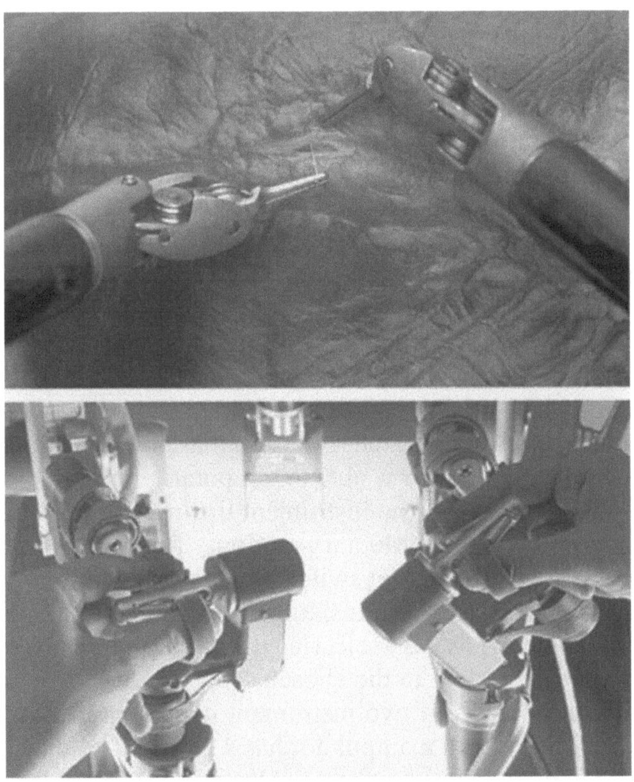

Fig. 2. Surgeon's view through viewer at the console (*top*) and orientation of master handles (*bottom*) demonstrating perfect hand–eye alignment.

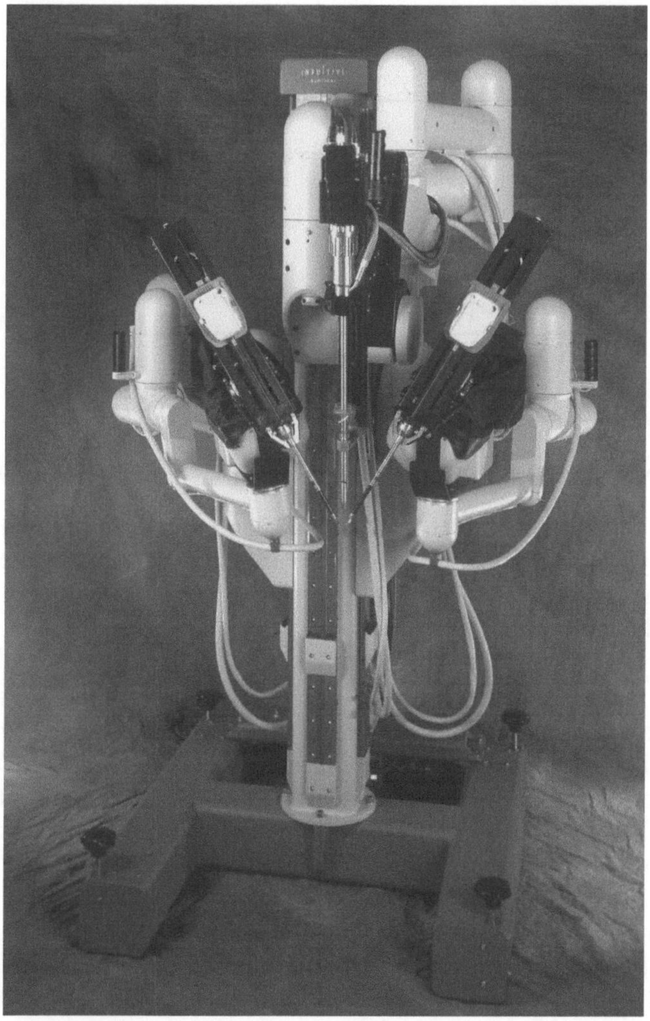

Fig. 3. Cart-mounted manipulator.

(rotation and two additional pitch and yaw axes at the tip). By means of this endowrist, a total of 6 DoF are provided, allowing for free motion and orientation of the tip in space. All three patient-side manipulators use remote-center technology to minimize shear stress at the site of insertion. The system setup on the patient side takes approx 15 min, and emergency removal of the manipulator from the patient can be performed in seconds. The ideal position for the setup joints of the instrument arms is 90° between the primary and secondary axis ("shoulder") and 45° between the secondary and tertiary axis ("elbow"). For the camera arm the net sum of angles should be 0°, resulting in straight alignment of the scope and the central column. With this setup there should be no necessity to move the setup joints during the procedure. The remote centers should be placed correctly within the ports to provide the highest precision and lowest friction. The system has been cleared by the U.S. Food and Drug Administration (FDA) for laparoscopic and thoracoscopic (ITA take-down) procedures and has received CE mark approval in Europe. Clinical trials to obtain FDA approval for coronary artery bypass surgery and mitral valve repair are currently underway.

Table 3
Worldwide Experience with the da Vinci System as of September 2001

Procedure	*n*
ITA[a] take-down	1337
TECAB[b] (arrested heart)	121
TECAB (beating heart)	80
Mitral valve repair	135
Atrial septal defect repair	42

[a]Internal thoracic artery.
[b]Total endoscopic coronary artery bypass.

EXPERIMENTAL AND CLINICAL EXPERIENCE

As of September 2002, more than 2000 cardiac procedures including endoscopic coronary artery bypass grafting, mitral valve repair, and atrial septal defect (ASD) closure have been performed—in part or completely—using the da Vinci system in some 45 centers around the world (Table 3).

Coronary Artery Bypass Surgery

Prior to clinical trials, a number of experimental studies were performed that demonstrated the feasibility of remote suturing of coronary anastomoses *(14–16)*. Other experimental studies demonstrated the superiority of 6- vs 4-DoF telemanipulator design and highlighted the importance of high-resolution three-dimensional vision to perform remote endoscopic procedures using a telemanipulation system *(17,18)*. A total endoscopic coronary artery bypass grafting procedure (TECAB) was first developed in a cadaver model through three ports and without assistance. In addition, a transabdominal, transdiaphragmatic endoscopic approach for double-vessel grafting was developed *(19)*.

In December 1998, the da Vinci system was introduced clinically, with the main focus on endoscopic coronary surgery *(20)*. In the majority of cases the system was used to harvest the internal thoracic artery endoscopically. After an initial learning curve that was similar in most centers using this technology, harvest times for the left internal thoracic artery (ITA) are now in the range of 30–40 min, and the technique is routinely performed in a number of centers *(21,22)*. For robotic-assisted ITA harvest, patients are placed in a supine position with the left chest slightly elevated and the left arm lowered. Single (right)-lung ventilation is performed. A 30° scope angled up is inserted at the fourth intercostal space. Continuous CO_2 insufflation is applied to enhance exposure by increasing the available space between the heart and the sternum. Although insufflation pressures up to 10 mmHg are usually well tolerated, hemodynamic studies have demonstrated an increase in right ventricular filling pressures, a decrease of intrathoracic blood volume index, and right ventricular ejection fraction with increasing insufflation pressures. As a result, cardiac index and MAP may decrease despite a compensatory increase in heart rate *(23)*. The instrument ports are created in the third and sixth intercostal spaces. Depending on the individual's body habitus, ports are created in a flat triangle (with the central camera port placed a little bit lower than the two instrument ports) or in an almost linear fashion following the anterior axillary line. The ITA is usually dissected as a pedicle from the first rib to the sixth inercostal space using low-energy cautery. Clips are rarely used. The precision of the instruments allows for a skeletonized take-down technique. As in conventional harvest, care must be taken to avoid injury of the subclavian vein and the phrenic nerve while dissecting the proximal part of the ITA. ITA harvesting is now performed routinely and allows tailoring the thoracotomy incision necessary for a MIDCAB procedure. As of this writing, 1350 cases of robotic ITA take-downs have been reported (Table 3). If the ITA is to be used for a TECAB procedure, the vessel is skeletonized distally, and cut and trimmed for the anastomosis *in situ*, using the native tissue for countertraction *(24)*. The pedicle is not detached from the chest wall until the anastomosis is finally performed, to avoid torsion of the graft and any interference during pericardiotomy. For bilateral ITA take-down, the right pleural space is opened and the right ITA is dissected first, which is sometimes facilitated by the use of a 0° scope.

The first successful TECAB procedure on the arrested heart was reported by Loulmet *(25)*. Following ITA take-down, the pericardial fat is removed and a pericardial window is created. After the LAD is identified, femorofemoral bypass is initiated using the Port-Access™ system for closed-chest cardiopulmonary bypass and antegrade cardioplegic cardiac arrest. The anastomosis is then performed in a running fashion on the arrested heart through the same ports. More than 100 cases have been reported in the literature, mostly single-vessel revascularizations of the ITA to the LAD. CPB time and crossclamp time are in the range of 80–120 and 40–60 min, respectively. The conversion rate to a sternotomy is now consistently less than 10%, and the reported patency rate for the TECAB procedure ranges from 95% to 100% prior to discharge and 96% at 3-mo follow-up angiography *(24,26–28)*. In a few patients, the right ITA was used to graft the RCA, and successful double-vessel TECAB to the LAD and RCA as well as sequential grafting of the LAD and a diagonal branch have been reported *(29,30)*. In addition, both ITAs may be harvested endoscopically, followed by a multivessel arterial revascularization on the arrested heart through a left parasternal minithoracotomy in the second interspace (Dresden technique) *(22,31)*.

The application of endoscopic coronary artery bypass grafting on the beating heart required the development of endoscopic stabilizers and methods for temporary vascular occlusion. Using a Nitinol-based self-expanding endoscopic stabilizer, complete endoscopic bypass grafting was first achieved in a canine model *(32,33)*. More advanced stabilizers have subsequently been developed, allowing articulation of the pads and providing easier placement. The latest generation of endoscopic stabilizers also features vacuum asssistance and an irrigation channel (**Fig. 4**).

Vascular occlusion can be achieved using vascular clamps or more commonly using silastic bands that are either locked into the pads of the stabilizer or are used in combination with a self-locking plate. Complete TECAB procedures on the beating heart have been reported by us and the Dresden group using the da Vinci system and an endoscopic stabilizer that was inserted through a subxiphoidal port (**Fig. 5**) *(34,35)*. After the site for the anstomosis is identified, occlusion snares are placed around the vessel. Rather than pushing the needle through, the motion of the heart is used to move the needle passively through the tissue. Before insertion of the stabilizer, all suture material to be used should be placed into the chest to avoid CO_2 leaks later during the procedure. Once the stabilizer is placed, the ITA is placed beneath the stabilizer. Alternatively, a first stitch can already be placed in the ITA while it is still attached to the chest wall. The irrigation is placed from behind, aiming at the site of the anastomosis. After occlusion (usually proximal and distal occlusion will be necessary, as even a little bleeding from the anastomotic site is not well tolerated), the anastomosis is performed in the usual fashion. About 80 closed-chest

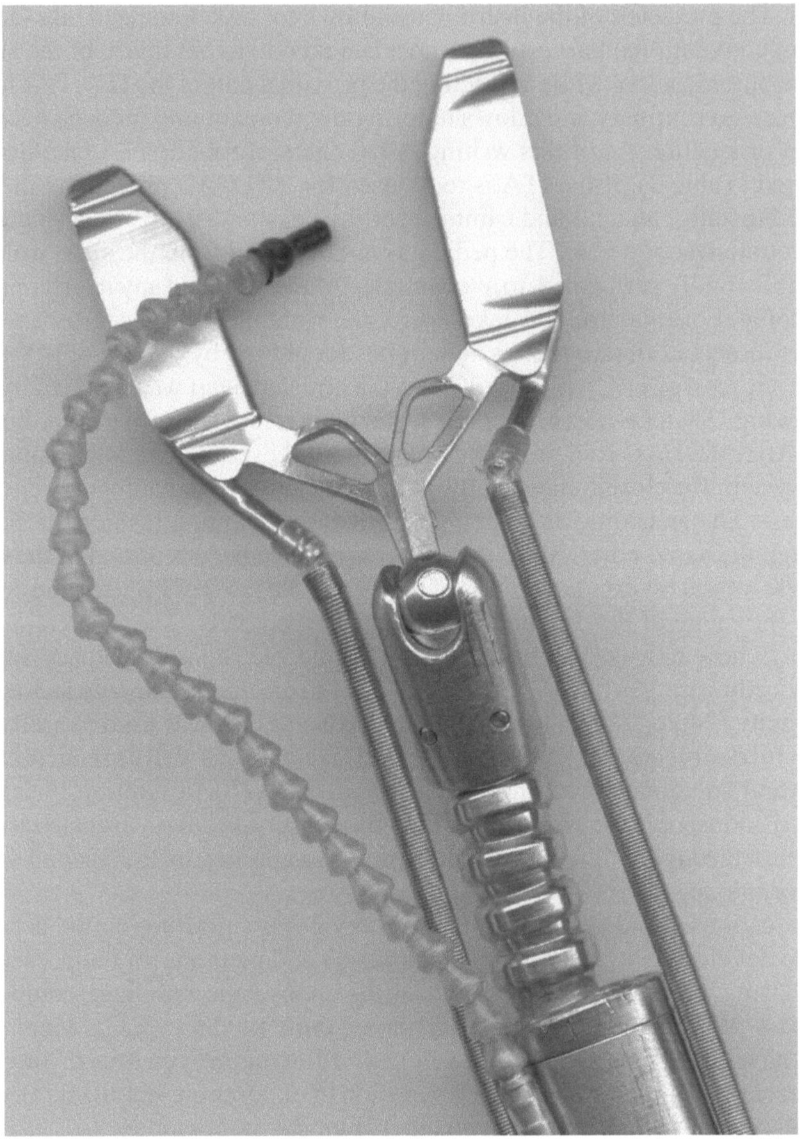

Fig. 4. Vacuum-assisted endoscopic stabilizer with irrigating channel.

beating-heart procedures including three double-vessel beating-heart TECAB's have been reported in the literature *(36,37)*. Based on an intention-to-treat analysis, the conversion rate (elective conversion to a MIDCAB procedure) with this approach is currently in the range of 20–30% in experienced centers *(26,36)*. LAD occlusion times are in the range of 25–40 min and thus exceed those reported for MIDCAB procedures. Among the difficulties reported are excessive epicardial fat, left ventricular dilatation, determination of optimal anastomotic site, target vessel calcification, and back-bleeding from septal branches. In addition, difficulties with positioning of the stabilizer, incomplete immobility of the target site, and the lack of assistance currently limit wider application of beating-heart closed-chest bypass grafting.

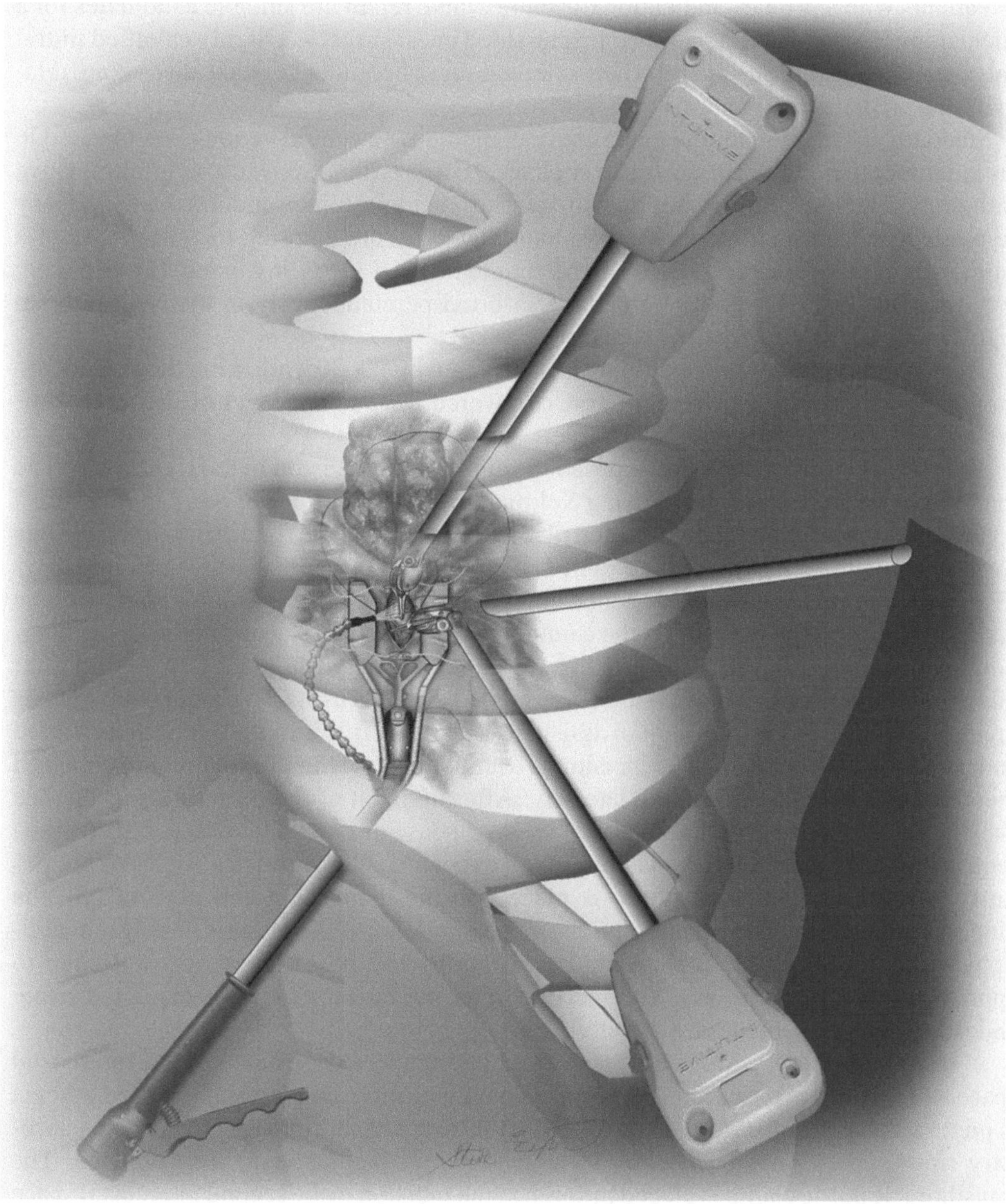

Fig. 5. Setup for endoscopic beating-heart bypass grafting. The stabilizer is inserted through a subxiphoidal port.

Mitral Valve Surgery

In 1998, a prototype of the da Vinci system was first used to perform part of a mitral valve repair procedure *(20)*. Thus far, access to the mitral valve is through a right anterolateral minithoracotomy similar to that used for most current techniques for minimally invasive mitral valve repair *(38–40)*. The actual mitral valve repair is then performed using the telemanipulation system *(41–43)*.

Patients with a primary indication for mitral valve repair are suitable candidates for a telemanipulator-assisted repair. Prior right-sided chest surgery, a highly calcified mitral valve annulus, severe peripheral atherosclerosis, or concomitant cardiac disease are relative contraindications

Standard anesthetic monitoring is applied, including a central venous line inserted in the left internal jugular vein and transesophageal echocardiography to assess mitral valve pathology. External defibrillator pads are placed. A single-lumen endotracheal tube may be used, since cardiopulmonary bypass is initiated before entering the chest. Use of a pulmonary artery catheter is optional and should be used according to individual patient requirements. A 17 fr venous cannula is inserted percutaneously in the right internal jugular vein for drainage of the superior vena cava.

The patient is placed with the right chest elevated by 20–30°, allowing the shoulder to drop as low as possible. The right arm is lowered beyond the level of the table, thus providing access to the mid-axillary line.

The right femoral vessels are exposed through a 3-cm incision in the right groin. The femoral vessels are cannulated using Seldinger technique. For venous cannulation, a 23 Fr. venous return cannula is used and placed at the level of the right atrial–inferior vena cava junction under TEE guidance (a PFO or small ASD should always be excluded by TEE prior to cannula insertion). Since some adjustments of the cannula may become neccessary during the procedure, the cannula is only loosely fixed. For arterial cannulation a 17 or 19 fr cannula is inserted in the femoral artery via a guide wire and after dilatation. Both venous cannulae are connected to the CPB using a Y-connector. Venous drainage is enhanced using vacuum assistance. Once CPB is initiated, cooling is started and both lungs are deflated. The incision is usually made in the inframammary crease in the mid-clavicular line extending laterally. After division of the pectoralis muscle, the chest is entered in the fourth intercostal space. In case of excess fat tissue, a soft-tissue retractor may be placed to provide improved exposure. A rib retractor is placed temporarily. A percutaneous stay suture is placed on the diaphragm and used to pull the diaphragm caudally. The pericardium is opened anterior to the phrenic nerve, and additional percutaneous stay sutures are placed along the posterior pericardial edge to approximate the heart toward the incision. The interatrial groove is dissected using endoscopic instruments under direct vision.

A straight cardioplegia needle is inserted percutaneously in the second intercostal space and inserted in the ascending aorta. At our institution, cold crystalloid cardioplegia is preferred, but blood cardioplegia as well as retrograde cardioplegia (provided a coronary sinus catheter has been placed via the internal jugular vein) may be used. The transthoracic aortic clamp is placed through a stab incision in the second intercostal space in the mid-axillary line. Placement of the clamp is ideally performed under video guidance and according to the guidelines described by Chitwood *(44)*. Alternatively, the port-access technique may be used.

The atriotomy is performed in the usual fashion beginning at the level of the right superior pulmonary vein and extending inferiorly just below the inferior vena cava. A pulmonary vent is inserted through the incision. Exposure of the mitral valve is achieved using a left atrial roof retractor inserted in the third intercostal space in close proximity to the sternal border. Once exposure of the mitral valve is achieved, the rib retractor is removed, since its blade may potentially interfere with the instruments. For deairing purposes, CO_2 insufflation is begun and maintained throughout the case until the left atrium is closed.

The manipulator is placed from the patient's left with the central camera arm aligned with the thoracotomy incision. The scope is inserted through the incision. A port is created in the same intercostal space below the incision and used for the right instrument. Although this position does not provide a perfect triangle, it avoids unintentional enlargement of the atrial incision, which has been described for a more rightward port *(41)*. A second port is created in the third intercostal space in the anterior axillary or mid-clavicular line above the transthoracic clamp. Potential problems can be caused by internal (scope and right instrument) or external (transthoracic clamp and left instrument) collisions and require careful attention of the table-side surgeon. A 30° scope angled up is preferred, because it allows easier access for the assisting surgeon. The table-side surgeon and the surgeon at the console should then check for potential collisions and nonintuitive behavior at all potential positions the instruments may encounter during the case.

The actual repair is performed remotely from the surgeon's console, applying standard repair techniques. Resection of leaflet segments, chordae shortening, sliding plasty, and annular decalcification can all be accomplished using the system. Suture material is provided by the table-side surgeon, who is also in charge of retrieving excised material or used needles using an endoscopic grasper or a magnet on a stick. Complete or partial rings may be implanted as indicated. Annuloplasty rings with a soft cuff are preferred. Knot tying is best performed using the sliding-square-knot technique. Motion scaling is set to 3:1 or 1:1 according to the surgeon's preference. After repair of the valve is accomplished, the instruments are withdrawn, the left atrium is closed manually, and the aortic clamp is released after de-airing through the aortic root needle. At our institution, 22 of 25 valves have been successfully repaired endoscopically using the da Vinci system, including complex repairs requiring chordal transfer, and complete ring insertion *(41,42)*. In 3 patients, manual repair became necessary. Cardiopulmonary bypass and crossclamp times exceed those for manual endoscopic techniques *(38)*.

Few cases of total closed-chest mitral valve repair have been reported [Lange R, personal communication]. After CPB is initiated, the instruments and camera ports are placed as described above. The atriotomy is performed with the system. Exposure of the valve is achieved by attaching the roof of the left atrium to the chest using patch enforced stay sutures. Until an exposure device (internal atrial expander) becomes available, this procedure is not recommended, however, as it is very time-consuming and requires long CPB and crossclamp times.

ASD Repair

For total endoscopic ASD repair, placement of the patient, system setup, and the technique for CPB are essentially the same as that described for mitral valve repair. After insertion of the ports in the third, fourth, and fifth interspaces, the pericardium is opened above the phrenic nerve. Both venae cavae are dissected and encircled with snare tapes, which can be occluded either inside (self-locking) or outside the chest (external snaring). A suction line is inserted percutaneously. The right atrium is then opened and the defect closed with a running suture or with a patch as required *(45,46)*. Details of this procedure are delineated in Chapter 32.

DISCUSSION

From the experience presented here, it can be concluded that the use of the da Vinci system is safe and allows for true endoscopic cardiac surgery. The use of the system is currently restricted to a few indications (single-vessel bypass grafting of the LAD, occasionally double-vessel grafting, and mitral valve repair, as well as some ASD closures), but it is conceivable that it may be used for additional procedures in the near future. An ergonomic human–machine interface and multilevel servo controlling allow for precise tissue handling despite the lack of fine tactile feedback. The three-dimensional vision technology provides enough optical resolution to visualize and manipulate small structures such as coronary arteries.

Importance of Training

As with all new technologies, a substantial learning curve has to be overcome and a structured training is considered essential for procedural success. This includes a principal understanding of telemanipulator technology and its components, the way it may expand our capabilities but also the limitations that are associated with its use. Mastering of the human–machine interface should be attained before any patient contact. This includes all maneuvers performed at the surgeon's console. Forces reflected at the master side as well as changes in dexterity need to be interpreted correctly, as they may indicate collisions or singularities (collapsing of 2 DoF into 1, reflecting joint limits at extreme articulations). Because fine force reflection is limited, visual cues become more important and need to be trained. Working with no assistance using natural tissue as a source for countertraction is a helpful concept that is best achieved in an animal model. Equally important is training of the patient-side surgeon. It is crucial that the table-side surgeon understand the basic mechanisms of joint motion of the manipulators in order to provide a setup that provides unrestricted range of motion during the case. With the use of the da Vinci system, another complex technical system is introduced into the surgical suite. Working in an endoscopic environment presents additional surgical challenges, including new anatomical orientation and no direct access to cardiac structures. A stepwise approach is therefore suggested. Initially, take-down of the ITA should be accomplished routinely, before aiming at a TECAB procedure. Several steps occur between ITA take-down and creation of the anastomosis. While these are trivial and automatic in an open scenario (removal of pericardial fat, identifying the target vessel, temporary vessel occlusion, delivering material inside the chest and others), they require sophisticated choreography to be mastered endoscopically. A low threshold for conversion is mandatory, to avoid any risk to the patient. Elective conversion is safe and should by no means be considered a failure. Importantly, algorithms for reacting to emergency situations should be familiar to everyone in the team.

FUTURE DEVELOPMENTS

The focus for developments in endoscopic coronary artery bypass grafting is twofold: (1) multivessel revascularization on the arrested heart using a percutaneous cardiopulmonary bypass system; and (2) improvements in endoscopic beating-heart bypass grafting. The latter will require the development of better endoscopic stabilizers as well as new methods for coronary occlusion and blood drainage.

For multivessel revascularization, endoscopic devices for exposure of the back wall of the heart need to be developed. Alternatively, different access routes (transabdominal, right chest) may be explored. To help identifying coronary pathology and to define the ideal location for an anastomosis in the absence of tactile feedback, endoscopic ultrasound probes may be useful *(47)*.

With refinements in telemanipulator technology and the development of adjunct devices to enhance exposure, the technique of computer-enhanced endoscopic cardiac surgery will evolve further and may prove beneficial for selected patients. Smaller and more flexible modular robotic arms will be developed, and new control algorithms will eventually allow one operator to control multiple arms. Three-dimension HDTV systems will provide even better optical resolution in the near future. The application of multimodal three-dimensional imaging and computational modeling of the range of motion of the robotic arms in an individual patient data set may optimize preoperative planning of the procedure *(48)*. The use of preoperative imaging may also help to better identify suitable candidates for an endoscopic approach. Multidetector CT scanning may help to identify intramyocardial LADs preoperatively and thus decrease the risk of conversion or erroneous grafting to a diagonal branch *(49)*. New devices for facilitated anastomosis (*see* Chapter 28), such as the Ventrica magnetic coupling device, may facilitate endoscopic coronary artery bypass grafting in the future *(50)*.

Endoscopic cardiac surgical simulation programs are currently being developed and may help to overcome the initial learning curve for beginners. One such system is based on the Karlsruhe Endoscopic Surgery Trainer, a virtual-reality training system for minimally invasive surgery. It provides several surgical interaction modules for deformable objects such as grasping, application of clips, cutting, coagulation, injection, and suturing. Additionally, it is possible to perform irrigation and suction in the operation area. Special attention is paid to elastodynamically deformable tissue models of the heart and vessels and geometric modeling techniques for graphical real-time performance. The system is currently programmed to run with the original da Vinci console as the user interface and thus allows a realistic simulation of beating-heart scenarios. Coupling of two consoles may serve as an educational tool, as it enables the introduction of the "driving school concept" into cardiac surgical training.

REFERENCES

1. Goertz RC. Fundamentals of general-purpose remote manipulators. Nucleonics 1952;10:36–45
2. Bejczy AK, Salisbury JK. Kinesthetic coupling for remote manipulators. Comput Med Eng 1983;2:48–62.
3. Taylor RH, Lavallee S, Burdea GC, Mösges R. Computer-Integrated Surgery. Technology and Clinical Applications. Cambridge, MA: MIT Press, 1996.
4. Taylor RH, Jensen M, Whitcomb L, et al. A steady-hand robotic system for microsurgical augmentation. Rob Res 1999;12:1201–1210.
5. Green PS, Hill JW, Jensen JF, Shah A. Telepresence surgery. Proc IEEE Eng Med Biol 1995:324–329.
6. Bowersox JC, Shah A, Jensen J, Hill J, Cordts PR, Green PS. Vascular applications of telepresence surgery: initial feasibility studies in swine. J Vasc Surg 1996;23:281–287.
7. Bowersox JC, Cordts PR, LaPorta AJ. Use of an intuitive telemanipulator system for remote trauma surgery: an experimental study. J Am Coll Surg 1998;186:615–621.
8. Schurr MO, Breitwieser H, Melzer A, et al. Experimental telemanipulation in endoscopic surgery. Surg Laparosc Endosc 1996;6:167–175.
9. Schurr MO, Arezzo A, Buess GF. Robotics and systems technology for advanced endoscopic procedures: experiences in general surgery. Eur J Cardiothorac Surg 1999;16(suppl II):S97–S105.
10. Guthart GS, Salisbury JK: The Intuitive™ telesurgery system: overview and application. Proc IEEE ICRA 2002; in press.
11. Falk V. Robotic surgery. In: Yim AP, Hazelrigg SR, Izzat MB, Landrenaeau RJ, Mack MJ, Naunheim KS, eds. Minimal Access Cardiothoracic Surgery. Philadelphia: Saunders, 1999:623–629.
12. Falk V, Diegeler A, Walther T, Autschbach R, Mohr FW. Developments in robotic cardiac surgery. Curr Opp Cardiol 2000;15:378–387.
13. Falk V, Swarup N. Robotic Cardiac surgery —technology and procedure development. Cardiovasc Eng 2001;6:39–43.

14. Falk V, Gummert J, Walther T, Hayesi M, Berry GJ, Mohr FW. Quality of computer enhanced endoscopic coronary artery bypass graft anastomosis—comparison to conventional technique. Eur J Cardiothorac Surg 1999;13:260–266.
15. Shennib H, Bastawisy A, Mack MJ, Moll FH. Computer-assisted telemanipulation: an enabling technology for endoscopic coronary artery bypass. Ann Thorac Surg 1998;66:1060–1063.
16. Shennib H, Bastawisy A, McLoughlin J, Moll F. Robotic computer-assisted telemanipulation enhances coronary artery bypass. J Thorac Cardiovasc Surg 1999;117:310–313.
17. Falk V, Mc Loughlin J, Guthart G, et al. Dexterity enhancement in endoscopic surgery by a computer controlled mechanical wrist. Min Inv Ther Allied Technol 1999;8:235–242.
18. Falk V, Mintz D, Grünenfelder J, Fann JI, Burdon TA. Influence of 3D vision on surgical telemanipulator performance. Surg Endosc 2001;15:1282–1288.
19. Falk V, Moll F, Rosa D, et al. Transabdominal endoscopic computer enhanced coronary artery bypass grafting. Ann Thorac Surg 1999;68:1555–1557.
20. Mohr FW, Falk V, Diegeler A, Autschbach R. Computer enhanced coronary artery bypass surgery. J Thorac Cardiovasc Surg 1999;117:1212–1213.
21. Kappert U, Cichon R, Schneider J, et al. Robotic coronary artery surgery—the evolution of a new minimally invasive approach in coronary artery surgery. Thorac Cardiovasc Surg 2000;48:193–197.
22. Cichon R, Kappert U, Schneider J, et al. Robotically enhanced "Dresden technique" with bilateral internal mammary artery grafting. Thorac Cardiovasc Surg 2000;48:189–192.
23. Raumanns J, Diegeler A, Falk V, Ender J, Petry A. Hemodynamic effects of CO_2 insufflation under one lung ventilation for robot-guided surgery. Anesth Analg 2000;90:SCA55.
24. Falk V, Diegeler A, Walther T, et al. Total endoscopic coronary artery bypass grafting. Eur J Cardiothorac Surg 2000;17:38–45.
25. Loulmet D, Carpentier A, d'Attellis N, et al. First endoscopic coronary artery bypass grafting using computer assisted instruments. J Thorac Cardiovasc Surg 1999;118:4–10.
26. Mohr FW, Falk V, Diegeler A, et al. Computer-enhanced robotic cardiac surgery—experience in 148 patients. J Thorac Cardiovasc Surg 2001;121:842–853.
27. Kappert U, Schneider J, Cichon R, et al. Development of robotic enhanced endoscopic surgery for the treatment of coronary artery disease. Circulation 2001;104(suppl I):I102–I107.
28. Dogan S, Aybek T, Andressen E, et al. Totally endoscopic coronary artery bypass grafting on cardiopulmonary bypass with robotically enhanced telemanipulation: report of forty-five cases. J Thorac Cardiovasc Surg 2002;123:1125–1131.
29. Aybek T, Dogan S, Andressen E, et al. Robotically enhanced totally endoscopic right internal thoracic coronary artery bypass to the right coronary artery. Heart Surg Forum 2000;3:322–324.
30. Dogan S, Aybek T, Westphal K, Mierdel S, Moritz A, Wimmer-Greinecker G. Computer enhanced totally endoscopic sequential arterial coronary artery bypass. Ann Thorac Surg 2001;72:610–611.
31. Kappert U, Cichon R, Schneider J Schramm I, Guliemos V, Schueler S. Closed chest bilateral mammary artery grafting in double vessel coronary artery disease. Ann Thorac Surg 2000;70:1699–1701.
32. Falk V, Diegeler A, Walther T, et al. Endoscopic coronary artery bypass grafting on the beating heart using a computer enhanced telemanipulation system. Heart Surg Forum 1999;2:199–205.
33. Falk V, Grünenfelder J, Fann JI, Daunt D, Burdon TA. Total endoscopic computer enhanced beating heart coronary artery bypass grafting. Ann Thorac Surg 2000;70:2029–2033.
34. Falk V, Diegeler A, Walther T, Jacobs S, Raumans J, Mohr FW. Total endoscopic off-pump coronary artery bypass grafting. Heart Surg Forum 2000;3:29–31.
35. Kappert U, Cichon R, Schneider J, et al. Closed chest coronary artery bypass surgery on the beating heart with the use of a robotic system. J Thorac Cardiovasc Surg 2000;120:809–811.
36. Kappert U, Cichon R, Schneider J, et al. Technique of closed chest coronary artery surgery on the beating heart. Eur J Cardiothorac Surg 2001:20:765–769.
37. Dogan S, Aybek T, Khan MF, et al. Computer enhanced telemanipulation enables a variety of totally endoscopic cardiac procedures. Thorac Cardiovasc Surg 2002;50:281–286.
38. Mohr FW, Onnasch JF, Falk V, et al. The evolution of minimally invasive mitral valve surgery—two years experience. Eur J Cardiothorac Surg 1999;13:233–239.
39. Falk V, Walther T, Autschbach R, Diegeler A, Battellini R, Mohr FW. Robot assisted minimally invasive solo mitral valve operation. J Thorac Cardiovasc Surg 1998;115:470–471.
40. Chitwood WR. State of the art review: videoscopic minimally invasive mitral valve surgery. Trekking to a totally endoscopic operation. Heart Surg Forum 1998;1:13–16.
41. Falk V, Autschbach R, Walther T, Diegeler A, Chitwood WR, Mohr FW. Computer enhanced mitral valve surgery—towards a total endoscopic procedure. Semin Thorac Surg 1999;11:244–249.

42. Autschbach R, Onnasch JF, Falk V, et al. The Leipzig experience with robotic mitral valve surgery. J Cardiac Surg 2000;15:82–87.
43. Chitwood WR, Nifong LW, Elbeery JE, et al. Robotic mitral valve repair: trapezoidal resection and prosthetic annuloplasty with the da Vinci™ surgical system. J Thorac Cardiovasc Surg 2000;120:1171–1172.
44. Chitwood WR. Video-assisted and robotic mitral valve surgery: toward an endoscopic surgery. Semin Thorac Cardiovasc Surg 1999;11:194–205.
45. Torracca L, Ismeno G, Alfieri O. Totally endoscopic atrial septal closure using robotic techniques: report of two cases. Ital Heart J 2000;1:698–701.
46. Dogan S, Wimmer-Greinecker G, Andressen E, Mierdl S, Westphal K, Moritz A. Totally endoscopic coronary artery bypass (TECAB) grafting and closure of an atrial septal defect using the da Vinci™ system. Thorac Cardiovasc Surg 1999;48(suppl. I):21.
47. Falk V, Fann JI, Grünenfelder J, Burdon TA: Endoscopic Doppler for detecting vessels in closed chest bypass grafting. Heart Surg Forum 2000;3:331–333.
48. Chiu AM, Dey DD, Drangova M, Boyd WD, Peters TM. 3-D Image guidance for minimally invasive robotic coronary artery surgery. Heart Surg Forum 2000;3:224–231.
49. Vogl TJ, Abolmaali ND, Diebold T, et al. Techniques for the detection of coronary atherosclerosis: multidetector row CT coronary angiography. Radiology 2002;223:212–220.
50. Falk V, Walther T, Stein H, et al. Facilitated endoscopic beating heart coronary bypass grafting using a magnetic coupling device. J Thorac Cardiovasc Surg, in press.

32 Totally Endoscopic Atrial Septal Defect Repair with Robotic Assistance

Michael Argenziano, MD, *Mehmet C. Oz*, MD, *and Craig R. Smith, Jr.*, MD

CONTENTS

INTRODUCTION
METHODS
RESULTS
CONCLUSIONS
REFERENCES

INTRODUCTION

In the past decade, the face of cardiac surgery has been changed by a number of advances, most notably the development of minimally invasive techniques, including minimally invasive direct coronary artery bypass (MIDCAB), off-pump coronary artery bypass (OPCAB), and minimal-access valve surgery. Initial attempts to perform cardiac operations through small incisions were hindered by the lack of appropriate accessory technology, such as visualization systems, retractors, stabilizers, and alternate methods of vascular cannulation and cardiopulmonary bypass. With the development of these enabling technologies, surgeons have been increasingly able to perform complex cardiac procedures, including coronary artery bypass, mitral and aortic valve replacement, and atrial septal defect (ASD) closure, through smaller-than-traditional incisions. Nonetheless, in many cases, the extent to which incision size has been reduced by these minimally invasive approaches has been matched by a corresponding increase in technical difficulty and operative time—and a potentially decreased safety margin—due to the constraints imposed by limited or incomplete cardiac exposure.

Computer (robotic) enhancement has emerged as a potential facilitator of minimally invasive surgical procedures. Initially, this technology was utilized to maximize visual-

From: *Contemporary Cardiology: Minimally Invasive Cardiac Surgery, Second Edition*
Edited by: D. J. Goldstein and M. C. Oz © Humana Press Inc., Totowa, NJ

ization of intracardiac structures by providing enhanced (including voice-activated) endoscopic camera control *(1)*. More recently, robotic surgical systems have permitted the manipulation of surgical instruments through limited thoracic incisions *(2)*. This chapter describes the next step in this progression: the performance of atrial septal defect repair entirely through thoracoscopic port incisions. Torracca and colleagues have recently reported a small series of patients undergoing this operation in Europe *(3)*. Our series of robotic ASD repairs supplements this experience and represents the first U.S. application of robotic technology for totally endoscopic open-heart surgery.

METHODS

Robotic Surgical System

The da Vinci™ surgical system (Intuitive Surgical, Inc., Mountainview, CA) consists of two primary components: the surgeon's viewing and control console and the surgical arm unit that positions and maneuvers detachable surgical EndoWrist instruments (**Fig. 1**). These pencil-sized instruments, which possess small mechanical wrists with seven degrees of motion, are designed to provide the dexterity of the surgeon's forearm and wrist at the operative site through entry ports less than 1 cm in size. One port allows access for the endoscope, and the other two ports provide access for surgical instruments. The wrists of the surgical instruments mimic the motions made by the operating surgeon, who sits at a console away from the operating table. The surgeon peers through an eyepiece that provides high-definition, full-color, magnified, three-dimensional images of the surgical site provided by the endoscope.

All patients in our series were enrolled in a U.S. Food and Drug Administration (FDA)-sanctioned trial, entitled "Atrial Septal Defect Closure Using Intuitive Surgical Inc.'s da Vinci™ Surgical System" and gave informed consent. This study was approved by the Columbia University Institutional Review Board and received an FDA Investigational Device Exemption (IDE # G010156).

Patient Selection

Inclusion criteria for the trial included age between 18 and 80 yr, and the presence of a secundum-type atrial septal defect with Qp:Qs ratio > 1.5, or patent foramen ovale with a documented neurological event. Patients were excluded if they could not tolerate single-lung ventilation or peripheral cardiopulmonary bypass, or otherwise were considered poor candidates for a thoracoscopic approach.

Surgical Technique

After induction of general anesthesia, a left-sided double-lumen endotracheal tube is positioned to allow single-lung ventilation. A transesophageal echocardiography probe and bilateral arterial pressure monitoring lines are inserted to facilitate monitoring of endoaortic balloon positioning later in the procedure. A 15 or 17 fr arterial cannula (Medtronic Bio-Medicus, Eden Prarie, MN) is placed percutaneously into the right internal jugular vein and passed into the superior vena cava with echocardiographic guidance. This cannula is heparinized before and after insertion to avoid thrombus formation. The patient is placed in a modified left lateral decubitus position, with the right arm either suspended above the head ($n = 7$) or tacked at the side ($n = 4$) and the pelvis relatively flat to facilitate femoral cannulation. After sterile preparation and draping, the right femoral vessels are accessed through a 2-cm oblique incision along the inguinal crease. After

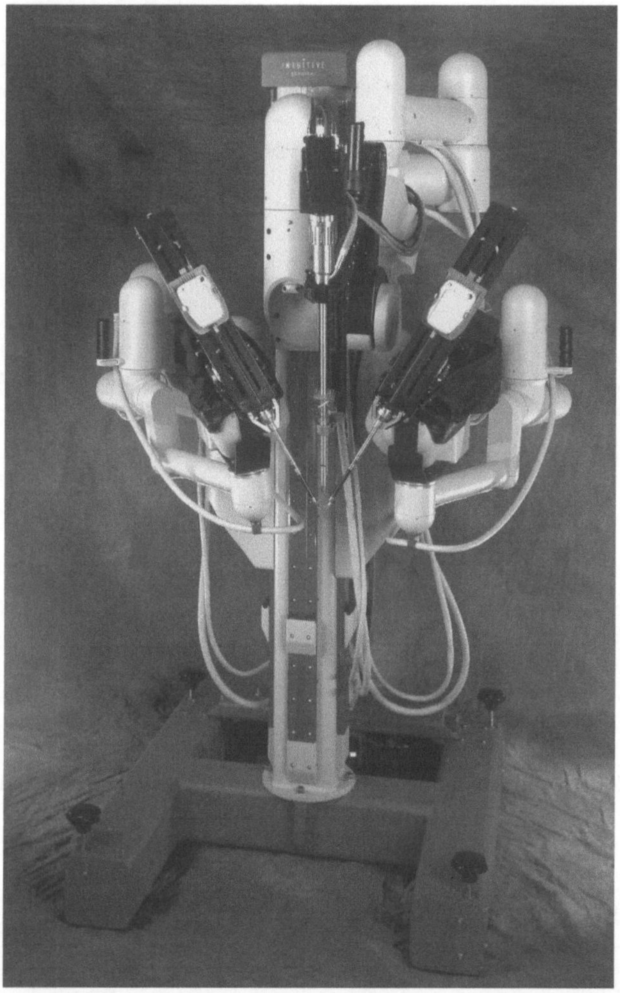

Fig. 1. The da Vinci surgical cart, with a central camera arm and two lateral instrument arms.

systemic heparinization, the right common femoral artery is cannulated with a 17 or 21 fr Remote Access Perfusion cannula with endoaortic balloon (ESTECH, Inc., Danville, CA) (**Fig. 2**). The distal tip of the arterial cannula is passed under echocardiographic guidance into the ascending aorta, approx 3 cm above the aortic valve. The bypass circuit is completed by inserting a 19 or 21 fr venous cannula (Medtronic Bio-Medicus, Eden Prarie, MN) into the right common femoral vein and passing it into the inferior vena cava, with its tip just inferior to the IVC-RA junction.

After establishment of selective left-lung ventilation, a port incision is made in the fourth intercostal space, in the midclavicular line, and a 12-mm endoscopic trocar (Ethicon, Inc., Somerville, NJ) is placed into the pleural space. The endoscopic camera is inserted and after pleural adhesions are ruled out, the pleural space is insufflated with carbon dioxide to a maximum pressure of 8 mmHg. Two additional 8-mm port incisions are made in the third and sixth intercostal spaces, in the anterior axillary line (**Fig. 3**). The da Vinci surgical cart is positioned at the operating table, and the left and right robotic arms are inserted into the pleural space. A fourth port incision (15 mm) is made in the fifth intercostal space, in the posterior axillary line, for use as a service entrance.

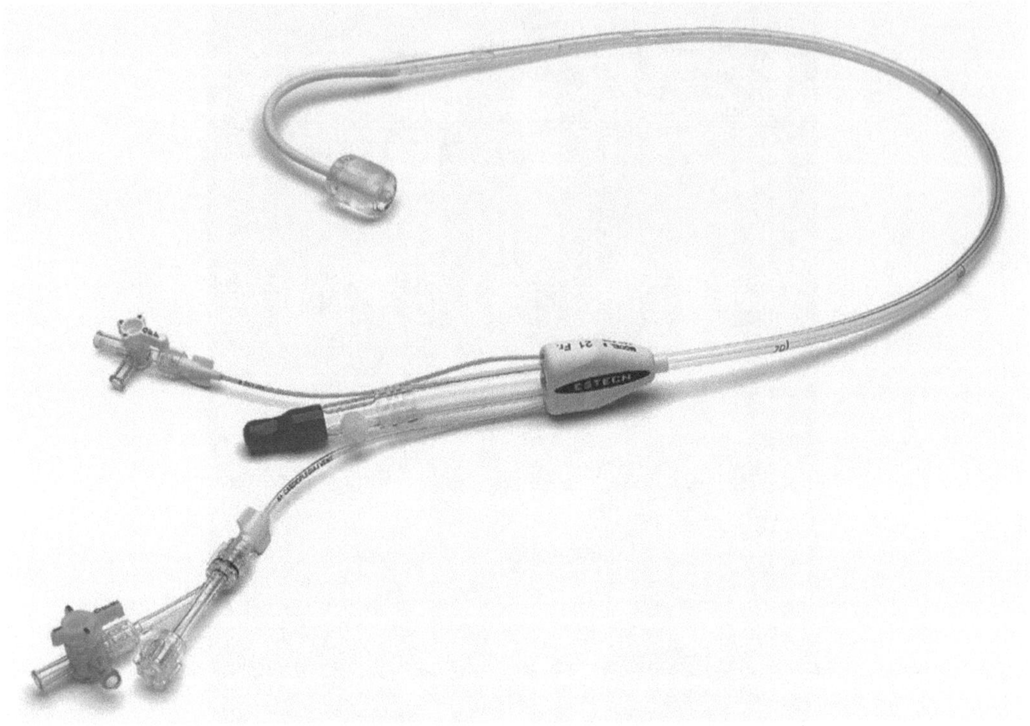

Fig. 2. The ESTECH arterial perfusion cannula, with endoaortic balloon and distal cardioplegia lumen.

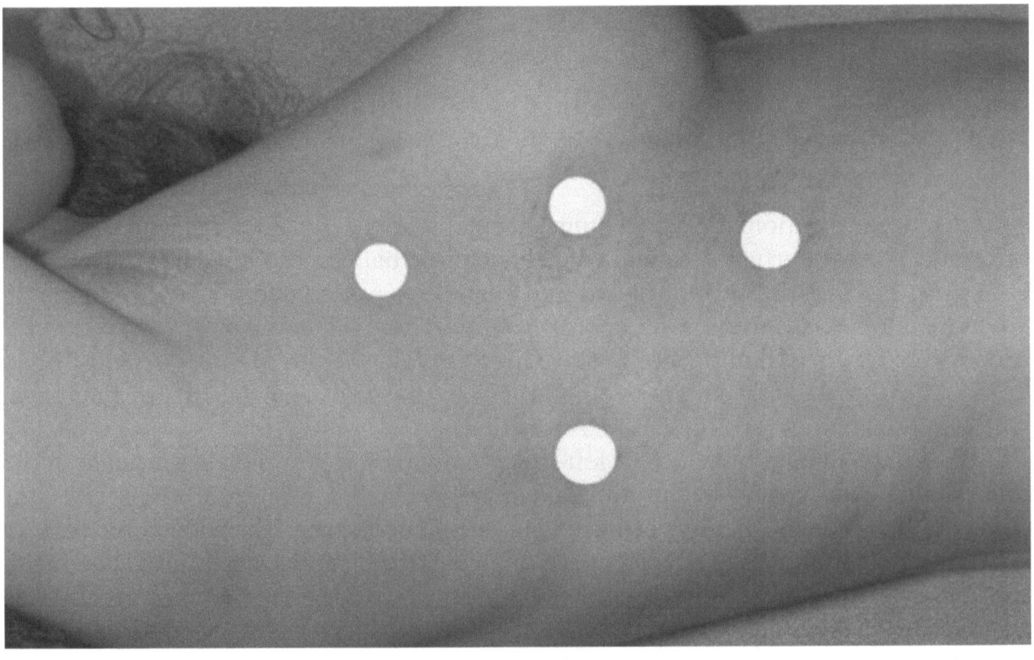

Fig. 3. Port sites for totally endoscopic, robotically assisted ASD repair.

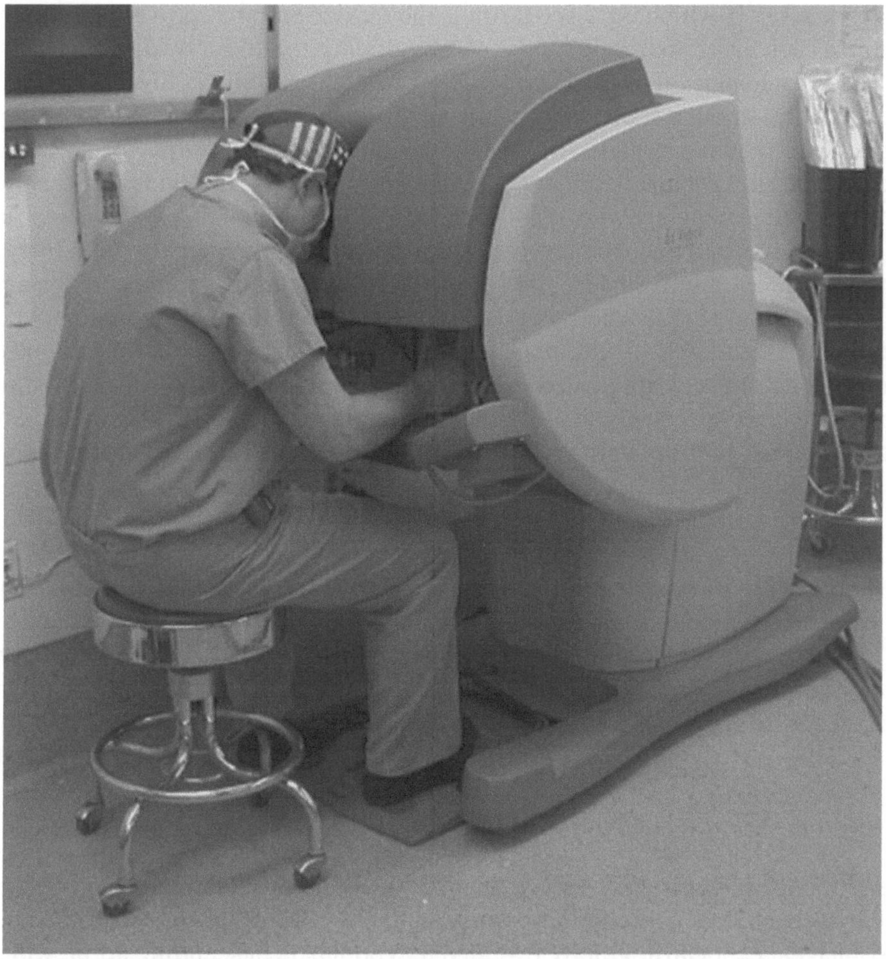

Fig. 4. The da Vinci surgeon's console, from which the robotic camera and instrument arms are controlled.

Next, the operating surgeon moves from the operating table to the surgeon's console, and begins the intrathoracic portion of the operation by controlling the robotic camera and surgical instrument arms (**Fig. 4**). A pericardiotomy is made using the "long tip forceps" and "cautery" attachments, and pericardial stay sutures placed, with traction provided by passing the sutures out of the chest through the service port (posteriorly) or by sewing the suture to the inside of the chest wall (anteriorly). Caval snares are placed using the "long tip forceps" and passed out of the service entrance port. Cardiopulmonary bypass with moderate hypothermia is initiated with kinetically assisted bicaval venous drainage. Atrial stay sutures are placed. The perfusion pressure is reduced, and the endoaortic balloon is inflated to a pressure of 250–300 mmHg. Antegrade cold blood cardioplegia (4:1) is administered through the distal cannula port, and a satisfactory cardiac arrest is confirmed.

Using the "round tip scissors" attachment, a right atriotomy is created, and the right atrium is explored. Cardiotomy suction is provided by a specially modified instrument (the "Flora sucker"), which is passed through the service entrance port by the patient-side surgeon. In each case, anatomic landmarks, including the fossa ovalis, coronary sinus ostium, and eustachian valve, are identified. Whether the pathology involves a large ASD or PFO with or without a septal aneurysm, we close the entire fossa with a double-layer primary suture technique. Before tying the atrial septopexy suture, the left atrium is de-aired by inflating the left lung. After the suture is tied, the endoaortic balloon is deflated, and the patient is rewarmed. The atriotomy is closed with two layers of running 4-0 polypropylene, and the patient is weaned from cardiopulmonary bypass. Integrity of the septal closure is confirmed by transesophageal echocardiography, and protamine is administered. After adequate hemostasis is achieved, the robotic arms are removed from the chest, and a small flexible drainage tube is placed in the pericardium and one or two conventional chest tubes are placed in the right pleural space, all through existing port incisions. The femoral vessels are decannulated, and the percutaneous catheter removed from the internal jugular vein. All incisions are closed in layers with absorbable suture material.

Postoperative Regimen

The patients are transported to the intensive care unit, where they remain until extubated. Upon extubation, patients are transferred to the general postoperative unit. Chest drains are removed when drainage subsides. Upon discharge, patients are given an appointment for a clinical visit and a transthoracic echocardiogram. Anticoagulants are administered only for patients with specific postoperative indications such as atrial fibrillation.

RESULTS

Demographics

Over 7 mo, 13 patients were enrolled in the study and provided informed consent. Of these, two were excluded intraoperatively prior to initiation of the procedure. In one case, transesophageal echocardiography revealed a hypoplastic descending aorta, which was considered a contraindication to passage of the endoaortic balloon cannula. This patient underwent ASD repair via a minithoracotomy, with central vessel cannulation. In another case, the patient had an anaphylactic reaction upon induction of anesthesia, with profound vasodilation, urticaria, and bronchospasm. After stabilization, this patient was awakened and the surgery deferred until appropriate allergic evaluation and testing were undertaken. The other 11 patients underwent the procedure robotically. The group of operated patients included 1 man and 10 women, with mean age 46.1 ± 14.2 (mean $\pm$ SD). Eight patients had secundum ASD, while 3 had PFO with septal aneurysm and a history of cerebrovascular accident not attributable to another cause.

Operative Results

All operations were completed robotically through four port incisions, with no intraoperative conversions to alternate techniques. All patients underwent primary suture repair of the ASD or PFO, and transesophageal echocardiography postoperatively confirmed successful closure in all cases. Median cardiopulmonary bypass time was 124 min, and median crossclamp time was 38 min. In the last five cases of our series, median values for cardiopulmonary bypass and crossclamp times were 121 and 28 min, respectively. Postoperatively all patients were extubated on the night of surgery, and median ICU length of stay was 20 h. One patient remained in the ICU for 3 d for treatment

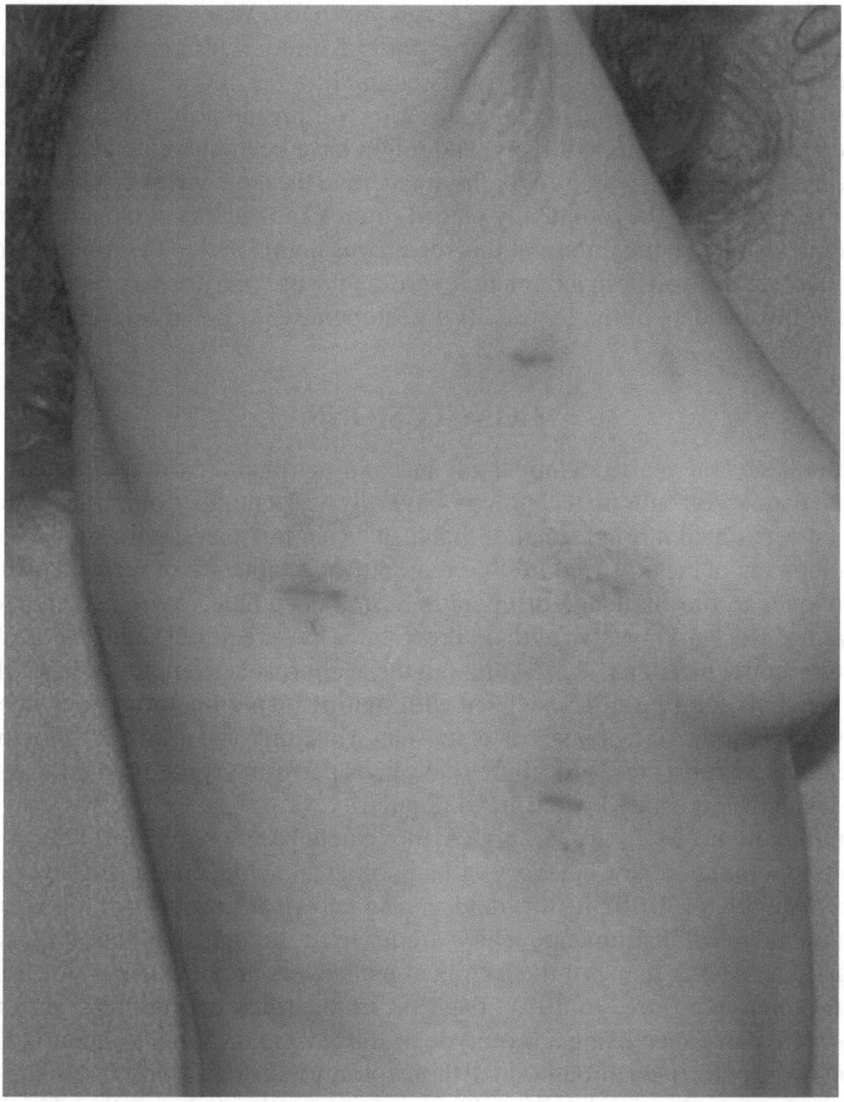

Fig. 5. A robotic ASD repair patient, 30 d after surgery, with four well-healed port incisions.

of a postoperative pneumonia that was presumed to be related to aspiration, and recovered without incident. Hospital length of stay ranged from 2.5 d (our first patient) to 10 d (a 68-yr-old patient who developed postoperative atrial fibrillation and required several days to establish effective rate control), with a median of 4 d. Cosmetic results were excellent in all cases (**Fig. 5**).

Complications

There were no deaths in our series. There were no cerebrovascular accidents, wound infections, reoperations for bleeding, or femoral vascular complications. There were two cases of perioperative atrial fibrillation, one case of pneumonia, and one patient with temporary arm discomfort due to intraoperative arm positioning. In one case, transthoracic echocardiography revealed a recurrent interatrial shunt on postoperative d 5, in a 58-yr-old patient who had had a large secundum ASD. When this was confirmed by transesophageal echocardiography, the patient underwent reoperation via right minithoracotomy. At operation, the primary suture line was found to be intact, but a tear was noted in the septum medial to the repair. This was presumably induced by excessive tension on the septum postoperatively, and might have been prevented by a patch technique. A pericardial patch was used for this repair, and the patient was discharged 4 d later without incident. Since the robotically placed sutures and the line of closure were intact, it is our conclusion that the failure of this repair was not related to the robotic procedure per se, but rather to an error in judgment regarding the use of a primary repair technique. In the other 10 patients in the series, 30-d postoperative echocardiography confirmed successful repair.

CONCLUSIONS

In the past several years, technical advances in peripheral cardiopulmonary bypass access and endoaortic balloon technology have allowed a number of intracardiac procedures to be performed through smaller than usual (but not necessarily small) incisions. The development of these procedures has required the adaptation of surgical instruments and techniques to the challenge of operating "in a deep hole," with less than optimal visualization. The least invasive of these procedures have required small thoracotomy or partial sternotomy incisions *(4,5)*. Although these approaches employ smaller than traditional incisions, they are still associated with significant perioperative pain, due largely to the division or retraction of intercostal muscles, ribs, and/or sternal bone. For these and other technical reasons, these procedures have been performed predominantly at selected centers, and have not gained widespread popularity.

The minimally invasive cardiac surgical movement has more recently been propelled by the introduction of a new category of technological achievement: the computerized telemicromanipulator. Utilizing this device, also known as the surgical robot, surgeons can manipulate small instruments, which are inserted through small chest incisions, in tight spaces, achieving many of the technical maneuvers previously possible only with traditional open exposure. In 1997, the first intracardiac procedures—mitral valve repairs—were performed using a prototype of the current da Vinci system *(6,7)*. These operations were performed through small thoracotomy incisions, since the "micro-wrists" allowed the surgeons to complete complex maneuvers without placing their hands within the chest. In December 2000, Chitwood and associates reported the first such mitral valve operation performed in the United States, using an inframammary mini-thoracotomy *(2)*. To date, over 100 such mitral valve repairs have subsequently been performed by Chitwood and others, under the auspices of an FDA-sanctioned multicenter trial. Details of this technique are outlined in Chapter 19. Our center is a participant in this trial, and we have performed 17 such repairs to date.

The success of robotically assisted operations through small thoracotomy incisions was a critical step in the evolution of minimally invasive open-heart surgery, because it proved that complex intracardiac procedures could be performed with robotically controlled instruments. The next step—a totally endoscopic intracardiac procedure—would wait until 2001, when closed-chest, robotically assisted atrial septal defect repairs would be performed, as described in this chapter. In addition to the 6 cases reported by Torracca and the 11 procedures performed by our group, an additional 5 procedures have been performed in Frankfurt, Germany (G. Wimmer-Greinecker, personal communication).

Our series of robotically assisted ASD repairs constitutes the first U.S. report of a totally endoscopic, robotically assisted open-heart procedure. By utilizing femoral cannulation and port incisions in the right chest, the da Vinci surgical system is utilized to perform every step of the repair. By avoiding thoracotomy incisions and rib spreading, this procedure results in minimal pain and postoperative recovery time. Despite the impressive results in our small series, and the potential advantages of this approach with regard to cosmesis and patient acceptance, it is currently unclear whether these benefits can be expected in all patients. For this reason, additional patients are being enrolled in our FDA-sanctioned clinical trial, in order to determine whether this technology will be of reproducible value in the management of patients with intracardiac disease on a larger scale. Furthermore, it is clear that the continued evolution of totally endoscopic cardiac surgery depends on the development of new accessory technology, such as retraction systems, perfusion catheters, noninvasive monitoring techniques, and sutureless anastomotic devices.

Thus, although the surgical robot allows unprecedented closed-chest access to the heart, it is only one of several tools that must be used in concert to achieve the technical goals of a particular operation. In this respect, the immediate future of closed-chest cardiac surgery depends on the ability of physicians and industry to work together to fill in the many technological gaps that are present in our current armamentarium of minimally invasive tools. With such advances, and continued success from pioneering centers, completely endoscopic cardiac surgery—literally an inconceivable notion only a few years ago—may become a widely available clinical reality in the near future.

REFERENCES

1. LaPietra A, Grossi EA, Derivaux CC, et al. Robotic-assisted instruments enhance minimally invasive mitral valve surgery. Ann Thorac Surg 2000;70(3):835–838.
2. Chitwood WR Jr, Nifong LW, Elbeery JE, et al. Robotic mitral valve repair: trapezoidal resection and prosthetic annuloplasty with the da vinci surgical system. J Thorac Cardiovasc Surg 2000;120(6):1171–1172.
3. Torracca L, Ismeno G, Alfieri O. Totally endoscopic computer-enhanced atrial septal defect closure in six patients. Ann Thor Surg 2001;72:1354–1357.
4. Reichenspurner H, Boehm DH, Gulbins H, et al. Three-dimensional video and robot-assisted port-access mitral valve operation. Ann Thorac Surg 2000;69(4):1176–1181.
5. Grossi EA, LaPietra A, Ribakove GH, et al. Minimally invasive versus sternotomy approaches for mitral reconstruction: comparison of intermediate-term results. J Thorac Cardiovasc Surg 2001;121(4):708–713.
6. Carpentier A, Loulmet D, Aupecle B, et al. Computer assisted open heart surgery. First case operated on with success. C R Acad Sci III 1998;321(5):437–442.
7. Falk V, Walther T, Autschbach R, Diegeler A, Battellini R, Mohr FW. Robot-assisted minimally invasive solo mitral valve operation. J Thorac Cardiovasc Surg 1998;115(2):470–471.

INDEX

A

Aesop 3000 system,
  congenital heart surgery, 320
  micro-mitral operation, 265
  mounting, 430
  popularity, 430
  voice commands, 430
AF, *see* Atrial fibrillation
Anastomosis,
  adhesives,
    BioGlue, 406
    gelatin–resorcin–formaldehyde glue, 406
  Guidant OPCAB System, 111
  laser welding, 406, 407
  mechanical systems,
    advantages, 394
    arcuate-legged clips, 396
    Automatic Anastomotic Device, 400, 401
    GraftConnector, 402, 403
    Heartflo device, 401, 402
    Magnetic Vascular Positioner, 403, 404
    Nitinol U-Clip device, 404, 406
    One Shot System, 401
    prospects, 408
    requirements, 394
    staplers, 394–396
    Symmetry Bypass System, 398
    vascular connectors, 396, 397
  minimally invasive direct coronary artery bypass, 133
  robotics, 408
Aortic valve surgery, minimally invasive,
  economic analysis, 361, 362
  historical perspective, 293, 294
  incisions,
    mini-sternotomy, 297–299
    right anterolateral thoracotomy, 296, 297
    right parasternal incision, 294–296
    transverse sternotomy, 297
  operative techniques, 300–303
  outcomes, 303–306
  preoperative preparation, 294
Aprotinin, attenuation of material-dependent activation in cardiopulmonary bypass, 11, 12
ASD, *see* Atrial septal defect
Atrial fibrillation (AF),
  atrial transection, 344
  epidemiology, 343
  left atrial isolation, 344
  Maze procedure,
    ablation techniques,
      chemical ablation, 352
      cryoablation, 346
      factors affecting, 345, 346
      hyperthermic ablation, 346
      laser ablation, 350, 351
      lesion characteristics, 345, 355
      microwave ablation, 348, 350
      radiofrequency ablation, 346–348
      ultrasound ablation, 352
    lesion sets, 353–355
    prospects, 356
    pulmonary vein isolation, 353
    success rate, 344, 355
  medical therapy, 343
  stroke, 343
  treatment goals, 344
Atrial septal defect (ASD),
  da Vinci system assistance,
    complications, 467–469
    outcomes, 455, 466, 467
    patient selection, 462, 466
    postoperative regimen, 466
    surgical technique, 462, 463, 465, 466
  hybrid closure of septal defects, 321
Automatic Anastomotic Device, features, 400, 401
Axius Stabilizer, *see* Guidant OPCAB System

B

BioGlue, anastomosis, 406
Bow-tie repair, *see* Percutaneous mitral valve repair

C

CABG, *see* Coronary artery bypass grafting
Cardiopulmonary bypass (CPB),
adhesion molecule response and effects, 8, 9
attenuation of material-dependent activation,
aprotinin, 11, 12
corticosteroids, 12, 13
surface coating of extracorporeal circuits, 10, 11
blood conservation strategies, 413
complement activation, 4, 5
cytokine response and effects, 6–8
elastase release and pulmonary dysfunction, 6
endothelial injury, 29, 30, 32, 33
extracorporeal circuit,
contact system activation, 4
milestones in development, 411, 412
traditional circuit features, 412
tolerance for morbidity, 412, 413
minimally invasive circuit design,
centrifugal pumps, 416–418
closed circuits, 418–423
CORx system, 414, 418, 420, 421, 423
prospects, 422
venous air removal, 414–416
venous reservoir, 416
improvement prospects, 16–18
material-dependent activation, 4
material-independent activation,
cardiotomy suction, 13
hemodilution, 14, 15, 413
heparin response, 16
hypothermia, 15, 16
ischemia-reperfusion injury, 13, 14
neurocognition effects,
assessment, 219, 220, 223
mechanisms, 218
stroke, 218
nitric oxide response, 9, 10
platelet defects, 32, 33
postperfusion syndrome, 4
stepwise logistic regression analysis of risk factors for untoward clinical outcomes, 142, 143
terminal complement complex recruitment, 4, 5
whole-body inflammatory reaction, 3, 411
Carotid artery disease, prevalence in cardiac patients, 218
Cognition, *see* Neurocognition
Complement,
activation in cardiopulmonary bypass, 4, 5
neutrophil binding effects, 5
terminal complement complex recruitment, 4, 5
Congenital heart surgery, *see also* Patent ductus arteriosus; Video-assisted thoracoscopic surgery,
hybrid closure of septal defects, 321
incisions,
lower sternotomy, 318
partial sternotomy, 316, 317
right anterolateral thoracotomy, 318, 319
thoracotomy, 315, 316
upper sternotomy, 317, 318
operative imaging and documentation, 315
robotics, 320
thoracotomy avoidance for palliative shunts, 314
Coronary artery bypass grafting (CABG),
endothelial effects, 28, 30, 36
fusing interventional cardiology and cardiac surgery to reduce trauma, 320, 321
minimally invasive surgery, *see also* Dresden technique; Minimally invasive direct coronary artery bypass; Off-pump coronary artery bypass grafting; Partial sternotomy coronary artery bypass grafting; Port access coronary artery bypass grafting; Snaring tourniquet; Total endoscopic coronary artery bypass,
access limitations, 49
circumflex artery revascularization, 50
definition, 53, 129, 130
historical perspective, 45–47, 129
learning curve, 54
popularity, 53
stabilizers, *see* Genzyme-OPCAB Elite system; Guidant OPCAB System; Octopus
percutaneous transluminal coronary angioplasty outcome comparison, 147, 148
prevalence, 75

prospects for minimally invasive surgery, 321–323
reoperation rates, 157
Corticosteroids, attenuation of material-dependent activation in cardiopulmonary bypass, 12, 13
CORx system, features, 414, 418, 420, 421, 423
CPB, *see* Cardiopulmonary bypass

D

da Vinci system,
atrial septal defect repair,
complications, 467–469
outcomes, 455, 466, 467
patient selection, 462, 466
postoperative regimen, 466
surgical technique, 462, 463, 465, 466
components, 447, 449
congenital heart surgery, 320
conventional endoscopy limitations, 446
historical perspective of telemanipulation, 445, 446
learning curve, 456
micro-mitral operation, 264, 265, 267, 468
mitral valve surgery outcomes, 453–455
prospects, 456, 457, 469
strengths and limitations compared with conventional surgery, 447
total endoscopic coronary artery bypass outcomes, 450, 451
Diaphragmatic pacing, video-assisted thoracoscopic surgery, 338–340
Direct limited-access vein harvesting, *see* Saphenous vein harvesting
Doppler ultrasound, intraoperative graft patency assessment, 182, 183
Dresden technique,
advantages, 62
disadvantages, 62, 63
indications, 62

E

Economic analysis,
minimally invasive direct coronary bypass grafting, 362, 363
minimally invasive valve surgery, 361, 362
off-pump coronary artery bypass grafting, 362–366
Elderly patients,
cardiovascular mortality, 241
demographics, 241
off-pump coronary artery bypass grafting,
mortality, 243, 247, 248, 249
multivessel grafting, 248, 249
operative technique, 242, 243
outcomes compared with conventional bypass grafting, 47
popularity, 246, 247
quality of life outcomes, 243, 249
stroke outcomes, 248, 249
study design, 242–245
Endoscopic vein harvesting, *see* Saphenous vein harvesting
Endothelium,
acute injury,
ischemia-reperfusion injury, 34, 35
mechanical trauma, 34
cardiopulmonary bypass activation, 28–30, 32, 33
cell–cell interactions, 33, 34
chronic injury,
atherosclerosis, 37
intimal hyperplasia, 36
functions,
coagulation regulation, 30–32
vasomotor function, 28, 29
injury response, 28, 29
intravascular homeostasis maintenance, 27
minimally invasive bypass grafting effects, 28, 30, 36
Extracorporeal circuit, *see* Cardiopulmonary bypass

F

Fulcrum effect, endoscopic surgery, 429, 433

G

Gelatin–resorcin–formaldehyde (GRF) glue, anastomosis, 406
Genzyme-OPCAB Elite system,
adverse hemodynamic effect mechanisms,
coronary insufficiency, 97
left ventricle, 96, 97
right ventricle, 97
exposure of inferior and lateral walls for multivessel grafting, 95, 96
exposure techniques,
apical suction devices, 102
deep pericardial sutures, 97, 98
right hemi-sternal elevation, 99–102

right pleurotomy and pericardiotomy, 98, 99
Heart Manipulation Device, 102
immobilizer platform,
coronary capture, 91, 92
development, 90
intracoronary shunt placement, 95
positioning, 93, 94
prototypes, 90
GraftConnector, automatic anastomosis, 402, 403
Graft harvesting, *see* Saphenous vein harvesting
GRF glue, *see* Gelatin–resorcin–formaldehyde glue
Guidant OPCAB System,
Lenox Hill Hospital experience, 111, 112
technical considerations,
cardiac anesthesia, 106
coronary artery anatomy, 106
heart displacement, 107, 110
proximal anastomosis, 111
sternotomy and pericardiotomy, 106, 107
vessel stabilization, 110, 111

H

Heartflo device, automatic anastomosis, 401, 402
Heartport, *see* Port-access mitral valve surgery
Heparin,
material-independent activation in cardiopulmonary bypass, 16
surface coating of extracorporeal circuits, 10, 11

I

ICAM, *see* Intercellular adhesion molecule,
IL-1, *see* Interleukin-1
IL-6, *see* Interleukin-6
IL-8, *see* Interleukin-8
IL-10, *see* Interleukin-10
Integrins, cardiopulmonary bypass induction and effects, 8, 9
Intercellular adhesion molecule (ICAM), cardiopulmonary bypass induction and effects, 8, 9
Interleukin-1 (IL-1), cardiopulmonary bypass induction and effects, 6, 7
Interleukin-6 (IL-6), cardiopulmonary bypass induction and effects, 7, 8
Interleukin-8 (IL-8), cardiopulmonary bypass induction and effects, 7, 8
Interleukin-10 (IL-10), cardiopulmonary bypass induction and effects, 7, 8

L

Laser welding, anastomosis, 406, 407
LAST, *see* Left anterior small thoracotomy
Left anterior small thoracotomy (LAST), *see* Minimally invasive direct coronary artery bypass

M

Magnetic resonance imaging (MRI), neurocognition assessment in heart patients, 220, 224
Magnetic Vascular Positioner (MVP), automatic anastomosis, 403, 404
Maze procedure, *see* Atrial fibrillation
Micro-mitral operation (MMO),
advantages, 269, 270
Aesop 3000 system, 265
annuloplasty rings and sutures, 262–264
camera placement, 260
cardioplegia, 260, 261
closure, 264
da Vinci robotic assistance, 264, 265, 267
incision, 258–260
insufflation, 261
learning curve, 270
outcomes, 265, 267, 268, 269, 272
preoperative preparation, 258
principles, 257, 258
MIDCAB, *see* Minimally invasive direct coronary artery bypass
Minimally invasive direct coronary artery bypass (MIDCAB),
access, 57, 58
advantages, 58, 59, 141
contraindications, 59–61, 114, 115, 131
definition, 113
economic analysis, 362, 363
endoscopic coronary artery bypass procedure, 58
historical perspective, 113, 114
hybrid revascularization,
case scenarios, 210–212
indications, 208, 213, 214
operative procedure, 208, 209
outcomes, 212–215
overview, 207, 208
percutaneous intervention, 209, 210

sequence of procedures, 214
indications, 57, 58–61, 64, 114, 115, 130, 131
limitations, 49, 59, 142
neurocognition outcomes, 223
open conversion rate, 136
outcomes, 125, 126, 134–136
patency rates, 59, 148
popularity, 57
postoperative course, 133, 134
quality-of-life outcomes, 374–380
reoperation,
anterior MIDCAB,
left anterior descending artery exposure, 163, 164
left internal mammary artery preparation, 62, 163
subclavian MIDCAB, 164–170
subxiphoid MIDCAB, 64, 170
transabdominal MIDCAB, 170, 172, 173
subxiphoid procedure,
advantages, 154, 155
approach, 58, 148, 149
mortality, 154
open conversion rate, 154
reoperation, 64, 170
technique, 119, 120, 123, 148, 149
technique,
anastomosis, 133
anesthesia, 131
endoscopic MIDCAB, 125
graft harvesting, 131, 142
heparin reversal, 133
H Graft, 119
intubation, 131
left anterior thoracotomy, 115–118
left anterior thoracotomy with axillary artery inflow, 118, 119
left posterior lateral thoracotomy, 123
stenting, 141
xiphoid approach, 119, 120, 123, 148, 149
Mitral regurgitation,
prognostic factors, 384
timing of surgery, 384
Mitral valve surgery, minimally invasive, *see also* Micro-mitral operation; Percutaneous mitral valve repair; Port-access mitral valve surgery,
Carpentier–Loulmet classification of degrees of surgical invasiveness, 256
da Vinci system assistance, 453–455
definition, 255
direct vision, 256
economic analysis, 361, 362
edge-to-edge technique, 384–386
evolution, 255, 256
micro-incision, 257
micro-or port-incision and video-directed robotic operation, 257
mini-incision, 256
video-assisted vision, 257
Zeus system assistance, 438, 439
MMO, *see* Micro-mitral operation
MRI, *see* Magnetic resonance imaging
MVP, *see* Magnetic Vascular Positioner

N

Neurocognition,
cardiopulmonary bypass effects,
assessment, 219, 220, 223
mechanisms, 218
stroke, 218
factors affecting, 219
minimally invasive direct coronary bypass grafting outcomes, 223
neuropsychological test batteries, 224, 225
off-pump coronary artery bypass grafting outcomes, 47, 48, 217–225
presurgical baseline and change definition, 221, 222
risk factors for deficits after heart surgery, 224
Neuron-specific enolase (NSE), neurocognition marker, 223
Nitinol U-Clip device, automatic anastomosis, 404, 406
Nitric oxide (NO),
atherosclerosis dysregulation, 37
cardiopulmonary bypass induction and effects, 9, 10
endothelial injury prevention, 33, 34
functions, 29
NO, *see* Nitric oxide
NSE, *see* Neuron-specific enolase

O

Octogenarians, *see* Elderly patients
Octopus,
comparison of prototypes, 81
development, 76, 78, 79
hemodynamic changes, 80, 82–84

histological changes, 82, 85, 88
off-pump coronary artery bypass grafting, clinical experience, 86–88
Octopus III, 70, 71
Off-pump coronary artery bypass grafting (OPCAB),
advantages, 50, 54, 67, 73
cardiac displacement and coronary target presentation, 70, 71
contraindications, 50, 55, 56, 58
coronary stabilization and grafting, 71, 72, 75, 76
economic analysis, 362–366
elderly patients,
mortality, 243, 247, 248, 249
multivessel grafting, 248, 249
operative technique, 242, 243
outcomes compared with conventional bypass grafting, 47
popularity, 246, 247
quality of life outcomes, 243, 249
stroke outcomes, 248, 249
study design, 242–245
exposure techniques,
apical suction devices, 102
deep pericardial sutures, 97, 98
median sternotomy, 136
right hemi-sternal elevation, 99–102
right pleurotomy and pericardiotomy, 98, 99
goals, 106
graft patency,
angiography, 183, 184
Doppler ultrasound, 182, 183
fluorescein angiography, 184
intraoperative assessment,
postoperative assessment,
early angiography, 185, 187
intermediate-term angiography, 187, 188
late angiography, 188
thermal coronary angiography, 184
transit time flow measurement, 180–182
prospects for postoperative evaluation, 188, 189
rates, 55, 139, 140, 142
grafting sequence, 69, 70
historical perspective, 46–48, 89
indications, 55, 56–58, 67, 68
inflammatory response, 48, 49
limitations, 54, 55
multivessel grafting, 95, 96, 142
neurocognitive outcomes, 47, 48, 217–225
Octopus stabilizer, 70, 71, 86–88
operative procedure, 68, 69, 136, 138
perfusion-assisted direct coronary artery bypass, 72, 73
popularity, 229, 230
postoperative course, 138
preoperative evaluation, 68
reoperation,
anesthesia, 159
indications, 158
intraoperative monitoring, 159
Lenox Hill Hospital outcomes, 173–177
pain control, 159, 160
preoperative planning, 158
resternotomy,
exposure of lateral and inferior wall, 160–162
median sternotomy, 160
mediastinal dissection, 160
surgical technique, 159, 160
severe left ventricular dysfunction patients,
operative technique, 231, 232
outcomes of multivessel revascularization, 232–237
patient selection, 230–232
quality of life outcomes, 235, 237
study design, 230, 231, 237
training, 238
stabilizers, *see* Genzyme-OPCAB Elite system; Guidant OPCAB System; Octopus
temporary intraluminal shunt, 49
verticalization of heart, 136, 138
One Shot System, automatic anastomosis, 401
OPCAB, *see* Off-pump coronary artery bypass grafting

P

Pacemaker, implantation with video-assisted thoracoscopic surgery, 338
PADCAB, *see* Perfusion-assisted direct coronary artery bypass
Partial sternotomy coronary artery bypass grafting,
access, 60, 61
advantages, 61
contraindications, 61, 62

disadvantages, 61
indications, 61, 62
Patent ductus arteriosus (PDA), video-assisted thoracoscopic surgery, 312, 313
PDA, *see* Patent ductus arteriosus
Percutaneous mitral valve repair,
bow-tie repair, 384–386
coil-fastening device, 388, 389
difficulty, 383–385
imaging, 391
indications, 389, 390
prospects, 391
Percutaneous transluminal coronary angioplasty (PTCA),
coronary artery bypass grafting outcome comparison, 147, 148
hybrid revascularization with minimally invasive direct coronary artery bypass, 207–215
Perfusion-assisted direct coronary artery bypass (PADCAB), off-pump coronary artery bypass grafting, 72, 73
Pericardial disease,
anatomy and physiology, 328, 329
etiology of pericarditis and effusion, 331, 333
historical perspective, 328
medical therapy, 327, 328
video-assisted thoracoscopic surgery,
advantages, 340
anesthesia, 329, 330
congenital defects, 335, 336
patient selection and preparation, 329
pericardial constriction, 334
pericardial cysts, 336, 338
pericardial effusion, 331–334
pericardial tamponade, 331–334
pericardial tumors, 335
surgical technique, 330, 331
Port access coronary artery bypass grafting,
advantages, 62
disadvantages, 62, 64
indications, 62
Port-access mitral valve surgery,
advantages, 289
aortic decannulation, 285
blood transfusion, 288
cardioplegia, 281, 282
central aortic cannulation, 279, 281
chest tube, 285
closure, 285
endoscopic instruments, 284
femoral artery cannulation, 277
Heartport system overview, 273
historical perspective, 273, 274
incisions, 275–277
intraoperative difficulties, 286
learning curve, 289
left atriotomy, 283
mitral valve repair, 284, 289
modifications, 285, 286
operative technique, 274, 275
outcomes,
hospital outcomes, 286, 288
intraoperative factors, 286
quality of life, 288, 289
pain, 289
patient selection, 274
postoperative care, 285
prospects, 290
rib repair, 285
robotics, 290
Prostacyclin, cardiopulmonary bypass induction and effects, 10
PTCA, *see* Percutaneous transluminal coronary angioplasty
Pulmonary artery stenosis hybrid therapy, 321

Q

QoL, *see* Quality-of-life
Quality-of-life (QoL),
Centro Cardiologico Monzino IRCCS experience with minimally invasive cardiac surgery,
early results, 376
late results, 376
measures of quality-of-life, 376–379
study design, 375, 376
cosmetic issues, 374, 375
definition, 369, 370
importance in overall health outcomes, 370, 371
minimally invasive cardiac surgery study abundance, 370
off-pump coronary artery bypass grafting outcomes, 235, 237, 243, 249
pain, 373, 374
port-access mitral valve surgery outcomes, 288, 289

prospects for study, 379–381
tools,
Nottingham Health Profile, 371, 373, 375, 379
physical activity score, 371, 376
Psychological General Well-Being Index, 373, 376, 378
table, 372

R

Radial artery harvesting, minimally invasive harvesting, 205
Robotics, *see* Aesop 3000 system; da Vinci system; Zeus system

S

S-100, neurocognition marker, 223
Saphenous vein harvesting,
angioscopy for intraluminal lesion monitoring, 204
complications, 193, 194
direct limited-access vein harvesting,
closure, 196
Genzyme retractor system, 195, 196
mid-calf incision, 196
popularity of grafting, 193
traditional technique, 193
video-assisted endoscopic vein harvesting,
complications, 201, 202, 204
disadvantages, 203, 204
dissection, 199–201
Guidant Vasoview Uniport Plus System, 198
insufflation, 199
learning curve, 197, 198
vein quality, 203
Selectins, cardiopulmonary bypass induction and effects, 8, 9
Snaring tourniquet, coronary artery trauma, 47
Stabilizers, *see* Genzyme-OPCAB Elite system; Guidant OPCAB System; Octopus
Staplers, anastomosis, 394–396
Symmetry Bypass System, automatic anastomosis, 398

T

TECAB, *see* Total endoscopic coronary artery bypass
Thromboxane B2 (TXB_2), cardiopulmonary bypass induction and effects, 10
TNF-α, *see* Tumor necrosis factor-α
Total endoscopic coronary artery bypass (TECAB),
access, 63
advantages, 63
contraindications, 63
da Vinci system assistance, 450, 451
disadvantages, 63
learning curve, 63
Transit time flow measurement (TTFM), intraoperative graft patency assessment, 180–182
TTFM, *see* Transit time flow measurement
Tumor necrosis factor-α (TNF-α), cardiopulmonary bypass induction and effects, 6–8
TXB_2, *see* Thromboxane B2

V

Vascular cell adhesion molecule (VCAM), cardiopulmonary bypass induction and effects, 8, 9
VATS, *see* Video-assisted thoracoscopic surgery
VCAM, *see* Vascular cell adhesion molecule
Verapamil, controlled hypotension in minimally invasive surgery, 46
Video-assisted endoscopic vein harvesting, *see* Saphenous vein harvesting
Video-assisted thoracoscopic surgery (VATS),
diaphragmatic pacing, 338–340
epicardial pacemaker implantation, 338
extracardiac congenital lesion repair, 314
patent ductus arteriosus repair, 312, 313
pericardial disease,
advantages, 340
anesthesia, 329, 330
congenital defects, 335, 336
patient selection and preparation, 329
pericardial constriction, 334
pericardial cysts, 336, 338
pericardial effusion, 331–334
pericardial tamponade, 331–334
pericardial tumors, 335
surgical technique, 330, 331
vascular ring division, 313, 314

X

Xpose, see Guidant OPCAB System

Z

Zeus system,

advantages of robotic systems, 431, 433
components, 430
computer integration, 440, 441
coronary artery surgery outcomes, 434–438
development, 430
endoscopic instruments, 434, 440
instrument handles, 430, 431
instrument rotation, 433
learning curve, 439, 440
mitral valve surgery outcomes, 438, 439
prospects for minimally invasive cardiac surgery, 440–442
robotic arms, 433, 434

MIX
Papier aus verantwortungsvollen Quellen
Paper from responsible sources
FSC® C105338

If you have any concerns about our products,
you can contact us on
ProductSafety@springernature.com

In case Publisher is established outside the EU,
the EU authorized representative is:
Springer Nature Customer Service Center GmbH
Europaplatz 3, 69115 Heidelberg, Germany

Printed by Libri Plureos GmbH
in Hamburg, Germany